Community-Based Nursing

AN INTRODUCTION

evolve

∴ To access your Student Resources, visit:

http://evolve.elsevier.com/McEwen

Evolve® Student Resources for **McEwen: *Community-Based Nursing: An Introduction,* Third edition,** offers the following features:

Student Resources

- **WebLinks**
  Links to hundreds of websites carefully chosen to supplement the content of the textbook.

- **Glossary**
  Key Terms and their definitions, with search engine.

- **Assessment Tools**
  Five health assessment tools related to book content.

THIRD EDITION

Community-Based Nursing

AN INTRODUCTION

Melanie McEwen, PhD, RN
Associate Professor
University of Texas Health Science Center at Houston
School of Nursing

Bridgette C. Pullis, PhD, RN
Assistant Professor
University of Texas Health Science Center at Houston
School of Nursing

SAUNDERS

ELSEVIER

SAUNDERS
ELSEVIER

11830 Westline Industrial Drive
St. Louis, Missouri 63146

COMMUNITY-BASED NURSING: AN INTRODUCTION,   ISBN: 978-1-4160-5771-0
THIRD EDITION

Previous editions copyrighted 1998, 2002

Library of Congress Cataloging-in-Publication Data

McEwen, Melanie.
  Community-based nursing: an introduction/Melanie McEwen, Bridgette C. Pullis. --3rd ed.
     p.; cm.
Includes bibliographical references and index.
ISBN 978-1-4160-5771-0 (pbk. : alk. paper)
1. Community health nursing. I. Pullis, Bridgett C. (Bridgette Crotwell) II. Tittle.
[DNLM: 1. Community Health Nursing. 2. Health Promotion. WY 106 M478c 2009]
RT98.M3 2009
610.73'43--dc22

                                          2008029882

Acquisitions Editor: Linda Thomas
Developmental Editor: Carlie Irwin
Publishing Services Manager: Jeff Patterson
Project Manager: Amy Rickles
Cover Design Direction: Paula Catalano
Interior Design Direction: Paula Catalano

Printed in Canada

Last digit is the print number: 9 8 7 6 5 4 3 2 1

About the Authors

Melanie McEwen, PhD, RN, is an Associate Professor at the University of Texas Health Science Center at Houston, School of Nursing. Dr. McEwen received her BSN from the University of Texas School of Nursing in Austin, her Master's in Community and Public Health Nursing from Louisiana State University Medical Center in New Orleans, and her PhD in Nursing at Texas Woman's University. Dr. McEwen is coauthor of *Theoretical Basis for Nursing,* which is targeted to graduate students, and an Elsevier publication, *Community/Public Health Nursing: Promoting the Health of Populations.*

Bridgette Crotwell Pullis, PhD, RN, is an Assistant Professor at the University of Texas Health Science Center at Houston, School of Nursing. Dr. Pullis received her BSN from Northeast Louisiana University and her Master's in Community Health Nursing and PhD in Health Studies from Texas Woman's University.

At the beginning of the twenty-first century, health care in the United States is still undergoing many changes. Cost consciousness among insurers, technology, and political decisions have altered *how* health care is provided, *who* is responsible for care delivery, *what* care is provided, and *when* clients are seen. One of the most significant changes, however, has been *where* care is given.

No longer is the hospital the central site for health care. Health care today is being provided in community-based settings such as homes, schools, clinics, offices, churches, and work sites, and even over the telephone or via e-mail. Correspondingly, there is a need for nurses who are prepared to practice in those settings. Therefore nursing education must include course content and clinical experiences that address community-based health care. *Community-Based Nursing: An Introduction* was written to be both a core and a supplemental textbook for nursing students who have an opportunity to deliver nursing care to clients in community-based settings.

ORGANIZATION

Community-Based Nursing: An Introduction, third edition, brings together the essential information necessary for nurses practicing in community settings. It includes content "hidden" in the major nursing textbooks that cover related material, information that may not be included in other resources, and content found in other books but presented from a different perspective.

For example, Chapter 2 discusses roles and interventions emphasized in community-based nursing care and describes how they differ from roles and interventions in acute care settings. Chapter 5 gives an overview of the health care delivery system, which is designed to help the reader understand why health care is becoming increasingly community based. Chapter 8 explores cultural influences on health and health care–seeking behaviors.

The chapters that focus on health care of major aggregates are presented from a different perspective from other major textbooks. In this textbook, the focus is on health promotion and illness prevention. For example, Chapter 12 discusses the care of infants, children, and adolescents. Information for community-based nursing care includes nutrition needs, growth and development guidelines, immunization schedules, and suggested screenings. This chapter also includes care of children with minor acute episodic illnesses, such as gastroenteritis, chicken pox, strep throat, and pediculosis (head lice), which are usually managed at home. In pediatric nursing textbooks, these topics are discussed largely from an acute-care perspective, and the information may be difficult to apply in community settings. This book presents the material in a format that emphasizes health teaching and care of the family.

The content of the book is organized into five units. Each unit covers different aspects of community-based nursing.

Unit 1, Foundations of Community-Based Nursing Practice, provides an overview of the many changes in the health care delivery system and corresponding opportunities for nurses to practice within the changing system. The unit also describes the roles and interventions used by nurses in community-based practice. Two new chapters are included in this unit. Chapter 3 explicitly presents Health Teaching information needed by nurses to better prepare them for this vital aspect of care in any setting. Also new, Chapter 4 covers "case management," an important skill needed by many nurses who work in community settings.

Unit 2, Factors That Influence Health and Health Care, presents data about the many issues and circumstances that may affect health and health care. Separate chapters describe the health care delivery system, epidemiology, environmental health issues, and culture. "Natural and Manmade Disasters" (Chapter 9) is a new chapter within this unit; it describes how and when nursing care might be delivered during emergency situations such as worksite violence incidents or major accidents, as well as natural or man-made disasters such as hurricanes or terrorist attacks.

Unit 3, Settings for Community-Based Nursing Care, describes the various settings for community-based care. In this unit, Chapter 10 presents an overview of a number of settings in which nurses practice (e.g., clinics, ambulatory surgery centers, parish health programs, occupational health programs); this gives the reader an idea of the various settings in which nurses may be employed in nonacute care settings. Chapter 11 outlines the work of home health nurses and includes information on various subspecialties (e.g., infusion therapy, perinatal home care) within this area of nursing.

Unit 4, Community-Based Nursing Care Across the Life Span, gives detailed information on health promotion activities and interventions appropriate for nursing care in community settings. Individual chapters cover the care of infants, children, adolescents, and adults. In addition, separate chapters describe the unique health needs of women, elders, and families.

Unit 5, Nursing Care of Clients with Special Needs in Community Settings, addresses nursing care for clients with special needs. In this unit, attention is given to vulnerable clients (i.e., those in poverty, the homeless, migrant farm workers, and disabled persons). This unit also has separate chapters on mental health care in the community and communicable disease prevention and intervention.

Community-Based Nursing: An Introduction includes material that will help direct nursing students in community-based practice, wherever the setting and whomever the population being served. For example, if the student is working with a home health care nurse providing skilled nursing services for older adults, helpful content would be found in Chapters 3 (Patient Education and Health Teaching), 4 (Case Management), and 15 (Health Promotion and Illness Prevention for Elders). If the student is working in an elementary school, the section in Chapter 10 (Nursing Care in Ambulatory Settings) describing school nursing and information from Chapter 12 (Health Promotion and Illness Prevention for Infants, Children, and Adolescents) would be beneficial. Or, if the student is working in a women's clinic, appropriate information is found in Chapters 13 (Health Promotion and Illness Preven-

tion for Adults), 14 (Issues in Women's Health Care), and 19 (Communicable Disease: Prevention and Intervention).

Much of the content of this text focuses on material that should be an integral part of client education (e.g., smoking cessation guidelines, fall prevention measures for elders). It includes guidelines for health promotion and illness prevention for all age groups (e.g., immunizations, screenings, risk identification); how to identify, intervene in, and refer various health problems and health threats in a variety of settings; and description, elaboration, and simplification of content the student needs to become community focused (e.g., cultural issues, the health care delivery system, and epidemiology).

KEY FEATURES

The following features are presented to enhance student learning:

Each chapter begins with **Learning Objectives** to explain the focus of the chapter.

Each chapter includes a list of **Key Terms** that are discussed in the chapter.

Each chapter is introduced by a **Case Study** illustrating how nurses in community-based practice use specific content covered within the chapter.

Goals, objectives, and information from *Healthy People 2010* are presented in *Healthy People 2010* boxes.

Research Highlight boxes present findings from research that is applicable to community-based practice.

Health Teaching boxes present specific information that the nurse can use for client education.

Community Application boxes give specific examples of how the content is relevant to nurses in community-based practice.

All chapters conclude with **Learning Activities & Application to Practice** exercises that students can use to gain more in-depth understanding of the content.

A **Glossary** at the end of the book presents the definitions of the Key Terms in every chapter.

NEW CONTENT IN THIS EDITION

Chapter 3, Patient Education and Health Teaching, gives information that will prepare nurses to present health-related information to clients in all settings.

This chapter describes processes, methods, theories, and tools that can be used by nurses to promote health education.

Chapter 4 describes the process of case management, a valuable tool used by many nurses caring for complex clients in community-based settings.

Chapter 9, Natural and Manmade Disasters, helps prepare nurses to respond appropriately in a variety of disaster situations. This includes recognition of potential threats to their community and knowledge of community resources.

TEACHING AND LEARNING WEBSITE

This edition includes a website with materials for both faculty and students. Visit the website at **http://evolve.elsevier.com/McEwen**.

MATERIALS AVAILABLE FOR THE INSTRUCTOR:

- Annotated Learning Objectives
- Chapter Outlines, which can be used to create PowerPoint presentations
- Additional Learning Activities
- Test Bank with 400 multiple-choice questions

MATERIALS AVAILABLE FOR THE INSTRUCTOR AND STUDENT

- WebLinks
- Glossary
- Assessment Tools

Acknowledgments

A *huge* "Thank You" goes to Linda Thomas, Managing Editor, Nursing Division, Elsevier, for her persistence and determination in pursuing this 3rd edition—it would not have happened without her support. Also, special thanks go to Elsevier Developmental Editor Carlie Bliss Irwin and Project Manager Amy Rickles for their diligence in keeping us on track and for the hours of assistance during the development and production processes.

Melanie McEwen and Bridgette Pullis

Once again, a great deal of appreciation, gratitude, respect,
and love go to my husband, Scott, for his many hours of help,
for keeping me supplied with the latest computer gadgetry and fast Internet
connections, and for putting up with the mess I made of his office.

Melanie McEwen

This work is dedicated to the memory of Jimmie Crotwell, RN, my mother,
my mentor, my friend. January 13, 1929, to January 8, 2008.

Bridgette Pullis

Contents

Unit Five

Nursing Care of Clients with Special Needs in Community Settings, *351*

Foundations of Community-Based Nursing Practice

Opportunities in Community-Based Nursing Practice

1. Define and discuss the focus of community-based nursing practice.

2. Discuss trends in employment for registered nurses and identify opportunities for their employment in community-based settings.

3. Describe the purpose of *Healthy People 2010* and give examples of the focus areas that encompass the national health objectives.

4. Explain the difference between primary, secondary, and tertiary care and give examples of how each may be provided in community-based settings.

key terms

Community-based nursing
Community health nursing
Healthy People 2010

Primary health care
Secondary health care
Tertiary health care

See Glossary for definitions.

case study

Martha McDonald will complete her nursing program and take the National Council Licensure Examination (NCLEX) in 3 months. Although she has enjoyed nursing school, Martha cannot wait to graduate and begin her new career. Anticipating graduation, she has begun the process of looking for employment and has been somewhat surprised by the variety of options available to her.

For the past year, Martha has worked two or three evenings each week as a "student nurse tech" on a general medical floor of a large, nonprofit hospital. Although she really enjoys working in the hospital, during the course of her studies, she became interested in the health promotion and illness prevention aspects of health care. Martha was particularly attracted to working with older adults and helping them achieve and maintain maximum wellness. She thought that a job in a community setting would be better suited to her.

Martha began her job search by reviewing the employment classified advertisements in the local Sunday paper. Surprisingly, many of the ads for registered nurses (RNs) were in the areas

Continued

of home health nursing, case management, and managed care groups, such as health maintenance organizations (HMOs). In addition, there were opportunities for RNs to work in nursing homes and a variety of outpatient settings, such as day surgery centers and minor emergency or primary care clinics.

Martha discussed employment opportunities with the job placement office and several of her nursing instructors. After a month of interviews and weighing options, Martha chose a position as a staff nurse in a geriatric clinic affiliated with one of the large nonprofit health care organizations in her city.

Over the past two decades, the health care delivery system has changed dramatically. Cost-consciousness among insurers at all levels has mandated massive alterations in health care delivery. This has resulted in a phenomenal decrease in the average length of hospital stays for virtually all illnesses and procedures. No one argues that patients are being discharged "sicker and quicker" now than in the past. In addition, emphasis on health promotion and illness prevention is increasing throughout society, with recognition of the impact of lifestyle choices and behavior on individual and population health. Table 1-1 lists some of the trends that have been observed in the health care delivery system in recent years.

There is little doubt that health care delivery is moving from an acute care focus and hospital-based delivery of care to illness prevention and management and community-based delivery of care. As a result, hospitals are reducing capacity and downsizing, becoming specialized, or closing altogether.

In the United States a significant shortage of nurses exists in virtually all areas, and this shortage is expected to continue and even expand over the next decade (AACN, 2007). As with the growing number of jobs in acute care facilities, there are many opportunities for nurses in community-based settings, whether in home care, HMOs, clinics, or other services.

The National League for Nursing (NLN) (1993) and nursing educators (Matteson, 2000; Zungolo 2000) have recognized the importance of moving much of the content and clinical focus in nursing education from acute care settings into community settings. Indeed, nursing educators in both associate and baccalaureate degree programs are aware of

TABLE **1-1** Change in Focus of Health Care Delivery Over the Last Two Decades

FROM	TO
Acute inpatient care	Out-patient and primary care
Disease focus	Health protection/illness prevention
Individual emphasis	Group, population and community emphasis
Population uniformity	Population diversity
Fragmented care	Managed care
Compliant patients	Educated consumers
Managing departments and organizations	Managing networks and systems
Service duplication	Continuum of care
Number of services provided	Documenting quality and outcomes

Sources: Mengel A, Donnelly G: Associate degree and baccalaureate nursing education. In Tagliareni ME, Marckx BB, editors: *Teaching in the community: preparing nurses for the 21st century,* Sudbury, Mass, 1999 and Jones & Bartlett. Shi L, Singh DA: *Delivering health care in America: a systems approach,* Boston, 2004, Jones and Bartlett.

the trends in health care and understand the need to incorporate community-based nursing (CBN) concepts and clinical experiences into curricula. In baccalaureate programs this often means expansion or integration of community content and clinical experiences throughout programs rather than confining them to the study of "community health nursing" (CHN) near the end of the program, as has been the traditional practice.

Associate degree nursing programs have also acknowledged the need to include community-based experiences and related content. Since the mid 1990s there has been an emphasis on promoting community-based clinical opportunities and learning experiences for students pursuing an associate degree in nursing (NLN/CADP, 1994) (Box 1-1).

COMMUNITY-BASED HEALTH CARE AND NURSING PRACTICE

For more than a decade, the nursing discipline has advocated an increasing emphasis on health promotion and illness prevention in all areas of the health care delivery system (American Nurses' Association [ANA], 1991; Heller, Oros, Durney-Crowley, 2004). Indeed, the ANA and many other organizations have recognized that homes, work sites, schools, churches, and neighborhood clinics are among the settings suggested to serve as "convenient familiar places" to enhance the delivery of preventive, systematic, and comprehensive health care. The emphasis on health care delivery in community-based settings has moved beyond **primary health care** (i.e., prevention activities, such as well-child check-ups, routine physical examinations, prenatal care, and diagnosis and treatment of common acute or episodic illnesses) and now encompasses secondary and tertiary care.

Secondary health care typically refers to relatively serious or complicated care that has historically been provided to patients in hospitals. However, recent changes in techniques, procedures, and medical practice have moved much of secondary health care into community settings. Examples of community-based secondary health care include the following:

- Outpatient surgery for complex procedures that would have required hospitalization just a few years ago (e.g., cholecystectomy, hysterectomy, appendectomy, herniorrhaphy)

BOX 1-1 Addressing the Nursing Shortage

The Tri-Council (2001), an organization comprising representatives from the American Association of Colleges of Nursing, ANA, American Organization of Nurse Executives, and NLN, has stated that the current nursing workforce shortage is complex and very different from any in the past. They explained that the problem is difficult to quantify and not simply an issue of there being too few RNs. Furthermore, concern that the shortage will grow more serious over the next 20 years is significant.

The Tri-Council cited the following concerns regarding the nursing shortage: fewer nurses are entering the workforce, nursing shortages in certain geographic areas are acute, and a shortage of nurses prepared to meet certain areas of client needs in the changing health care environment exists. In addition, they explained that although low pay rates continue to be cited by nurses as a professional drawback, the leading factor for nurse turnover is "increased market demand" exacerbated by "dissatisfaction with the job, the supervisor or career prospects" (Tri-Council, 2001, 1). The second most cited reason for turnover is workload and staffing. They also reported serious concerns over the increased need for more nurses because of the increasing age of the general population and the growing need for management of chronic disease conditions.

Recommendations from the Tri-Council are that health care environments must recognize and reward educational and practice competencies by defining nurses' roles and by utilizing and compensating nurses according to their educational preparation and competencies. They suggest that health care organizations need to implement specific strategies to retain experienced nurses in the provision of direct client care, create a partnership environment that advances the practice of nursing by establishing appropriate management structures within the health care system, and ensure adequate nurse staffing. Finally, they should provide nurses with sufficient autonomy over their practice in all settings.

- Treatment of serious illnesses (e.g., chemotherapy, radiotherapy)
- A wide variety of diagnostic testing procedures (e.g., computed tomography, magnetic resonance imaging, angiography)

Similarly, **tertiary health care** (management of chronic, complicated, long-term health problems) is now frequently delivered in community settings. Rehabilitation centers for clients with neurological conditions (e.g., spinal cord injuries, multiple sclerosis, amyotrophic lateral sclerosis), centers for cardiac rehabilitation, home health care for bed-bound older people, home care for respirator-dependent infants, and hospice care for the terminally ill are examples of tertiary health care commonly provided in non-hospital settings.

Nursing care is an essential component in each of these settings and for each level of care described. Nursing practice in community settings is similar to nursing practice in acute care facilities because nurses perform assessments, administer procedures, teach clients and their caregivers, counsel, and work to ensure that clients receive needed care and services.

Nursing practice in community settings, however, may differ significantly from nursing practice in the hospital. The community setting is often characterized by less structure, less formality, and more independence. Reliance on technology and a "controlled" environment is greatly reduced, and recognition of the importance of knowing and understanding the client's unique situation and individual needs is enhanced. Thus the application of the nursing process (assessment, analysis, planning, intervention, evaluation) must take into account information beyond the immediate physical and psychosocial needs that are addressed in the formal and controlled hospital setting. In community-based practice, environmental threats, availability of resources, financial burdens, family concerns, lifestyle choices, and various management issues for clients and their caregivers are often of primary concern.

COMMUNITY-BASED NURSING AND COMMUNITY HEALTH NURSING

Within the discipline of nursing, confusion regarding what comprises CBN practice and how it differs from CHN is common. **Community-based nursing** (CBN) practice refers to the application of the nursing process in caring for individuals, families, and groups where they live, work, or go to school or as they move through the health care system. In CBN, all levels of prevention are emphasized (i.e., primary, secondary, and tertiary), but its focus is more on secondary and tertiary levels. Home health nursing and nursing in outpatient or ambulatory settings are examples of CBN.

Community health nursing (CHN) is a synthesis of nursing practice and public health practice applied to promoting and preserving the health of populations (ANA, 1986). The CHN practice is continuous and comprehensive and considers the impact of the environment on health. In CHN the dominant responsibility is to the population as a whole, but care is directed to individuals, families, or groups, thus contributing to the health of the total aggregate or population. Public health nursing, school nursing, and occupational health nursing are examples of CHN.

In an excellent discussion, Zotti, Brown, and Stotts (1996) compared CBN and CHN. They explained that the goals of the two are different because CHN emphasizes preservation and protection of health, whereas in CBN, the emphasis is on managing acute or chronic conditions. In CHN the primary client is the community, and in CBN the primary clients are the individual and the family. Also, services in CBN are largely direct, and in CHN services are both direct and indirect. Thus although both community-based nurses and community health nurses work in the community, they have different goals, methods, and purposes in delivering nursing care.

EDUCATION FOCUS

As mentioned, nursing educators have recognized the need to enhance community content and clinical experiences for nursing students. Matteson (2000) and Hamner (1999) identified several content areas that should be enhanced in all programs to address the need for CBN education. This content includes knowledge of health-promotion strategies, concepts of risk reduction and disease prevention, illness and disease management, continuum of health services, family health care, self-care, community resources, collaboration, delegation, health care systems, and policy development. Areas for expanded clinical experiences include ambulatory care facilities, college health facilities, correctional facilities, genetic clinics, geriatric clinics, and home health nursing.

DIFFERENTIATED PRACTICE ISSUES

The movement of nursing out of traditional, structured roles found in acute care settings has given new direction to the debate on "differentiated practice," sparking questions on whether associate degree or diploma-prepared nurses are educationally equipped to practice in less structured community-based settings. Although the ANA's published 1965 and 1984 position statements outlining two entry levels for nursing practice (the "technical" nurse and the "professional" nurse) were widely debated, little action has been taken toward an official distinction in levels of practice. Indeed, despite repeated calls for this change, no U.S. states require a baccalaureate degree for a professional nurse's license.

Discussion of the merits of differentiated practice is beyond the scope of this book. When appropriate, however, specific educational requirements and recommendations for nurses using advanced knowledge or working with designated populations or in specialized settings are included.

EMPLOYMENT OPPORTUNITIES IN COMMUNITY SETTINGS

CURRENT TRENDS IN NURSING EMPLOYMENT

In the case study at the beginning of the chapter, what Martha discovered when she began her job search is not unusual. As a result of cost-containment measures and medical practice modifications, nursing employment has changed over the past several years. The Public Health Service's Division of Nursing has chronicled this change in practice settings through periodic surveys of RNs. The 2004 National Sample Survey of Registered Nurses (U.S. Department of Health and Human Services/Division of Nursing [USDHHS/DON] 2006) discovered the following:

- The rate for RNs who worked outside of hospitals in 2004 was 43.8% (up from 33.5% in 1992 and an increase of 2.9% since 2000).
- Although the number of RNs working in hospitals increased, the proportion of nurses working in hospitals declined significantly between 1992 and 2004.
- The number of nurses employed in ambulatory care settings showed a 168.7% increase between 1980 and 2004, and the number of RNs employed in public health and community health settings increased by 128.8% during the same period.

Reforms in health care delivery appear to dictate that these trends will continue well into the twenty-first century. Table 1-2 presents data detailing employment settings for RNs practicing in the United States.

Another finding of the National Nursing Survey (USDHHS/DON, 2006) was that the supply of RNs, like that of other health care providers, has a problem with geographic maldistribution. States in the Southwest, Pacific, and mountain regions have approximately half the number of employed nurses per 100,000 people as states in New England and the Midwest.

For example, California, Nevada, Idaho, Oklahoma, and Texas have 589 to 646 employed RNs per 100,000 people. In contrast, Massachusetts, Rhode Island, and

TABLE **1-2** Summary of Employment Settings for All Registered Nurses—2004

SETTING	ESTIMATED PERCENT
Hospitals	56.2
Nursing home/extended care facilities	6.3
Nursing education	2.6
Community/public health settings (includes home health agencies, school health, occupational health, correctional facility)	15.5
Ambulatory care settings	11.5
Other (includes insurance claims/benefits, policy or regulatory agency, private duty, clinical research, unknown)	7.9

From U.S. Department of Health and Human Services Division of Nursing, Bureau of Health Professions: The registered nurse population: national sample survey of registered nurses, March 2004, Washington, DC, 2006, Government Printing Office.

the Dakotas have 1175 to 1283 RNs per 100,000 people. It is interesting to note that the District of Columbia has the greatest per capita concentration, with 2093 RNs per 100,000 people. Rural areas in particular are understaffed with RNs because about 80% of all nurses work in urban areas (USDHHS/DON, 2006).

EMPLOYMENT OPPORTUNITIES

The movement from an illness-oriented "cure" perspective in hospitals to a focus on health promotion and primary health care in community-based settings—combined with changing demographics (i.e., an aging population), cost-consciousness, and changes in medical technology and treatments—has dramatically changed employment opportunities for today's RNs. This shift of emphasis to primary care and outpatient treatment and management of both acute and chronic health conditions will continue. As a result employment growth in a variety of ambulatory care settings, home health care, nursing homes, occupational health, school health, and parish care programs can be expected. Box 1-2 lists current and future employment options for RNs in nonacute-care settings.

As shown in Box 1-2, nursing opportunities in community settings are extensive and varied. New graduates and experienced nurses should have a number of alternatives to explore to meet individual professional interests. For instance:

- If pediatrics is the nurse's primary area of interest, employment choices include working in a pediatrician's office, a pediatric hospital-based clinic, a school health program, and a well-child clinic.
- If the nurse enjoys working with older people, there are many options, including adult day care, geriatric clinics, home health, and nursing homes.
- If surgery is an interest, the nurse should realize that almost half of all surgical procedures are performed on an outpatient basis.

As a result, employment opportunities in both freestanding and hospital-based day surgery centers have increased and include not only operating room nursing, but also postanesthesia care, intake/admissions, and patient education positions. In addition, postday surgery home care is becoming increasingly popular (see the Research Highlight "Future of Nursing Employment").

CHARACTERISTICS OF COMMUNITY-BASED NURSING

Although opportunities for employment in community-based settings are impressive, a baccalaureate degree may be required for some positions. Many school health programs and most public health departments, for example, will hire only nurses with a Bachelor of Science in nursing (BSN) degree. Similarly, experience may be necessary for some nursing positions in nonhospital settings. Home health agencies, for example, typically prefer 1 to 2 years of recent acute care experience for new-hire RNs.

Practicing in community settings has several advantages. Many nurses prefer the emphasis on health promotion and illness prevention that is a major focus of primary health care. The opportunity to get to know clients and their families by seeing them in their own homes, workplaces, schools, or communities and to provide more holistic care has also been cited as an advantage of nursing in the community setting. Another advantage has been the customary Monday-to-Friday daytime work schedule. Although a hospital must be staffed 24/7, few nonacute-care facilities require staffing for night shifts, weekends, and holidays. As more services are provided in the community, however, hours may expand.

Wages and salaries have tended to be somewhat lower for RNs in community-based practice. This is, in part, reflective of the lack of evening, night, and weekend differential payment. Also, some nurses report concern over the relative lack of a controlled environment and lack of immediate access to support from other nurses when providing nursing care in some community-based settings. This lack of support, or structure, may be a difficult adjustment for some nurses.

NATIONAL HEALTH GOALS

Healthy People: The Surgeon General's Report on Health Promotion and Disease Prevention was initially published in 1979 as a national prevention initiative of the U.S. Department of Health and Human Services (USDHHS) (2000). The 1979 version included a set of goals: reduce mortality among four different age groups—infants, children, adolescents and young adults, and adults—and increase independence among older adults.

1-2 Community-Based Employment Opportunities for Registered Nurses

AMBULATORY CARE

Physicians' offices (solo, partnership, or private group practice)
Managed health care organizations/insurers
HMOs
Utilization review
Case management
Hospital-based ambulatory services
Hospital clinics
Day surgery
Freestanding ambulatory surgery centers
Freestanding emergi-centers
Categorical clinics and services (may be hospital-based or freestanding)
Intravenous therapy and chemotherapy clinics
Dialysis units
Adult day care centers
Day care centers for ill children
Mental health clinics
Family planning clinics
Cardiac rehabilitation programs
Neurological rehabilitation programs (spinal cord injuries, multiple sclerosis, amyotrophic lateral sclerosis)
Geriatric clinics
Migrant health clinics
AIDS clinics
Diabetes management and education services
Pulmonary clinics (asthma, chronic obstructive pulmonary disease, cystic fibrosis)
Genetic screening and counseling services
Bloodmobiles
Freestanding diagnostic centers
Diagnostic imaging centers
Mobile mammography centers

HEALTH DEPARTMENT SERVICES

Maternal/child health clinics
Family planning clinics

Communicable disease control programs
HIV/AIDS (testing, counseling, and treatment)
Tuberculosis (testing, treatment, and surveillance)
Sexually transmitted diseases (testing, counseling, and treatment)
Immunization clinics
Neighborhood clinics serving disenfranchised populations
Mobile clinics serving disenfranchised populations
Substance abuse programs
Jails and prisons
Indian health service (American Indians and Alaska natives)

HOME HEALTH CARE SERVICES

Skilled nursing care
Intravenous therapy
High-risk pregnancy/neonate care
Maternal/child newborn care
Private duty (hourly care)
Respite care
Hospice care

LONG-TERM CARE

Skilled nursing facilities
Hospital-based facilities
Freestanding/nursing home-based facilities
Hospice facilities
Nursing homes
Skilled nursing care
Assisted living

OTHER COMMUNITY HEALTH SETTINGS

School health programs
Occupational health programs
Parish nursing programs
Summer camp programs
Childbirth education programs

AIDS, Acquired immunodeficiency syndrome; *HIV*, human immunodeficiency virus.

An updated version, *Healthy People 2000,* was published in 1990. *Healthy People 2000* contained three broad goals:

1. Increase the span of healthy life for Americans.
2. Reduce health disparities among Americans.
3. Achieve access to preventive services for all Americans (USDHHS, 1990).

Healthy People 2000 was developed to provide direction for individuals in changing personal behaviors and to guide organizations and communities in improving health through health-promotion policies. It was organized under the broad approaches of health promotion, health protection, and preventive

services and contained more than 300 objectives organized into 22 priority areas.

A third edition, **Healthy People 2010,** was introduced in January 2000. It expands on the objectives from *Healthy People 2000* through a broadened scientific base and improved surveillance and data systems. There is also a heightened awareness of preventive health services, which is reflective of changes in demographics, science, technology, and disease. *Healthy People 2010* lists two broad goals:

Goal 1: Increase quality and years of healthy life.
Goal 2: Eliminate health disparities.

Research Highlight

Future of Nursing Employment

Ongoing analyses indicate that the current and projected nursing shortage contributes to the challenge of an already demanding profession. In a review of studies of nursing service reports, Marrelli explained that the shortage of fulltime RNs is anticipated to grow from 6% in 2000 to 29% by 2020. In addition to simply requiring *more* nurses to provide care, she noted that nurses will need (1) to be better educated, (2) to be prepared to work in a wide variety of settings and situations from schools to hospitals (universal skill set), (3) specialized education and training to acquire the skills and knowledge to respond to changes in technology and evidence-based practice guidelines, (4) to understand the impact of the aging population (baby boomers) on the health care system, and (5) to be prepared to practice in a variety of settings.

Marrelli concluded that although hospitals will continue to be a major site for RN employment, the demand for RNs to work in nursing homes and home health care will grow significantly. Further, case management/care management and telehealth opportunities will increase dramatically. She challenged all RNs to recognize these changes and to respond to them by seeking educational programs, advanced training, and service opportunities.

Marrelli T: Nursing in flux: are you ready to meet the challenge of the future?, *Am J Nurs* 106(1):19, 2006.

Goal 1 moves beyond the idea of increasing life expectancy to incorporate the concept of "health-related-quality-of-life" (HRQOL), a concept of health that includes aspects of both physical and mental health and their determinants and measures functional status and well-being. By integrating mental and physical health concepts, it provides a way to expand the definition of health beyond simply being the opposite of the negative concepts of disease and death (USDHHS, 2000).

In *Healthy People 2010* some 467 objectives are divided into 28 focus areas (see the *Healthy People 2010* box). The objectives may be used as a framework to guide health-promotion activities in schools, clinics, worksites, and so forth and for community-wide initiatives (USDHHS, 2000). All health care practitioners should review *Healthy People 2010* objectives, focusing on those areas relevant to their practice. Whenever possible, objectives should be incorporated into programs, events, and publications and should be used to promote healthy individuals, families, groups, and communities.

Leading health indicators used to measure progress toward the *Healthy People 2010* goals focus on positively impacting physical activity, overweight and obesity, tobacco use, substance abuse, responsible sexual behavior, mental health, injury and violence, environmental quality, immunizations, and access to health care. These indicators are intended to help all Americans understand the importance of health promotion and disease prevention and to

healthy people 2010

Priority Areas

1. Access to quality health services
2. Arthritis, osteoporosis, and chronic back conditions
3. Cancer
4. Chronic kidney disease
5. Diabetes
6. Disability and secondary conditions
7. Educational and community-based programs
8. Environmental health
9. Family planning and sexual health
10. Food safety
11. Health communication
12. Heart disease and stroke
13. HIV
14. Immunizations and infectious diseases
15. Injury and violence prevention
16. Maternal, infant, and child health
17. Medical product safety
18. Mental health and mental disorders
19. Nutrition and overweight
20. Occupational safety and health
21. Oral health
22. Physical activity and fitness
23. Public health infrastructure
24. Respiratory diseases
25. Sexually transmitted diseases
26. Substance abuse
27. Tobacco use
28. Vision and hearing

From U.S. Department of Health and Human Services: *Healthy People 2010: National health promotion and disease prevention objectives*, Washington, DC, 2000, Government Printing Office.

encourage participation in improving health in the next decade.

Implementation of activities and interventions to achieve most of the goals for *Healthy People 2010* rests on health care providers in community-based practice. Furthermore, meeting these objectives requires changing the focus of practice from illness and cure to health promotion and illness prevention. Throughout this book, related objectives from *Healthy People 2010* and updates from the 2010 Midcourse Review (DHHS, 2007) are presented, and practical methods to achieve them are discussed (see the Research Highlight "*Healthy People 2010*").

SUMMARY

Health care at all levels is becoming increasingly community based. In response, nurses, such as Martha from the chapter-opening case study, must be educationally and experientially prepared to provide care in very diverse settings. Indeed, like Martha, nurses are learning that in most localities, RNs are desperately needed to fill positions in home health agencies, managed care organizations, and a large variety of outpatient clinics, as well as in acute care settings.

This chapter introduces the recognition of, and rationale for, enhancing educational opportunities for all nurses in community-based settings. Related information is presented in Chapter 2, which discusses differences and similarities between nursing roles and interventions in acute care and community settings.

KEY POINTS

- The health care delivery system is changing; care is becoming more focused on health promotion and illness prevention and moving from acute care and hospital-based delivery to prevention and management in community-based settings.
- Nurses have recognized the need to adapt delivery of care and nursing education to meet the needs of the population and the changing health care system.
- Like primary health care (preventive services and diagnosis and treatment of common acute episodic illnesses), secondary health care (relatively serious or complicated care traditionally provided in hospitals), and tertiary health care (management of chronic, complicated, long-term health problems) are increasingly being delivered in community-based settings.
- Although most nurses still work in hospitals, the proportion is changing, with nurses increasingly being employed in community-based settings. This trend is expected to continue.
- Opportunities for nurses to work in community-based settings are numerous and diverse.
- *Healthy People 2010* has two goals: (1) to increase quality and years of healthy life for U.S. residents and (2) to eliminate health disparities. Community-based health care providers are responsible for the implementation of activities and interventions to achieve most of the goals.

Research Highlight

Healthy People 2010

Albrecht and colleagues reported on a review of the literature documenting efforts to meet *Healthy People 2010* objectives for reducing smoking among pregnant women. They noted that to meet the *Healthy People 2010* objectives, 30% of pregnant women who smoke must stop smoking (up from a baseline of 14% of pregnant women) during the course of their pregnancy. To help prepare health providers to address this issue, the researchers reviewed almost 100 articles that described methods and programs aimed at reducing smoking among pregnant women. From their analysis, the team concluded that "health care professionals should routinely screen pregnant clients and women of childbearing age for tobacco use and should implement evidence-based smoking cessation strategies appropriate for pregnant women and women who may become pregnant" (p. 304). The authors explained that this literature review will be used to develop a research-based protocol, data collection tools, and instructions to encourage effective methods that could be used by providers and educators to reduce smoking among pregnant women.

Albrecht SA, Maloni JA, Thomas KK et al: Smoking cessation counseling for pregnant women who smoke: scientific basis for practice for AWHONN's SUCCESS project, J Obstet Gynecol Neonatal Nurs 33(3):298, 2004.

Learning Activities & Application to Practice

1. Obtain a copy of *The Registered Nurse Population: National Sample Survey of Registered Nurses* (USDHHS, 2006). Review changes in your geographic region. Compare local statistics with those of other regions of the United States.
2. Access the *Healthy People 2010* website (www.healthypeople.gov). With classmates, discuss the document and the implications for nursing practice.
3. Research employment opportunities for RNs in both hospital and community-based settings in your area. Where are more opportunities? Are there differences in salaries? Hours? Experience requirements? Share your findings with classmates.

REFERENCES

American Association of Colleges of Nursing (2007): *Nursing shortage fact sheet* (online): http://www.aacn.nche.edu/Media/FactSheets/NursingShortage.htm. Accessed June 11, 2007.

American Nurses Association: *Standards of community health nursing practice*, Washington, DC, 2004, American Nurses Association.

American Nurses Association: *Nursing's agenda for health care reform*, Washington, DC, 1991, American Nurses Association.

Hamner MB: Associate and baccalaureate degree preparation for home health care in an era of managed care. In Tagliareni ME, Marckx BB, editors: *Teaching in the community: preparing nurses for the 21st century*, Sudbury, Mass, 1999, Jones & Bartlett.

Heller BR, Oros MT, Durney-Crowley J: *The future of nursing education: ten trends to watch*, 2004, National League for Nursing website: www.nln.org/nlnjournal/infotrends.htm#1. Accessed June 11, 2007.

Marrelli T: Nursing in flux: are you ready to meet the challenge of the future?, *Am J Nurs* 106(1):19, 2006.

Matteson P: Preparing nurses for the future. In Matteson PS, editor: *Community-based nursing education*, New York, 2000, Springer.

Mengel A, Donnelly G: Associate degree and baccalaureate nursing education. In Tagliareni ME, Marckx BB, editors: *Teaching in the community: preparing nurses for the 21st century*, Sudbury, Mass, 1999, Jones & Bartlett.

National League for Nursing: *A vision for nursing education*, New York, 1993, National League for Nursing.

National League for Nursing/Council of Associate Degree Programs: *Web of inclusion: faculty helping faculty—evaluation summary*, National Video Conference October 14, 1994, New York, 1994, National League for Nursing.

Shi L, Singh DA: *Delivering health care in America: a systems approach*, Boston, 2004, Jones and Bartlett.

Tagliareni ME, Murray JP: Community-focused experiences in the ADN curriculum, *J Nurs Educ* 34(8):366, 1995.

Tri-Council (American Association of Colleges of Nursing, American Nurses Association, American Organization of Nurse Executives, National League for Nursing) 2001 White paper: Strategies to reverse the new nursing shortage (online): http://www.ana.org/pressrel/2001/sta0205.htm. Accessed July 26, 2001.

U.S. Department of Health and Human Services, Division of Nursing, Bureau of Health Professions, Public Health Service: *The registered nurse population: national sample survey of registered nurses, March 2004*, Washington, DC, 2006, Government Printing Office.

U.S. Department of Health and Human Services: *Healthy people 2000. national health promotion and disease prevention objectives*, Washington, DC, 1990, Government Printing Office.

U.S. Department of Health and Human Services: *Healthy people 2010*, Washington, DC, 2000, Government Printing Office.

U.S. Department of Health and Human Services: *Healthy people 2010 midcourse review*, 2006 (online): http://www.healthypeople.gov/data/midcourse/. Accessed June 11, 2007.

Zotti ME, Brown P, Stotts RC: Community-based nursing versus community health nursing: what does it all mean?, *Nurs Outlook* 44(5):211, 1996.

Zungolo E: Changing nursing education. In Matteson PS, editor: *Community-based nursing education*, New York, 2000, Springer.

Chapter 2

Roles and Interventions in Community-Based Nursing Practice

objectives

Upon completion of this chapter, the reader will be able to:

1. Discuss the various roles played by registered nurses in community-based practice.

2. Compare and contrast the emphasis placed on various roles in community-based practice and practice in acute care settings.

3. Give examples of nursing interventions used in various community-based settings and explain how they are similar to and different from nursing interventions in acute care settings.

key terms

Advocate
Collaborator
Counselor
Direct care provider
Educator

Leader
Manager
Nursing Interventions
    Classification (NIC) system
Researcher

Role model

See Glossary for definitions.

case study

Sally Smith is a home health nurse for a hospital-based agency in a small city. Last Tuesday Sally saw five clients: (1) Mrs. Black, to perform a fasting blood glucose tolerance test and to teach about type 2 diabetes; (2) Mr. Johnson, for twice-a-day dressing changes following amputation of his left great toe; (3) Mrs. Garcia, to teach about anticoagulant therapy and to draw blood to monitor clotting times; (4) Mrs. Gray, who has a diagnosis of Alzheimer's disease, and her family, who are considering placing her in a nursing home because they can no longer care for her at home; and (5) Mr. Jones, who was recently discharged from the hospital following an episode of congestive heart failure (CHF) and who needs to be evaluated for fluid retention, hypertension, and heart and lung function.

Sally performs several roles and interventions in her practice as a home health care nurse. In preparation, Sally must schedule the day's visits on the basis of several factors. For example, she needs to see Mrs. Black before breakfast to obtain an accurate fasting glucose value and allow her to maintain her normal insulin and breakfast schedule. Mr. Johnson must be seen

Continued

fairly early too because his dressing changes are scheduled for early to midmorning and early evening. To ensure accuracy, Mrs. Garcia's blood sample must be taken to the laboratory within 30 minutes, and the results should be reported to her physician by 3:00 pm. Finally, the visit to Mrs. Gray and her family is to be coordinated with one of the agency's medical social workers. Sally must consider each of these factors, calculate the distance that must be covered between the clients' residences, ensure that all supplies are available (dressing materials, laboratory supplies), and schedule with other providers when planning the day's visits. Therefore management of self, time, client's care needs and schedules, and resources is a key component of Sally's workday.

In addition to her management roles, Sally performs numerous skilled nursing interventions, such as physical assessment, wound care, blood glucose monitoring, and venipuncture. She continually teaches her clients about their health and health care management. She also collaborates closely with clients, their caregivers, the social worker, physicians, other home health care nurses, and various other providers (e.g., aides, therapists, laboratory technicians), and she routinely acts as a counselor, advocate, and role model for her clients, their families, and other caregivers.

Nursing practice in community settings differs considerably from practice in the hospital. Just as nursing practice in acute care institutions varies greatly from one area to another (the operating room differs from the intensive care unit [ICU], which differs from postpartum care, which differs from acute psychiatric care), it can be very different between community settings. Home health nursing is very different from school nursing, which in turn is very different from working in a health maintenance organization (HMO) or clinic. But just as there are similarities in nursing practice in acute care settings (i.e., following physician orders, medication administration, and taking vital signs), there are similarities throughout community settings (i.e., emphasis on health promotion, teaching, counseling, advocacy, and ensuring continuity of care).

NURSING ROLES IN COMMUNITY SETTINGS

Shortened hospital stays, proliferation of day surgery, emphasis on health promotion, recognition of the unique health care needs of older clients and the underserved, and the desire to decrease costs have changed the health care system and nursing practice (see Chapter 1). Performing traditional nursing skills (e.g., administering injections, taking vital signs, changing dressings) in the role of "direct care provider" is still an integral part of nursing practice, but the importance of other roles is increasing. Although the variety of roles that make up nursing practice is

the same no matter what the setting, the emphasis varies greatly. This chapter describes some of the roles common to nursing practice and explains how these roles differ in community-based practice compared with hospital-based practice and how they differ among community settings.

DIRECT CARE PROVIDER

The **direct care provider** role involves the direct delivery of care. Performing tasks or skills for which the nurse has been trained and that are typically associated with nursing practice (e.g., client assessment, taking vital signs, medication administration, changing dressings, and inserting catheters) is the essence of the role of direct care provider.

This role constitutes much of nursing practice in acute care settings, where patients are typically hospitalized after surgery or for treatment of serious or complex medical conditions. For example, most of an ICU nurse's time (about 70% to 80%) is spent in direct care provision. A nurse working on a "general medicine" floor devotes about 50% of the time in direct delivery of care. In contrast, the amount of time a nurse working in a postpartum unit spends in direct care delivery is 40% to 50%; for the nurse working in an inpatient psychiatric unit, it is 20% to 30%.

Although direct care provision is an important part of community-based nursing practice, this task tends to occupy less time than in acute care settings. In community settings direct care provision might be most time-intensive for the nurse in home health

(35% to 40%). It is less significant in occupational health or school health (10% to 15%), and it might be minimal at an HMO practice. As a result many nursing students and registered nurses (RNs) new to community-based practice often discount the nurse's importance in health care delivery in these settings because the nurses are not observed giving direct care (i.e., giving medication, performing hygiene procedures, managing intravenous lines). It is important that nurses recognize the difference in emphasis on roles in the various settings.

EDUCATOR

Regardless of the setting, health education is an essential component of quality nursing care. Education in hospitals typically focuses on patient instructions for posthospital discharge and is often severely restricted because of time limitations as hospital stays have become shortened. The limited amount of time for teaching, coupled with the acuity level of the patient and stress on the family, often means that health teaching is marginally effective. Incorporation of written discharge instructions with verbal explanations and other techniques, including postdischarge telephone calls, has helped improve the assimilation of information by clients and caregivers in acute care settings.

Although health education is an important nursing role in acute care settings, it is often the most significant role of the nurse working in community settings. Teaching individuals, families, and groups about maintenance of health, threats to health, and relevant lifestyle choices that affect health is integral in all community settings. The information presented should allow clients to make informed decisions on health matters and to direct self-care to follow treatment regimens.

The **educator** role makes up much of community-based nursing practice, as noted by the following:

- School nurses often spend 30% to 40% of their time providing health education in areas such as prevention of sexually transmitted diseases (STDs), basic hygiene, and dental care.
- Occupational health nurses instruct clients on issues such as accident prevention, ergonomics, smoking cessation strategies, and the importance of physical fitness.
- Home health nurses spend much of their time teaching clients and families self-care strategies

(e.g., dressing changes, diabetes management, colostomy care).
- Nurses in ambulatory clinic settings teach infant nutrition to new parents, signs and symptoms of infection to clients with acquired immunodeficiency syndrome (AIDS), principles of a low-fat diet to clients with coronary artery disease, and medication management to clients with CHF.

Health education goes beyond simple dissemination of information. Whether the information is instruction concerning the schedule and potential side effects of a prescribed medication, nutritional principles to reduce blood lipids, or breastfeeding, it must be presented appropriately for the individual client. As health educators, nurses should consider such factors as the client's developmental stage, learning readiness, language, educational level, and perceived learning needs. In addition, the nurse must accurately evaluate the learner's level of understanding and reinforce it accordingly.

All RNs should be familiar with the basics of client teaching. Theories, models, principles of teaching, and experience in applying principles need to be part of every introductory or nursing fundamentals course. Various tools (e.g., written materials, visual aids, models) and techniques (e.g., demonstration, observation, repetition) should be incorporated into the teaching plan. Use of terminology familiar to clients (i.e., avoidance of medical jargon), consideration of cultural variables, and encouraging or enabling clients to ask questions are essential nursing approaches. Evaluation of the client's level of understanding is accomplished through questioning, the use of return demonstration, or both. Chapter 3 provides detailed information related to patient education and health teaching.

COUNSELOR

A nurse in the role of **counselor** listens to clients and their families, encourages them to explore issues and options, and enables them to manage their personal situations. Assistance with identification of problems and possible solutions and guidance through the problem-solving process are functions of nurses in most community-based settings. Indeed, counseling represents a significant component of quality community-based nursing care. For example, a clinic nurse may discuss contraception options with a young mother; a school nurse might talk with a high school student perceived to be "at risk" for using drugs or alcohol; or a hospice nurse might discuss the importance of respite care (caring for the caregiver) with the family of a terminally ill client.

In contrast, nurses in acute care settings typically spend considerably less time counseling clients. Because much of the care in hospitals is directed by hospital procedure or physician orders, there tends to be less emphasis on this role. Exceptions may include nursing care in psychiatric settings, where counseling might constitute the greatest percentage of the nurse's time, and nursing care for families of very seriously ill clients for whom the family must weigh options for treatment and long-term care.

ADVOCATE

A nurse **advocate** is one who acts on behalf of, or intercedes for, the client. Frequently clients—particularly children, elderly people, and the disadvantaged—are unable to obtain needed care and services within today's health care system. Advocates ensure that clients receive necessary care and services.

Nurses act as client advocates in all settings. In hospitals, nurses work as advocates through creative interventions such as:

- Ensuring that patients are as pain free as possible, even if it means phoning a physician at 1:00 co to change a medication.
- Working with administrators to plan visiting hours to accommodate individual and family needs.
- Helping parents to stay in hospital rooms with small children.
- Protecting a client's desires regarding advanced directives.

In community settings, the nurse's role as an advocate is vital. Because they often work with vulnerable populations, nurses in community settings serve as client advocates constantly (Box 2-1). For example, it is often the school nurse who identifies a source of funding to pay for eyeglasses for the child whose parents cannot afford them or who identifies and reports suspected child abuse or neglect. The occupational health nurse's responsibility is to ensure that Occupational Safety and Health Administration (OSHA) guidelines for employee safety are carried out. The home health nurse may be the one

BOX **2-1** The Nurse as Advocate

According to Schroeter, advocacy refers to the act of pleading for, supporting, urging by argument, recommending publicly, and active espousal. Advocacy implies taking action to achieve a goal on behalf of another, and in nursing it is directly related to client care. As client advocates, nurses should continually strive to ensure the quality and continuity of care and to make certain that clients' needs are being met. Nurses must also be advocates for each other, coworkers, family members, and students. The following concepts are keys to advocacy:

- Understanding advocacy as an ethical concept. In nursing, advocacy is an ethical practice based on individual values and nursing's code of ethics.
- Understanding the place of advocacy within nursing practice. Nurses must recognize that advocacy is an important component of basic practice standards.
- Analyzing personal communication skills. Nurses should recognize their own strengths and weaknesses in interpersonal skills and develop them as needed.
- Identifying situations in which advocacy is necessary. Nurses should follow their own values and ethical perspectives in identifying advocacy situations, but they should also recognize differing perspectives and adapt accordingly.
- Taking action. Advocacy involves taking some type of action (physical, written, verbal), and nurses should be willing to take action when appropriate.

From Schroeter K: Advocacy in perioperative nursing practice, *AORN J* 71(6):1207-10, 1213, 1215-18, 2000.

who finds a way to provide glucose monitoring strips for an older client who cannot afford to buy them, and the nurse in the homeless shelter clinic might ensure that clients receive blankets and coats in the winter.

MANAGER

Possibly most similar to the role of the nurse in an acute care setting is the role of the nurse as **manager** in a community-based practice. Nursing care in both hospital and community settings involves management of the nurse's time, limited resources, other personnel, program organization and coordination, and management of the client's care. The management role includes planning, organizing, coordinating, marketing, controlling, and evaluating care and care delivery.

For example, in community settings school nurses do the following:

- Manage clinics.
- Ensure that student records are complete.

- Perform and document legally mandated services, such as vision and hearing screenings.
- Direct clinic volunteers.

As described in the case study earlier, home health nurses:

- Coordinate scheduled visits based on client needs (i.e., fasting blood glucose or three times daily intravenous administration), estimating distances between client's homes and services to be provided.
- Ensure that other professional services are delivered when necessary and monitor or oversee the practice of a home health aide.
- Use each client's resources to develop a plan of care.

Nurses in clinics or physician offices perform triage so that clients in need of immediate help are treated first, ensure that supplies and equipment are available, and assist in ensuring that clients are seen in a timely fashion.

OTHER ROLES IN COMMUNITY-BASED NURSING

Direct care provider, educator, manager, counselor, and advocate are the roles most often performed by nurses. Additional roles all nurses should perform routinely or occasionally are the following:

- Collaborator
- Role model
- Researcher
- Leader

Each role is described briefly, and examples for application of each role to community-based nursing practice are presented.

Collaborator

Changes in health care delivery have included a move from reliance on an individual physician as the sole director of care (who is thereby responsible for all aspects of care) to a more comprehensive, interdisciplinary approach wherein several health care team members are responsible for various facets of care. The nurse in the role of **collaborator** participates in health care management decision making with individuals from various professions and works with the client and family or caregivers to jointly determine the course of care. Through interaction, discussion, and coordination, goals are set and a plan of care is formed to meet those goals.

For clients with a complex or chronic health problem, such as coronary artery disease, Alzheimer's disease, or renal failure, the nurse must work with other health providers to deliver the most comprehensive, effective, cost-conscious care possible. Caring for a stroke victim, for example, may involve collaboration between physicians, nurses, physical therapists, occupational therapists, speech therapists, and possibly others in both community and hospital settings.

Similarly, health-promotion interventions need to be collaborative. For example, a team of professionals in a senior health clinic might work with an elderly client with diabetes to teach principles of nutrition, medication management, and foot care. The nurse in this setting might collaborate with a dietitian, pharmacist, diabetes educator, and others to seek the best management of client care (Box 2-2).

Role Model

A **role model** is a person who demonstrates an action or behavior that is learned by others. Role modeling is both conscious and unconscious, and nurses in all settings, whether "on the job" or at home, are in a position to demonstrate to others both positive and negative actions and attitudes related to health and health care.

BOX 2-2 The Nurse as Collaborator

In a recent article Strawhacker and Wellendorf examined the importance of collaboration among nurses, families, and clinicians while caring for school-aged children with cystic fibrosis. The authors noted several factors that promote collaboration between school staff, families and clinical providers. These include frequent and explicit communication between and among all who help care for the child, establishment and maintenance of a trusting relationship, sharing of goals and plans across all settings, seeking clarification from fellow professionals whenever in doubt, and addressing misunderstandings quickly and thoroughly. It was reiterated that these principles can be applied in many situations in which nurses in school settings must collaborate with multiple individuals in order to promote optimal health and assist academic achievement for all children.

From Strawhacker MT, Wellendorf J: Caring for children with cystic fibrosis: a collaborative clinical and school approach, *J Sch Nurs* 20(1):5-15, 2004..

In community-based practice, nurses serve as role models to clients, their caregivers, and other health professionals. For example, a student receiving helpful, therapeutic, understanding care from the school nurse might be motivated to become a nurse; the caregiver of an elderly woman watching the professional, matter-of-fact changing of a sterile dressing may be convinced that he or she, too, may be able to learn to perform this task. In another example, a nurse working with immigrant families in a community clinic can demonstrate care, empathy, and appreciation for cultural differences of clients to new employees and nursing students working in the clinic.

Researcher

Nurses, whatever their practice setting or primary population served, must remain informed of developments that are relative to their individual practice. Nurses should be careful, discriminating consumers of research. In the role of **researcher** they should critically review research findings for merit and applicability to practice and should determine care accordingly. Nurses in obstetric clinics, for example, should be aware of the latest recommendations regarding dietary guidelines during pregnancy and the rationale behind these recommendations. Similarly, nurses working with new families should share findings about sleeping positions for newborns, and nurses who work with adults should be aware of new guidelines and rationale for prostate and breast screenings and exercise and diet recommendations. Often the client is unaware of recent discoveries and innovations related to health, and it is the nurse's responsibility to share them when relevant.

Occasionally a nurse in community-based practice may be a part of a research study. Identifying problems or questions for investigation, participating in approved research studies, and disseminating research findings to clients and other professionals are appropriate actions for all nurses.

Leader

Leadership refers to the ability to influence the behavior of others. In community settings the nurse may assume the role of a leader with clients and their families, other health care providers, public officials, local leaders, or employers.

As a **leader** the nurse may work with others to identify and assess threats to health and intervene to remove or lessen these threats. For example, a nurse employed in a manufacturing setting might direct a group in establishing a health-promotion program; a school nurse might lead a coalition of concerned parents to improve the nutritional value of hot lunches; and a nurse working in a clinic for low-income families might undertake the establishment of evening hours to meet the scheduling needs of the working poor.

COMPARISON OF NURSING ROLES IN HOSPITALS AND COMMUNITY SETTINGS

Although each of the many roles should be part of quality comprehensive nursing care in any setting, role emphasis varies according to each client's needs and from setting to setting. Figure 2-1 visually depicts estimates of time spent by nurses in various roles in selected community and acute care settings. The time spent in any role varies according to each client's specific needs. Remember, these are estimates and are not meant to be examples of ideal amounts of time spent in each role. Furthermore, they are not necessarily accurate for each nurse in each setting. Instead, the purpose of the diagrams is to illustrate the variety of nursing roles in different settings.

NURSING INTERVENTIONS IN COMMUNITY SETTINGS

Nursing interventions have been defined as "any treatment, based upon clinical judgment and knowledge, that a nurse performs to enhance patient/client outcomes," and they include both direct and indirect care and treatments that may be nurse-initiated, physician-initiated, or other provider-initiated (Bulechek et al, 2008, p. xxi). Because nursing roles vary, often dramatically, between acute care and community settings and among different community settings, nursing interventions also vary.

The **Nursing Interventions Classification (NIC) system** (Bulechek et al, 2008) is the most comprehensively developed taxonomy of nursing interventions. The NIC system lists 542 nursing interventions that have been defined and developed to include thousands of appropriate nursing activities (behaviors or actions that implement the intervention) for

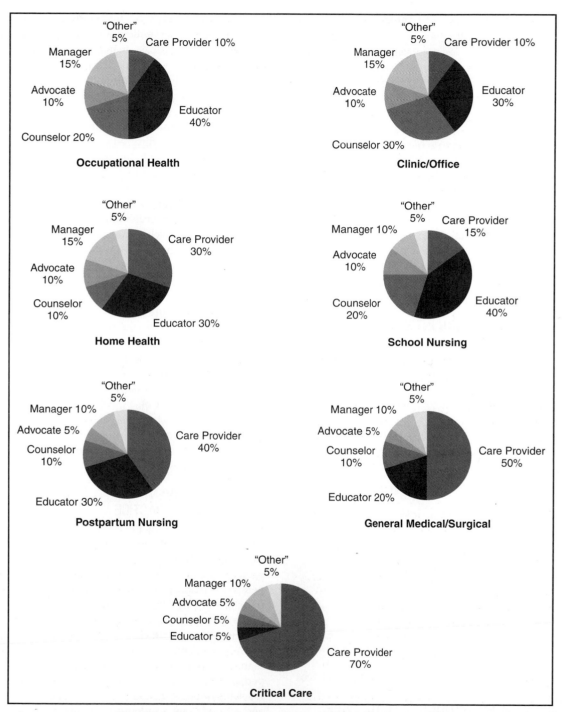

Figure 2-1. Comparison of nursing roles in selected settings.

each. The identified nursing interventions are divided into seven "domains":

1. *Physiological (basic): care that supports physical functioning.*
2. *Physiological (complex): care that supports homeostatic regulation.*
3. *Behavioral: care that supports psychosocial functioning and facilitates lifestyle changes.*
4. *Safety: care that supports protection against harm.*
5. *Family: care that supports the family.*
6. *Health system: care that supports effective use of the health care delivery system.*
7. *Community: care that supports the health of the community.*

Bulechek et al, 2008

Each domain is further divided into "classes" into which individual interventions are grouped. Some interventions fall into more than one class or domain. The remainder of the chapter describes some of the similarities and differences in nursing interventions in community and acute care settings.

"UNIVERSAL" NURSING INTERVENTIONS

Certain nursing interventions are required of virtually all nurses in almost all settings (Bulechek et al, 2008). Examples of universal nursing interventions are as follows:

- *Documentation: recording of pertinent patient data in a clinical record.*
- *Environmental management (safety): monitoring and manipulation of the physical environment to promote safety.*
- *Anticipatory guidance: preparation of patient for an anticipated developmental and/or situational crisis.*
- *Infection control: minimizing the acquisition and transmission of infectious agents.*
- *Laboratory data interpretation: critical analysis of patient laboratory data in order to assist with clinical decision making.*
- *Learning facilitation: promoting the ability to process and comprehend information.*
- *Patient rights protection: protection of health care rights of a patient, especially a minor, incapacitated or incompetent patient unable to make decisions.*
- *Physician support: collaborating with physicians to provide quality patient care.*
- *Vital signs monitoring: collection and analysis of cardiovascular, respiratory, and body temperature data to determine and prevent complications.*

Bulechek et al, 2008

NURSING INTERVENTIONS IN ACUTE CARE

Some nursing interventions are very specialized, and nurses would provide related activities only when delivering care in certain settings. For example, in critical care settings nurses frequently perform many of the nursing interventions termed "physiological complex" (e.g., acid-base management, cerebral edema management, circulatory care, mechanical assist device), but rarely perform many from the "behavioral" domain (e.g., behavior modification, learning readiness enhancement, health education).

Alternatively, many of the interventions in the "family" domain are directed specifically to the practice of perinatal nursing, including the following:

- Cesarean section care
- Electronic fetal monitoring: intrapartum care
- High-risk pregnancy care

Some nursing interventions are performed only rarely outside the acute care or emergency setting, as illustrated by the following examples:

- Anesthesia administration
- Autotransfusion
- Artificial airway management
- Cardiac care: acute
- Cerebral edema management
- Circulatory care
- Electronic fetal monitoring
- Endotracheal extubation
- Gastrointestinal intubation
- Hemorrhage control
- Intrapartal care: high-risk delivery
- Mechanical ventilation
- Traction and immobilization care
- Tube care: chest

NURSING INTERVENTIONS FREQUENTLY USED IN COMMUNITY PRACTICE

A number of nursing interventions are commonly used throughout all community settings and more often than in acute care settings. For example, abuse protection support (identification of high-risk dependent relationships and actions to prevent further infliction of physical or emotional harm) is appropriate for home health nurses who see caregivers of seriously ill or infirm clients and are in a position to identify who may need respite care. In the same manner, school nurses and nurses in geriatric or pediatric clinics and similar settings should monitor for signs of neglect or unexplained illness or injury and should seek to identify parents or caregivers who might be at risk of being abusers (i.e., alcoholics or substance abusers or those abused as children) (Bulechek et al, 2008).

Bulechek et al (2008) also identified other nursing interventions commonly found throughout community-based practice:

- *Health education: developing and providing instruction and learning experiences to facilitate voluntary adaptation of behavior conductive to health in individuals, families, groups, or communities.*
- *Health screening: detecting health risks or problems by means of history, examination, and other procedures.*
- *Health system guidance: facilitating a patient's location and use of appropriate health services.*
- *Medication administration: preparing, giving, and evaluating the effectiveness of prescription and nonprescription drugs.*
- *Teaching (prescribed medication): preparing a patient to safely take prescribed medications and monitoring for their effects.*
- *Nutritional counseling: use of an interactive helping process focusing on the need for diet modification.*
- *Referral: arrangement for services by another care provider or agency.*
- *Risk identification: analysis of potential risk factors, determination of health risks, and prioritization of risk reduction strategies for an individual or group.*
- *Teaching (individual): planning, implementation, and evaluation of a teaching program designed to address a patient's particular needs.*

- *Telephone consultation: eliciting patient's concerns; listening and providing support, information, or teaching in response to patient's stated concerns, over the telephone. [See the Community Application box about telephone consultation.]*

Bulechek et al, 2008

Although not all of these interventions are implemented by all nurses working in community settings, they are performed by most nurses.

Table 2-1 compares typical nursing interventions for several settings, both hospital-based and community-based. As with the comparison of nursing roles in various settings, these are examples only, and the lists are by no means comprehensive or exclusive. Nursing in each area involves many more interventions than are presented here, and there may be significant overlap and exceptions in all areas.

SUMMARY

To deliver comprehensive, competent, appropriate, and effective client care in any setting, a number of nursing roles and nursing interventions are required. As a home health nurse, Sally from the

---

COMMUNITY APPLICATION
Nursing Intervention: Telephone Consultation

Robinson, Anderson, and Acheson described the process for implementing a telephone health advice program. They suggested the following steps:

- Define the scope of the problem. Conduct a descriptive prospective study of trends in telephone calls, including chief complaints, temporal distribution of calls (e.g., are calls heaviest in the morning, evening, weekends), the profile of the caller (gender, age, client or family member), and type of problem(s).
- Identify problems to be addressed via telephone. Prepare a list of the chief symptoms reported by callers, and determine whether advice can be provided over the telephone.
- Develop protocols or guidelines. Telephone protocols or guidelines should be developed to evaluate, classify, advise, educate, and intervene in advice calls. Nurses may develop their own protocols or use those marketed for telephone consultation. If existing protocols are used, the standards of care for the community should be incorporated. Protocols should be comprehensive, current, authoritative, user friendly, symptom based, and conservative.

- Develop a file system for protocols. Protocols should be filed alphabetically according to the symptom(s) addressed. A computer database that can search and find the appropriate protocol on the basis of key words is ideal. A copy of the protocols and reference material should be placed at the telephone station.
- Determine a method for documentation. A log of calls and advice given should be maintained to minimize legal risk. Documentation should include date and time of call, name of caller/client, demographic information about the caller/client, brief statement of illness history and signs and symptoms, statement of advice given/protocol followed, any warning given regarding time frame within which the caller should be seen, and any warnings regarding the severity of the illness.
- Set quality controls. Formal orientation should be provided for those providing telephone consultation. Phone logs should be audited periodically to track trends and critique the quality of information given by the RN.

From Robinson DL, Anderson MM, Acheson PM: Telephone advice: lessons learned and considerations for stating programs, *J Emerg Nurs* 22(5):409-415, 1996.

TABLE **2-1** Commonly Used Nursing Interventions in Selected Settings

PHYSIOLOGIC	BEHAVIORAL	SAFETY
HOME HEALTH		
Wound care Cardiac care: rehabilitative Phlebotomy: venous blood sample IV therapy Medication administration Chemotherapy management	Anxiety reduction Teaching: disease process Teaching: preoperative Teaching: prescribed medication Teaching: prescribed activity/ exercise Teaching: prescribed diet	Risk identification Fall prevention Abuse protection support: elder
SCHOOL NURSING		
Oral health promotion Medication administration: oral Heat/cold application Exercise promotion	Substance use prevention Behavior management: overactivity/ inattention Teaching: group Teaching: sexuality Distraction	First aid Abuse protection: child Immunization/ vaccination administration Risk identification
AMBULATORY CARE NURSING (CLINIC OR PHYSICIAN'S OFFICE)		
Phlebotomy: venous blood sample Exercise promotion Weight management Weight reduction assistance Medication administration	Self-responsibility facilitation Smoking cessation assistance Substance use prevention Substance use treatment Communication enhancement: hearing deficit Coping enhancement Decision-making support Teaching: disease process Teaching: preoperative Teaching: prescribed diet Teaching: safe sex	First aid Triage Abuse protector: child Abuse protector: elder Health screening Immunization/ vaccination administration Risk identification
OCCUPATIONAL HEALTH NURSING		
Weight management Exercise promotion Weight reduction assistance Stress management	Health education Self-responsibility facilitation Smoking cessation assistance Substance use prevention Coping enhancement Decision-making support Teaching: safe sex	Environmental management: worker safety First aid Emergency care Health screening Risk identification Surveillance: safety

FAMILY	HEALTH SYSTEM	COMMUNITY
Caregiver support Home maintenance assistance Normalization promotion Family involvement Respite care	Culture brokerage Discharge planning Health system guidance Insurance authorization Supply management Multidisciplinary care conference Referral Telephone consultation	Case management Risk identification
Developmental enhancement Family involvement Family integrity promotion Parent education: childbearing family Parent education: adolescent	Health policy monitoring Supply management Multidisciplinary care conference Referral	Health screening Health education Program development
Caregiver support Family mobilization Developmental enhancement Family involvement Family integrity promotion Parent education: childbearing family	Referral Telephone consultation Insurance authorization Health system guidance Controlled substance checking Supply management Health care information exchange	Community disaster preparedness Surveillance: community
Role enhancement Family integrity promotion Parent education: childbearing family Family support	Referral Telephone consultation Insurance authorization Health system guidance Controlled substance checking Supply management Health policy monitoring	Community disaster preparedness Environmental risk protection Program development

Continued

TABLE **2-1** Commonly Used Nursing Interventions in Selected Settings—cont'd

PHYSIOLOGIC	BEHAVIORAL	SAFETY
CRITICAL CARE NURSING		
Acid-based management	Dying care	Code management
Airway suctioning	Emotional support	Area restriction
Artificial airway management	Presence	
Bowel management		
Cardiac care: acute		
Cerebral edema management		
Circulatory care		
Electrolyte management		
Phlebotomy: arterial blood sample		
Tube care: chest		
IV therapy		
Embolus precautions		
Pain management		
GENERAL MEDICAL/SURGICAL NURSING		
Exercise therapy: ambulation	Anxiety reduciton	Code management
Self-care assistance	Teaching: disease process	
Cough enhancement	Teaching: preoperative	
IV therapy	Teaching: prescribed medication	
Incision site care	Teaching: prescribed activity/	
Venous access device maintenance	exercise	
Self-care assistance	Teaching: prescribed diet	
POSTPARTUM NURSING		
Perineal care	Grief work facilitation: perinatal	Code management
Constipation management	death	Area restriction
Pelvic floor exercise	Support system enhancement	
Self-care assistance	Family planning: contraception	
Pain management	Parent education: childbearing	
Bleeding reduction: postpartum	family	
uterus	Teaching: infant care	

Data from Bulechek GM, Butcher HK, Dochterman JM (editors): *Nursing interventions classification (NIC)* ed 5, St. Louis, 2008, Mosby.

opening case study is an advocate and role model in addition to a direct care provider. In these roles she performs multiple nursing interventions.

This chapter describes some functions—manager, health educator, counselor—associated with the most important nursing roles and has shown how they are distinctive in both acute care and commu-nity settings. Likewise, nursing interventions are numerous and diverse and their implementation may vary significantly from setting to setting. Similarities and differences are discussed to encourage nurses to recognize and appreciate some of the unique characteristics of nursing care in a wide variety of settings.

FAMILY	HEALTH SYSTEM	COMMUNITY
Family involvement Family process maintenance Family mobilization	Delegation Emergency cart checking Order transcription Shift report Visitation facilitation Bedside laboratory testing Technology management	Environmental risk protection Environmental management: worker safety
Family involvement Family process maintenance Family mobilization Normalization promotion	Admission care Discharge planning Bedside laboratory testing Delegation Emergency cart checking Order transcription Shift report	Case management Environmental management: worker safety
Postpartum care Attachment promotion Breastfeeding assistance Environmental management: attachment process Infant care Newborn monitoring Caregiver support Family integrity promotion	Admission care Discharge planning Bedside laboratory testing Delegation Emergency cart checking Order transcription Shift report	Environmental management: worker safety

KEY POINTS

- Nursing practice in community-based settings differs considerably from practice in the hospital, and nursing practice also differs across various community settings.
- Nursing roles that are most frequently played in community-based practice are educator, counselor, manager, advocate, and care provider. The amount of time spent in each role varies from setting to setting, client to client, and day to day.
- Nursing interventions vary, often dramatically, between acute care and community-based settings and among different community settings.

Learning Activities & Application to Practice
In Class

1. With classmates, discuss or debate how the various roles of the nurse differ from setting to setting. What role or roles are seen as most important in each setting? Why?

2. Obtain a copy of *Nursing Interventions Classification (NIC)*, 5th edition (Bulechek, Butcher, & Dochterman,, 2008). Outline examples of nursing interventions that would be appropriate in several situations in both hospital and community settings. Discuss similarities and differences.

In Clinical

3. Estimate the amount of time you spend during your clinical day in each of the nursing roles described. Keep track of these estimates in a log or diary. Do nursing roles change between settings? How and why? Compare observations with classmates in other settings.

4. List nursing interventions you have performed in each clinical setting in a log or diary. How are interventions different in each setting? Do you feel some interventions are more important or necessary than others? Why or why not?

REFERENCES

Bulechek GM, Butcher HK, Dochterman JM (editors): *Nursing interventions classification (NIC)*, ed 5, St. Louis, 2008, Mosby.

Robinson DL, Anderson MM, Acheson PM: Telephone advice: lessons learned and considerations for stating programs, *J Emerg Nurs* 22(5):409, 1996.

Schroeter K: Advocacy in perioperative nursing practice, *AORN J* 71(6):1207, 2000.

Strawhacker MT, Wellendorf J: Caring for children with cystic fibrosis: a collaborative clinical and school approach, *J Sch Nurs* 20(1):5, 2004.

Client Education and Health Teaching

Upon completion of this chapter, the reader will be able to:

1. Define health education.

2. Apply the Health Belief Model and the Transtheoretical Model to enhance the health education of individuals or groups in a community setting.

3. Assess the learning needs of clients in a community setting.

4. Plan client-centered health education programs for individuals, families or groups in a community setting.

5. Create learning objectives for a health education program.

6. Use appropriate teaching methods in health education.

7. Apply principles of education while teaching low–literacy learners about health.

8. Evaluate a health education plan.

Chunking	Learning	
Health Belief Model	Literacy	
Health communication	Objectives	
Health education	Transtheoretical Model	*See Glossary for definitions*

Erin Short, RN, works in a public health department caring for young children and their families. She is responsible for assessing the children's health, their growth and development, and their family's health and response to parenting. One important component of Erin's practice is teaching parents and caregivers about child health promotion and strategies for illness prevention.

Recently Erin conducted a well-child visit with Sylvia Martinez, a 6-year-old brought to the clinic by her mother. During assessment Erin noted that Sylvia is 48 inches tall and weighs 88 pounds, making her body mass index (BMI) 26.6, according to published guidelines. These
Continued

measurements put Sylvia in the 99th percentile of BMI for her age, height, and gender, indicating that she is overweight. In addition, Erin noted darkening of the skin on Sylvia's neck and in both axilla, suggesting acanthosis nigricans. Fortunately Sylvia's blood pressure is within normal limits for her age and gender, but her high BMI and acanthosis nigricans concerned Erin.

Erin questioned Mrs. Martinez about her impression of Sylvia's weight. Mrs. Martinez responded that she thought Sylvia is "a little chubby, but healthy, and we are all heavy. Besides," Mrs. Martinez remarked, "there is nothing that I can do about her weight."

During the health history, Mrs. Martinez reported that Sylvia eats about nine tortillas and drinks several glasses of fruit juice each day in addition to eating three meals and snacks. Her mother also explained that Sylvia doesn't like to play outside, but "sits in front of the TV all of the time."

Erin recalls that Mrs. Martinez is a stay-at-home mom with four children: Tony, 13; Maria, 11; Eddie, 9; and Sylvia, 6. Though all of their children are doing well in school, Mr. and Mrs. Martinez have only 6 to 8 years of formal education and are not native English speakers. Mr. Martinez works long hours as a store owner, and the family struggles financially. Mrs. Martinez states that her husband "wants a big dinner when he gets home," and that "we all like the foods that we are used to, and we don't want to eat new stuff."

What education needs are evident in this case study?

What barriers to patient education can be discerned?

What strategies could Erin use to teach the Martinez family to achieve a more healthy weight for Sylvia and other family members?

More on the Case Study will follow.

INTRODUCTION TO HEALTH EDUCATION

Health education has always been a part of nursing care. Early nurse leaders such as Florence Nightingale, Mary Breckinridge, and Lillian Wald understood that that an individual's actions, or the lack thereof, can have a profound effect on health. Accordingly they sought to improve the lives and health of their clients through health education.

Education is empowering. Through education individuals and families gain the knowledge and skills necessary to make decisions (good or bad) regarding their health. Knowledgeable clients can then make informed choices, rather than merely responding to circumstances or being acted upon by external forces in their environment. Education rejects the idea that people are deficient; it is their knowledge that is deficient. Through education clients themselves can manage their health and make behavioral changes, which may positively influence well-being.

Nurses teach their clients in whatever setting they find them. For example, a school nurse may teach a child with diabetes to administer her own insulin; a public health nurse may teach a young mother how to feed her infant and how to use contraception; an occupational health nurse may teach factory workers about back safety; or a nurse working in a prison may teach inmates how to avoid contracting a bloodborne illness.

On some occasions, education is planned and delivered in formal classroom-type settings. Most often, however, it is delivered as nurses interact with clients in informal face-to-face encounters. Increasingly clients are well-informed after receiving health education from the internet, television, or written materials. These clients may ask many questions about their health.

During the course of daily practice, every nurse will consider such questions as: "Why does this person continue to smoke, even after the diagnosis of lung cancer?" or "Why doesn't this parent seek immunizations for her children?" The frustrations associated with seeing clients continue to smoke or overeat or fail to control chronic health conditions such as diabetes and hypertension are familiar to health professionals. Why people fail to follow known and established health recommendations is one of the most perplexing aspects of health promotion. Although education alone does not always produce constructive changes in behavior, it is an essential component that must be addressed if desired behavior change is to take place.

Health education seeks to close the gap between what people know about optimum health practice and what they actually do (Griffiths, 1972). Health education is defined as "any planned combination of **learning** experiences designed to predispose, enable, and reinforce voluntary behavior conducive to health in individuals, groups, or communities" (Green and Kreuter, 1991, p. 432). The broad goal of health education is to assist individuals, families, groups, and communities to achieve optimum health by providing information regarding health risks, tools, motivation, and support needed to produce a change in behavior that will reduce these risks. As research continues to find associations between behavior and health risks, "closing the gap" between knowledge and behavior assumes new urgency.

This aspect of patient care is recognized in *Healthy People 2010* as Focus Area 11, which covers the practice of **health communication**. *Health communication* refers to the use of communication strategies to inform and influence individuals and communities in making decisions regarding their health (U.S. DHHS, 2000). The health communication focus is concerned with evaluating access to health information resources such as internet resources, written materials, face-to-face encounters with health care professionals, and exposure to public service announcements and other health information carried on public media. Attributes of effective health communication are found in Box 3-1. Like health education, health communication covers the continuum of health promotion across the lifespan and uses all levels of prevention. Anticipatory guidance for parents of young children and information regarding health promotion in adulthood (primary prevention), screening to detect early disease (secondary prevention), and rehabilitation (tertiary prevention) are addressed in this focus of *Healthy People 2010*.

THEORETICAL FOUNDATIONS FOR HEALTH EDUCATION

Health education is rooted in community-based efforts in communities, schools, and worksites. As a result, the theories that form the foundation for its practice and application are quite diverse. A working

---

BOX 3-1 National Center for Health Statistics

ATTRIBUTES OF EFFECTIVE HEALTH COMMUNICATION

- **Accuracy:** The content is valid and without errors of fact, interpretation, or judgment.
- **Availability:** The content (whether targeted message or other information) is delivered or placed where the audience can access it. Placement varies according to audience, message complexity, and purpose, ranging from interpersonal and social networks to billboards, and mass transit signs to prime-time TV or radio, to public kiosks (print or electronic), to the internet.
- **Balance:** Where appropriate, the content presents the benefits and risks of potential actions or recognizes different and valid perspectives on the issue.
- **Consistency:** The content remains internally consistent over time and also is consistent with information from other sources (the latter is a problem when other widely available content is not accurate or reliable).
- **Cultural competence:** The design, implementation, and evaluation process that accounts for special issues for select population groups (for example, ethnic, racial, and linguistic) and also educational levels and disability.
- **Evidence base:** Relevant scientific evidence that has undergone comprehensive review and rigorous analysis to formulate practice guidelines, performance measures, review criteria, and technology assessments for telehealth applications.
- **Reach:** The content gets to or is available to the largest possible number of people in the target population.
- **Reliability:** The source of the content is credible, and the content itself is kept up to date.
- **Repetition:** The delivery of/access to the content is continued or repeated over time, both to reinforce the impact with a given audience and to reach new generations.
- **Timeliness:** The content is provided or available when the audience is most receptive to, or in need of, the specific information.
- **Understandability:** The reading or language level and format (including multimedia) are appropriate for the specific audience.

From U.S. Department of Health and Human Services (2000): *Healthy People 2010* (website): http://www.healthypeople.gov/Document/pdf/Volume1/1HealthCom.pdf. Accessed September 10, 2007.

---

knowledge of relevant theory is essential to promoting an understanding of why clients act as they do and to help them progress from knowledge to behavior change. Two theories that are used frequently in health education, the Health Belief Model and the Transtheoretical Model, are discussed here.

THE HEALTH BELIEF MODEL

Initially proposed in 1958, The **Health Belief Model** (HBM) provides the basis for much of the practice of health education today. The HBM was developed by a group of social psychologists to explain why the public failed to participate in screening for tuberculosis (Hochbaum, 1958). Hochbaum and his associates had the same questions that perplex many health professionals today: Why do people who may have a disease reject health screening? Why do individuals participate in screening if it may lead to the diagnosis of disease? Through their work, this group found that information alone is rarely enough to motivate one to act. Individuals must know what to do and how to do it before they can take action. Also, the information must be related in some way to the individual's needs. One of the most widely-used conceptual frameworks in health behavior, the HBM has been used to explain behavior change, maintain behavior change, and guide health promotion interventions (Janz et al, 2002).

The HBM has several constructs: perceived seriousness, perceived susceptibility, perceived benefits of treatment, perceived barriers to treatment, cues to action, and self-efficacy. These components are found in Table 3-1. All of these constructs relate to the *client's* perception. How does the client perceive: The seriousness of the condition? His susceptibility to the condition? The benefits of prevention or treatment? The barriers to prevention or treatment?

Consider the Martinez Family

Does Mrs. Martinez perceive that Sylvia is susceptible to problems associated with being overweight? Her comment that "we are all heavy" indicates that she knows Sylvia has a weight problem. Sylvia's overweight status is also an observable fact. What about Sylvia's susceptibility to the complications of being overweight? Mrs. Martinez thinks that Sylvia is "a little chubby, but healthy" and has remarked that her weight is not bad for her health, so she probably does not perceive that there are serious health complications related to overweight.

On the other hand, Erin fears that Sylvia may be susceptible to development of Type 2 diabetes. The fact that Mrs. Martinez states "there is nothing that I can do about her weight" could indicate that she may not perceive benefits to treating Sylvia or that she feels Sylvia's condition is beyond prevention efforts.

Mrs. Martinez faces several perceived barriers to weight management for her daughter. For example, Mrs. Martinez's lack of knowledge about proper diet, including serving sizes and appropriate food

TABLE **3-1** Key Concepts and Definitions of the Health Belief Model

CONCEPT	DEFINITION
Perceived susceptibility	One's belief regarding the chance of getting a given condition
Perceived seriousness	One's belief regarding the seriousness of a given condition
Perceived benefits	One's belief in the ability of an advised action to reduce the health risk or seriousness of a given condition
Perceived barriers	One's belief regarding the tangible and psychological costs of an advised action
Cues to action	Strategies or conditions in one's environment that activate readiness to take action.
Self-efficacy	One's confidence in one's ability to take action to reduce health risks.

From Janz NK, Champion VL, Stretcher VJ: The health belief model. In Glanz K, Rimer BK, Lewis FM, editors: *Health behavior and health education: theory, research, and practice*, San Francisco, 2002, Jossey-Bass, Table 3-3.

choices for a 6-year-old, is a barrier to reducing Sylvia's BMI and preventing the health complications of obesity. In addition, Mr. and Mrs. Martinez have limited formal education and are not native English speakers; this limits their access to health information, as health education materials are often written at a level that exceeds the Martinezes' English-language reading ability. Finally, Mrs. Martinez must also feed her family on a limited income and considering cultural and personal preferences. Also, access to fresh food may be limited due to transportation issues.

A lack of self-efficacy is also a barrier to behavior change. Mrs. Martinez's statement that she cannot do anything about Sylvia's weight may indicate that she does not have confidence in her ability to effect change in her daughter's health (self-efficacy). Understandably the Martinez family is comfortable with their routines and choices; this provides few cues to action in their environment to motivate changes in their behavior.

THE TRANSTHEORETICAL MODEL

The **Transtheoretical Model** (TTM) combines several theories of intervention, thus the name *transtheoretical*. Table 3-2 lists the core constructs of the model, which also includes the constructs of self-efficacy and the processes of change.

The TTM is based on the assumption that behavior change takes place over time, progressing through a sequence of stages. It also assumes that each of the stages is both stable and open to change. In other words, one may stop in one stage, progress to the next stage, or return to the previous stage.

The Martinez family is firmly in the precontemplation phase. They have no intention of changing their diet or incorporating more exercise into their routine. The Martinez family also lacks information regarding the potential health risks related to their lifestyle. They may be underinformed about ways to integrate healthier foods into their diet, and they may be unaware of foods and drinks to avoid and how to initiate exercise for each family member. *In their perception, the costs outweigh the benefits of behavior change.*

The Transtheoretical Model and Change

Change is difficult, even for the most motivated of individuals. People resist change for many reasons. Change may:

- *Be unpleasant (exercising)*
- *Require giving up pleasure (eating deserts or watching TV)*
- *Be painful (insulin injections)*
- *Be stressful (eating new foods)*
- *Jeopardize social relationships (gatherings with friends and family involve food)*
- *Not seem important anymore (older individuals or those suffering the ill effects of lifestyle choices such as diabetes and hypertension)*
- *Require change in self-image (from couch potato to athlete)*

Westberg and Jason, 1996

TABLE **3-2** The Transtheoretical Model

CONSTRUCTS	DESCRIPTION
STAGES OF CHANGE	
Precontemplation	The individual has no intention to take action toward behavior change in the next 6 months. May be in this phase because of lack of information about the consequences of the behavior or failure in previous attempts at change.
Contemplation	The individual has some intention to take action toward behavior change in the next 6 months. Weighing pros and cons to change.
Preparation	The individual intends to take action within the next month and has taken steps toward behavior change. Has a plan of action.
Action	The individual has changed overt behavior for less than 6 months. Has changed behavior sufficiently to reduce risk of disease.
Maintenance	The individual has changed overt behavior for more than 6 months. Strives to prevent relapse. This phase may last months to years.
DECISIONAL BALANCE	
Pros	The benefits of behavior change
Cons	The costs of behavior change

From Prochaska JO, Redding CA, Evers KE: The Transtheoretical model and stages of change. In Glanz K, Rimer BK, Lewis FM, editors: *Health behavior and health education: theory, research, and practice*, San Francisco, 2002, Jossey-Bass.

Change also takes place in many contexts. For example, each individual has a peer group that affects how and if they achieve change. Teenagers and adolescents are the groups most often considered in regard to peer influence, but everyone has a valued peer group. The businessman who is trying to decrease his alcohol intake must face telling his friends that he is not going to be joining them for "happy hour." One's peers can also be a useful support system. Alcoholics Anonymous is an example of positive peer influence.

The family is a powerful influence for or against change. In addressing the health risks of children, the family is an essential component of change because children are unable to control much of their environment alone. Family influence must also be addressed while working with adults. Imagine the difficulties a working mother must face in her attempts to prepare healthful family meals at home rather than feeding the family their favorite fast food.

In another example, community norms can challenge efforts to help clients achieve lasting behavior change. Unsafe neighborhoods or those without sidewalks or parks make it difficult for many clients to maintain an exercise regimen. A community that values good air quality and encourages mass transit and walking over the use of automobiles helps its residents to achieve better health.

Finally, the media has enormous influence. Women and teenage girls grapple with images of thin, perfect women; men and boys see rich, powerful athletes. Such influences make change difficult. An overweight teen may feel that there is "no hope" for her to "ever look that good, so why try?" The abundance of sedentary entertainment available through the media is contributing to the increase in overweight throughout the country, with more people spending hours in front of televisions or computers each day. Conversely the media can also encourage positive health behaviors. Information from television shows and public service announcements provides information on weight reduction, exercise, smoking cessation, and addiction recovery.

How can clients be encouraged to achieve and sustain behavior change? Merely telling them that they eat too much fatty food, drink too much alcohol, exercise too little, or engage in other unhealthful behaviors is insufficient. According to Westburg and Jason (1996), individuals take several steps toward making changes in the way they care for themselves. These are:

- Acknowledging that a problem exists. (This may take months or even years due to a natural inclination toward denial.)
- Deciding to make a change. (Mrs. Martinez must recognize the potential threats and understand the benefits of action.)
- Setting a goal (e.g., Sylvia will not gain weight during the next 3 months).
- Exploring options to achieve the goal. (Mrs. Martinez can add more fruits and vegetables to the family diet and reduce the number of tortillas. She can limit TV time.)
- Deciding upon and implementing a plan. (Sylvia will not drink more than one 8-ounce glass of juice or more than one soda per day. She will engage in 30 minutes of vigorous exercise per day.)
- Assessing progress toward achieving the goal. (Sylvia will weigh weekly.)
- Guarding against backsliding. (How can Mrs. Martinez modify the plan to keep Sylvia interested?)

MOVING TOWARD CHANGE

How can Erin help the Martinez family move from precontemplation to contemplation? To achieve lasting behavior change, individuals must experience ownership of the need for change. They must want to make the change for themselves, not because "that nurse is nagging me." Most people realize the harmful effects of their behaviors; smokers will exclaim that "this will kill me if I don't stop," or the overweight businessman will observe "I need to stop eating so much and get to the gym." *Individuals facing change must feel that the benefits of the change outweigh the costs; they must feel that they have more to gain than to lose.*

The best way to help clients achieve ownership is through collaboration. For successful and sustained change to take place, the client must be a partner with the nurse in the change process. Change should be gradual, and patience is essential on the part of both client and nurse. No one wants to be told only what they are doing wrong, so in presenting a plan for changing unhealthy behavior, it is helpful to be positive and empathetic, emphasizing what behaviors to continue. The beneficial aspects of new behaviors to be adopted should also be emphasized. For example, clients may complain less about a new exercise regimen if they can look forward to being more energetic or needing less medication for their diabetes or hypertension. Less emphasis should be placed on the behaviors that must be stopped. The smoker knows that he faces "kicking the habit," and the client with type 2 diabetes is aware that she must give up the chocolate mocha latte.

MOTIVATION

Though clients may readily see that the end results of their behaviors are not desirable, and that they have much to gain from ceasing to smoke, ceasing to overeat, or becoming more active, they may lack the needed motivation to proceed with the change process. Motivational Interviewing may be a helpful tool in this situation.

Motivational Interviewing is a way of interacting with clients to assist them to evaluate their health, the reasons for and against behavior change, and their own motivation to change (Miller and Rollnick, 2002). The goal is not to teach new skills, but to allow the nurse and the client to explore a health concern and the behaviors associated with it. During the motivational interview, the nurse develops a collaborative relationship, partnering with the client, rather than taking the role of an authority figure. The client's values, perceptions, and experiences are considered, as are the client's resources and motivation to effect change. The nurse should facilitate informed choices and respect the client's right to make decisions and to act as he or she sees fit. Motivational interviewing can be used during any encounter with a client, but it is most effective when the nurse and client have significant time to discuss potentially detrimental behaviors. Carving a few minutes of time from a busy day to focus on the client and discuss concerns can help move the client toward change.

How might Erin use this motivational strategy in her interaction with Mrs. Martinez? She might say, "I am concerned about Sylvia's weight and the effect it might have on her health. May we discuss this for a moment?" Note that if Erin states her concern in a nonjudgmental way, without blaming the family for Sylvia's condition, she might enlist Mrs. Martinez's permission to focus on the matter.

Erin can then go on to explain the implications of acanthosis nigricans and ask, "Does anyone in your family have diabetes?" If Mrs. Martinez has any personal experience with the disease (e.g., a parent, sibling, or grandparent), she may be more likely to respond with concern and willingness to change. Once Erin has engaged Mrs. Martinez, she can direct the interview to the point at hand: "Tell me more about your diet. I know that Sylvia eats a lot of tortillas and drinks a lot of juice. How does the rest of your family eat?" She can then lead the discussion to what changes Mrs. Martinez would be willing to make: "To help Sylvia and the rest of the family to be healthier, what changes could you try?" At this point, if Mrs. Martinez is fully engaged in the conversation and her input is being sought, Erin can continue to build on this foundation and develop the conversation to include exercise and other changes.

PRINCIPLES OF TEACHING AND LEARNING

For most clients like the Martinez family, change begins with education. As stated previously, many clients remain in the precontemplation stage because of a lack of information. Presentation of information regarding unhealthful behavior is essential; some clients may not consider their behavior to be unhealthful. Similarly, information on positive and/or preventative steps that can be taken can be extremely valuable.

Learning is defined as "a relatively permanent change in mental processing, emotional functioning and/or behavior as a result of experience" (Braungart and Braungart, 2003). Individuals learn by interacting with their environment and by incorporating new information with past experiences or current knowledge. Individuals have a preferred learning style: visual, auditory or tactile (see Table 3-3). To facilitate learning across groups of clients, nurses should be adept at presenting information in a variety of ways and not merely assume that people learn by being told (auditory learning).

The individual's developmental stage, culture, society, past experiences, motivation, self-concept, and personality all impact the learning process and

TABLE **3-3** Learning Styles

LEARNING STYLE	APPLICATIONS
Visual	Visual learners remember the details of what they see. They learn best by reading or watching demonstrations or videos.
Auditory	Auditory learners remember what they hear. They learn best through the use of discussion, oral instructions, and audio-enhanced websites.
Tactile	Tactile learners remember what they feel or manipulate. They learn best through interactive experiences such as practice and return demonstration.

have implications for those providing health education. Nurses must be knowledgeable about the content to be taught, the learner's needs and background, basic teaching and learning principles, and the environmental and social aspects of the learning experience. Nurses should also be flexible and imaginative in their presentation styles and have well-developed communication skills (Braungart and Braungart, 2003).

How does one know how a client learns best? Learning style can be assessed by asking questions such as: "When you get new information, do you prefer it to be written down, or do you remember more if you see pictures?" or "Do you remember better what you hear or what you see?" or "When someone asks you how to do something, do you tell them or show them?" In many cases, a nurse will not know the preferred learning style of the client; thus a variety of teaching tools should be used.

In addition to the differing learning styles, learning takes place in three domains or categories: the cognitive domain, the affective domain, and the psychomotor domain (Bloom et al, 1956). The cognitive domain involves recall and understanding of new information and ideas. In this domain a newly diagnosed diabetic will remember that he is supposed to perform blood glucose checks prior to eating. In the affective domain the individual will

exhibit changes in interests, attitudes, values, and adjustment. For example, if a newly diagnosed diabetic believes that performing blood glucose checks is important to his health, he will overcome his fear of performing them. In the psychomotor domain, the individual will practice and accomplish the physical tasks and motor skills required. In the example, the diabetic will correctly perform his fingerstick and use of his glucometer to obtain accurate blood glucose measurement.

When faced with an educational need, it is not sufficient to simply offer a pamphlet or show a video without regard to how the client learns best. To achieve lasting change in behavior, learning must be enhanced through a combination of teaching tools and consideration of the client's developmental stage. Because of their changing developmental stages, pediatric populations can be challenging to any health educator. For example, preschool children cannot think abstractly; they experience the world in concrete, tangible terms. Only those things they can see, hear, feel, or experience are real to them. They learn quickly when they can feel, smell, taste, or manipulate objects, and they learn from interacting with and watching others. Because young children learn so much from watching others, role models are powerful influences (for good or bad). Stories and games are useful tools for presenting health information to preschool-age children. Younger children are egocentric and see the world from only their point of view, so any information must be presented in the context of its usefulness to the child.

Young school-age children are capable of problem solving and can understand the concept of permanence. Though they still think and function in concrete terms, they can now see a problem from several aspects and are no longer so self-centered. They are learning how to read and write, want to achieve new skills, and are anxious to demonstrate new mastery in crafts and projects. Games, show and tell, and manipulative activities are important tools for school-aged children. They also enjoy using technology and are comfortable with computers and computer-based learning. Lastly, school-aged children are concerned about friends who have an illness that makes them different from the group (such as cancer or diabetes) and are eager to learn basic aspects of illness and health.

Adolescents are able to think in abstract terms and draw logical conclusions from their observations (e.g., passing an exam requires study). Adolescents can develop and test hypotheses and consider theoretical and practical matters. Likewise, many adolescents are able to understand anatomy, physiology, and biology, and they find textbooks, pamphlets, and experiments useful tools. Concrete learning experiences can be effective with this age group. Visits to the emergency department of the local hospital or to jail can help to make a point about the consequences of decisions. Adolescents are present-oriented, however, and are not necessarily concerned about the effects of today's habits on their future health. Discussion of health topics should be related to the present and to the immediate consequences of their behavior on their well-being (Saewyc, 2007).

Adults too have developmental stages, although not as discrete. Further, the various life stages adults encounter have implications for health education. A young mother, for example, may not be receptive to education presented from the perspective of a retired person, and conversely, empty-nesters may not be interested in the health problems of young parents.

Whatever the developmental stage, it is essential to take advantage of *learning readiness*, that time when the client is open to learning the information needed to maintain optimal health or to reduce health risks. An individual suffering from bronchitis will be interested in learning how to prevent a relapse; the parent of a newborn will be acutely interested in learning how to protect their child's health. Lichtenthal (cited in Kitchie, 2003) suggests a systematic way of assessing a client's readiness to learn, dividing readiness into four categories: physical readiness, emotional readiness, experiential readiness, and knowledge readiness (Box 3-2).

Physical readiness assessment identifies those attributes of the client's physical abilities (or lack thereof) that could act as either a barrier or an attribute to learning. This includes vision, hearing, strength, endurance, and pain. The difficulty of the task to be performed in relation to the client's physical ability to perform it is also evaluated. No matter how much the client would like to learn to inject insulin, she will not be able to perform this skill if she is unable to see the dosage lines on the syringe.

The cognitive and psychomotor complexity of a given task, as well as the affective component,

---

BOX 3-2 Assessment of Learning Readiness

PHYSICAL READINESS

- Physical ability
- Difficulty of the task to be performed
- Environmental impact on learning
- Health status
- Gender

EMOTIONAL READINESS

- Anxiety level
- Support system
- Motivation
- Risk-taking behavior
- Frame of mind
- Developmental stage

EXPERIENTIAL READINESS

- Level of aspiration
- Past coping mechanisms
- Locus of control
- Cultural background
- Orientation

KNOWLEDGE READINESS

- Present knowledge base
- Cognitive ability
- Learning disabilities
- Learning styles

---

should also be assessed. For example, the impact of the physical environment on the learning process is considered: Is the room noisy, too hot, or too cold? The client's health status is an important factor in the progress of learning. A decreased energy level or discomfort can deter the client's ability to mentally process new information and perform new skills. The client's gender may also affect the outcome of the learning process. Women tend to be more receptive to health information than men and tend to take fewer risks with their health than do men.

The client's emotional readiness to learn can also hinder or enhance the learning process. Anxiety is often encountered as clients learn new information and adjust to a newly diagnosed illness. Some anxiety can be motivating, but too much anxiety can deter learning and too little may prevent learning. A strong support system decreases anxiety and fear, but the lack of adequate support may contribute to increased anxiety and fear. The client must also be motivated to learn. Every nurse has had the experience of teaching a client who is not motivated. Often in these cases, the information is presented and skills are demonstrated, yet the client does not retain the information. When the client disregards health advice, the nurse must accept the client's right to act as he sees fit. The nurse must inform the client of the possible consequences of his actions, but the choice is the client's.

When assessing emotional readiness, the client's *frame of mind* refers to whether the client is more oriented to the present or the future. When the client is not concerned about meeting basic needs of survival, he is better able to learn than one who is worried about how he will meet those needs. Children are notable for their present orientation; egocentricity and concrete thinking make them focus on what will make them happy *now*.

As previously discussed, a client's developmental stage impacts what and how the client will learn. Adults have past experiences and prior knowledge that supplements the new knowledge and skills to be learned. Considerations for teaching adults are listed in Table 3-4. Children, on the other hand, do not have the varied and complex life experiences or the knowledge base that can enhance the acquisition of new knowledge; however, this lack of experience may contribute to less bias and resistance to learning.

Experiential readiness refers to the client's past experiences with learning and whether these have been positive or negative. If a client has had negative experiences with learning new skills and solving problems in the past, he may be poorly motivated to attempt learning again. A client's *level of aspiration* is the degree to which he is driven to achieve set goals. This can be mediated by past successes and failures and the degree of satisfaction attained from achieving successes. An individual's coping mechanisms help him deal with the stressors of life. Those who have effective coping mechanisms are more successful in dealing with life's problems than those who do not cope as well. If possible, the nurse should determine what coping skills and mechanisms have worked for the client in the past and evaluate whether these coping mechanisms will be useful in the present situation.

As discussed previously, high levels of anxiety decrease learning; the better a client's coping mechanisms, the less anxiety he is likely to have and the more likely teaching will be successful. A client's cultural background often determines the meaning of health, illness, and suffering. Many personal health care practices are learned from family traditions and

TABLE **3-4** Needs of Adult Learners

LEARNING NEED	APPLICATION STRATEGIES
Adults must be actively involved in the learning process.	Interactive learning strategies and return demonstrations keep adults on task.
Adults need to have information repeated.	Adults have a lot on their minds and have varied learning styles, so presenting the same information in different ways, such as through audio-visual aids, computer programs, demonstration, and pamphlets, enhances learning for adults.
Adults want prompt feedback on their performance.	They want to know if they are "doing it right" or if they "have the right idea," so provide verbal feedback often. Encouraging words mean a lot to every learner.
Adults do not tolerate having their time wasted.	Concentrate on the important, essential information. Offer more if the client asks.
Adults want the content to relate to their real life experiences.	Helping adults understand why the information is important and useful to them encourages them to integrate the new knowledge into their lives.
Adults want to focus on real world problems.	Adults want to know how to solve problems here and now. Keep the information pertinent to the health issue currently facing the client.

are culturally based. The nurse should convey acceptance of these cultural differences rather than express judgments about whether they are good or bad. Often, asking "What have you tried to help you get better? Did that help?" will elicit conversation about cultural health care practices in which the client may engage.

Locus of control refers to whether the client is motivated to learn as a result of internal or external stimuli. Clients who ask questions about their illness and indicate a desire for information are motivated by an internal drive to learn. These clients have an internal locus of control and will indicate their readiness to learn by asking questions. Clients who learn only when motivated by others or by external stimuli (e.g., complications of uncontrolled diabetes) have an external locus of control. It is the nurse's responsibility to find creative ways to motivate these clients to learn and to assure follow up to keep the client motivated and learning. Engaging family members in the learning process or providing telephoned or written reminders often keeps these clients on track with change.

Orientation refers to the client's tendency to conform to a "parochial" or a "cosmopolitan" point of reference. Those who conform to the parochial point of reference tend to be reticent to learn new skills and self-care information, deferring to authoritarian figures such as the physician or family members rather than making health care decisions on their own. Clients with a parochial orientation typically come from small rural towns or tight-knit families or cultural groups and have less education with fewer experiences outside of their cultural or family group than their peers. Clients with a cosmopolitan point of reference tend to be better educated urban dwellers with experiences outside of their culture or family group. These clients are generally more open to learning new skills and information and are more independent in making health care decisions.

Knowledge readiness encompasses the client's learning style, knowledge base, and level of learning capability. The nurse enhances learning by building upon present knowledge rather than repeating what the client already knows. Besides wasting valuable time, repeating information known to the client can be insulting and boring. *Cognitive ability* refers to the level at which the client is capable of learning. The client may be able to state reasons why she must

minimize sugar in her diet, but she may not be capable of transferring this knowledge into planning and implementing a diabetic diet.

In many settings it is difficult for the nurse to determine the client's cognitive ability. In these cases, involving a supportive family member or friend is often helpful. Clients with lower literacy levels or learning disabilities can be challenging to the most determined nurse. In these instances, involvement of the client's support system is essential to ensure the client's health. As previously mentioned, learning disabilities will affect the level at which the client is able to learn, and the client's support system must be enlisted in the learning process. Clients with low literacy skills can readily learn and apply health care information when the information is presented correctly. Teaching these clients is discussed in detail later in the chapter.

APPLYING LEARNER ASSESSMENT

Erin's assessment of the Martinez family's knowledge of proper diet, exercise, and the complications of overweight revealed that the Martinez family knew very little about these topics. Through previous experiences with the Martinezes, Erin learned that Mr. and Mrs. Martinez are auditory learners, and the children are both auditory and visual learners. She also recognized that Mr. and Mrs. Martinez's low literacy level and the ages of the children influence their preferred learning style.

Erin is aware that because of their lack of knowledge, she must begin educating the Martinezes in the cognitive domain. They must learn why being overweight is a serious health problem before they can begin to value the changes they must make to achieve a better diet and reduce sedentary behaviors. Once the Martinezes understand important concepts and value the changes they must make, they can then embark on the effort to learn psychomotor skills such as new cooking methods and family exercise options.

The individuals in the Martinez family are all at differing developmental levels and have diverse priorities and concerns. The adults are concerned with meeting the basic needs of the family and are largely present—rather than future—oriented because of financial issues. The children are all school-aged and concerned with friends, school, and fun; they have few prior experiences on which to build new health knowledge. To be effective the education program for the family must relate to multiple differing developmental needs and concerns. Further, Erin recognizes that culture is a consideration in educating the Martinez family. This family, like most families, eats what is customary in their culture, with food being a core part of family gatherings and celebrations. Expectations of physical size and appearance differ from culture to culture, and "normal" size in the Martinez's traditional Hispanic culture is heavier than the thinner ideal of Caucasian culture.

Mr. and Mrs. Martinez tend to be externally motivated in matters of health, making it a challenge to sustain change. On the other hand, they have a high level of aspiration for the success and well-being of their children. Their aspirations can be addressed in teaching and follow-up sessions and used to maintain motivation. As with many clients facing health concerns, the Martinez family has no past coping mechanisms to help them in this instance, requiring them to learn new coping behaviors as they progress. When a client must learn new methods of coping, the process of change will proceed at a slower pace, requiring patience from both the client and the nurse. Erin will set up home visits with the Martinez family and will teach many of the concepts and skills in the Martinezes' kitchen. She knows the familiar environment will be a positive influence in the change process.

WRITING GOALS AND OBJECTIVES FOR PATIENT EDUCATION

Goals and objectives provide (1) an outline of the content to be covered in a teaching event and (2) teaching strategies that will be employed. In differentiating the two, it can be noted that goals are the broader, more general, final outcome of the educational experience. Goals are accomplished over a longer time period—weeks or months (e.g., the client will effectively self-manage her diabetes). Conversely, **objectives** are specific and can be assessed in the short term—minutes or days (e.g., the client will correctly state the cause of diabetes). Simply put, the goal is the destination, and objectives are

the specific steps one must take to arrive at the destination. Redman (1993) observed that learning objectives have some important characteristics:

- They are derived from a goal. This ensures that the objectives are related to the end goal and will contribute to achieving it.
- Objectives describe a precise behavior or change that is required. Objectives must be precise and focus on only one behavior in order to be measurable. Examples of precise terms that may be used in objectives are state, discuss, identify, list, compare and contrast, decrease by x%, and demonstrate.
- Objectives focus on the learner. The objectives should state what the learner will achieve in order to measure the progress of the learner toward the goal.
- Objectives state what changes the learner can expect. The objective stated thus will guide both the nurse and the learner in achieving behavior change.
- Behavioral objectives are action-oriented. The client will do or say something measurable or will make an overt, measurable change.

In summary, learning objectives should be SMART:

- Specific: the more specifically an objective is stated, the better it will guide interventions. Address only one outcome to be achieved per objective.
- Measurable: the objective must be measurable to provide an assessment of progress.
- Achievable: the client must be able to actually perform the skill or learn the information presented in the objective.
- Related to the goal: all objectives should be moving the client toward the goal.
- Time-limited: in order to assess progress toward the goal, the objective must state when the client is to achieve an outcome. This may be long-term or short-term in nature, but must be time-limited.

Goals should be determined in collaboration with the client. As previously discussed, for change to occur and for the change to be enduring, the client must be engaged in the process. Goals set without input from the client negates his or her role as a partner in change, and the client is likely to fail to meet these goals.

Knowing that the entire family must be involved for interventions to be effective and for change to be enduring, Erin met with the Martinez family to determine their priorities regarding their health. Although they agreed that losing weight would be good for all family members, they were very concerned about achieving the lifestyle changes that would result in lasting weight loss. Together, Erin and the Martinez family agreed upon this goal: *The members of the Martinez family will have the knowledge to achieve and to maintain a healthy weight.* This is a broad statement of the desired final outcome of the teaching plan.

To meet the goal, Erin identified several simple objectives that were important to the goal and would enable the Martinez family to experience success early in the process. Success in mastering new content helps instigate change and provides momentum to keep it going. Examples of objectives Erin expected the Martinezes to meet by the end of the first teaching session are as follows:

- *Mr. and Mrs. Martinez will state the correct definition of "overweight."*
- *The members of the Martinez family will state two causes of overweight.*
- *The members of the Martinez family will identify at least three ways they might modify their diet to reduce caloric intake.*

With assessment data, goals, and objectives in hand, Erin was able to choose content to present. In most cases nurses have a limited amount of time to present large amounts of information, necessitating prioritization of the information to be covered. In setting priorities for teaching content, the nurse must decide what information the client needs to maintain health for the immediate time period. Information that will allow the client to provide self-care until further teaching is given in follow-up visits should be presented.

Bruner (1960) points out that the teaching strategy chosen greatly impacts learning. Though lecture is one of the favorite teaching strategies and can be used effectively in many instances, learners retain only about 5% of what is taught through lecture. In contrast, the experiential techniques of practice and teaching others help the learner retain 75% to 90%, respectively (Figure 3-1). The client's physical or mental condition may preclude teaching or extensive

Figure 3-1. Learning Pyramid. From NTL Institute for Applied Behavioral Science, 300 N. Lee Street, Suite 300, Alexandria, VA 22314. 1-800-777-5227.

practicing, but participative learning should be included as much as possible.

Providing the client with pamphlets, websites, and information about support groups will support and reinforce new material. Visuals and "take-away" information will give clients tangible resources for building upon what has been taught. Finally, involving the client's family may increase the amount of information that can be presented at one time without overwhelming the client.

As the content is planned, one must state the *teaching objectives*. Teaching objectives state what the *educator* hopes to achieve during the teaching experience, and what actions the educator will take to achieve desired outcomes. Like learning objectives, teaching objectives conform to the SMART criteria, focus on the client, and are derived from the goal or goals that have been set with the client. Teaching objectives are useful in organizing the content to be taught and coordinating the teaching methods to be used. Teaching objectives relevant for the Martinez family would be:

- *The nurse will begin the teaching experience by engaging the clients in a game to stimulate interest in the topic of overweight.*
- *The nurse will create an effective learning environment by reducing or eliminating distractions (e.g., turning off the TV, radio, and electronic games) and gathering the family members around the kitchen table.*

To effectively provide patient education, the nurse should:

- Send a clear message. Inform the client of the objectives to be addressed in the learning experience and follow them. Discuss one concept at a time, encouraging the client to ask questions as needed for clarification.
- Select the best learning format. Considering variables such as the amount of time available for teaching, the content to be taught, and the personal aspects of the client (e.g., learning style, education level), select the most effective way to present the material.
- Create an environment conducive to learning. A poor teaching environment can disrupt the most carefully planned learning experience. When the environment cannot be modified or controlled, it may be best to forego teaching until the environment is less disruptive or a better setting can be identified.
- Provide evaluation and feedback. Everyone needs to know if "I'm doing this right." Praise and encouragement will motivate the most reluctant learner. Give positive feedback often, and offer correction in a manner that is not critical or judgmental.
- Assure follow-up teaching experiences. In most circumstances, the nurse will only be able to cover a part of the information that is needed in

one session. Follow-up teaching is often vital for presentation of the material, to allow the client to practice new skills, and to reinforce important facts.

- Tell clients what will be taught; teach them; and repeat what they were told. Restating information in differing ways increases retention and may help answer unasked questions.
- Evaluate the teaching experience. Questions to consider: What worked? What flopped badly? What can you do to improve next time? What was the client's reaction to the teaching? Were the objectives SMART? Will the client be able to improve his health and make behavioral changes based on the material taught? Were the client's concerns and learning priorities addressed?

TEACHING CLIENTS WITH LOW LITERACY SKILLS

An estimated seven million adults in the United States are considered "nonliterate" in English, and another 30 million lack the literacy skills to read drug or food labels or to recognize information on paychecks, schedules, or maps. Though most people with low literacy skills are native-born Americans, individuals who were not born in the United States, or who speak another language in addition to English, tend to have lower literacy rates than individuals who were born in the United States or who speak only English. Older Americans are less literate as well; nearly half of the people in the elderly population have low reading skills.

Individuals with lower rates of literacy have substantially lower incomes than those who are more literate, and they are more likely to be unemployed or underemployed than their more literate peers. The inability to read and understand health information and to navigate the health care system is related to disparities in health. Individuals with lower literacy levels are more likely to report poor health, have a poor understanding of their condition and treatment, and are more likely to be hospitalized. These individuals also have higher health care costs than do more literate persons (U.S. DHHS, 2000).

Literacy is defined as "using printed and written information and material to function in society, to achieve one's goals, and to develop one's knowledge and potential." (Kutner et al, 2007, p. 2). This definition emphasizes that literacy is more than just being able to pronounce or recognize words; it is a tool that adults use to achieve an objective, and without it one's ability to be successful in life pursuits will suffer. Literacy increases with each increasing grade in school. Exceptions can be observed for individuals who take longer than 12 years to graduate from high school and those who attain a GED; these individuals tend to have lower literacy than persons who graduate from high school within 12 years (Kutner et al, 2007).

Nurses often do not know the literacy level of clients in their care. Clean, well-dressed individuals may have poor reading skills, and the stated level of education may not accurately depict a client's literacy level. People with low literacy skills are not likely to reveal that they cannot read. They may claim to have forgotten their glasses or may have a family member present to complete forms or read pamphlets and instructions. Despite the pervasive inability to understand health information, most patient information literature is presented without considering the client's ability to read and understand it. Health histories and patient intake interviews, for example, proceed under the assumption that clients can understand the questions and are able to provide the requested information. Nurses deliver oral education at levels well above what many laypersons are capable of understanding. Most troubling of all, clients are regularly presented with consent forms they do not understand, undermining the informed consent process.

Comprehension of written or oral information is a complex process involving logic, language, and experience. This process involves transferring symbols or images into knowledge and takes place more slowly for someone with low literacy skills (Doak et al, 1985). Persons who are not fluent readers may have to read one letter at a time in order to recognize the word. They may be able to read or to recognize words that are presented in print but not those that are in handwriting, **bold** print, or in all CAPITAL letters. Reading simple abbreviations, such as those for the days of the week or the months of the year, or telling time from a clock may also be problematic for those who do not read well.

Common terms used in patient instruction (e.g., "alternate," "grasp," "position") are not familiar to poor readers and may cause them to lose interest and

stop paying attention during health teaching. Many people who do not read well have had negative experiences with education and try to avoid frustration and embarrassment by agreeing with whatever is asked of them. If asked if they understand, many will respond in the affirmative, even if they do not understand; they may not have the vocabulary or knowledge to explain what it is they do not know.

Though many clients read at a seventh-grade level or below, most health education materials are written at the tenth-grade level or higher (Doak et al, 1985). Table 3-5 lists some common barriers encountered by illiterate persons when seeking or receiving health care.

Clients who struggle with reading are not able to perform a skill called *chunking*. **Chunking** refers to being able to read and understand an entire sentence or idea at one time. Poor readers must read each word individually, often loosing the meaning of the information in the process. For example, look at the list of words below and try to remember as many as possible:

cat	feed
each	twice
the	day
tomorrow	after

Without context, a list of words is difficult to remember and has no meaning. "Feed the cat twice each day after tomorrow" makes much more sense and is easier to remember.

Chunking is a concept that is taken for granted in most patient education literature.

"Excessive body temperature will necessitate forcing fluids to restore the fluid and electrolyte balance." The client will need to read each word individually and probably will not understand most of them. A better approach is to put the sentence in everyday terms rather than complicated medical jargon: "When the baby has a fever, you will need to give him more water to drink."

"Masking" is also a concern in teaching clients with low literacy skills. Masking is when a word has a different meaning in the medical vocabulary than it generally has in the client's vocabulary. For example, for most people "stool" is something you sit on, but a health provider might use the term referring to a bowel movement. Another example would be "diet" which might refer to a weight-loss regimen or the type and amount of food consumed.

TABLE **3-5** Barriers to Health Care Related to Low Literacy

BARRIER TO HEALTH CARE	EXAMPLE
A client's perspective is limited to his personal experience. Descriptions of events or information are perceived to be important only through their meaning to the client.	The patient responds to information regarding infant car seats by saying, "I didn't listen to that stuff. I don't have a car."
A poor reader may not realize the need to provide information to health care providers. He may not understand the need to clarify information.	A client's response to questions regarding his medical history may be: "Why does that nurse need to know about stuff that doesn't bother me anymore?"
A client may not think in terms of classes or categories of information. Poor readers think in terms of concrete concepts and are not accustomed to dealing with large amounts of information.	Placing items in categories such as fruits, cereals, or fats confuses the client.
Clients may give information in bits and pieces, with one word acting as the trigger for another idea.	When asked about breast feeding, the client responded with a long story of her past five deliveries. The nurse only wanted to know if she knew how to breastfeed her infant.

From Doak CC, Doak LG, Root JH: *Teaching patients with low literacy skills*, Philadelphia, 1985, JB Lippincott.

STRATEGIES FOR TEACHING CLIENTS WITH LOW LITERACY SKILLS

Four steps are recommended in teaching clients with low literacy skills(Doaket al, 1985):

1. Teach the smallest amount possible at one time. The nurse should impart enough instruction for the client to be free of pain and safely carry out needed self-care until further information can be given during a follow-up appointment. The client should know enough about his condition to understand the type of treatment and how long it will last.

2. Make the information as vivid as possible. As previously discussed, learning takes place in a variety of ways; use of a combination of teaching strategies will help the client understand vital information. Illustrate the point with simple drawings, examples, or case studies the client can identify with. Use simple language, taking the client's knowledge into account. Avoid medical jargon and technical terms the client may not understand. Use active voice: "Take your medicine before breakfast, lunch, and dinner" is more vivid than "Medication should be taken with meals."

3. Have the client restate and demonstrate the information learned. As previously discussed,

retention is increased by experiential learning. If the client can teach you or others, the information is being retained.

4. Review information repeatedly. No matter what the literacy level, the stress of illness can decrease how much is learned and increase the time needed to take in new information.

SUMMARY

Health education is a vital component of nursing care, no matter what the setting. Like Erin's work with the Martinez family, nurses in community settings must take into account multiple factors beyond what information to provide when planning to teach clients about health and health issues. Learning styles, learning needs, literacy levels, education, developmental stage, motivation, and culture are some of the factors that should be considered.

To be effective, a teaching plan should include both goals for outcomes and teaching and learning objectives. Finally, to summarize, when planning for health education:

- Don't overstuff.
- Give a little, get a little.

- Three or four items of instruction are enough at one time.
- Space the learning.
- Anxiety is the enemy.
- Reward every accomplishment with encouraging words.

A helpful booklet for educating clients with low literacy skills is available at http://www.cdc.gov/od/oc/simpput.pdf

Learning Activities and Application to Practice

In Class

1. With classmates, use the models presented in the chapter (The Health Belief Model or the Transtheoretical Model) to discuss factors that influence or determine why people choose (or not) to follow teaching or advice related to health. Recall actions of yourself, family members, or patients encountered in clinical who followed or did not follow health recommendations. Suggest strategies that nurses might use to reduce negative influences and enhance positive ones to help patients comply with health teaching.

2. Discuss personal learning styles with classmates. Have each member describe how he or she learns. Using the "Learning Pyramid" (Figure 3-1, p. 39) describe different teaching methodologies and strategies. Which teaching strategies are the most effective? Which are the least effective?

3. Collect examples of patient teaching materials from various clinical settings and analyze their reading level. How useful are the materials for patients with low literacy levels? Discuss what can be done to improve the teaching materials.

In Clinical

4. Identify an actual or potential health problem that can be addressed through education. In groups of four to six develop a teaching plan to present appropriate information. In the plan consider characteristics and learning needs of the clients, create goals and write learning objectives, and identify the teaching methods to be used.

5. Present and evaluate the teaching plan. Consider the following: What worked and why? What should be changed for future presentations?

REFERENCES

Bloom SB, Engelhart MD, Furst EJ and others: *Taxonomy of educational objectives: the classification of educational goals, handbook I: cognitive domain*, New York, 1956, David McKay.

Braungart M, Braungart R: Applying learning theories to healthcare practice. In Bastable SB: *Nurse as educator: principles of teaching and learning for nursing practice*, Sudbury, Mass, 2003, Jones and Bartlett.

Bruner, J: *The process of education*, Cambridge, Mass, 1960, Harvard University Press.

Doak CC, Doak LG, Root JH: *Teaching patients with low literacy skills*, Philadelphia, 1985, JB Lippincott.

Green LW, Kreuter MW: *Health promotion planning: an educational and environmental approach*, Mountain View, Calif, 1991, Mayfield.

Griffiths W: Health education definitions, problems, and philosophies, *Health Educ Monogr* 31:12, 1972.

Hochbaum G: *Public participation in medical screening programs: a socio-psychological study*, Washington, DC, 1958, U. S. Public Health Service.

Janz NK, Champion VL, Stretcher VJ: The health belief model. In Glanz K, Rimer BK, Lewis FM, editors: *Health behavior and health education: theory, research, and practice*, San Francisco, 2002, Jossey-Bass.

Kitchie S: Determinants of learning. In Bastable SB: *Nurse as educator: principles of teaching and learning for nursing practice*, Sudbury, Mass, 2003, Jones and Bartlett.

Kutner M, Greenberg E, Ying J and others: *Literacy in everyday life: results from the 2003 national assessment of adult literacy*, Jessup, Md, 2007, U.S. Dept of Education.

Miller WR, Rollnick S: *Motivational interviewing: preparing people for change*, ed 2, New York, 2002, Guilford Press.

Prochaska JO, Redding CA, Evers KE: The Transtheoretical model and stages of change. In Glanz K, Rimer BK, Lewis FM, editors: *Health behavior and health education: theory, research, and practice*, San Francisco, 2002, Jossey-Bass.

Redman BK: *The process of patient education*, St Louis, 1993, Mosby.

Saewyc EM: Health promotion of the adolescent and family. In Hockenberry MJ and Wilson D, editors: *Wong's nursing care of infants and children*, edition 8, St Louis, 2007, Mosby.

U.S. Department of Health and Human Services: *Healthy people 2010*(website): http://www.healthypeople.gov/document/HTML1/11HealthCom.htm. Accessed July 24, 2007.

Westberg J, Jason H: Fostering healthy behavior: the process. In Woolf SH, Jonas S, Lawrence RS, editors: *Health promotion and disease prevention in clinical practice*, Baltimore, 1996, Williams & Wilkins.

Case Management

1. Define and describe case management.

2. Explain roles used and skills needed by nursing case managers.

3. Compare various settings for internal and external case management.

4. Describe how case managers can use clinical pathways to improve patient care.

key terms

Case management
Clinical pathway
Disease management
Managed care

Nursing case management
Utilization management

See Glossary for definitions.

case study

Kathy Lambert is a nurse for a large urban school district. For several years Kathy has been in a specialized role as a case manager for pregnant students. In this role she oversees and coordinates all of the services provided by the school district for these students. This includes such interventions as monitoring the pregnancies, providing health education on issues related to pregnancy and infant care, ensuring that nutritional guidelines are followed, referral for social services (e.g., Medicaid, WIC) as needed, and collaborating with teachers to ensure that progress is made in schoolwork.

Kathy's caseload consists of all of the district's students who have been identified as pregnant. As soon as one of the district's school nurses becomes aware that a student is pregnant, the nurse contacts Kathy. At that time, Kathy sets up an appointment for the student at the girl's convenience. At the initial meeting, Kathy completes comprehensive physical, social, and environmental assessments. Using that information, she sets up a personal plan of care for the girl, following a clinical pathway that was developed by a team of school nurses, social workers, teachers, counselors, and administrators. The clinical pathway outlines what services and interventions each girl should receive at defined intervals,
Continued

based on the number of weeks of her pregnancy. It also defines specific goals and expected outcomes, which are measured on an ongoing basis, and a method to record care given. As case manager, Kathy holds conferences every other week with a designated school counselor, teacher, and social worker. These professionals are responsible for monitoring aspects of each girl's care.

On a recent Monday, Kathy saw Paige Summerfield, a 16-year-old sophomore whose pregnancy is in its twenty-eighth week. She has monitored Paige's progress for nearly 4 months, and she is aware that Paige receives prenatal care from a family health clinic associated with a local medical school and that her pregnancy is progressing normally. Based on the parameters of the clinical pathway, at 28 weeks Paige should receive a blood pressure check, a test for anemia, and a urine test. Also, her nutritional status and fetal growth should be assessed, and she should be given information on prepared childbirth classes.

In her assessment, Kathy learned that Paige has gained a total of 15 pounds. She reported that she is eating a good diet and tries to exercise at least three times per week. The baby is active, but Paige stated that she is able to rest. She denied other problems. Paige's blood pressure was 112/72, her hemoglobin was 12.5, and her urine test was negative for protein, glucose, and blood.

In previous conversations Paige had informed Kathy that she plans to keep the baby. According to the clinical pathway, between the twenty-fourth and twenty-eighth week, girls are referred to low-cost prepared childbirth classes, and an appointment was made with the social worker to help Paige work out childcare arrangements for the baby while she is in school. Also, Kathy confirmed with the school office that Paige's schoolwork is satisfactory and that she has only been absent 2 days during the past 8 weeks.

Kathy carefully documented the care provided. She concluded that based on the goals and expected outcomes outlined in the clinical pathway, Paige's progress is on schedule. Before she left, Kathy made an appointment for her next visit in 2 weeks.

Although nursing case management is seen as relatively new, in reality nurses have been providing case management services for many years. Indeed, rather than being a new role, case management is a redefinition and restructuring of an already existing practice strategy in which nurses assume overall responsibility for client care management, oversee coordination of care, and serve as client advocates. In this manner they work to decrease fragmentation of health care and increase its quality while managing costs.

BACKGROUND OF CASE MANAGEMENT

As early as the 1920s, aspects of case management were used in psychiatry and social work to direct the long-term care of persons with chronic illnesses. Then in the 1930s, visiting nurses began using case management principles to care for sick patients in the home (Cesta and Tahan, 2003). Beginning in the 1940s, insurance companies used case management strategies as a cost-containment measure for worker's compensation cases, and in the 1960s, mental health care emphasized case management to avoid client service fragmentation. More recently, in community settings case management concepts have been applied to caring for elders who are home-bound or have complex health problems and to individuals with high-cost illnesses (e.g., COPD, CHF) (Lyon, 2007).

In the 1970s and 1980s, explosive growth in the cost of health care led to efforts to contain expenditures. In 1983 PL 98-21 of the Social Security Amendments introduced the Prospective Payment System (PPS) (Hunt and Knickman, 2005). Under the PPS, health care providers receive a fixed amount of money based on the relative cost of resources they use to treat Medicare clients within a diagnosis-related group (DRG). Other third party payers followed this example in contracts with managed care organizations (MCOs) and negotiated reimbursement schedules based on disease or procedure classification. Health care costs continue to escalate, and the population is aging, with a concurrent increase in chronic disease, so case management has come to be viewed as an essential service that can help control costs and distribute health care resources equitably (Lyon, 2007).

Recent trends that have fostered the need for case management include managed care, enhanced information systems, changes in Medicare and Medicaid, insurance company requirements, decentralization of care, and the growing number of persons with chronic health problems. As a result Lowery (2008) notes that there are more than 100,000 case managers working in the U.S. health care system.

This chapter discusses a number of issues in case management. These include the roles of the case manager, skills needed by case managers, and activities they perform. It also describes settings and models of case management, focusing on those that are community-based. Finally, it explains the process of utilization management and the use and development of clinical pathways.

OVERVIEW OF CASE MANAGEMENT

Because case management has only recently become widespread in the health care system, there has been some confusion about what it is. Furthermore, definitions of case management and nursing case management abound in the literature. This section clarifies information on case management.

WHAT CASE MANAGEMENT IS *NOT*

Case management is *not* utilization review (UR), although it may contain elements of UR. UR is a program, usually established by an acute care facility or insurance company, which works to control the amount of health care services used. The goal of UR is to decrease the number of unnecessary or inappropriate health care services while maintaining quality. UR typically includes precertification for nonemergent admissions, continued-stay review, retrospective review, and hospital bill audit (Siefker et al, 1998). Utilization management, an enhanced version of traditional UR, is described later in the chapter.

Also, case management is *not* managed care, although it may be a component of managed care. **Managed care** is a system of cost-containment programs, such as HMOs and PPOs, which strive to manage costs and quality of health care. Managed care features financial incentives to reduce utilization and streamline services through limiting access. It may include UR services and may include case management (Siefker et al, 1998).

WHAT CASE MANAGEMENT *IS*

Case management can be a position, a role, or an intervention that is practiced by professionals from several different disciplines. Nurses, social workers, counselors, and vocational counselors can all serve as case managers (More and Mandell, 1997).

Case management has been defined as:

- "a collaborative process of assessment, planning, facilitation, and advocacy for options and services to meet an individual's health needs through communication and available resources to promote quality, cost-effective outcomes" (Case Management Society of America, 2002, p. 2).
- "a health care delivery process whose goals are to provide quality health care, decrease fragmentation, enhance the client's quality of life, and contain costs" (ANA, 1994, p. 2)
- "an enduring process in which a population manager establishes systems and processes to monitor the health status, resources and outcomes for a targeted aggregate of the population" (Cary, 2004, 447)

Case management is client-focused and outcome-oriented. It works to facilitate and promote coordination of care while minimizing fragmentation. Further, it is ongoing rather than episodic, and it is collaborative in nature. In short, case managers seek to provide cost-efficient, coordinated, and individualized services to clients with chronic illnesses and disabilities. Their focus is twofold: (1) assisting with obtaining and organizing resources and (2) streamlining care to ensure the best outcome possible (Mullahy, 2004).

GOALS OF CASE MANAGEMENT

Case management has several specific goals. It is used to: (1) enhance the quality of health care, (2) decrease fragmentation of care across settings, (3) ensure appropriate use of resources, (4) contain costs, and (5) allow patients to make informed decisions. These activities improve care coordination and increase client satisfaction through achieving the maximum level of wellness (Lowery, 2008).

Research has shown that case management benefits both the client and the health care system. For the client it provides better coordination of care, assistance in negotiating a complex health care system, access to acceptable and affordable health care services, attention to multiple health care needs, improved health outcomes, and increased satisfaction with care. For the health care system it provides reduced cost of care, minimization of hospitalization, prevention of re-hospitalization, and elimination of service duplication (Clark, 2008).

APPROPRIATE USE OF CASE MANAGEMENT

Case management is time-intensive and can be costly. When it is used inappropriately, rather than saving health care dollars, it may in fact cost more. It is not necessary or desirable to use case management principles for all clients in all settings. Case management should be considered for clients with serious long-term illnesses or conditions that will necessitate services across settings and across disciplines. Examples of diagnoses or conditions that might benefit from case management services include some types of cancer, stroke, chemical dependency, COPD and asthma, congenital defects and neonatal complications, neurodegenerative disorders (e.g., ALS, MS), organ transplant, chronic pain, AIDS, complications of pregnancy, severe psychiatric disorders, spinal cord injury, and severe trauma (Brooks and Younce, 2007; Levy, Heffner, Stewart, et al, 2006; Metcalfe, 2006; Palsbo, Mastal, and O'Donnell, 2006; Raderstorf and Kurtz, 2007).

NURSING CASE MANAGEMENT

As mentioned, case management services may be provided by several disciplines. Nursing, however, is particularly suited to case management because nursing practice is holistic and family-focused. In addition, a nurse's clinical background enhances attention to biological and physical conditions that may go undetected in counseling or social work.

Nursing case management is nursing care that focuses on the coordination, integration, and direct delivery of client services. It places internal controls on the resources used for care and emphasizes early assessment and intervention, comprehensive care planning, inclusive services, and necessary referrals. Also, it incorporates consideration of the relationships among cost, quality, and health care (Cohen and Cesta, 2005).

Nursing case management can be described as:
- A *system* in which elements include assessment and problem identification, planning, procurement and coordination of services, and monitoring of services.
- A *role* because case managers actively coordinate care through negotiation with providers and management of care, both directly and indirectly.
- A *technology* because case managers generate tools and techniques to organize complex care delivered by multiple providers.
- A *process* that expands on the nursing process and views health care needs along a continuum and often across multiple settings.
- A *service* in that case managers act as facilitators and gatekeepers while helping clients and their caregivers make informed decisions.

Nursing case managers are RNs who are accountable for managing a defined group of clients to optimize clinical and cost outcomes. The outcomes are achieved by establishing and maintaining partnerships with clients, families, and providers over time and across settings. This is accomplished through the coordination of services, enhanced communication and collaborative skills, and adherence to population-specific guidelines and practice protocols (Mahn and Zazworsky, 2000). The Research Highlight box describes a study involving the case management process.

COMPONENTS OF NURSING CASE MANAGEMENT

Nurse case managers work with the client, the client's family, and professionals from several different disciplines in planning and providing care. In addition, care may involve more than one organization or setting and frequently must consider insurance requirements and limitations. To be prepared to practice as a case manager, a nurse must have requisite knowledge, be competent in various roles, and possess certain skills. In addition, the case manager should understand the types of activities common to this specialty area.

Research Highlight

Levy and colleagues (2006) described the results of a study that examined the efficacy of a school-based case management program to address childhood asthma among urban children. The study found that students who were case managed had half the number of absences of their counterparts who were in a control group and significantly fewer urgent care or emergency department visits. Finally, students who were in the case management program evidenced significantly fewer hospital days and significant improvements in asthma knowledge.

The study's authors concluded that school-based nurse case management worked for several reasons. For one,

the nurses were able to teach and reinforce principles of self-care and asthma management (e.g., correct use of medications, use of the peak flow meter, and trigger avoidance). In addition, interactions with the children and school personnel helped with coordination of care and removal of triggers such as mold, chalk dust, and chemical irritants in the classroom. They noted that implementation of "best practices" related to asthma management is not consistent, particularly among underserved populations, and concluded that school-based nurse case management in urban schools can significantly reduce the burden of asthma in this aggregate.

KNOWLEDGE DOMAINS FOR CASE MANAGERS

The Commission for Case Manager Certification (CCMC) (CCMC, 2005) has identified six "knowledge domains" for effective case management. These are discussed briefly here and summarized in Box 4-1.

- *Case management concepts*—refers to knowledge of accreditation standards and requirements, case management models, processes and tools, and case recording and documentation strategies. It also includes knowledge of goals and objectives of case management and methods for program evaluation and quality improvement.
- *Case management principles and strategies*—includes such concepts as confidentially, conflict resolution strategies, and negotiation. It also includes knowledge of legal and ethical responsibilities and regulatory requirements.
- *Psychosocial and support systems*—involves knowledge of concepts such as behavioral health, psychiatric disability, and management of clients with substance abuse or addictive disorders. Recognition of the impact of family dynamics, cultural issues, beliefs and practices, and spirituality on client health and well-being are important. Knowledge of community resources, support programs, and crisis intervention are essential.

- *Health care management and delivery*—focuses on understanding the roles and functions of various care providers during the planning and implementation of care. It includes applying assistive technology and clinical pathways or practice guidelines to care delivery across various settings.
- *Health care reimbursement*—denotes understanding strategies used in managed care, cost containment principles, health insurance principles, reimbursement methodologies, the prospective payment system, and utilization management, among other concepts and processes. It also includes knowledge of managerial techniques such as cost-benefit analysis.
- *Vocational concepts and strategies*—includes understanding of management and modifications of homes and workplaces to accommodate disabilities. Job development, placement, life care planning, and ergonomics are related concepts case managers may need to apply.

NURSING CASE MANAGEMENT ROLES

Nurse case managers are responsible for coordinating the care delivered to a group of clients. This is carried out through applying the nursing process in a

---

BOX **4-1** Case Management Knowledge Domains

- Case management concepts
- Case management principles and strategies
- Psychosocial and support systems

- Health care management and delivery
- Health care reimbursement
- Vocational concepts and strategies

Commission for Case Manager Certification: *CCM Certification Guide*, 2005 (website): http://www.ccmcertification.org/pages/22frame_set.html. Accessed November 1, 2007.

manner that ensures the delivery of cost-effective, outcome-oriented, quality care and promotes access to health care. To accomplish this objective, many roles must be used by nursing case managers. Box 4-2 lists and describes some of these roles. Many of them (e.g., clinical expert, educator, advocate, outcome manager) are used by most nurses in most settings. A few, however, (e.g., coordinator or care negotiator/broker, risk manager, utilization manager) are less common to other areas of nursing practice and more specific to this nursing specialty.

SKILLS NEEDED BY NURSE CASE MANAGERS

Nurse case managers need to possess a number of skills. Some of the most essential, as explained by More and Mandell (1997), are described here.

Communication

Communication is constantly needed between and among all parties involved in care, and the case manager is responsible for giving all of the health care providers information they need to ensure coordinated care. Methods for communication include person-to-person, telephone, written correspondence, and e-mail. In case management, written communication is particularly key and may include reports, contracts, letters, proposals, and/or client records. As a result, it is important that case managers have a good vocabulary, good grammar, and the ability to summarize data without distortion or judgment. They should be able to provide information in a written report that is clear, concise, accurate, and as nontechnical as possible.

Teaching

Excellent theory-based teaching skills are vital because the case manager is a knowledge and information broker. Teaching should relate to treatment options, possible adverse effects, medications, health care system issues, and insurance issues, among others, to assist the client and family in making informed decisions and to enhance self-care.

Management

Management is an essential component of case management. As noted previously some of the skills related to management include delegation, negotiation, problem solving, organization and time management, and networking.

Delegation involves sharing responsibility and authority with subordinates and holding them accountable for their actions. When delegating, the case manager must make sure that the person receiving the task is capable and competent to carry it out. Oversight is a component of delegation.

Negotiation is the act of arriving at a compromise in a situation where persons on one side of an issue try to persuade persons on the other side to accept a given viewpoint. Qualities that enhance negotiation include good interpersonal skills and flexibility. The case manager negotiates on behalf of the client, insurance carrier, physician and/or other health care providers.

BOX 4-2 Case Manager Roles

- Clinical expert: Knowledgeable regarding clinical conditions and best evidence-based practice
- Consultant: Provides assistance to clients and other health care professionals regarding client needs and available services
- Coordinator of care: Arranges seamless care across systems and agencies to meet client needs; makes referrals for needed services; serves as liaison to community agencies
- Manger of care: Controls use of resources and coordinates activities of care team members to assure quality outcomes
- Educator: Educates clients, families, health care providers, and the public regarding health issues and interventions
- Negotiator/broker: Negotiates appropriate care to meet client needs in the most cost-effective settings
- Advocate: Serves as liaison between client and health care system and advocates for services to meet client needs
- Outcome and quality manager: Monitors and evaluates client care outcomes and quality of care provided

- Researcher: Engages in research related to interventions and outcomes
- Risk manager: Minimizes financial risk to the organization by identifying and dealing with threats to client or staff safety
- Change agent: Promotes change in client behaviors and/or health care delivery systems
- Holistic care provider: Provides care to address the client's needs in a holistic rather than a fragmented way
- Counselor: Addresses the emotional and spiritual needs of clients and their families
- Utilization manager: Reviews services to determine medical necessity, appropriateness of setting, and quality of care
- Transition/discharge planner: Assists with smooth transition between elements of the health care system
- Ethicist: Brings ethical dilemmas to the attention of the health care team and facilitates their resolution

Adapted from Cesta TG, Tahan HA: *The case manager's survival guide: winning strategies for clinical practice*, ed 2, St Louis, 2003, Mosby.

Problem solving is essential, and case managers must be able to anticipate problems and work to remediate or prevent them. Steps in the problem solving process include identification of the problem, classification of the problem (actual, potential, critical), gathering and analyzing information, developing a solution that considers consequences, making and implementing a decision or plan, and then evaluating the solution.

Organization and time management are compulsory in case management. Indeed, the case manager must be aware of treatment plans and recommended time frames for appropriate care implementation. Prioritization of the needs of each client is crucial and ongoing. In addition, it is important that the case manager's time be used efficiently.

Networking is the development and maintenance of professional contacts and relationships, and it is crucial in case management. Case managers must form positive relationships within the multidisciplinary team and must establish contact with additional agencies and providers whose services might be needed by clients.

Advocacy

In case management, advocacy is provided for all parties (i.e., client, providers, insurers) to promote both cost containment and appropriate, quality care. The desire is to reach mutually agreeable decisions that will address needs and constraints of all involved. Advocacy also involves supporting or upholding a client's right to make a choice and to act on the choice. Often this might include informing clients about choices and potential consequences.

Collaboration

Collaboration is very important and refers to when two or more persons work together toward a common goal; input is equal, and responsibility is shared. Case managers should encourage open dialogue and input from all team members.

ACTIVITIES OF NURSING CASE MANAGERS

Nursing case managers work to maximize the client's outcomes in the most cost-effective way. To accomplish this, the nurse case manager is responsible for developing a plan of care that is appropriate, high quality, and cost effective. The nursing process is used and expanded on to include components of coordination and monitoring of care. Important elements of each component are listed below (Tahan, 2008a).

- *Assessment.* Assessment is comprehensive and ongoing. All relevant client/family needs must be identified and assessed. This includes identification of actual or potential issues related to health, financial status, social and family support, vocational/work issues, and other concerns as appropriate.

- *Planning.* In the planning process, research may be necessary to determine available and appropriate options for patient care. The case manager may need to review available benefits under the client's insurance coverage, negotiate with insurance adjusters and providers, and write a plan of care including goals or outcomes and noting the anticipated time frame. Prioritization of patient needs and determination of the types of services and resources that will be necessary to meet the defined goals or outcomes are part of this step.

- *Implementation.* In the implementation phase, the plan is executed to achieve the identified goals and outcomes. The case manager coordinates the activities prescribed in the plan. The implementation phase also includes empowerment of the client/family to participate in care through education, advocacy, and enhancing communication among the patient/family and all providers and other parties.

- *Coordination.* Coordination involves identifying, organizing, securing, integrating, and modifying resources to accomplish goals. Reassessment of the client and his/her response to the plan of care is ongoing, and obtaining certifications/authorizations for care and services may be necessary. As mentioned, coordination is key to case management.

- *Monitoring.* Monitoring of care is done to assure goal attainment, identify new problems, and provide the basis for revision or alteration of the plan as needed.

- *Evaluation.* Evaluation is done to determine if desired outcomes and goals have been achieved. It involves constant communication with the client and family, providers, and others associated with provision or financing of care. During this phase a case manager identifies any variances or delays in care and addresses them as indicated.

Box 4-3 summarizes some of the many activities provided by nurse case managers.

SETTINGS FOR NURSING CASE MANAGEMENT

Case managers work in many different settings, and as a result their practice can be quite variable. Case managers can be found in hospitals, rehabilitation facilities, subacute facilities, community-based programs, home care, ambulatory care clinics, emergency departments, palliative care/hospice agencies, worker's compensation offices, occupational health settings, and insurance companies, among others (Tahan, 2008b). These are often categorized as "within-the-walls" or *internal case management*, and "beyond-the-walls" or *external case management* (Cohen and Cesta, 2005).

SETTINGS FOR INTERNAL CASE MANAGEMENT

Case managers in acute care (hospital) settings typically focus on the physical, psychological, social, financial, and discharge planning needs of a specific group of clients (e.g., cardiac, pediatric oncology). In addition to the comprehensive physical and psychosocial assessment, client assessment generally includes the ability to perform activities of daily living

---

BOX 4-3 Activities of Nurse Case Managers

- Collaboration with administrative, management, and clinical staff who are responsible for specified client groups
- Assessment, planning, implementation, coordination, referral, and evaluation of clients and families in assigned target populations
- Provision of internal consultation to other disciplines and departments with the goal of expeditiously managing care of clients and families
- Participation in the development of documentation systems and tools (i.e., clinical pathways or practice guidelines) to monitor clinical and fiscal outcomes
- Collecting, analyzing, and sharing of data and information to influence process improvements and to support integration of core systems and processes within the care environment
- Development of partnerships with physicians to achieve clinical and fiscal outcomes
- Teaching and coaching other caregivers on the health care team regarding clinical, fiscal, and system processes related to client care management
- Serving as a role model of professional nursing practice

From Mahn VA, Zazworsky D: Nurse case management as an advance practice role. In Hamric BA, Spross JA, Hanson CM, editors: *Advance nursing practice: an integrative approach*, ed 2, Philadelphia, 2000, Saunders, p . 549.

(ADLs), nutrition and exercise, sleep, substance use, mental status, and emotional health (Cohen and Cesta, 2005). According to Daniels (2008) hospital case management programs have evolved to include: (1) working with physicians to enhance the quality of patient outcomes, (2) overcoming process obstacles to allow patients to move smoothly and efficiently through the acute care episode, and (3) minimizing the occurrence of unwanted clinical events that increase risks to the patient.

Several different types of internal case management models can be identified. One example is the *collaborative practice model* (dyad or triad model), which is most commonly found in large tertiary care facilities. In this model a team comprising a case manager, a UR specialist, and a social worker oversee care for complex patients. A *functional model*, in which UR and discharge planning are integrated, is more commonly found in smaller community-based hospitals.

The *clinical resource management* (CRM) model focuses on "disease management." In CRM a case manager is assigned to high-volume or high-risk patient populations. The case manager monitors resource utilization and assists with coordination of post-acute services (Daniels, 2008).

Primary nurse case management (the "New England model") is another model for hospital-based case management. In this model a staff nurse or primary nurse is the case manager and is responsible for direct and indirect care, including discharge planning, outcomes management, and monitoring of utilization. Typically, primary nurse case managers use clinical pathways (critical paths/care maps), coordinate care across units, and devise and implement a discharge plan (Cohen and Cesta, 2005; Lyon, 2007).

UR nurse case managers review medical records to determine appropriateness of care based on documentation. UR case managers are employed by hospitals and insurance companies to ensure appropriate and cost-effective utilization of services. Nurses performing UR provide precertification approval, concurrent review, and retrospective review of selected cases (Cohen and Cesta, 2005).

SETTINGS FOR EXTERNAL CASE MANAGEMENT

Outside of acute care hospitals, case management services can be provided in long-term care settings, home health, MCOs, and other settings. In long-term care settings (i.e., nursing homes, rehabilitation facilities, skilled nursing facilities) case managers work to coordinate care of severely injured or catastrophically ill clients, with the goal of returning them to an independent lifestyle. In these settings case managers provide preventative care, assistance with maintenance of function, monitoring, and evaluation of progress. They often coordinate the multidisciplinary team, typically consisting of a physician, therapists, vocational counselors, and social workers.

Case management is very common in home health care. In home health the case manager provides oversight of all aspects of care from participating in discharge planning and home care intake through discharge from services. This involves completing comprehensive assessments, developing a treatment plan, and implementing the plan; much of the care may be direct. Other activities of the home health care case manager include obtaining durable medical equipment and supplies, obtaining services (e.g., OT, PT, speech therapy) as needed, determining frequency of skilled nursing care, supervising care of ancillary providers, documenting care, and developing the clinical pathway (Alvarado and Sunderland, 2008).

In managed care organizations (e.g., HMOs, PPOs) case managers provide a number of services, including working to improve the organization of services, promoting efforts to decrease costs, UR and utilization management, and assisting clients to access care not covered in their benefits package. Activities include acting as gatekeeper, conducting onsite visits, developing provider networks, assessing high-risk clients, and monitoring care.

Chronic care case management is often termed *disease management* and is becoming increasingly common in some community-based settings such as MCOs. **Disease management** controls both quality and expenditures by integrating activities associated with chronic and costly disease conditions (e.g., AIDS, diabetes) and coordinating interdisciplinary health care across settings or delivery systems. Disease management addresses the entire cycle of a disease process, incorporating primary, secondary, and tertiary care interventions and promoting self-care management. It usually requires active involvement by the client as well as various health care providers. Disease management programs provide long-term oversight of care and health education,

encourage health promotion and illness prevention interventions, and closely monitor symptoms to minimize or prevent exacerbations and complications of severe chronic illnesses (Koch, Beck, Norris, 1998; Powell and Tahan, 2008).

Lind (2005) points out that to enhance success, disease management providers should:
- Understand the course of the disease
- Target patients likely to benefit from the intervention
- Focus on prevention and resolution
- Increase patient compliance through education
- Provide continuity across health care settings
- Establish integrated data management systems
- Align incentives

Case managers are sometimes employed by insurers to coordinate benefits and services and to monitor recovery and rehabilitation. Activities of case managers employed by insurance companies focus on analysis of claims to determine coverage. This includes assessment of the claim and review of the policy to determine type of coverage, benefit period, exclusions, exceptions, covered benefits, and limits. It also involves precertification for surgery and other procedures, meeting with physicians and other providers, meeting with the client and family, and making benefits decisions (Tahan, 2008b).

Occupational health case managers coordinate health services for seriously ill or injured employees. Sometimes the occupational health nurse will be called upon to assist with disability management. The goal of disability management is to reduce financial costs associated with disabilities by providing information and coordinating access to employer-provider benefit plans and services (e.g., workers compensation, sick leave, short-term and long-term disability, medical leaves of absence, and social security disability) (Provine and Vierling, 2008).

Workers' compensation programs are federally mandated social insurance plans that provide financial assistance with medical care and wage replacement to employees with work-related injuries and illnesses. Case managers in workers' compensation programs seek to lower medical costs, improve communication, and manage claims. Case managers can enhance workers' compensation programs by assisting the injured worker, the provider, the employer, and the carrier/third-party administrator. In general, case managers are advocates for the worker and his/her family, but with competing issues and circumstances, the case manager may serve as a sponsor or advocate for the other stakeholders (i.e., insurance carrier, medical provider, or employer) (DiBenedetto, 2008).

Finally, case managers may be employed in other community-based settings such as schools, public health agencies, and churches. In these settings the nurse case manager focuses on primary care and prevention for well individuals who are at risk or who have the potential for needing health care services. The goal in these settings is to support and empower individuals to maximize their optimal level of wellness through the use of community resources and health promotion. Ongoing education and support are provided by community-based case managers.

TOOLS AND STRATEGIES USED BY CASE MANAGERS

Two tools or strategies commonly associated with case management are utilization management (utilization review) and clinical pathways. These will be briefly described in this section.

Utilization Management

Utilization management (UM) has existed for more than three decades as hospitals and third party payers have sought ways to manage costs while improving the appropriateness and quality of care. Initially UM focused on reviewing hospital care, but it gradually grew to include outpatient services and home care. UM refers to the formal and comprehensive review of services used by a patient to ensure the services are: (1) medically necessary, (2) provided in the most appropriate care setting, and (3) at or above quality standards (Lattimer and Garrett, 2008).

Generally UM programs focus on such areas as precertification, preadmission review, concurrent review of care, review of outpatient and ancillary services, and pharmacy management (Cohen and Cesta, 2005). Goals of UM programs are listed in Box 4-4.

During the UM review process the case manager will initially verify the patient's eligibility for services and determine whether a requested service is a covered benefit. The case manager collects demographic and clinical information to certify the requested service or length of stay; this should include the current medical situation and anticipated treatment plan. The clinical information will be reviewed against evidence-based decision criteria or guidelines, and the case manager will determine if the case meets the criteria. If the criteria are met, the provider will be notified of approval; if the criteria are not met, the review is typically sent for peer review. All activities are documented within the organization/agency's medical record keeping process. Case managers who provide UM services must be very familiar with the appeals processes in place and respond appropriately when a request is denied (Lattimer and Garrett, 2008).

Clinical Pathways

Case Managers often use support tools such as protocols, algorithms, or pathways to manage the organization, quality, and costs of services. These tools can assist in planning and coordinating care and determining whether the services are indicated and provided at the appropriate level of care.

One approach frequently used by case managers to lower health care costs is known as the *clinical pathway* (also called *clinical path, critical path or pathway, care map, collaborative plan of care, multidisciplinary action plan [MAP], care path, guidelines,*

BOX 4-4 Goals of Utilization Management Programs

- Ensure effective utilization of health care resources through ongoing monitoring
- Determine medical necessity and appropriateness of care
- Identify patterns of overutilization, underutilization, and inefficient scheduling of resources
- Promote quality patient care and optimal outcomes
- Assist in the identification of coordination of care options for members and providers

- Facilitate appropriate, safe, timely, and effective discharge to the most appropriate level of care
- Provide education concerning the UM program to providers and department staff
- Identify potential participants in disease management and case management programs.

From Lattimer C, Garrett MB: Utilization management and resource management. In Powell SK, Tahan HA, editors: *CMSA core curriculum for case management*, ed 2, Philadelphia, 2008, Lippincott, p. 208.

protocols, algorithm, and anticipated recovery path). **Clinical pathways** are written tools that specify activities that providers use in a timely sequence to achieve desired outcomes for care. Clinical pathways are guidelines for care of clients who have a predictable course of illness, surgery, or event, and are typically developed for high-volume, high-cost, or high-risk diagnoses, procedures, or symptoms. They are designed to minimize delays and use of resources while maximizing the quality of client care (Cohen and Cesta, 2005; McKendry, 2008).

Clinical pathways are generally developed around a specific diagnosis using an International Classification of Diseases-9, Clinical Modification (ICD-9-CM) code or a Current Procedural Terminology (CPT) code. The ICD-9-CM is a statistical classification system that organizes disease and injuries into groups according to standardized criteria. Each diagnosis is assigned a code number. These codes are used by insurance carriers to reimburse providers. Similarly the CPT code is a systematic listing of procedures and services performed by physicians. Each specific procedure has an assigned five-digit code that reports services provided to insurance carriers.

For the identified diagnosis or procedure, the clinical pathway defines the most common or preferred courses of treatment (best practices). The pathway organizes, sequences, and specifies timelines for interventions and establishes specific goals and outcomes for the client. If the expected outcome is not met, the outlying outcome is called a *variance*. The variance can also be a deviation from an activity or key aspect of care listed on the clinical pathway.

The clinical pathway consists of a grid outlining treatment along a timeline with expected outcomes. Categories may include assessment and evaluation, tests and procedures, consults, medications, diet, activity, patient/family education, therapy, pain management, and discharge planning (McKendry, 2008). Timelines are essential and can be measured in hours or minutes (in the emergency department), in days (in the acute care setting), or in months (in MCOs or long-term care facilities). The case manager continuously assesses whether the client is meeting the expected outcomes. If the outcome is not achieved, the case manager documents this as a variance (McKendry, 2008; More and Mandell, 1997). Bassett (1998) described several phases to be explored during the process of developing a clinical pathway. Table 4-1 summarizes that process.

Clinical pathways have been successful in many settings and appear to benefit all parties. Benefits to the client include consumer involvement, improved education, mutual goal setting, and increased satisfaction. Benefits for health team members include standardized and organized care, improved communication, reflection of best practices, increased staff satisfaction, and an educational tool for students and new graduates. Benefits for the health care organization include support by the Joint Commission, support by third party payers, integration of quality improvement, utilization management and risk management, improved communication, decreased costs, and availability of data for evaluating care.

SUMMARY

Although case management in health care is not new, it has received increased interest during the past decade. Expansion of case management has been noteworthy and has been seen in multiple settings. This growth is attributed to the high costs associated with health care and anticipated needs related to an aging population, along with an increase in chronic illnesses.

Many nurses, such as Kathy in the opening case study, act as case managers or use case management principles in community-based settings. As the health care delivery system continues to evolve, with more emphasis being placed on coordination of services across settings, as well as cost-effective, high-quality care, the role of the nurse as case manager will continue to grow.

KEY POINTS

- Aspects of case management have been used in health care since the 1920s. Since the mid-1980s, however, case management has become increasingly common as a means to help control health care costs and promote coordinated, cost-effective care.
- Case management is a collaborative process that plans, implements, coordinates, monitors, and evaluates services to meet health needs. Goals of case management are to enhance the quality of health care, decrease fragmentation, ensure appropriate use of resources, and contain costs.

TABLE **4-1** Developing a Clinical Pathway

PHASE	ACTIVITIES
Planning	Select team members (should have experience in development of pathways if possible).
	Identify high-volume, recurring diagnoses or procedures (problems should be those that are prevalent and relatively expensive to manage).
	Determine who will collect data, how it will be collected, and how it will be used.
Current Practice	Perform record reviews of the diagnoses/procedures to identify and understand current practices (25 to 50 cases).
	Document contacts with the client and outcome of care on a grid or worksheet.
	Summarize interventions by day or visit and identify best practices.
Designing	Design pathway to include basic information such as client name, diagnosis or procedure (corresponding with ICD-9 or CPT codes), age, race, sex, date of entry into pathway, and date of discharge.
	Using best practices of care, develop goals, interventions, and outcomes on a day-to-day, visit-by-visit, or week-by-week basis, as appropriate (goals should be specific and measurable, and interventions are bound by time).
	Devise a method for documentation; documentation may be incorporated in the actual pathway tool or in the providers' notes.
	Outline specific information regarding the disease process (e.g., nutrition, fluid and electrolytes, functional activities, and community resources).
	Identify education interventions (e.g., understanding medication regimen, infant care, nutrition guidelines).
	Include process that will be used for discharge planning.
Testing	Involve all team members in implementation.
	Adjust components of the pathway as needed.
	Implement with a small number of clients.
	Evaluate continually.
Variance	Identify variances among care team members, clients, and physicians.
	Examine variances to determine if components of the pathway need adjusting.
	Categorize variances as system-, client-, or clinically related.
	Determine if variances are positive or negative.
	Devise a way to communicate variances.
Evaluation	Consider both quality and cost in evaluation.
	Determine outcomes based on client's physiological progression for functionality.

From Bassett S: Clinical pathways. In Price SA, Koch MW, Bassett S, editors: *Health care resource management: present and future challenges* St Louis, 1998, Mosby, p. 103.

- Nursing case managers are typically accountable for managing a defined group of clients in order to optimize clinical and cost outcomes through partnership with clients and their families. Case managers coordinate services with other health care providers and often use specific tools or guidelines such as clinical pathways.
- In the clinical role nursing case managers assess clients and identify existing or potential health problems. Working with an interdisciplinary team, they develop a plan of care to meet those needs. In the managerial role the nurse case manager facilitates and coordinates the care of clients during the course of their illness. In the financial role the nurse case manager works to ensure that clients receive quality care that is appropriate, while taking into account issues of resource allocation and cost containment.
- Skills needed by nurse case managers include excellent communication skills (in person, on the

telephone, and written), teaching skills, management skills (i.e., delegation, negotiation, problem solving, organization, networking), advocacy, and collaboration.

- Activities provided by nurse case managers center on the nursing process (assessment, planning, implementation, evaluation), but include the additional components of coordination and monitoring of care.
- In acute care settings, case managers generally work as primary nurse case managers, advanced practice case managers, or in UR. In external (outside the hospital) settings, nurse case managers work in long-term care settings, home health, managed care organizations, and disease management. Case managers are often employed by insurance companies, and case management may be a component of the practice of school nurses, parish nurses, or occupational health nurses.
- Clinical pathways are written tools that specify activities that providers use to achieve desired outcomes of care. For a particular diagnosis or procedure a clinical pathway defines a course of treatment and organizes, sequences, and specifies timelines for interventions. If specific goals or outcomes are not met, the result is called a *variance*.

Learning Activities & Application to Practice
In Class

1. With classmates, review examples of clinical pathways that are used in community-based settings. How can they be used to standardize practice? What are potential benefits? What are potential problems?

In Clinical

2. Spend a day with a case manager in a community setting. Options include home health care, a community mental health clinic, or an insurance office. How does case management expand on routine nursing care?
3. Attend an interdisciplinary conference for client care management. Who is the coordinator of care for the client? What disciplines are represented? Share findings with classmates.

REFERENCES

Alvarado E and Sunderland E: Case management in the home care setting. In Powell SK, Tahan HA, editors: *CMSA core curriculum for case management*, ed 2, Philadelphia, 2008, Lippincott.

American Nurses Association: *Nursing case management*, Kansas City, Mo, 1994, ANA.

Bassett S: Clinical pathways. In Price SA, Koch MW, Bassett S, editors: *Health care resource management: present and future challenges*, St Louis, 1998, Mosby.

Brooks E, Younce J: A case management model for the ambulatory care patient experiencing chronic pain, *AAACN Viewpoint* 29(1):3, 2007.

Carey AH: Case management. In Stanhope M, Lancaster J, editors, *Community & public health nursing*, ed 6, St Louis, 2004, Mosby.

Case Management Society of America: *Standards of practice for case management*, Little Rock,, 2002, CMSA.

Cesta TG, Tahan HA: *The case manager's survival guide: winning strategies for clinical practice*, ed 2, St Louis, 2003, Mosby.

Clark MJ: Case management. In Clark MJ, editor: *Community health nursing: advocacy for population health*, ed 3, Upper Saddle River, NJ, 2008, Prentice Hall.

Cohen EL, Cesta TG: *Nursing case management: from essentials to advanced practice applications*, ed 4, St Louis, 2005, Mosby.

Commission for Case Manager Certification: *CCM certification guide*, 2005 (website): http://www.ccmcertification.org/pages/22frame_set.html. Accessed November 1, 2007.

Daniels S: Case management in the acute care setting. In Powell SK, Tahan HA, editors: *CMSA core curriculum for case management*, ed 2, Philadelphia, 2008, Lippincott.

DiBenedetto DV: Workers' compensation case management. In Powell SK, Tahan HA, editors: *CMSA core curriculum for case management*, ed 2, Philadelphia, 2008, Lippincott.

Hunt KA, Knickman JR: Financing for health care. In Kovner AR, Knickman JR, editors: *Jonas and Kovner's health care delivery in the United States*, ed 8, New York, 2005, Springer.

Koch RW, Beck KL, Norris TL: Case management. In Price SA, Koch MW, Bassett S, editors: *Health care resource management: present and future challenges*, St Louis, 1998, Mosby.

Lattimer C, Garrett MB: Utilization management and resource management. In Powell SK, Tahan HA, editors: *CMSA core curriculum for case management*, ed 2, Philadelphia, 2008, Lippincott.

Levy M, Heffner B, Stewart T and others: The efficacy of asthma case management in an urban school district in reducing school absences and hospitalizations for asthma, *J Sch Health* 76(6):320, 2006.

Lind PH: Disease management: applying systems thinking to quality patient care delivery. In Cohen EL, Cesta TG, editors: *Nursing case management: from essentials to advanced practice applications*, ed 4, St Louis, 2005, Mosby.

Lowery S: History and evolution of case management. In Powell SK, Tahan HA, editors: *CMSA core curriculum for case management*, ed 2, Philadelphia, 2008, Lippincott.

Lyon JC: Case management. In Nies MA, McEwen M, editors: *Community/public health nursing: promoting the health of populations*, ed 4, St Louis, 2007, Saunders.

Mahn VA, Zazworsky D: Nurse case management as an advance practice role. In Hamric AB, Spross JA, Hanson CM, editors: *Advance nursing practice: an integrative approach*, ed 2, Philadelphia, 2000, Saunders.

McKendry MJ: Case management plans, clinical pathways and protocols. In Powell SK, Tahan HA, editors: *CMSA core curriculum for case management*, ed 2, Philadelphia, 2008, Lippincott.

Metcalfe J: Enhancing the care of older people in the community, *Nurs Stand* 21(7):35, 2006.

More PK, Mandell S: *Nursing case management: an evolving practice*, New York, 1997, McGraw-Hill.

Mullahy CM: *The case manager's handbook*, ed 3, Sudbury, Mass, 2004, Jones and Bartlett.

Palsbo SE, Mastal MF, O'Donnell LT: Disability care coordination organizations: improving health and function in people with disabilities, *Lippincotts Case Manag* 11(5):255, 2006.

Powell SK, Tahan HA: Disease management and case management. In Powell SK Tahan HA, editors: *CMSA core curriculum for case management*, ed 2, Philadelphia, 2008, Lippincott.

Provine KN, Vierling LE: Disability and occupational health case management. In Powell SK, Tahan HA, editors: *CMSA core curriculum for case management*, ed 2, Philadelphia, 2008, Lippincott.

Raderstorf M, Kurtz J: Managing mental health issues in the workplace, *Prof Case Manag* 12(4):242, 2007.

Siefker JM, Garrett MB, Van Genderen A and others: *Fundamentals of case management: guidelines for practicing case managers*, St Louis, 1998, Mosby.

Tahan HA (2008a): The case management process. In Powell SK, Tahan HA, editors: *CMSA core curriculum for case management*, ed 2, Philadelphia, 2008, Lippincott.

Tahan HA (2008b): Case management practice settings and throughput. In Powell SK, Tahan HA, editors: *CMSA core curriculum for case management*, ed 2, Philadelphia, 2008, Lippincott.

Two

Factors that Influence Health and Health Care

Chapter 5

Overview of the Health Care Delivery System

objectives

Upon completion of this chapter, the reader will be able to:

1. Describe the public sector and private sector components of the health care delivery system.

2. Explain the different organizations (e.g., hospitals, ambulatory health centers, nursing homes, home health) and providers (e.g., nurses, physicians, therapists, pharmacists) that make up the health care system.

3. Describe financing of health care delivery, including third party payers, managed care options (i.e., health maintenance organizations, preferred provider organizations), Medicare, and Medicaid.

4. Compare and contrast Medicare and Medicaid.

5. Discuss factors that have contributed to the high costs of health care.

key terms

Capitation
Coinsurance
Copayments
Deductibles
Diagnosis-related groups (DRGs)
Gatekeeper

Health maintenance organization (HMO)
Independent practice association (IPA)
Managed care
Medicaid
Medicare

Preferred provider organizations (PPOs)
Third party reimbursement
Utilization review

See Glossary for definitions.

case study

Carol Clark is employed as a head nurse for the evening shift in the emergency department of a large, nonprofit hospital in an urban area. Carol has been a nurse for 20 years, and during that time she has witnessed dramatic changes in health care provision and in the health care delivery system. Carol knows that reimbursement issues are extremely important to the hospital, but she finds it confusing and even unfair that a client's care is often affected by health care insurance coverage or lack of it. It concerns her that one of the first questions she must ask clients as they come into the emergency department is "Do you have health insurance?"

Continued

One recent Monday, Carol saw Melissa Mills, a 34-year-old woman experiencing lower abdominal pain; George Green, a 76-year-old man with chest pain; Beth Bell, a 12-year-old girl who had sprained her ankle; Nancy Nelson, a 19-year-old prima gravida in active labor; and Andy Adams, a 46-year-old man suffering an acute asthma attack. During the evening Carol wondered whether the care given each of these clients was influenced by insurance coverage and insurer requirements. Following the shift Carol reviewed the disposition of each case from a financial standpoint, and following is what she learned.

Ms. Mills is insured through a large health maintenance organization (HMO). It was determined that her pain was caused by ovulation, and she was sent home with pain medication. Because she was not referred to the emergency department by her primary care provider, it is unlikely that the HMO will pay for the visit.

Mr. Green is insured by Medicare parts A and B. He was admitted into the coronary care unit for observation. Hospital coverage is comprehensive and based on the prospective payment system. Medical coverage is at 80% following a deductible.

Beth Bell's health care is insured by a Preferred Provider Organization (PPO) through her father's employer. Hospital and medical coverage will be 80% to 100% after a predetermined deductible.

Ms. Nelson has no health insurance. Because it was determined that delivery was not imminent, she was sent to the local public hospital, which provides care for indigent clients. She is eligible for Medicaid but has not applied.

Mr. Adams has no health insurance. Because his asthma attack was severe and he was in danger of respiratory arrest, he was kept for treatment and observation. Although Mr. Adams has no insurance, he is responsible for the costs of his health care and will be billed. Because he is only sporadically employed, he will be unable to pay most of the bill, which totals several thousand dollars, and the hospital will incur the cost of his care as "bad debt."

Carol, like many other health care providers, is struggling to understand the health care delivery system and trying to be informed about financing of health care and differing health plans and reimbursement methods. She, along with other providers, must learn to practice within the context of constant change and work with multiple insurance plans and providers.

To better understand the context in which they practice, it is essential that all nurses—particularly nurses working in primary care or community-based settings (including emergency departments, as in the case study)—acquire a working knowledge of the health care delivery system (HCDS). This chapter presents basic concepts, information, illustrations, and tables to reinforce the nurse's understanding of the HCDS, including its structure, health care settings and organizations, provider roles, and health care financing. Understanding these concepts will assist the nurse to deliver the highest quality, most cost-effective care possible.

Like the Holy Roman Empire, which was neither Holy nor Roman nor an Empire, the Health Care System refers not to health, nor to care, nor is it a system. Ninety-five percent of the medical effort in the United States goes to disease, not health; provides medical treatment, not care; and is in no way a system. Rather it is a vast haphazard conglomeration of medical entrepreneurs, be they doctors, pharmacies, pharmaceutical manufacturers, hospitals or insurance companies.

Earl Ubell, 1974

STRUCTURE OF THE HEALTH CARE DELIVERY SYSTEM

Organizationally the HCDS can be divided into public sector and private sector components. The public sector of the HCDS can be subdivided into federal, state, and local level divisions and is typically concerned with the health of populations and the provision of a healthy environment. The private sector includes nonprofit and proprietary organizations (e.g., hospitals, clinics, home health agencies, voluntary groups) and providers (e.g., physicians, dentists, therapists) whose primary focus is health care for individuals and families.

PUBLIC SECTOR

The U.S. Department of Health and Human Services (USDHHS) is the federal cabinet department that directly or indirectly oversees most components of the HCDS. Most USDHHS agencies have regional, state, or local offices that may be contacted for specific needs or questions. For example, regional or local offices of the Social Security Administration, the Administration on Aging, and Aid to Families with Dependent Children (AFDC) should be accessed to obtain information on services, eligibility, and other issues.

Agencies within the USDHHS include the Centers for Disease Control and Prevention (CDC), the Food and Drug Administration (FDA), and the National Institutes of Health (NIH). Each of these agencies and organizations is responsible for oversight or regulation of differing issues related to health and health care delivery. The NIH, for example, finances a significant amount of research related to health; the FDA is responsible for monitoring and regulating the safety of pharmaceuticals, food additives, other consumer goods, and health care products and equipment; and the CDC monitors infectious diseases and directs programs to control and prevent diseases. The impact of these agencies and other components of the USDHHS on health and the health care system cannot be overstated, and all nurses should be familiar with the various components of the USDHHS. Listings and functions of most of the offices and agencies within the USDHHS are presented in Table 5-1.

TABLE **5-1** U.S. Department of Health and Human Services—Selected Agencies and Units

AGENCY OR ORGANIZATION	FUNCTION
Department of Health and Human Services	Oversees, manages, and finances most of the products, organizations, and interests related to health.
Centers for Disease Control and Prevention	Monitors and supports programs to prevent and control infectious diseases and promote health.
Food and Drug Administration	Provides surveillance for the safety of pharmaceuticals and other consumer goods.
Health Resources and Services Administration	Provides health care for medically underserved populations and maintains the National Health Service Corps.
National Institutes of Health	Conducts and funds health-related research.
Substance Abuse and Mental Health Services Administration	Supports research and programs related to substance abuse and mental health.
Agency for Health Care Research and Quality	Provides evidence-based information on health care outcomes, quality, cost, use, and access.
Office of Disease Prevention and Health Promotion	Carries out the goals of *Healthy People 2010* and provides other information services.
Centers for Medicare and Medicaid Services	Administers Medicare, Medicaid, and Child Health Insurance Program.
Administration for Children and Families	Coordinates efforts for children and families, including Head Start, Job Opportunities and Basic Skills Training (JOBS), and Aid to Families with Dependent Children (AFDC).
Indian Health Services	Supports hospitals and health centers that provide services to 1.5 million Native Americans.
Administration on Aging	Represents the concerns of older U.S. residents.

Direct links to the website for each agency can be accessed through www.dhhs.gov.

Each state maintains a state health department, usually located in the state capital. Most state health departments are headed by a health officer or commissioner and funded through state taxes and federal monies (e.g., grants, matching funds). Local health departments may reside within a city, county, municipality, or district. State legislatures generally define the responsibilities and roles of the local health agency. Funding for local activities comes from a combination of local and state taxes and federal grants. Although roles, functions, and services vary, state and local health departments are typically responsible for the activities listed in Box 5-1.

PRIVATE SECTOR

The private sector of the HCDS is composed of various providers (e.g., physicians, nurses, dentists, pharmacists), organizations (e.g., American Red Cross, American Heart Association, American Cancer Society), institutions (e.g., hospitals, clinics), industries and corporations (e.g., pharmaceutical companies, hospital equipment manufacturers), and insurers (e.g., Blue Cross/ Blue Shield, Aetna). Although most components of the private sector of the HCDS are income producing or for profit, others are designated nonprofit and thus tax exempt. Nonprofit private sector organizations include voluntary agencies, such as the Red Cross and the American Cancer Society, and direct care providers, including the visiting nurses' associations and many hospitals and community clinics.

The individuals and organizations that compose the private sector of the HCDS work more or less independently to produce goods and services to promote the health of U.S. residents and to treat and manage health threats, diseases, and related conditions. However, the public component of the HCDS maintains a degree of control over the private sector through a variety of means, as described previously. Examples of how the public sector of the HCDS directly affects the private sector in health care delivery are as follows: licensure of most direct providers (e.g., physicians, nurses, dentists) is required by all states; federal approval is needed before marketing all new medications and devices used in medical treatment; and recommendations and federal and state requirements exist for communicable disease prevention, management, and reporting. The following sections provide more examples and details about various organizations and providers.

HEALTH CARE PROVIDER ORGANIZATIONS

The U.S. HCDS is composed of a multitude of providers and organizations serving the population at many levels and for a vast array of needs. Chapter 1 included a discussion of primary, secondary, and tertiary health care. Recall that *primary health care* refers to basic care for preventive services or treatment of common acute illnesses and conditions (e.g., sore throat, otitis media, pregnancy) or routine chronic conditions (e.g., diabetes, hypertension, arthritis) in ambulatory settings. *Secondary health care* refers to more intensive or complicated care, usually provided in acute care settings (typically a hospital [e.g., open-heart surgery, treatment of complications of diabetes]). Finally, *tertiary health care* is long-term care for complex, chronic, and complicated health problems (e.g., burn units, skilled nursing facilities, nursing homes). Facilities, organizations, and providers for each of these levels are described here.

BOX **5-1** Functions and Services of State and Local Health Departments

STATE HEALTH DEPARTMENTS
- Administer Medicaid
- Operate state mental hospitals
- Provide licensure and regulation of health practitioners and health facilities
- Regulate insurance companies
- Control and monitor communicable diseases
- Enforce and oversee environmental programs
- Direct health planning and development
- Maintain vital records for the state

LOCAL HEALTH DEPARTMENTS
- Provide direct health services (e.g., family planning and Women, Infants, and Children [WIC])
- Record local vital statistical data and report them to the state
- Control and prevent communicable diseases
- Direct environmental services (e.g., monitor water quality, inspect food services, vector control)

AMBULATORY HEALTH CARE

Primary health care is provided to ambulatory clients in community-based settings. Ambulatory care is commonly thought of as health care provided to an individual who is not a bed patient in a health care institution.

The numbers and types of ambulatory care settings and providers are rapidly growing. There are two basic types of ambulatory care: (1) care provided by private physicians in solo, partnership, or group practice on a fee-for-service basis or preferred provider organization (PPO) arrangement; and (2) care provided in organized or institutional settings, such as some types of HMOs, hospital-based ambulatory services, hospital-sponsored group practices, surgicenters, urgicenters or emergicenters, neighborhood health centers, organized home care, and school and workplace health services (Gourevitch, Caronna, and Kalkut, 2005).

Providers of care in ambulatory settings include physicians, dentists, nurses, nurse practitioners (NPs), physician assistants (PAs), social workers, therapists, pharmacists, optometrists, and chiropractors. Specific information regarding some of the many health care providers is presented later in this chapter.

According to a survey performed in 2005, U.S. residents averaged four visits to ambulatory care facilties each year (USDHHS 2007). The number of yearly physician visits varied greatly based on age (approximately 9.5 visits per year for infants; 4 visits per year for small children; 2-3 visits per year for adolescents and young and middle-aged adults; and 7-9 visits per year for those older than 65 years), gender (males had 3.4 visits per year; females, 4.5 visits per year) and race/ethnicity (white people had 4.2 visits per year; black people had 3.7 visits per year; Hispanics had 3.0 visits per year). The 10 most common principal diagnoses/reasons for office visits in 2005 were the following:

1. Essential hypertension
2. Health supervision of infant or child
3. Acute upper respiratory infection
4. Arthritis and related disorders
5. Malignant neoplasms
6. Diabetes mellitus
7. Spinal disorders (back pain)
8. Normal pregnancy
9. Otitis media
10. General medical examination

Residents of the United States average about two visits each year for dental care. In contrast to physician care, dental visits are fewest for small children (less than one visit per year) and greatest between the ages of 5 and 14 and 45 and 64 (2.3 visits per year on average). Although the number of yearly dental visits varies little between men and women, there is marked difference between races (whites, 2.1 visits per year; blacks, 1.3 visits per year). Most dental visits are for preventive care (e.g., cleaning and fluoride treatment) and to obtain fillings.

Innovations in anesthesiology and surgical techniques have led to rapid growth in the number of outpatient surgery and day surgery procedures. Begun in the early 1970s as a cost-cutting measure, ambulatory surgery is now very common. Indeed, it is estimated that more than half of all surgical procedures are performed on an outpatient basis.

Likewise, the growth of freestanding emergicenters is attributed to attempts to lower costs by decreasing the use of expensive hospital emergency rooms for nonurgent primary care. Emergicenters offer convenient locations, flexible hours, and short waiting periods at significantly lower costs for services. As emergicenters have increased in number and in acceptance by clients, they have evolved to offer a combination of walk-in and appointment services. They provide a wide range of primary care, including preventive care (e.g., physical examinations) and diagnosis and treatment of acute, episodic illnesses (e.g., bronchitis, influenza) and injuries (e.g., minor lacerations, sprains, and strains).

HOSPITALS

Acute care hospitals are the principal settings for provision of secondary health care. Hospitals differ based on such factors as size, mission, ownership, complexity, population served, financing, physical facilities, and costs per day for care (Sultz and Young, 2006). Hospitals may range in size from less than 30 beds to more than 500 beds, serve special populations (e.g., children, elders, disabled), care for clients with specific diagnoses (e.g., acquired immunodeficiency syndrome [AIDS], tuberculosis, cancer), and/or support a defined mission of service (e.g., hospice, rehabilitation). Hospitals in which the average stay is less than 30 days are called *short-term hospitals*.

Collectively, hospitals are among the largest industries in the United States in terms of the number of employees and revenue. About half of health care personnel work in hospitals and about 30% of health care expenditures are to hospitals (CMS, 2007a).

Hospitals may be publicly or privately funded. Those that are privately funded may be nonprofit or proprietary. Examples of each are found in Table 5-2. The distinction between public and privately funded institutions is not absolute because virtually all public facilities accept private-pay clients and many private hospitals will take uninsured clients and/or may be reimbursed by public monies.

It is important to note that the total number of hospitals decreased rather significantly during the past several decades. Cost containment strategies, the increasing use of outpatient care, and many other factors have resulted in hospital closures throughout the nation. These same factors have prompted a reduction in hospital beds in many other hospitals.

Table 5-3 illustrates the trend in reduction in the number of hospitals over the past decade.

LONG-TERM CARE FACILITIES

Tertiary, or long-term, care includes institutional health services, mental health services, and residential services provided to temporarily or chronically disabled persons over an extended period. The goal of long-term care is to provide services that enhance the functional ability of these individuals.

Functional ability refers to a person's capacity to perform basic self-care activities such as eating, dressing, and personal care (e.g., bathing, showering, oral care, and maintenance of bowel and bladder control). These activities are generally termed activities of daily living (ADL). Long-term care may also assist the client in performance of instrumental activities of daily living (IADL) (e.g., shopping, housekeeping, preparing meals, managing of monetary affairs).

The need for long-term care may be temporary (e.g., an older person's recovery from joint

TABLE **5-2** Types of Hospitals

Public			Private	
FEDERAL	**STATE**	**LOCAL**	**NONPROFIT**	**PROPRIETARY**
Veterans Administration hospitals	State mental facilities	City/county general or charity hospitals	Religious-based (e.g., Catholic, Christian, or Jewish)	Corporately owned (e.g., Humana, Columbia/HCA, National Medical Enterprises)
Federal prison hospitals	Tuberculosis hospitals		Foundation, charity, or voluntary (e.g., many children's hospitals, Masonic hospitals)	Group owned (typically physician groups)
Military hospitals	Teaching hospitals associated with state universities (also local)			
Special hospitals (e.g., Native Americans, Hansen's disease)				

TABLE **5-3** Hospital Facts: 1981, 1991, 1999, 2005

TYPE OF HOSPITALS	HOSPITALS 1981 (n)	HOSPITALS 1991 (n)	HOSPITALS 1999 (n)	HOSPITALS 2005 (n)
PUBLIC				
Federal	348	334	264	226
State psychiatric	549	800	649	456
State respiratory	11	4	NA	NA
Long-term general	146	124	NA	118
State and local government	1744	1429	1197	1110
PRIVATE				
Nonprofit	3340	3175	3012	2958
Proprietary	729	738	747	868

NA, Not available.
From American Hospital Association: *Hospital Statistics 2006*, Chicago, 2006, American Hospital Association; American Hospital Association: *Facts on US Hospitals*, 2006 (website): http://www.aha.org/aha/resource-center/Statistics-and-Studies/fast-facts.html.

replacement surgery or rehabilitative care for a client with a spinal cord injury) or permanent (e.g., institutional care for an individual who is profoundly mentally retarded or for a bed-bound, frail, older person). Functional disability, particularly in the elderly, often results from chronic conditions such as arthritis, hearing impairment, vision impairment, diabetes, and respiratory or cardiac disease. The need for more and higher quality long-term care facilities and providers is evident with the increase in the number of elderly and chronically ill. Examples of long-term care facilities and some of the services they provide are listed in Box 5-2.

In general, long-term care is financed through governmental programs (Medicaid, Medicare, and state funding for care of the mentally ill) and out-of-pocket payment. Nursing home care of the elderly, for example, is largely financed through a combination of Medicaid, Medicare, and out-of-pocket payment. It is important to note that approximately 42% of long term care—largely for care of elders—is financed through Medicaid (CMS, 2006). Detailed information on financing of health care services is discussed later in this chapter.

HEALTH CARE PROFESSIONALS

When people consider health care professionals, they most often think of nurses and doctors; however, in reality, health care in the United States is provided by more than 200 different occupational groups. Consumers have a general understanding of the roles and functions of providers, but there remains much room for misunderstanding. For example, what are the educational requirements for a nurse? What is the difference between a psychologist, a psychiatrist, and a psychotherapist or between an MD and a doctor of osteopathy (DO)? Does a specific client need to see an audiologist or a speech therapist?

Because of the importance of collaboration and coordination in their practice, nurses working in community settings need to understand the practice parameters, roles, education, and credentialing requirements of the many health care providers. Knowledge of the different disciplines can assist the nurse in the planning and implementation of health care. Information on education, practice, and licensure for many health care providers is described here. The *Healthy People 2010* box presents information about objectives related to increasing the

BOX 5-2 Examples of Long-Term Care Facilities and Services

NURSING HOMES

Generic term that includes a wide spectrum of facilities such as retirement centers, convalescent homes, and skilled nursing facilities. Nursing homes are utilized by individuals who are not able to remain at home because of physical health problems, mental health problems, or functional disabilities.

SKILLED NURSING FACILITIES

Long-term care establishments that are designed to provide a higher level of care than custodial care facilities but at a level less intensive than care provided in short-term, acute care hospitals. Skilled nursing facilities must have a licensed nurse available at all times and are eligible for Medicare reimbursement.

HOME HEALTH CARE

Consists of a variety of nursing, therapy, and social support services provided to individuals and their families at their place of residence. Home health care can include skilled nursing care, nurse's aide services, physical therapy, occupational therapy, and speech therapy. For Medicare reimbursement, home health care must include a plan of care prescribed by a physician.

ADULT DAY CARE

Refers to a variety of health and social services for the elderly during the day and out of the home. Adult day care provides caregiver respite care to delay or prevent institutionalization, particularly for elders in families in which the caregivers work or when the elder lives alone.

RESPITE CARE

Provides a temporary respite, or break, for caregivers of the frail elderly or disabled chronically ill. Respite care may be provided in or out of the client's home and may include homemaker services and/or assistance with ADL. Medicaid and Medicare will pay for respite care in some circumstances.

HOSPICE

Refers to the provision of care for the terminally ill. Hospice care may be delivered at home or in an institutional setting and is directed toward symptom management, pain control, and psychological, social, and spiritual care for the client and the family.

ASSISTED LIVING ARRANGEMENTS

Refers to a group or residential setting (licensed or unlicensed) that provides personal care and meets unscheduled needs for older disabled persons. Assisted living facilities vary greatly with regard to size, funding sources, target populations, services, and staffing. There are several models, including:

Congregate living arrangements – provide group-living and supportive service facilities; typically multiunit apartment complexes where residents can live and eat independently.

Board-and-care homes – provide rooms, meals, assistance with ADL, and some protective oversight; may be licensed or unlicensed.

Continuing care communities – comprehensive service settings providing three levels of living: (1) independent, (2) assisted, and (3) nursing home care. A resident can join a continuing care community as an independent resident and progress through the services if physical or mental disabilities dictate.

Data from Evashwick CJ: The continuum of long-term care. In Williams SJ, Torrens PR, editors: *Introduction to health services*, ed 7, Clifton Park, NY, 2008, Thomson/Delmar Learning, p. 210; Feldman PH, Nadash P, Gursen MD: Long-term care. In Kovner AR, Knickman JR, editors: *Jonas & Kovner's health care delivery in the United States*, ed 8, New York, 2005, Springer, p. 274.

number of health professionals from racial and ethnic minority groups, which hopefully will contribute to better health care access for those groups.

PHYSICIANS, PHYSICIAN ASSISTANTS, AND DENTISTS
Doctor of Medicine

Allopathic doctors of medicine (MDs) prevent, diagnose, and treat disease and injury. They prescribe medications, perform surgery, and direct many other health services (e.g., laboratory services, hospital use) and providers. Education requirements are 3 to 4 years of college (most have a bachelor's degree) and 4 years of medical school, followed by a 1-year internship. The MDs who stop training at this point are nonspecialists, or general practitioners. However, most MDs (80% to 90%) specialize. Specialization requires 3 to 4 years of additional residency training. Medical specialties include internal medicine, general surgery, obstetrics, pediatrics, and radiology.

healthy people **2010**

Health Professions and *Healthy People 2010*

The USDHHS has recognized that certain racial and ethnic groups and low-income communities lag behind the overall U.S. population on virtually all health status indicators. Among other factors, this can be tied to lack of a specific source of care. One way to help achieve the goal of eliminating health disparities is proposed in Objective 1-8 of *Healthy People 2010*—to increase the proportion of all health professions' degrees awarded to members of racial and ethnic minority groups. Although members of racial and ethnic minority groups make up about 25% of the U.S. population, only about 10% of health professionals are from these groups. Many believe that increasing the number of health professionals from racial and ethnic minority groups will help improve access to care.

Several suggestions have been proposed to help accomplish this. First, enhanced efforts are needed to provide financial assistance for students from underrepresented racial and ethnic groups to pursue health care degrees. Second, health care practitioners, particularly those from minority groups, should encourage mentor relationships with health profession students. Third, efforts should be made to promote early recruiting of students from certain racial and ethnic groups. Finally, the number of minority faculty members in schools that train health care professionals needs to be increased.

Subspecialties include hematology, oncology, cardiology, orthopedic surgery, and thoracic surgery.

All states require physicians to be licensed. Requirements for licensure include graduation from an accredited professional school, passage of a licensing examination administered by the National Board of Medical Examiners, and successful completion of an accredited graduate medical education program (internship or residency).

Doctor of Osteopathy

Like MDs, DOs prevent, diagnose, and treat diseases. Osteopathy, however, emphasizes that the body can make its own remedies, given normal structural relationship, environmental conditions, and nutrition. Education requirements and specialties are similar to those for an MD and include instruction in body mechanics and manipulative methods in diagnosis and treatment and medicinal and surgical treatments.

Physician Assistant

The role of the PA developed in the 1960s in response to a shortage of primary care physicians in certain areas. The PA's practice includes physical examination, ordering and interpretation of laboratory tests, and making tentative diagnoses and prescribing treatments under protocol and direct and/or indirect supervision of physicians. Education requirements are 3 to 4 years of college (a bachelor's degree is usually required) and 2 years of PA school. The PA programs are located in medical schools, universities, or schools of allied health. Most offer a bachelor's degree as the basic degree, although some offer a master's degree.

All states require licensure to practice as a PA. Graduation from an accredited professional school is necessary for licensure. Specialization is possible and specialty areas include surgery, emergency medicine, and orthopedics.

Doctor of Dental Surgery and Doctor of Dental Medicine

Dentists may obtain one of two degrees: doctor of dental surgery (DDS) and doctor of dental medicine (DDM). Dentists prevent, diagnose, and treat problems of the teeth and tissues of the mouth. Education requirements are similar to those for an MD, with an additional 4 academic years in dental school. Most dentists (85%) are generalists. Specialization requires 2 years or more of additional training and includes endodontics (treatment of the roots of teeth), orthodontics (straightening of teeth), periodontics (treatment of the gums and bone supporting the teeth), and pedodontics (children's dentistry).

All states require dentists to be licensed. Licensure requires graduation from an accredited dental school and successful completion of a licensing examination, including written and practical components.

NURSES

Nurses use the nursing process in the promotion and maintenance of health; management of illness, injury, or infirmity; restoration of optimum function; or achievement of a dignified death. Nursing practice varies depending on education, licensure, and credentialing.

Licensed Practical Nurse or Licensed Vocational Nurse

Education programs for licensed practical nurses (LPNs) or licensed vocational nurses (LVNs) are 12 to 18 months and are available in trade, technical, and vocational schools and community colleges. All states require LPNs/LVNs to be licensed, and requirements include graduation from a state-approved program in practical nursing or vocational nursing and successful completion of a licensing examination.

Registered Nurses

Education for a registered nurse (RN) may be an associate degree (2 years of community college), diploma (2- to 3-year hospital-based training), or baccalaureate degree (4 to 5 years at a college or university). All states require RNs to be licensed. Requirements include graduation from a state-approved nursing program and successful completion of the National Council Licensure Examination (NCLEX), a written examination administered by each state.

Advanced Practice Nurses

Advanced practice nurses (APNs) may be NPs, clinical nurse specialists (CNSs), certified nurse-midwives (CNMs), or certified RN-anesthetists (CRNAs). They conduct assessments and diagnose and treat clients, usually following a predefined protocol. Most APNs are in specialty practices such as anesthesia, pediatrics, geriatrics, gynecology, and obstetrics. Education requirements generally include a basic undergraduate degree in nursing, with additional graduate education. Most APN programs award master's degrees. Licensure requirements vary between states, but typically include graduation from an accredited APN program, completion of a certification examination conducted by a nationally recognized organization, and completion of a requisite number of hours in advanced practice. Scope of practice parameters for APNs in such areas as prescriptive authority and third party reimbursement also vary between states and are detailed in each state's Nurse Practice Act.

THERAPISTS

A number of different types of therapists practice in the U.S. HCDS. Some of those more commonly encountered in community-based practice are described.

Physical Therapists

Physical therapists (PTs) plan, organize, and administer treatments to restore functional mobility, relieve pain, and prevent or limit permanent disability. In addition, some PTs perform diagnostic testing to determine joint measurement, functional activity, and voluntary muscle power. Although education requirements vary somewhat, the minimum educational requirement for practice is a bachelor's degree. Some programs confer a certificate (for those who hold a degree in another field) and others confer a master's degree. All states require PTs to be licensed, and requirements include graduation from an accredited professional school and successful completion of a licensing examination. Specialization requires additional educational preparation, 2 years or more of practice experience, and successful completion of a certification examination. Specialization areas include pediatrics, sports therapy, geriatrics, and orthopedics. Physical therapy technicians usually have a 2-year associate degree education.

Occupational Therapists

Occupational therapists (OTs) employ a number of techniques to help clients who are mentally, physically, developmentally, or emotionally disabled to maintain daily living skills and cope with physical and emotional effects of disability. The OTs assist clients in learning or relearning ADL and help them establish as independent, productive, and satisfying a lifestyle as possible. Educational preparation requires a bachelor's degree. Some programs confer a master's degree if the student is postbaccalaureate. Most states regulate OTs through licensure. Requirements include degree or certificate from an accredited program and successful completion of the OT National Certification Examination.

Speech Therapists and Audiologists

Speech therapists (STs), or language pathologists, diagnose and treat persons experiencing speech or language problems resulting from conditions such as hearing loss, brain injury (cerebrovascular accident), cleft palate, and voice pathology. Audiologists assess, diagnose, treat, and work to prevent hearing problems. Educational preparation for STs and audiologists is generally at the graduate level. Specialty areas include pediatrics, geriatrics, and linguistics. Most states mandate licensure for STs and audiologists, and requirements include graduation from an accredited master's degree program, completion of a licensing examination, and supervised clinical experience.

OTHER HEALTH CARE PROVIDERS

Nurses in community-based practice may work with several other health care providers. These include optometrists, pharmacists, psychologists, dietitians, and social workers.

Optometrists

Optometrists are primary eye care providers who diagnose and treat common vision problems and prescribe eye glasses, contact lenses, and vision therapy. Most optometrist programs require 2 to 3 years of undergraduate study (most optometrists have a bachelor's degree) followed by completion of a 4-year program to obtain a doctor of optometry degree. All states require optometrists to be licensed.

Psychologists

Psychologists study the behavior of individuals to understand and identify fundamental processes of behavior; develop, administer, and score a variety of psychological tests; provide counseling and therapy to persons suffering emotional or adjustment problems; conduct research to improve diagnosis and treatment of mental and emotional disorders; and study human and animal behavior. A psychologist's education is 7 years or more. Typically a psychologist has an undergraduate degree in psychology and 3 to 5 years of graduate study. A master's degree (master of arts, master of science, or master of education) allows for provision of supervised psychological services, whereas a doctoral degree (doctor of philosophy [PhD], doctor of psychiatry, or doctor of education) is the standard entry-level degree required for independent practice. A psychiatrist is a physician who has completed a 3-year residency in psychiatry and can diagnose and treat mental illness using a variety of therapies, including pharmacotherapeutics. All states require licensure or certification of psychologists, although requirements vary.

Pharmacists

Pharmacists dispense medicines prescribed by physicians, podiatrists, and dentists, and in some states, PAs and NPs; they also advise health professionals on medication selection and use. A bachelor's degree is the standard entry-level requirement for the practice of pharmacy. Graduate preparation confers a master's degree, doctor of pharmacy (PharmD), or a PhD and is necessary for educators, researchers, and specialists. All states require pharmacists to be licensed. Requirements include graduation from an accredited program, successful completion of a licensing examination, supervised clinical experience or internship, and that the pharmacist be over 21 years of age. Pharmacology technicians generally have an associate degree and work under the supervision of a pharmacist.

Dietitians

Dietitians teach individuals and health professionals about the science of food and nutrition. The entry level for practice as a dietitian is a bachelor's degree. A 6- to 12-month supervised internship is required if the graduate desires licensure.

Social Workers

Social workers work with individuals and families to address a wide variety of social problems and issues. Medical social workers refer clients to community resources, assist clients in attaining needed social and health care services, and help plan for institutional community placement (e.g., nursing home or extended-care facility). Identification of community resources, financial assistance, and referral for additional services are part of the practice of many social workers. A bachelor's degree is the minimum entry level for practice as a social worker. Master's and advanced master's degrees (e.g., doctoral level training) are necessary for licensure in some states and for the provision of some interventions, such as counseling. Licensure for practicing social workers is required by all states, and most states recognize more than one category of social worker based on education and work experience.

HEALTH CARE FINANCING

Financing of health care is becoming increasingly complex and confusing. Over the past 50 years, the HCDS has evolved from being a simple, fee-for-service enterprise to a very complex entity in which various individuals, groups, corporations, and/or insurers contract with providers and organizations to deliver care to individuals, families, and groups. Because of their important role in coordination and management of care, all nurses should be aware of the payment structure for health care. Understanding of eligibility requirements, copayments, deductibles, and the variety of third party reimbursement strategies can assist nurses in planning and implementing appropriate, cost-effective, and reimbursable care.

THE HIGH COST OF HEALTH CARE

The National Center for Health Statistics (NCHS, 2006) reported that in 2004, health care expenditures represented an estimated 16% of the U.S. gross national product (up from 13.8% in 2000, 12.4% in 1990, and 9.1% in 1980). This represents about $5219 per capita, compared with $3968 in 2000 and $2389 in 1990. This per capita expenditure is by far the highest in the world. By comparison, France, Germany, and Canada spent 9.8% to 10.6% of their gross national products on health care during 2004, and Japan and Great Britain spent about 7.8% and 8.1%, respectively (WHO, 2007). In other words, health care costs in the U.S. are almost double the costs of other highly developed countries.

Reasons for the expenditures and the phenomenal growth of the cost of health care are numerous and interrelated. The growth in private insurance and **third party reimbursement** for services and general economic inflation are two of the most often cited reasons for rising health care costs. In addition, the rapid increase in the income of health care providers, most notably physicians, has profoundly affected health care expenditures. During the past 25 years, for example, physician income grew faster than most professions. Although this growth has slowed in

recent years and even reversed in some cases, mean physician net income ranges remain very high. Indeed, the average net income for physicians in 2003 was between $146,000 and $203,000 for primary care physicians and almost $236,000 for specialists (Tu and Ginsburg, 2006).

Another factor that affects the cost of health care is America's changing demography. As people age, more expensive and intensive health care is required; and lifestyle choices, including smoking, alcohol consumption, high-fat diets, obesity, lack of exercise, use of legal (e.g., alcohol) and illegal (e.g., cocaine) substances, and indiscriminate sexual practices have contributed to an increase in chronic diseases such as lung cancer, heart disease, diabetes, and AIDS. Growth in the number of uninsured individuals has contributed indirectly to higher health care costs because to offset bad debt health care providers raise charges and fees for those able to pay.

> The American public has been warned that medical care may soon have to be rationed.... The truth is that medical care is already rationed, and it always has been. One of the disgraces of national policy is that the poor and unemployed who cannot afford to pay for medical care or have no medical insurance must often accept inferior treatment, if they can get it at all.
>
> John P. Bunker, Stanford University, from Lee and Estes, 1994, p. 273.

Dependence by health care providers on technology and insistence on high-tech care by consumers contribute to misuse and abuse of technology. Overuse of expensive care and procedures (e.g., cesarean section, hysterectomy, cataract surgery, prostatectomy), medications (e.g., use of a very expensive antibiotic when penicillin would produce the same result), and failure to encourage preventive interventions such as immunizations and health-promotion activities (e.g., stopping smoking, lowering cholesterol, exercising regularly) have also contributed to inefficiency, waste, and overuse of care. The increase in costs of health care include the costs incurred in research and development; manufacture and marketing; and profits made on new medications, equipment, and techniques. Finally, malpractice insurance premiums and alterations in practice to address potential litigation and forestall malpractice claims (defensive medicine) have been cited as factors contributing to the rapid increase in health care costs.

The current system of health care financing is composed of a combination of fee-for-service, public sector payment, and third party (e.g., health insurance) reimbursement. Financing sources and distribution of health care expenditures are presented in Figure 5-1. As indicated in this illustration, payment for health care services comes from a combination of government sources (e.g., Medicare, Medicaid, Veteran's Administration, military service) and private sources (e.g., private health insurance, direct payment). In addition, the greatest percentage of payment went to hospital care (30%), followed by "other spending" (25%) (e.g., dental care, other professional services, home health, durable medical products, over-the-counter medicines, research and construction) and physicians and clinical services (21%).

PUBLIC FINANCING

As discussed, local, state, and federal governments combine to finance about 46% of health care. Because Medicare and Medicaid are very important sources of health care financing, it is imperative that nurses be aware of specific components of these programs, including eligibility parameters, reimbursement requirements, and which services are and are not covered.

Medicare

Medicare is a federal health insurance program for people age 65 and older, people with end-stage renal disease, and certain disabled people (CMS, 2007b). Medicare was established by Title XVIII of the Social Security Act in 1965 and is financed through taxes on employers and employees, administered by the Social Security Administration (responsible for application and determining eligibility), and funded through the Centers for Medicare and Medicaid Services (CMS) (see www.cms.gov for additional information).

Medicare is divided into Part A, Part B, and Part D. Medicare Part A insures qualified individuals for hospital and skilled nursing facility care and for home health, hospice care, and blood. Part A has **deductibles** and **coinsurance**. Most U.S. residents (about 98%) are eligible for premium-free Medicare Part A benefits when they reach age 65, based on their own or their spouse's employment. Medicare Part A benefits are also available for individuals who rely on

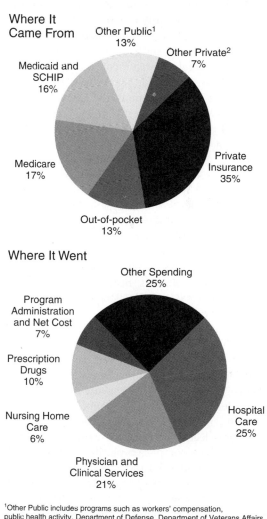

The Nation's Health Dollar, Calender Year 2005

Where It Came From

Other Public[1] 13%

Other Private[2] 7%

Medicaid and SCHIP 16%

Private Insurance 35%

Medicare 17%

Out-of-pocket 13%

Where It Went

Other Spending 25%

Program Administration and Net Cost 7%

Prescription Drugs 10%

Nursing Home Care 6%

Hospital Care 25%

Physician and Clinical Services 21%

[1]Other Public includes programs such as workers' compensation, public health activity, Department of Defense, Department of Veterans Affairs, Indian Health Service, State and local hospital subsidies and school health.
[2]Other Private includes industrial in-plant, privately funded construction, and non-patient revenues, including philanthropy.
NOTE: Numbers shown may not add to 100.0 because of rounding.
NOTE: Other Spending includes dentist services, other professional services, home health, durable medical products, over-the-counter medicines and sundries, public health, other personal health care, research and structures and equipment.

Figure 5-1. Health care funding sources and expenditures. From Centers for Medicare & Medicaid Services, Office of the Actuary, National Health Statistics Group, 2006 (website): http://www.cms.hhs.gov/NationalHealthExpendData/downloads/PieChart-SourcesExpenditures2005.pdf. Accessed July 25, 2007.

dialysis for permanent kidney failure or have had a kidney transplant and for those who are disabled and eligible for Social Security benefits.

Medicare Part B insures qualified individuals for physician services, outpatient hospital services, home health care, durable medical equipment, and other medical services and supplies not covered by Part A. Part B requires monthly premiums for all subscribers ($93.50 per month in 2007) and deductibles ($131 per year in 2007) and coinsurance (20% of the Medicare-approved amount), for which the individual is responsible (CMS, 2007b).

Medicare Part B also helps pay for ambulance services; artificial limbs and eyes; arm, leg, back and neck braces; limited chiropractic services; emergency care; medical supplies; and transplants. Services that Medicare does not cover include dental care and dentures, cosmetic surgery, custodial care at home, health care received while traveling outside of the United States, hearing aids, routine eye care, routine or yearly physical examinations, and some screening tests.

Medicare Part D was initiated in 2006 to help cover the costs of prescription drugs for Medicare enrollees. Participation is optional, and eligible Medicare recipients must enroll in an approved prescription drug plan. Most will pay a monthly premium, a yearly deductible (typically around $250), and copayments, with these out-of-pocket costs based on the plan selected and drugs used. The payment schedule can be complex; typically enrollees pay the deductible (about $250) and a percentage of the costs between $250 and $2250 (usually 25%). One hundred percent of the costs between $2250 and $5100 are the responsibility of the enrollee. This is termed the *coverage gap* or *donut hole*. Once the out-of-pocket costs for drugs reaches $3850, Medicare will pay 95% of the costs of prescription drugs (CMS, 2007c). This financing structure can be hugely problematic for elders and others on fixed incomes. Many elders who can afford to purchase "Medigap" insurance plans will do so to help defray the costs of high deductibles, copayments, and the "donut hole."

Before 1983 Medicare paid physicians and other providers on a fee-for-services basis and hospitals on a cost-based retrospective basis (Sultz and Young, 2006). In an attempt to better manage costs and stop the rapid increase in expenditures, Congress enacted the Social Security Amendment of 1983 (Public Law 98-21). This act ended the cost-plus, fee-for-service system and introduced the prospective payment system for hospital coverage. The prospective payment system uses 468 **diagnosis-related groups (DRGs)** to classify cases for payment, and reimbursement is based on a fixed price per case, a fee known as **capitation**. The prospective payment system requires that all providers bill Medicare directly for reimbursement for services. A few years later the Omnibus Budget Reconciliation Act of 1989 (OBRA) established the "Resource-based Relative Value Scale" to revise the fee-for-service reimbursement system for physicians. The new system was implemented to contain costs and better equalize payments between and among generalists and specialists. The intent of this Act was to help contain costs by reducing the number of expensive procedures and to increase the number of physicians electing to practice primary care rather than specialize.

Medicare claims are paid indirectly by the CMS through the use of fiscal intermediaries. These intermediaries are typically insurance companies who contract with Medicare to review, process, and pay all claims (see the Community Application box "Medigap Insurance").

Medicaid

The Medicaid program was initiated in 1965 by Title XIX of the Social Security Act. **Medicaid** is a public assistance welfare program that provides financial assistance to pay for health care for the poor, blind, disabled, and families with dependent children. Medicaid is funded jointly by the federal government and each state. Eligibility, coverage, and payment for services vary greatly from state to state.

Although covered services vary, federal requirements dictate that Medicaid cover certain services in all states. These include inpatient and outpatient hospital care; skilled nursing care; physician services; family planning services; home health care; and early and periodic screening, diagnosis, and treatment (EPSDT) services for eligible children. Additional services that may be covered in some states include dental care, eye care, and medications. Box 5-3 provides detailed information on Medicaid beneficiaries and services. A comparison of Medicare and Medicaid appears in Table 5-4.

COMMUNITY APPLICATION
Medigap Insurance

A Medigap plan is a health insurance plan that helps fill the gaps in Medicare coverage. Medigap may help a beneficiary lower their out-of-pocket costs and get more health insurance coverage. When purchasing a Medigap policy, the individual will pay a premium to the insurance company but must still pay his or her monthly Medicare Part B and Part D premiums. Medigap plans are not sold or serviced by the state or federal government; they are sold by private insurance companies. Medigap plans must meet requirements of the state, and each state has a different required set of benefits in its Medigap plans.

Services and items typically covered by Medigap policies include a portion of coinsurance for hospital and skilled nursing stays, the Medicare Part B and Part D yearly deductibles, and routine yearly checkups. Medigap plans do not generally cover long-term care, vision or dental care, hearing aids, or private duty nursing care.

Other helpful information about Medigap plans includes the following:
- Medigap plans are designed to not duplicate coverage provided by Medicare.
- The front of the Medigap policy must identify it as "Medicare Supplement Insurance."
- There may be preexisting condition exclusions in Medigap plans.
- It is illegal for an insurance company to sell a second Medigap plan.
- It is illegal to sell a Medigap plan to someone in a Medicare managed care plan.
- It is illegal for an insurance company or agent to use high pressure tactics to force or frighten someone into buying a Medigap plan
- It is illegal to make false or misleading comparisons to promote switching from one company or plan to another.

Data from Centers for Medicare & Medicaid Services: *Medicare & you: Medicare supplement health insurance (Medigap)*, Washington, DC, 2007, Centers for Medicare & Medicaid Services (website): http://www.cms.hhs.gov/Medigap/. Accessed July 23, 2007.

It is important to note that both the legislative and executive branches of the federal government are exploring ways to decrease health care costs. Several states, including Arizona, Massachusetts, Hawaii, Wisconsin, and Oregon are experimenting with plans to reduce costs through a variety of changes. Reduction of coverage for certain services, prioritizing care based on specified criteria such as effectiveness and benefit, refusal to pay for certain procedures or services, encouraging participants to use managed care, and other efforts have been proposed and are being tested. All health providers and consumers are advised to closely monitor the ongoing debates and support legislative efforts that control costs and maintain quality.

PRIVATE FINANCING

The greatest percentage of health care is financed by private health insurance (Figure 5-1). At present, the structure of the private sector health insurance system is very complex. In the United States, health care insurance is frequently provided by employers and has become an expected benefit of employment. Typically employer-provided health insurance covers both the employee and the employee's family, and both employer and employee contribute to the cost of premiums.

As insurance premium costs have increased dramatically over the past two decades, alterations in the structure and coverage parameters of this system have been and continue to be made. The result has been an increase in **managed care** plans; changes in premiums, coinsurance, and deductibles; limits to coverage; and refusal to pay for preexisting conditions. Health care insurance programs and options include various financial arrangements such as traditional indemnity health insurance coverage, PPOs, and HMOs.

Traditional Health Insurance

In the United States, health insurance began when teachers in Dallas, Texas, devised a way to finance and share the costs of health care. In 1929 Dallas public school teachers contracted with Baylor Hospital to provide specified health care services for a predetermined cost. By 1939 this insurance plan had grown to include many other groups and became Blue Cross-Blue Shield (Koch, 2008; Shi and

BOX 5-3 Medicaid Beneficiaries and Services

FEDERALLY DICTATED RECIPIENTS

- Families who meet state's Aid to Families with Dependent Children (AFDC) eligibility requirements
- Supplemental Security Income (SSI) recipients
- Pregnant women and children up to 6 years of age with a family income below 133% of the poverty level
- Children 6 to 19 years of age with a family income below the federal poverty level
- Caretakers (relatives or legal guardians who take care of children younger than age 18)
- Individuals and couples who are living in medical institutions and who have monthly income up to 300% of the SSI income standard

OPTIONAL RECIPIENTS

- Pregnant women and infants to age 1 whose family income is below 185% of the poverty level (percentage set by the state)
- Optional targeted low-income children
- Certain aged, blind, or disabled adults who have incomes above those requiring mandatory coverage but below the federal poverty level
- Medically needy older persons not qualified for income assistance (welfare)

STATE-DETERMINED OPTIONAL SERVICES

- Prescription drugs
- Dental care
- Optometry and eyeglasses
- Residential intermediate care facilities for the mentally retarded
- Nursing facility services for people under 21 years of age
- Prescription drugs
- Prosthetic devices

FEDERALLY REQUIRED SERVICES

- Inpatient and outpatient hospital care
- Physician services
- Medical and surgical dental services
- Skilled nursing home care
- Home health care for persons eligible for nursing facility services
- Family planning services and supplies
- Rural health clinic services
- Laboratory and X-ray services
- Pediatric and family nurse practitioner (NP) services
- Ambulatory services offered by a federally qualified health center
- Nurse-midwife services (as authorized under state law)
- The EPSDT service for individuals younger than age 21
- Prenatal care and delivery services for pregnant women

From Centers for Medicare & Medicaid Services: *Medicaid at-a-glance: 2005*(website): http://www.cms.hhs.gov/MedicaidEligibility/downloads/MedGlance05.pdf. Accessed July 25, 2007.

Singh, 2004). The idea of health insurance grew very rapidly, and currently about 73% of U.S. residents are covered by health insurance.

Health insurance organizations may be nonprofit (e.g., Blue Cross-Blue Shield) or commercial for-profit (e.g., Aetna, Prudential). Under traditional contracts the insurance company finances care for enrollees. Premiums, deductibles, and copayments or coinsurance are required by indemnity policies. Premiums have increased dramatically since the 1980s, prompting cost-containment strategies by most employers. These strategies include encouraging the use of managed care, reducing reliance on traditional insurers through increasing self-funding of health benefits, and increasing the share of health care expenses paid by employees. Many insurers now provide options for enrollees whereby they may choose traditional coverage or care through an HMO or PPO.

Preferred Provider Organizations

Preferred provider organizations (PPOs) are business arrangements, or contracts, between a group of health care providers (e.g., hospitals or physicians) and a purchaser of health care services (e.g., employers or insurance companies). The PPOs began during the mid-1980s to decrease the costs of health care insurance. In these arrangements the providers agree to supply services to a defined group of patients (e.g., employees of company "X") at a discounted fee-for-service cost. According to Koch (2008), PPOs have five elements:

1. A limited number of physicians and hospitals
2. Negotiated fee schedules
3. Utilization review or utilization management
4. Consumer choice of providers with incentives to use participating providers
5. Expedient settlement of claims

As of 2003 about 54% of private insurance was through PPOs—up from 28% in 1996 (Hunt and Knickman, 2005).

Health Maintenance Organizations

A **health maintenance organization (HMO)** is an organized health care system that provides health services to enrolled individuals for a fixed, prepaid fee. HMOs typically possess an organized system to provide health care in a particular geographical area, an agreed-upon set of services for health maintenance

TABLE **5-4** Comparison of Medicare and Medicaid

MEDICARE	MEDICAID
• A federal health insurance program for persons 65 years and older, disabled persons, and persons with end-stage renal disease	• A welfare assistance program for the poor; those eligible for Medicaid include families receiving AFDC, individuals receiving benefits for the SSI Program because of age or disability, and the medically needy whose incomes fall below a certain percentage of the poverty level. Each state determines eligibility requirements, payment for services, and type of services provided (with some federal restrictions)
• Financed through Social Security taxes and monthly premiums	• Jointly funded by the states and the federal government
• Administered by the CMS within the USDHHS	• Administered by a designated state agency and CMS
• The CMS contracts with insurance companies to process and pay claims submitted by beneficiaries	
• Medicare Part A covers inpatient hospital care, home health care, hospice care, and skilled nursing care • Medicare Part B covers physicians' services; covered services provided by other health professions, including RNs, NPs, chiropractors, psychologists, and social workers; outpatient hospital services; ambulance services; ambulatory surgery; outpatient physical, occupational, and speech therapy; radiation therapy; durable medical equipment; surgical dressing; and screening examinations • Medicare Part D provides coverage for prescription drugs	• Medicaid benefits include inpatient and outpatient hospital services; prenatal care; outpatient diagnostic and laboratory services; home health care; physicians' services; screening, diagnosis, and treatment of children; and family planning services; states may add additional benefits, including prescription medications, dental services, ambulance services, psychiatric care, medical supplies, optometrists' services, and eyeglasses
• Medicare enrollees in Parts B and D pay monthly premiums, deductibles, and copayments	• There is no cost to those eligible for Medicaid
• Payment may be fee-for-service or option of enrolling in an HMO or comprehensive medical plan	• Payment to providers is a combination of fee-for-service based on "reasonable charges" and a state-defined "Medicaid fee schedule"
• Payment to hospitals is based on DRGs or audited costs	• Payment to hospitals is based on DRGs, with some exceptions

From Centers for Medicare & Medicaid Services (www.cms.gov).

and treatment, voluntarily enrolled membership, and rates similar to those of providers in the community. An HMO provides fairly comprehensive coverage in return for the prepaid fee, usually without deductibles and with minimal **copayments** ($10 to $20 per visit is common). By encouraging illness prevention

and health maintenance and reducing inappropriate care, HMOs are intended to reduce hospitalizations and health care costs.

Koch (2008) noted that in the United States, the concept of the HMO began in 1929 at a private health clinic in Los Angeles, which expanded in

1930 as the Kaiser company provided coverage for workers building the Grand Coulee Dam. During the same year (1929), in Oklahoma, the Farmer's Union started a "cooperative health association" providing health care for members. The number of prepaid insurance plans, however, grew very slowly until the 1970s. The cost of health care had already become a concern, and in response the HMO Act of 1973 (Public Law 93-222) was passed. Subsequent amendments have encouraged rapid growth through the 1980s by offering incentives to employers and providers. Members enrolled in HMO plans expanded dramatically, growing from 9.1 million (1980), to 18.9 million (1985), to 36.5 million (1990), to 63.3 million (1996). Over the last decade HMO enrollments have dropped somewhat and currently account for about 24% of enrollment in group health plans (Hunt and Knickman, 2005).

Some basic HMO models are the staff model, the group model, and the **independent practice association (IPA)**, with some variations in each. In the traditional, or staff model, the HMO is an organization that employs physicians and other providers to deliver services to the HMO's enrollees. In the group model, a group or association of physicians contracts with the fiscal agent to provide services to enrollees. Finally, in the IPA model, the fiscal agent contracts with a range of physicians who are not associated with each other and work in independent practices to provide services on a capitated basis.

Because of capitated payments, physicians working in HMOs usually have incentives to use resources efficiently. Reportedly some HMOs offer bonuses to physicians if services such as specialists and expensive procedures are not significantly utilized, and HMOs might reprimand providers for overuse of services and specialists.

An HMO usually requires that enrollees designate one primary care provider as a **gatekeeper**. The gatekeeper may be a family practitioner, internist, pediatrician, or in some cases an obstetrician/gynecologist. This primary care physician determines when referral to a specialist is needed and provides oversight for all of the client's health care needs.

Other cost-containment strategies employed by managed care organizations and health care insurers include second surgical opinions, preauthorization for most hospital admissions, case management,

and **utilization review** (Torrens and Williams, 2002). Preauthorization requirements and second surgical opinions were developed to correct the practice of unnecessary surgeries and unneeded hospitalizations.

Table 5-5 presents a simplified comparison of HMOs, PPOs, and traditional health insurance. An understanding of the requirements of each increases the nurse's awareness of the similarities and differences in the programs so that care planning that is sensitive to the financial needs and resources of the client may be established.

CARING FOR THE UNINSURED

In the United States more than 46 million individuals were without health insurance coverage in 2005 (US Census Bureau, 2006). Furthermore, at any given time in the United States, as many as 25% of Americans have no or inadequate health care coverage. The typical uninsured individual is a member of a family in which the adults are unemployed or underemployed and thereby ineligible for employee/employer-paid health insurance coverage. Children, young adults, members of minorities, and noncitizens are disproportionately represented among uninsured persons.

The lack of insurance affects health and well-being in many ways. Lack of access to timely and affordable health care discourages use of preventive services and seeking early treatment for acute, episodic illnesses. Failure to seek preventive care (e.g., prenatal care) contributes to an increase in complications of pregnancy, such as low-birth-weight infants. Likewise, failure to adequately immunize infants and small children puts them at risk for a variety of illnesses. People who have no health care coverage often wait to seek care until the illness has progressed to a stage requiring more extensive, and therefore more costly, treatment. Emergency departments are more accessible to the uninsured and are often their only source of health care.

By default the lack of accessible health care services for those who are uninsured or underinsured has created health care rationing, in which only those who can afford treatment receive it. Uncompensated care continues to drain many regional and public hospitals and also affects private health providers and society at large. Public hospitals must

TABLE **5-5** Comparison of Private Insurance Plans

TRADITIONAL INDEMNITY	PREFERRED PROVIDER ORGANIZATION	HEALTH MAINTENANCE ORGANIZATION: STAFF MODEL	HEALTH MAINTENANCE ORGANIZATION: INDIVIDUAL PRACTICE ASSOCIATION AND GROUP MODELS
Free choice of providers without any restrictions	Free choice of providers; lower costs if providers are within network of preferred providers	Choice of providers limited to physicians and other providers employed by the HMO	Choice of providers limited to physicians under contract with the HMO
No referral necessary for specialty care	No referral necessary for specialty care; use of specialists within PPO encouraged through financial incentives	Designated primary care provider (gatekeeper) must approve treatment and determines when referrals are made to specialists; specialists within the HMO are used whenever possible	Designated primary care provider (gatekeeper) must approve treatment and determines when referrals are made to specialists; Individual Practice Association specialists are used whenever possible
Providers use their own office; referrals for specialized care may not be conveniently located	Providers use their own offices	Centralized facility allows for convenience and coordination of care	Providers use their own offices
Costs of premiums highest of all insurance plans; deductibles required; copayments 20% to 30% of total medical care	Premiums and deductible are lower than traditional insurance; copayment or coinsurance is usually required; costs to the insured if providers are outside of the PPO	Premiums and copayments are lower than traditional indemnity and PPOs	Premiums and copayments are lower than traditional indemnity and PPOs
No coordination of care; each provider works independently	Limited coordination of care	Care coordinated through primary care provider; case management may be utilized	Care coordinated through primary care provider; case management may be utilized
Provider or insured must file claim forms for reimbursement; processing time may be lengthy	May require additional paperwork or approval for some services	No paperwork required for basic services	No paperwork required for basic services
Preventive care may or may not be covered	Preventive care may or may not be covered	Preventive care encouraged	Preventive care encouraged

incur a very large share of uncompensated care, resulting in increased taxes and higher insurance costs for everyone. Recognition of these problems has motivated efforts to reform the HCDS, and many proposals have been made to address these issues and institute some form of universal coverage. Nurses are encouraged to stay informed of legislative efforts at all levels and to support efforts to provide care to all.

SUMMARY

Like Carol, the nurse in the chapter case study, nurses across the country have recognized that it is essential for all health care providers to have a basic understanding of the HCDS. Although it may not seem to fit with predetermined perceptions of nursing practice, nurses must learn to work within the context of change and to understand the different health care reimbursement mechanisms.

Indeed, it has been widely recognized that financial and reimbursement considerations, current and anticipated need for health care, practice parameters for providers, and various other factors influence how health care is delivered in the United States. Each of these issues bears further reflection and study as nurses learn to work within the system to deliver the best possible care.

KEY POINTS

- The HCDS is divided into public sector and private sector components.
- The public sector is subdivided into federal, state, and local levels and is typically concerned with the health of populations and maintaining a healthy environment. At the federal level, the USDHHS oversees many of the issues related to health. Each state maintains a state health department and defines what services will be offered at the state level and at the local level.
- The private sector system is composed of a variety of providers, institutions, industries, corporations, and insurers. It can be further divided into nonprofit or proprietary components.
- The HCDS contains a multitude of organizations that serve the population at many levels and for many needs. These include ambulatory health care settings, hospitals, and long-term care facilities (e.g., nursing homes, skilled nursing units, hospice care).
- Numerous different health care professionals provide care to members of the population. These include physicians, PAs, dentists, nurses, NPs, therapists, optometrists, psychologists and counselors, pharmacists, social workers, and many others.
- In the United States, health care is very expensive, representing about 16% of the gross national product. Reasons for the high cost of health care include growth in insurance and third party payment for services, general economic inflation, increases in the income of health care providers, changes in population demography (e.g., aging of U.S. residents), lifestyle choices that are detrimental to health (e.g., smoking, drug abuse, poor diet, indiscriminate sexual practices), and dependence on technology.
- Financing of health care is very complex and consists of a combination of fee-for-service, public sector payment, and third party reimbursement. Payment for health care comes from a combination of governmental sources (e.g., Medicare, Medicaid, Veteran's Administration) and private sources (e.g., private health insurance, direct payment).
- Medicare is the federal health insurance program for people 65 years of age and older and persons with certain disabilities. It is divided into Parts A, B, and D. Medicare Part A insures individuals for hospital and skilled nursing facility care, home health, and hospice care. Part A has deductibles and coinsurance, but most people do not pay premiums for coverage. Medicare Part B insures individuals for physician services, outpatient hospital services, medical equipment, and other medical services and supplies not covered by Part A; a monthly premium is required. Part D helps reduce the high costs of prescription drugs; participants must enroll in a Medicare Approved Plan and pay a premium, deductible, and copayments.
- Medicaid is a public assistance welfare program that pays for health care for the poor, blind, and disabled and families with dependent children. Medicaid is funded jointly by the federal government and each state. Eligibility, coverage, and payment for services are set by each state and

vary greatly. Medicaid covers inpatient and out-patient hospital care; skilled nursing care; physician services; family planning services; home health care; and early periodic screening, diagnosis, and treatment services for eligible children. Other services that may be covered in some states include dental care, eye care, and medications.

- The greatest percentage of health care is financed by private health insurance. The health insurance system is very complex and typically provided by an individual's employer; both the employer and the employee contribute to the cost of premiums. Health care insurance programs consist of a variety of financial arrangements, including indemnity health insurance, PPOs, and HMOs.
- Approximately 25% of U.S. residents have no or inadequate health care coverage. Children, young adults, and members of minorities are disproportionately represented among the uninsured and underinsured.

Learning Activities & Application to Practice

In Class

1. Obtain a copy of the current Medicare Handbook (CMS, 2007). With classmates, discuss Medicare coverage and related fees. Discuss the importance of Medicare requirements, guidelines, and reimbursement parameters in directing health care payment for services (e.g., DRGs).
2. With classmates, create a list of local health care organizations (e.g., ambulatory care agencies, hospitals, voluntary organizations) according to source of payment (public or private) and whether they are nonprofit or for profit. Identify actual or perceived differences in mission and services provided.
3. Discuss personal sources of health care insurance with other students. Compare coverage, costs, deductibles, and copayments. Share personal experiences with the costs of health care (e.g., recent pregnancy, chronic illness, having a checkup, medications). What are some experiences with managed care?

In Clinical

4. In each setting gather information on the sources of and procedure for reimbursement. What is covered by insurance, Medicare, or Medicaid and what is not? How can services be provided efficiently and be cost-effective?
5. Interview a health care professional from another discipline (e.g., PT, medical technologist, pharmacist) encountered during clinical. Question the professional on issues such as education and licensure or certification requirements, practice, salary range, and related information. If possible, spend a few hours observing this individual in practice, and share observations with the other students.

REFERENCES

Centers for Medicare & Medicaid Services (2007a): *National health expenditure data* (website): http://www.cms.hhs.gov/NationalHealthExpendData/. Accessed July 23, 2007.

Centers for Medicare & Medicaid Services (2007b): *Medicare & you* (website): http://www.medicare.gov/Publications/Pubs/pdf/10050.pdf. Accessed July 23, 2007.

Centers for Medicare & Medicaid Services (2007c): *Quick facts about Medicare's coverage for prescription drugs* (website): http://www.medicare.gov/Publications/Pubs/pdf/11102.pdf. Accessed July 23, 2007.

Centers for Medicare & Medicaid Services: *Brief summaries of Medicare & Medicaid, 2006* (website): http://www.cms.hhs.gov/MedicareProgramRatesStats/downloads/Medicare-MedicaidSummaries2006.pdf. Accessed July 22, 2007.

Evashwick CJ: The continuum of long-term care. In Williams SJ, Torrens PR, editors: *Introduction to health services*, ed 7, Clifton Park, NY, 2008, Thomson/Delmar Learning

Gourevitch MN, Caronna CA, Kalkut G: Acute care. In Kovner AR, Knickman JR, editors: *Jonas & Kovner's health care delivery in the United States*, ed 8, New York, 2005, Springer.

Hunt KA, Knickman JR: Financing for health care. In Kovner AR, Knickman JR, editors: *Jonas & Kovner's health care delivery in the United States*, ed 8, New York, 2005 Springer.

Koch AL: Financing health services. In Williams SJ, Torrens PR, editors: *Introduction to health services*, ed 7, Clifton Park, NY, 2008, Thomson/Delmar Learning.

Lee PR, Estes CL, editors: *The nation's health*, ed 4, Boston, 1994, Jones and Bartlett.

Mezey AP: Ambulatory care. In Kovner AR, Jonas S, editors: *Jonas & Kovner's health care delivery in the United States*, ed 6, New York, 1999, Springer.

National Center for Health Statistics: *Health, United States, 2006*, Hyattsville, Md, 2006, NCHS.

National Heritage Insurance Company: *Medicaid provider procedures manual: Texas Department of Human Services*, Austin, Tex, 1995, National Heritage Insurance Company.

Shi L, Singh DA: *Delivering health care in America: a systems approach*, ed 3, Sudbury, Mass, 2004, Jones & Bartlett.

Sultz HA, Young KM: *Health care USA: Understanding its organization and delivery*, ed 5, Sudbury, MA, 2006, Jones and Bartlett.

Torrens PR, Williams SJ: Managed care: restructuring the system. In Williams SJ, Torrens PR, editors: *Introduction to health services*, ed 6, Albany, NY, 2002, Delmar.

Tu HT, Ginsburg PB: *Losing Ground: physician income 1995-2003*, Center for Studying Health System Change Tracking Report, June 2006 (website): http://www.hschange.org/CONTENT/851/. Accessed July 23, 2007.

U.S. Census Bureau: *Income, poverty and health insurance coverage in the United States: 2005* (website): http://www.census.gov/prod/2006pubs/p60-231.pdf. Accessed July 25, 2007.

U.S. Department of Health and Human Services: *National ambulatory medical care survey, 2005 summary* (website): http://www.cdc.gov/nchs/data/ad/ad387.pdf. Accessed July 25, 2007.

U.S. Department of Health and Human Services: *Healthy people 2010. National health promotion and disease prevention objectives*, Washington, DC, 2000, Government Printing Office.

World Health Organization: *Core Health Indicators, 2007* (website): http://www.who.int/whosis/database/core/core_select_process.cfm?countries=all&indicators=nha. Accessed July 22, 2007.

Epidemiology

objectives

Upon completion of this chapter, the reader will be able to:

1. Explain ways in which concepts of epidemiology can be used in community-based nursing practice.

2. Apply models of disease causation in examining diseases and health problems.

3. Develop primary, secondary, and tertiary prevention strategies for selected health threats.

4. Discuss commonly used rates such as mortality rates, incidence rates, and prevalence rates, and give examples of when they are used.

5. Identify sources of information related to disease occurrence that may be accessed by nurses in community settings.

6. Describe the difference between descriptive epidemiology and analytic epidemiology and give examples of each.

key terms

Agent
Analytical epidemiology
Descriptive epidemiology
Epidemiology
Host

Incidence rate
Morbidity rates
Mortality rates
Natural history of disease
Prevalence rate

See Glossary for definitions.

case study

Meg Henderson is a school nurse who cares for children of elementary school age in a small city. One of her primary responsibilities is prevention of communicable diseases. In addition to monitoring each child's immunization status, her duties include identifying children with communicable diseases, excluding them from school, and then reinstating them, according to school district policy.

One recent Monday Meg saw Elizabeth Ellis, a third grader, whose teacher sent her to the clinic because she was seen scratching her head repeatedly. Using applicators, Meg carefully
Continued

examined Elizabeth's hair and saw evidence of head lice. When questioned, Elizabeth replied that her head had been itching "about 2 or 3 days." Meg learned that Elizabeth lives with her parents and older brother and younger sister, who are also students at the school. Following district guidelines, Meg examined both of Elizabeth's siblings and determined that they were also infected. She called Mrs. Ellis and informed her that she must come to school to get her children and treat the entire family for lice.

When Mrs. Ellis arrived to pick up her children, she was obviously embarrassed. Meg explained that lice are a very contagious parasite, easily passed between children through sharing of brushes, combs, hats, or other items, and not an indicator of poor hygiene. She also stated that head lice are easily treatable and gave Mrs. Ellis an information packet describing the transmission, identification, and treatment of head lice. She reviewed the information with Mrs. Ellis, informed her that the children could return to school after they had all been treated, and pointed out that they should be treated again in 2 weeks.

After the Ellis family left, Meg examined all of the students from each of the Ellis children's classes for head lice. From the three classes, she identified five more children with lice and then called their parents. These children had siblings in three more classes and the children in each of these classes were also examined. At the end of the day, a total of 15 children had been excluded from school.

The following week, Meg reexamined all of the children in every class that had an infected student. Two weeks after the incident, she examined all of the excluded children and determined that they had been successfully treated. No more cases of lice were identified that semester.

Much of nursing practice, particularly in community settings, involves prevention, early identification, and prompt treatment of health problems, and monitoring for emerging threats and unidentified patterns that might signify health problems. For example, a nurse working in an inner-city women's clinic might note that the diagnosis of cervical dysplasia among teenagers and women in their early 20s has increased over a period associated with increases in human papillomavirus (HPV) infection. In addition to assisting with treatment of the clients involved, she would inform officials from the county health department's sexually transmitted disease (STD) program or a regional medical school to initiate further investigation.

Another example would be a nurse working in a manufacturing plant who notes an unusual increase in complaints of back strain. After assisting the workers with reducing their back pain, the nurse should collect data on cases of back strain during the past 6 months and look for trends. Further, the nurse should inform the plant management and work with them to take appropriate steps to identify the cause of the problems and develop plant policy to minimize risks. Recording problems, keeping track of patterns, and working to identify causes are all part of the science and practice of epidemiology.

Epidemiology is the basic science of public health and refers to "the study of the distribution and determinants of health-related states or events in a specified population, and the application of this study to the control of health problems" (Centers for Disease Control and Prevention [CDC], 1992). The science of epidemiology is based on the idea that disease, illness, and ill health are not randomly distributed in a population, but rather that "each of us has certain characteristics that predispose us to, or protect us against, a variety of different diseases" (Gordis, 2004). Identifying these characteristics and removing or minimizing them if they are harmful, or enhancing or transferring them if helpful, are basic goals in epidemiology.

Nurses who work with clients in community settings are frequently in a position to assist in identification, management, treatment, and prevention of health problems, and as a result they need a general understanding of the basic principles, theories, and concepts of epidemiology. In addition, a nurse needs to be able to read and interpret data about trends in diseases to carry out responsibilities in client teaching. Valanis (1999) outlines seven uses of epidemiology, which are shown in Box 6-1.

Healthy People 2010 (U.S. Department of Health and Human Services, 2000), introduced in Chapter 1,

6-1 Uses of Epidemiology

- Investigation of disease etiology
- Identification of risks
- Identification of syndromes and classification of disease
- Differential diagnoses and planning clinical treatment
- Surveillance of population health status
- Community diagnosis and planning of health services
- Evaluation of health services and public health interventions

Data from Valanis B: *Epidemiology in nursing and health care,* ed 3, Norwalk, Conn, 1999, Appleton & Lange.

was written based on epidemiological principles. This document presents health statistics and data; describes health threats; discusses interventions and plans; and sets goals and objectives directed toward prevention, management, minimization, or elimination of the identified health threats. The *Healthy People 2010* box presents examples of *Healthy People 2010*'s objectives related to epidemiological concepts (e.g., primary prevention, rates) described in this chapter.

This chapter presents basic concepts of epidemiology and describes how understanding the course or progression of a disease or health condition is important for nurses who practice in community settings. The use of epidemiological concepts and principles to identify risks and to assist in the prevention and management of disease also is discussed. Box 6-2 defines some common terms used in epidemiology.

MODELS OF DISEASE CAUSATION

Several theories and models describe disease causation and the properties that relate to disease processes and prevention. Four of the most frequently encountered models are briefly discussed in the following sections.

THE EPIDEMIOLOGICAL TRIANGLE

The classic epidemiological model, particularly useful in the depiction of communicable disease, is the epidemiological triangle (Figure 6-1). This

healthy people **2010**

Objectives Related to Epidemiology

OBJECTIVE	BASELINE (1998)	TARGET
3.1: Reduce the overall cancer death rate	201.4 per 100,000	158.7 per 100,000
9.7: Reduce pregnancies among adolescent females	72 pregnancies per 1000	46 pregnancies per 1000
10.1b: Reduce infections caused by *E. coli* 0157:H7	2.1 per 100,000	1.0 per 100,000
12.13: Reduce the mean total blood cholesterol levels among adults	206 mg/dL	199 mg/dL
13.1: Reduce AIDS among adolescents and adults (incidence)	19.5 new cases per 100,000	1.0 new cases per 100,000
14.3a: Reduce hepatitis B among adults 19-24 years (incidence)	24 new cases per 100,000	2.4 new cases per 100,000
16.1b: Reduce fetal and infant deaths during perinatal period	7.5 per 1000 live births	4.5 per 1000 live births
19.2: Reduce the proportion of adults who are obese (prevalence)	23%	15%
27.1a: Reduce cigarette smoking by adults (prevalence)	24%	12%

Data from U.S. Department of Health and Human Services: *Healthy people 2010,* conference ed, Washington, DC, 2000, Government Printing Office.

BOX 6-2 Epidemiological Terms and Concepts

Epidemiology is derived from three Greek words: *epi* (upon), *demos* (the people), and *logos* (science). *Epidemiology* is defined as "The study of the distribution and determinants of health-related states or events in a specified population, and the application of this study to the control of health problems" (CDC, 1992, p. 430). The following terms are related to epidemiology but are not discussed in this chapter:

- *Carrier:* A person or animal without apparent disease who harbors a specific infectious agent and is capable of transmitting the agent to others.
- *Cohort:* A well-defined group of people who have had a common experience or exposure, who are then followed up for the incidence of new diseases or events, as in a cohort or prospective study.
- *Common source outbreak (point source):* An outbreak that results from a group of persons being exposed to a common noxious influence, such as an infectious agent or toxin. If the group is exposed over a relatively brief time so that all cases occur within one incubation period, then the common source outbreak is further classified as a point source outbreak.
- *Crude mortality rate:* The mortality rate from all causes of death for a population.
- *Direct transmission:* The immediate transfer of an agent from a reservoir to a susceptible host by direct contact of droplet spread.
- *Endemic disease:* The constant presence of a disease or infectious agent within a given geographical area or population group; it may also refer to the usual prevalence of a given disease within such an area or a group.
- *Epidemic:* The occurrence of more cases of disease than expected in a given area or among a specific group of people over a particular period.
- *Herd immunity:* The resistance of a group to invasion and spread of an infectious agent, based on the resistance to

infection of a high proportion of individual members of the group.
- *Indirect transmission:* The transmission of an agent carried from a reservoir to a susceptible host by suspended air particles or by animate (vector) or inanimate (vehicle) intermediaries.
- *Pandemic:* An epidemic occurring over a very wide area (several countries or continents) and usually affecting a large proportion of the population.
- *Propagated outbreak:* An outbreak that does not have a common source but instead spreads from person to person.
- *Risk:* The probability that an event will occur (e.g., that an individual will become ill or die within a stated period or age).
- *Risk factor:* An aspect of personal behavior or lifestyle, an environmental exposure, or an inborn or inherited characteristic that is associated with an increased occurrence of disease or other health-related event or condition.
- *Universal precautions:* Recommendations issued by the CDC to minimize the risk of transmission of bloodborne pathogens, particularly HIV and hepatitis B virus, by health care and public safety workers. Barrier precautions are to be used to prevent exposure to blood and certain body fluids of all clients.
- *Vector:* An animate intermediary that carries the agent from a reservoir to a susceptible host in the indirect transmission of an agent.
- *Vehicle:* An inanimate intermediary that carries the agent from a reservoir to a susceptible host in the indirect transmission of an agent.
- *Years of potential life lost:* A measure of the impact of premature mortality on a population, calculated as the sum of the differences between some predetermined minimum or desired life span and the age of death for individuals who died earlier than that predetermined age.
- *Zoonosis:* An infectious disease that under normal conditions is transmissible from animals to humans.

From Centers for Disease Control and prevention: *Principles of epidemiology,* ed 2, Atlanta, 1992, Centers for Disease Control and prevention.

model is often used to illustrate the interrelationships among the essential components of **host**, **agent**, and environment with regard to disease causation. A change in any of the three components can result in the disease process. For example, exposure (environment) of a child who has

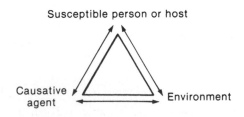

Figure 6-1. The epidemiological triangle.

not been immunized (host) to the measles virus (agent) will probably result in a case of measles. Another example would be respiratory difficulties resulting after an adult with chronic bronchitis (host) drives to work during rush hour (environment) on a day with excessive atmospheric ozone (agent).

Within the epidemiological triangle, prevention of the disease lies in preventing exposure to the agent, enhancing the physical attributes of the host to resist the disease, and minimizing any environmental factors that might contribute to disease development. Box 6-3 outlines host, agent, and environmental factors that affect health and could influence progression of the disease process.

BOX 6-3 Some Host, Agent, and Environmental Factors that Affect Health

HOST FACTORS

- Demographic data: Age, gender, ethnic background, race, marital status, religion, education, economic status
- Level of health: Genetic risk factors, physiological states, anatomical factors, response to stress, previous disease, nutrition, fitness
- Body defenses: Autoimmune system, lymphatic system
- State of immunity: Susceptibility versus active or passive immunity
- Human behavior: Diet, exercise, hygiene, substance abuse, occupation, personal and sexual contact, use of health resources, food handling

AGENT FACTORS (PRESENCE OR ABSENCE)

- Biologic: Viruses, bacteria, and fungi, and their mode of transmission, life cycle, virulence
- Physical: Radiation, temperature, noise
- Chemical: Gas, liquids, poisons, allergens

ENVIRONMENTAL FACTORS

- Physical properties: Water, air, climate, season, weather, geology, geography, pollution
- Biological entities: Animals, plants, insects, food, drugs, food source
- Social and economic considerations: Family, community, political organization, public policy, regulations, institutions, workplace, occupation, economic status, technology, mobility, housing, population density, attitudes, customs, culture, health practices, health services

From Tarzian AJ: Epidemiology: unraveling the mysteries of disease and health. In Maurer FA, Smith CM, editors: *Community/public health nursing: health for families and populations*, ed 3, St. Louis, 2005, Saunders, p. 150.

THE WEB OF CAUSATION

The causes of most diseases are more complex than simply an interaction between a host, agent, and environment. To explain disease and disability caused by multiple factors, MacMahon and Pugh (1970) developed the concept of "chain of causation," later termed the *web of causation*. Chronic diseases such as coronary artery disease and most types of cancer are not attributable to one or two factors alone. Rather, the interaction of multiple factors is necessary to produce the disease. An example of the application of the web of causation to the development of coronary heart disease is presented in Figure 6-2.

The web of causation can also be applied to many health-related threats and conditions. The problem of teenage pregnancy, for example, is attributable to a complex interaction between a number of causative and contributing factors, including lack of knowledge about sexuality and pregnancy prevention, lack of easily accessible contraception, peer pressure to engage in sex, low self-esteem, social patterns that encourage early motherhood, and use of alcohol or other drugs. Patterns of family violence, cocaine use, and gang membership are examples of other threats to health and well-being that can be more accurately explained through a multiple-causation model.

Recognition that many health problems have multiple causes leads to the recognition that simple solutions to these health problems rarely exist. When trying to manage teenage pregnancy, for example, the solution is not as simple as addressing a "knowledge deficit" about sexuality and contraception. Many (if not most) teens are well informed about contraception and the mechanics of how one gets pregnant yet still fail to take preventative measures.

To prevent heart disease in an individual at risk, intervention should begin with health education that addresses a number of areas, including smoking cessation, reduction of blood pressure, weight loss, cholesterol reduction, and exercise. Interventions might also need to address lifestyle, stress management, social support, and personality traits, among others. Likewise, to prevent teenage pregnancy, interventions should include health teaching on improving self-esteem, role-playing exercises on how to say "no," encouraging an orientation to the future, enhancing parental supervision, and providing recreational alternatives (sports and other after-school activities) in addition to giving information on sexuality, the mechanics of reproduction, and methods of contraception.

THE ICEBERG MODEL

The "iceberg model" or "iceberg principle" (Figure 6-3) describes the phenomenon that at any given time there are a small number of known cases of a disease or condition at the early and advanced stages. These

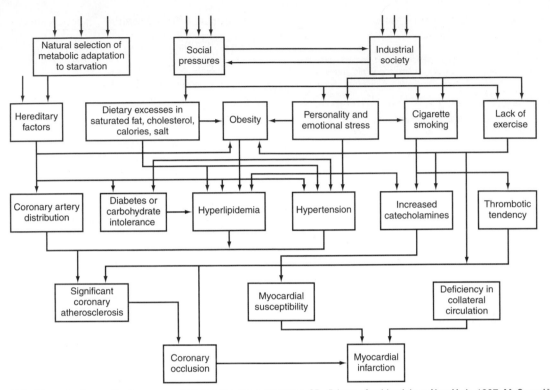

Figure 6-2. The web of causation for myocardial infarction. From Frideman GD: *Primer of epidemiology*, New York, 1987, McGraw-Hill.

known cases are those that are visible. However, like the iceberg, the larger threat comes from the greater amount of unknown cases (i.e., those that are not identified).

Infection with human immunodeficiency virus (HIV) is an excellent illustration of this principle. The clinically diagnosed cases of acquired immunodeficiency syndrome (AIDS) (manifest disease) represent only a small fraction of all cases of those infected. Those known to have HIV infection (mild, atypical disease) make up a more significant part of the whole, but the greatest concern, and possibly the greatest threat, comes from those individuals who have not been diagnosed and may be transmitting HIV unknowingly.

NATURAL HISTORY OF DISEASE

The **natural history of disease** refers to the progress of a disease process in an individual over time. In what is now a classic model, Leavell and Clark (1965) described two periods in the natural history of disease, prepathogenesis and pathogenesis. In this model, the prepathogenesis stage occurs before interaction of the disease agent and human host, when the individual is susceptible. For example, an adult man may smoke, a teenage girl might consider becoming sexually active, or a preschooler attends a party also attended by a sick child. After exposure or interaction, the period of pathogenesis proceeds to early pathogenesis (e.g., alterations in lung tissue, pregnancy, or chicken pox) and on through the disease course to resolution—death, disability, or recovery (e.g., lung cancer, teenage motherhood, immunity to chicken pox).

LEVELS OF PREVENTION

In addition to the description of the natural history of disease progression, Leavell and Clark (1965) also outlined three levels of prevention that correlate with the stages of disease progression: (1) primary prevention, (2) secondary prevention, and (3) tertiary prevention. These levels are described as follows:

- *Primary prevention* consists of activities directed at preventing a problem before it occurs. Altering

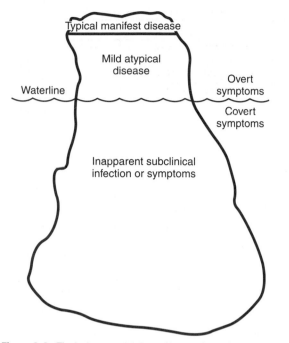

Figure 6-3. The iceberg model. From Clemen-Stone S, Eigsti DG, McGuire SL: *Comprehensive community health nursing*, ed 4, St Louis, 1995, Mosby.

susceptibility or reducing exposure for susceptible individuals in the period of prepathogenesis is primary prevention. Primary prevention has two categories: (1) general health promotion (e.g., good nutrition, adequate shelter, rest, exercise) and (2) specific protection (e.g., immunization, water purification).

- *Secondary prevention* refers to early detection and prompt intervention in a disease or health threat during the period of early pathogenesis. Screening for disease and prompt referral and treatment are secondary prevention. Mammography, blood pressure screening, scoliosis screening, and Papanicolaou smears are examples of secondary prevention.

- *Tertiary prevention* consists of limiting disability and fostering rehabilitation during the period of advanced disease and convalescence, where the disease has occurred and resulted in a degree of damage. Teaching a diabetic the principles of disease management and how to perform insulin injections, referring a head injury victim for occupational and physical therapy, and leading a

support group for grieving parents are examples of tertiary prevention.

Much of nursing practice in community settings is intended to prevent the progression of disease at the earliest period or phase, using the appropriate level or levels of prevention. Thus when applying "levels of prevention" to AIDS, a nurse would do the following:

- Educate clients on the practice of sexual abstinence or "safer sex" (primary prevention in the period of prepathogenesis).

- Encourage testing and counseling for clients with known exposure or who are in high-risk groups; provide referrals for follow-up for clients who test positive for HIV (secondary prevention in the period of early pathogenesis for early diagnosis and prompt treatment).

- Provide education on management of HIV infection, advocacy, case management, and other interventions (tertiary prevention to limit disability through the periods of advanced disease).

Figure 6-4 illustrates the relationship between the levels of prevention and the natural history of disease, as described by Leavell and Clark (1965).

EPIDEMIOLOGICAL TOOLS
RATES—DESCRIPTION, CALCULATION, AND INTERPRETATION

In epidemiology, rates are used to make comparisons among groups or populations or to compare a subgroup of the population with the total population. Rates are essential tools in identifying actual and potential problems in a given community or population. Rates from a given aggregate or community can be compared with international, national, state, local, or regional rates; age-specific rates; gender-specific rates; or race-specific rates. Just as a nurse working in a hospital compares a complete blood count with a given norm or standard, nurses who work in community settings use rates to compare information on morbidity and mortality in their practice setting or aggregate with "norms," "standards," or "goals."

The use of rates allows the nurse working in any setting to recognize when a health threat or disease encountered is normal or typical, or if a problem or concern that warrants further investigation or intervention exists. For example, an

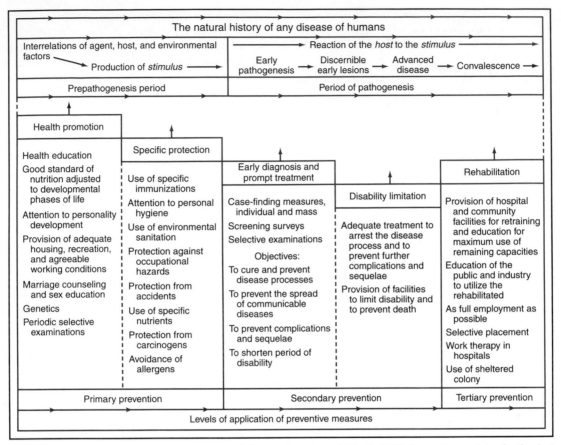

Figure 6-4. Levels of prevention in the natural history of disease. From Leavell HR, Clark EG: *Preventive medicine for the doctor in his community: an epidemiologic approach*, New York, 1965, McGraw-Hill.

elementary school nurse found that five children in her school of 500 have chicken pox (a rate of 10 children per 1000). Should school be closed to prevent further infection? The nurse called the local health department and discovered that the current state incidence rate was 25 per 1000 children, and the county incidence rate was 20 per 1000. Thus she determined that the rate of chicken pox in her school was actually much lower than rates in comparison groups, so there was no reason to be alarmed.

In calculating a rate, the numerator is the number of events and the denominator is the total population at risk. The rate is usually converted to a standard base denominator (1000; 10,000; or 100,000) to permit comparisons between various groups.

Measures of Morbidity

Measurement of morbidity and mortality is an integral part of public health. Different types of **morbidity rates** are used to measure and monitor illnesses. The **incidence rate** refers to the number of new cases of an illness or injury that occur within a specified time. The **prevalence rate** refers to all of the existing cases of an illness at a given point in time. Incidence rates are most helpful in detecting and describing fluctuations in acute diseases, and prevalence rates are important in measuring chronic illness.

Table 6-1 provides an example of disease prevalence in describing arthritis in persons 18 years and older. As the table indicates, approximately 22% of Americans report having arthritis. In addi-

TABLE **6-1** Example of Disease Prevalence: Prevalence by Sex and Age of Doctor-Diagnosed Arthritis Among Persons 18 Years and Older

CHARACTERISTIC	PREVALENCE
SEX	
Women	25.4%
Men	17.6
AGE GROUP (YEARS)	
18-44	7.9%
45-64	29.3%
>65	50.6%
Total	21.6%

From Centers for Disease Control and Prevention: Prevalence of doctor-diagnosed arthritis and arthritis-attributable activity limitation–United States, 2003-2005, *MMWR Morb Mortal Wkly Rep* 55(40):1089, 2006.

tion, arthritis is strongly associated with age, and there is a weaker association with gender (i.e., women have a higher prevalence than do men) (CDC, 2006).

Figure 6-5 presents an example of disease incidence (new cases) by visually depicting the rates of reported AIDS cases for 2005. In reviewing this map it is interesting to note that the areas with the highest incidence of AIDS are located in Southeastern states (Florida, Georgia, and Louisiana), Mid Atlantic states (Maryland, Delaware, District of Columbia), and Illinois. Further, states with the lowest rates were generally located in the central and northern part of the country (Minnesota, Nebraska, Iowa, the Dakotas) and upper New England. The figure shows where problems with AIDS persist, and this allows for better targeting with prevention programs.

Measures of Mortality

Just as different types of morbidity rates are used to measure and monitor illnesses, a number of different rates are used to measure attributes regarding death (**mortality rates**). Measures of mortality frequently used in public health are listed in Table 6-2. Of particular interest to nurses working in community settings are the infant mortality rate, crude death rate, and the cause-specific death rate (e.g., how many individuals have died from AIDS or automobile accidents). Table 6-3 presents an example of mortality data.

COLLECTION OF DATA: THE CENSUS, VITAL STATISTICS, AND HEALTH STATISTICS

Sources of population-focused data for nurses in community-based practice include the census and local, state, and national vital statistics and health statistics. Each of these is discussed briefly. Much of the relevant information for nurses is available at local or state health departments and the local library.

The Census

The Bureau of the Census is responsible for collection of data on the U.S. population. A census of the population to assess its characteristics has been conducted every 10 years since 1790 as mandated by the Constitution of the United States. Among other reasons, the census is undertaken to establish each state's representation in the House of Representatives.

The methodology of census taking has evolved over the decades. To make the task more manageable and the data more meaningful, census tracts were developed. Census tracts are relatively small, usually homogenous, geographic areas that allow for analysis of small units within communities. Maps outlining boundaries for census tracts can be obtained from a local public library.

Census tract information can be extremely valuable for nurses and others involved in health program planning. Information elicited from the census questionnaire includes:
* Name, sex, race, age, ethnicity, and marital status of everyone living in the household (including housemates, foster children, boarders, and live-in employees)
* Housing characteristics, including the type of dwelling (e.g., mobile home, single-family detached, duplex, apartment); age of the dwelling; number of rooms; number of bedrooms; presence of plumbing facilities; kitchen facilities; source of fuel; source of water; sewage system; yearly costs for electricity, gas, and water

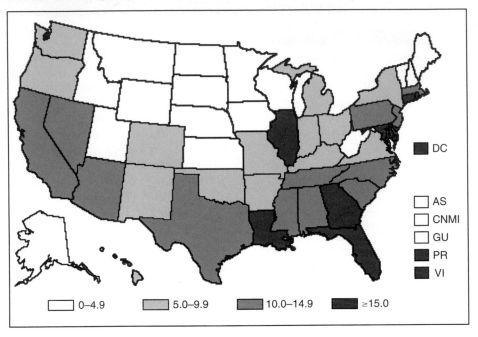

**ACQUIRED IMMUNODEFICIENCY SYNDROME (AIDS). Incidence* — United States†
and U.S. territories, 2005**

DC

AS
CNMI
GU
PR
VI

0–4.9   5.0–9.9   10.0–14.9   ≥15.0

*Per 100,000 population.
†Includes 209 persons with unknown state of residence.

The highest AIDS rates were observed in the northeastern part of the country. High incidence (i.e.,
≥15 cases per 100,000 population) also was reported in the southeastern states, the U.S. Virgin
Islands, and Puerto Rico.

Figure 6-5. Example of disease incidence: acquired immunodeficiency syndrome (AIDS), Incidence United States and U.S. Territories, 2005. From Centers for Disease Control and Prevention: Summary of notifiable diseases–United States, 2005, *MMWR Morb Mortal Wkly Rep* 54(53):1-96 (serial online): http://www.cdc.gov/mmwr/PDF/wk/mm5453.pdf. Accessed August 21, 2007.

- Information on the ownership of the home (e.g., owned by the resident, rented, mortgaged), estimated value, monthly rent, length of time in residence, property taxes
- Education attainment of all in the household
- Language spoken in the home
- Information related to occupation and work, including location of work, transportation to work (e.g., car, bus, subway, ferry, motorcycle), estimated time to get to work and home, employment information, type of work (e.g., manufacturing, wholesale trade, retail trade, agriculture, construction, service, government), retirement benefits, and income

This information is gathered during April of each new decade (i.e., 1990, 2000, 2010) for all individuals residing in the United States. Information

on numerous divisions (e.g., U.S. geographical areas) and subdivisions (e.g., states, metropolitan areas, census tract) of the census can be obtained at a regional public library and from the Bureau of the Census (www.census.gov).

Vital Statistics

The term *vital statistics* refers to data collected about the significant events that occur within a population over a period. These data are systematically gathered by agencies at local, state, national, and international levels. Vital statistics data include the data collected from ongoing recording, or registration, of all vital events—births and adoptions; deaths and fetal deaths; and marriages, divorces, legal separations, and annulments. Data on vital events are collected locally and reported to area and state offices through channels

TABLE **6-2** Frequently Used Measures of Mortality

MEASURE	NUMERATOR (X)	DENOMINATOR (Y)	EXPRESSED PER NUMBER AT RISK (10N)
Crude death rate	Total number of deaths reported during a given time interval	Estimated midinterval population	1000 or 100,000
Cause-specific death rate	Number of deaths assigned to a specific cause during a given time interval	Estimated midinterval population	100,000
Neonatal mortality rate	Number of deaths under 28 days of age during a given time interval	Number of live births during the same time interval	1000
Postneonatal mortality rate	Number of deaths from 28 days to, but not including, 1 year of age, during a given time interval	Number of live births during the same time interval	1000
Infant mortality rate	Number of deaths under 1 year of age during a given time interval	Number of live births during the same time interval	1000
Maternal mortality rate	Number of deaths assigned to pregnancy-related causes during a given time interval	Number of live births during the same time interval	100,000

From Centers for Disease Control and Prevention: *Principles of epidemiology*, ed 2, Atlanta, 1992, Centers for Disease Control and Prevention.

dictated by each state. Local vital statistics data can typically be obtained from the county or district records office and are often available at public libraries. State vital statistic information can be gathered from state records departments and national information from the National Center for Health Statistics (NCHS) (http://www.cdc.gov/nchs/).

Health Statistics

The CDC, the National Institutes of Health (NIH), and the NCHS are the primary sources for morbidity and mortality data in the United States. Each of these organizations is a component of the Department of Health and Human Services, as discussed in Chapter 5.

The CDC has primary responsibility for monitoring communicable diseases and other actual and potential health threats. The CDC publishes information for health providers in the *Morbidity and Mortality Weekly Report* (*MMWR*). Included in this periodical are weekly updates on selected reportable diseases; brief articles on a variety of topics; periodic recommendations for prevention, detection, and treatment of diseases; and field reports detailing current and completed investigations

into disease outbreaks. The *MMWR* can be found in most medical libraries, in public libraries with significant public document collections, at local health departments, or online through the CDC's website (www.cdc.gov).

The NIH is essentially concerned with research into numerous areas related to health. Information from NIH primarily covers federally funded research projects. Information generated from the various studies is typically published in professional journals. In addition, selected major studies, reports, guidelines, and recommendations are published and available from the Government Printing Office. Besides maintaining information on vital statistics (births, deaths, marriages, migrations) as discussed, the NCHS also monitors and publishes causes of morbidity and mortality.

DESCRIPTIVE AND ANALYTICAL EPIDEMIOLOGY

There are two basic types of epidemiology. **Descriptive epidemiology** examines the amount and distribution of a disease in terms of person, place, and time to distinguish characteristics of individuals

TABLE **6-3** Mortality Rate Example: Deaths, Death Rates, and Percent of Total Deaths for the 15 Leading Causes of Death: United States, 2004

RANK	CAUSE OF DEATH	NUMBER	DEATH RATE	TOTAL DEATHS (%)
___	All causes	2,397,615	816.5	100.0
1	Diseases of heart	652,486	222.2	27.2
2	Malignant neoplasms	553,888	188.6	23.1
3	Cerebrovascular diseases	150,074	51.1	6.3
4	Chronic lower respiratory diseases	121,987	41.5	5.1
5	Accidents (unintentional injuries)	112,012	37.7	4.7
6	Diabetes	73,138	24.9	3.1
7	Alzheimer's disease	65,965	22.5	2.8
8	Pneumonia and influenza	59,664	19.8	2.5
9	Nephritis, nephrotic syndrome, and nephrosis	42,480	14.5	1.8
10	Septicemia	33,373	11.4	1.4
11	Intentional self-harm (suicide)	32,439	11.0	1.4
12	Chronic liver disease and cirrhosis	27,013	9.2	1.1
13	Essential hypertension and hypertensive renal disease	23,076	7.9	1.0
14	Parkinson's Disease	17,989	6.1	0.8
15	Assault (homicide)	17,357	5.9	0.7
___	All other causes	414,674	141.2	17.3

From National Center for Health Statistics: Deaths: final data for 2004, *National Vital Statistics Report* 55(19), 2007 (website): http://www .cdc.gov/nchs/data/nvsr/nvsr55/nvsr55_19.pdf. Accessed August 22, 2007.

who have a specific disease from those who do not. **Analytical epidemiology** investigates the etiology of disease. In analytical epidemiology, observational and experimental studies are used to establish a causal relationship between identified threats and development of disease or disability.

DESCRIPTIVE EPIDEMIOLOGY

Descriptive epidemiology, as stated earlier, considers the amount and distribution of disease within a population by person, place, and time. As implied by the name, it is predominantly used to describe patterns of disease rather than considering or speculating on causality. Table 6-4 details characteristics or descriptors commonly used in the study of the amount and distribution of disease.

In many health reports and records, health problems are often presented with accompanying information on characteristics of those who have the health problem (i.e., data on person, place, and time). Table 6-5, for example, describes characteristics of young

smokers by grade (high school, middle school), sex, and race/ethnicity. As Table 6-5 illustrates, epidemiological data are often presented in a manner that allows for interpretation and application to other populations and provide information that can be re-gathered and compared to analyze trends over time.

ANALYTICAL EPIDEMIOLOGY

Analytical epidemiology focuses on the determinants of disease or a health-related event in a given population. The search for causes and effects, or the attempt to quantify the association between exposures and outcomes and test hypotheses about causal relationships, is the purpose of analytical epidemiology. The process of identifying the etiology of a disease occurs following comparison of groups through epidemiological studies (see the Community Application box, "Preventing Emerging Infectious Diseases"). Epidemiological studies are typically experimental or observational and may involve significant amounts of time.

TABLE **6-4** Characteristics Assessed in Descriptive Epidemiology: Person, Place, and Time

PERSON	PLACE	TIME
Age	Natural boundaries	Secular trends
Sex	Political subdivisions	Cyclic changes
Ethnic group and race	Environmental factors	Clusters in time and place
Social class	Urban-rural differences	
Occupation	International comparisons	
Marital status		
Family variables (e.g., family size, birth order, maternal age, parental deprivation)		
Personal variables (e.g., blood type, environmental exposure, personality traits)		

Data from Mausner JS, Kramer S: *Epidemiology–an introductory text*, Philadelphia, 1985, W.B. Saunders

One example of analytic epidemiology was a CDC (2007) report that examined sports and recreation-related traumatic brain injuries (TBIs). It was noted that thousands of people visit Emergency Departments (EDs) each year with TBIs obtained during sports or recreational activities. Among other findings, it was learned that males accounted for more than 70% of the ED visits, and children/adolescents between 10 and 19 years had the highest incidence. Activities with the greatest *number* of TBI-related ED visits included bicycling, football, playground activities, basketball, and riding all-terrain vehicles (ATVs). The greatest *percentages* of TBIs were from horseback riding, ice skating, riding ATVs, and bicycling (indicating that the chance of serious injury for these activities is higher). It was concluded that persons aged 5 to 18 accounted for 65% of ED visits for sports/recreation-related TBIs. Prevention measures, therefore, should be targeted to this group and focus on use of appropriate protective equipment, following of all safety policies, and adherence to the rules of the sport.

Another example of analytic epidemiology is a study of suicide data (CDC, 2006). In this work, investigators examined multiple circumstances and factors contributing to suicide among Americans. Included in the findings was the observation that the highest suicide rates were among persons 35 years and older, with the highest rate among older (65+) males. Further, almost half the suicides involved individuals with diagnosed mental illness, predominately depression. Other health problems, conflict with significant others, and alcohol abuse were also frequently reported contributing factors (Figure 6-6). The report highlighted the importance of recognizing underlying causes and circumstances leading to suicide. This will, in turn, allow providers and others to improve risk-factor identification and design programs to reduce the number of suicide victims.

SUMMARY

This chapter presents some of the basic elements of epidemiology. Recognition of the causes and course of a disease or health problem and identification of methods to prevent progression of the disease are very important components of nursing practice in any setting, and they are essential when practicing in the community. Indeed, this principle was illustrated by the case study in which Meg, a school nurse, was called upon to deal with an outbreak of head lice.

Many of the concepts included here are carried throughout the remainder of this book. Each of the chapters describing health promotion across

TABLE **6-5** Percentage of Middle School and High School Students Who Are Current Users of Cigarettes and Smokeless Tobacco, 2002

STUDENT CHARACTERISTIC	ANY TOBACCO	CIGARETTES	SMOKELESS TOBACCO
Middle School			
SEX			
Male	14.7	9.8	5.3
Female	11.7	9.7	1.6
RACE/ETHNICITY			
White	13.2	10.1	3.8
Black	13.5	9.0	2.3
Hispanic	12.5	8.7	2.7
Asian	8.6	7.4	3.5
Total, Middle School	13.3	9.8	3.5
High School			
SEX			
Male	32.6	23.9	10.5
Female	23.7	21.0	1.2
RACE/ETHNICITY			
White	30.9	25.2	7.3
Black	21.7	13.8	1.8
Hispanic	24.1	19.8	3.3
Asian	14.6	12.2	2.1
Total, High School	28.2	22.5	5.9

From Centers for Disease Control and Prevention: Youth tobacco surveillance–United States, 2001-2002, *MMWR Morb Mortal Wkly Report* 55(SS-3):1, 2006.

the life span (Chapters 12, 13, 15, and 16), for example, includes several primary, secondary, and tertiary prevention interventions. In addition, Chapter 19 takes a closer look at disease transmission and epidemiology when discussing communicable disease.

KEY POINTS

- *Epidemiology* is defined as the study of the distribution and determinants of disease in humans and application of this information to control health problems. Identifying characteristics or risk factors that predispose persons to or protect them against disease, then removing or minimizing

them if harmful and enhancing them if helpful are basic goals in epidemiology. The use of epidemiological concepts and principles to identify risks and assist in the prevention and management of disease is important for nurses working in community-based practice.

- A basic understanding of disease causation is important to identifying risk factors and developing prevention strategies. Models of disease causation include the *epidemiological triangle* (host, agent, and environment triad), the *web of causation* (explains diseases of multiple causation), and the *natural history of disease* (demonstrates how a disease progresses through stages of prepathogenesis and pathogenesis).

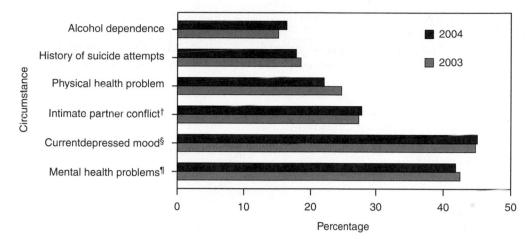

*Percantage might total to more than 100% because certain incidents involve multiple circumstances.
†Include separation, major argument, or violence.
§Current depressed mood was based on the family or friends' impression of the decedent's mood.
¶Includes any mental illness diagnosis of the decedent (e.g., clinical depression, dysthymia, bipolar disorder, or schizophrenia).

Figure 6-6. Example of analytic epidemiology. Percentage of suicide cases by selected circumstances. From Centers for Disease Control and Prevention: Homicides and suicides, National Violent Death Reporting System–United States, 2003-2004, *MMWR Morb Mortal Wkly Rep* 55(26):721, 2006.

COMMUNITY APPLICATION
Preventing Emerging Infectious Diseases

The CDC has recognized that infectious diseases are a continuing threat to all persons, regardless of age, sex, lifestyle, ethnic background, and socioeconomic status. In recognition of the potential problem of emerging infections, the CDC (1998) has identified these emerging threats:

- New variant Creutzfeldt-Jakob disease, which is possibly transmitted by ingestion of beef from animals afflicted with bovine spongiform encephalopathy (mad cow disease)
- A new and virulent strain of influenza in Hong Kong
- Several multistate foodborne outbreaks including hepatitis A on frozen strawberries and *Escherichia coli* 0157:H7 in apple cider, lettuce, alfalfa sprouts, and ground beef

- *Staphylococcus aureus* with reduced susceptibility to vancomycin
- A new strain of multidrug-resistant tuberculosis (strain W); appears more frequently in persons with HIV infection and has become endemic in New York

A set of goals was established to address these emerging infections. These goals include strategies for surveillance and response, applied research, infrastructure and training, and prevention and control. It is hoped that achieving these goals will promote understanding of infectious diseases and enhance their detection, control, and prevention.

- Much of nursing practice in community settings is intended to prevent the progression of disease at the earliest period or phase, using the appropriate level of prevention. Nursing interventions can be delivered at three different levels of prevention: (1) *primary prevention* (activities that prevent a problem before it occurs), (2) *secondary prevention* (early detection and prompt intervention during the period of early pathogenesis), and (3) *tertiary prevention* (efforts to limit disability and promote rehabilitation during the period of advanced disease and convalescence).

- *Rates* are statistical tools used to make comparisons between groups or populations or compare a subgroup of a population with the total population. Rates that measure the amount of morbidity associated with a particular illness include incidence and prevalence rates. Commonly used measures of mortality include the infant mortality rate, crude death rate, and cause-specific death rates.

- Sources of data on health-related issues include the *census* (population characteristics such as sex, race or ethnicity, age, housing characteristics, education levels, occupation information), *vital statistics* (e.g., registration of births, deaths), and *health statistics* (maintained by state health departments and the CDC).
- *Descriptive epidemiology* refers to the amount and distribution of a disease in terms of person, place, and time. *Analytical epidemiology* investigates the etiology of disease through observational and experimental studies to identify causal relationships between identified threats and development of subsequent disease or disability.

Learning Activities & Application to Practice
In Class

1. Select one or two timely illnesses or syndromes (e.g., bovine spongiform encephalopathy [BSE], autism, AIDS, skin cancer). Examine the illness using the models of disease causation described. Which model best fits each illness? Are the models useful for determining appropriate interventions?
2. For the illnesses or health conditions discussed in the previous exercise or other similar conditions, discuss primary-, secondary-, and tertiary-level interventions that nurses might be expected to deliver in community-based settings. With classmates, come up with examples of each level of prevention.
3. Complete the calculation exercises in Box 6-4.

In Clinical

4. With a small group of classmates, obtain selected census and vital statistics data on a local community or group. Determine what data are pertinent to the health of members of the community or to management of health care resources (e.g., presence or absence of running water, number of persons in the household, number of small children, number of elders, number of deaths, number of live births). Share findings with other groups and compare.

5. Observe for clusters of health problems that might indicate the need for comparison with other groups. For example, if working in a school, observe how many children seem to be having breathing difficulties or are being diagnosed with asthma. A comparison should be done with another school to see if one has higher rates of asthma than the other.

BOX **6-4** Exercises for Calculation of Rates

During 2007, 215 new cases of AIDS were reported in Grand River, a city of 500,000. This brought the total number of active cases of AIDS to 2280. During that time, 105 deaths were attributable to the disease.
1. What is the incidence rate per 100,000 for AIDS during 2007?
2. What was the prevalence rate of AIDS per 100,000?
3. What is the cause-specific death rate for AIDS per 100,000?
   Sun City is a small city with a mid-2007 population of 120,000. During 2007, 342 live births and 515 deaths were reported. Sun City has a large elderly population, with approximately 24,000 individuals older than 65 years. Of the 515 deaths during 2007, 425 were persons older than 65.
4. What is the crude birth rate for Sun City for 2007 per 1000?
5. What is the crude death rate for Sun City for 2007 per 1000?
6. What is the age-specific death rate for individuals older than 65 for Sun City for 2007 per 1000?
(Answers at end of chapter after the References.)

REFERENCES

Centers for Disease Control and Prevention: *Principles of epidemiology*, ed 2, Atlanta, 1992, Centers for Disease Control and Prevention.

Centers for Disease Control and Prevention: Nonfatal traumatic brain injuries from sports and recreation activities–United States, 2001-2005, *MMWR Morb Mortal Wkly Rep* 56(29):733, 2007.

Centers for Disease Control and Prevention: Summary of notifiable diseases–United States, 2005, *MMWR Morb Mortal Wkly Rep* 54(53):1-96, 2007.

Centers for Disease Control and Prevention: Homicides and suicides–National Violent Death Reporting System, United States, 2003-2004, *MMWR Morb Mortal Wkly Rep* 55 (26):721, 2006.

Centers for Disease Control and Prevention: Prevalence of doctor-diagnosed arthritis and arthritis-attributable activity limitation–United States, 2003-2005, *MMWR Morb Mortal Wkly Rep* 55(40):1089, 2006.

Centers for Disease Control and Prevention: Youth tobacco surveillance–United States, 2001-2002, *MMWR Morb Mortal Wkly Rep* 55(SS-3):1-60, 2006.

Centers for Disease Control and Prevention: Preventing emerging infectious diseases: a strategy for the 21st century, overview of the updated CDC plan, *MMWR Morb Mortal Wkly Rep* 47(RR15):1-14, 1998.

Clemen-Stone S, Eigsti DG, McGuire S.L: *Comprehensive community health nursing*, ed 4, St Louis, 1995, Mosby.

Frideman GD: *Primer of epidemiology*, New York, 1987, McGraw-Hill.

Gordis L: *Epidemiology*, ed 3, Philadelphia, 2004, Saunders.

Leavell HR, Clark EG: *Preventive medicine for the doctor in his community: an epidemiologic approach*, ed 2, New York, 1965, McGraw-Hill.

MacMahon B, Pugh TF: *Epidemiologic principles and methods*, Boston, 1970, Little, Brown.

Mausner JS, Kramer S: *Epidemiology: an introductory text*, Philadelphia, 1985, W.B. Saunders.

National Center for Health Statistics: Deaths: final data for 2004, *Nat Vital Stat Rep* 55(19), 2007 (online): http://www.cdc.gov/nchs/data/nvsr/nvsr55/nvsr55_19.pdf. Accessed August 22, 2007.

Tarzian AJ: Epidemiology: unraveling the mysteries of disease and health. In Maurer FA, Smith CM, editors: *Community/public health nursing: health for families and populations*, ed 3, St. Louis, 2005, Saunders.

U.S. Department of Health and Human Services: *Healthy people 2010*, conference ed, Washington, DC, 2000, Government Printing Office.

Valanis B: *Epidemiology in nursing and health care*, ed 3, Norwalk, Conn, 1999, Appleton & Lange.

Answers to Calculations for Box 6-4

1. $215/500,000 \times 100,000 = 43$ cases per 100,000
2. $2280/500,000 \times 100,000 = 456$ cases per 100,000
3. $105/500,000 \times 100,000 = 21$ deaths per 100,000
4. $342/120,000 \times 1000 = 2.85$ births per 1000
5. $515/120,000 \times 1000 = 4.29$ deaths per 1000
6. $425/24,000 \times 1000 = 17.71$ deaths over age 65 per 1000

Environmental Health Issues

objectives

Upon completion of this chapter, the reader will be able to:

1. Discuss potential environmental health threats related to housing and living patterns.

2. Discuss potential environmental health threats related to air pollution.

3. Discuss potential environmental health threats related to water pollution.

4. Discuss potential environmental health threats related to food quality.

5. Discuss potential environmental health threats related to radiation.

6. Discuss environmental problems related to solid waste.

7. Describe primary, secondary, and tertiary prevention strategies for individuals, families, and communities for each of the areas presented above.

key terms

Atmospheric quality
Carbon monoxide (CO)
Chlorofluorocarbons (CFCs)
Foodborne pathogens
Hazardous waste
Indoor biological
  contaminants

Intentional food additives
Lead poisoning
Occupational health risk
Ozone
Ozone depletion
Radon
Secondhand smoke

Ultraviolet radiation
Unintentional food
  additives

See Glossary for definitions.

case study

Susan Baldwin is a registered nurse working in a pediatric primary care clinic in an inner city. On Tuesday of this week, Susan assisted the pediatric nurse practitioner with a routine well-child examination on Billy Benson, a 2-year-old boy who lives with his mother and three siblings in an area housing project. The health care professionals at the clinic follow guidelines from the American Academy of Pediatrics for preventative care. In addition to overall physical assessment, the health professionals perform various screenings on the children (height and weight, vision and hearing testing, for example), based on these recommendations.

Continued

One of the recommended screening examinations is a test of the level of lead in blood of children who are considered at risk. These recommendations have been established because a significant number of inner-city children have serum lead levels above acceptable safe limits, and lead has been cited as the most common cause of mental impairment and mental retardation in children.

Susan understands the importance of lead screening and explained the problem of lead exposure and the rationale for testing to Billy's mother. She provided Mrs. Benson with clinic pamphlets explaining the basics of lead poisoning and prevention measures. While discussing the written materials with Mrs. Benson, Susan reviewed some of the main sources of lead contamination. These include paint in homes built before 1960, lead smelters, battery recycling plants, and hobbies that expose individuals to lead (e.g., ceramics, furniture refinishing, and stained glass work). Susan questioned Mrs. Benson and discovered that their residence was built in the late 1970s, which is not a problem, but learned that Billy regularly visits his grandmother, whose home was built in the 1940s. Mrs. Benson stated that she does not participate in any of the mentioned hobbies and knows of no area lead smelters or battery recycling plants.

Following guidelines set by the state health department, Susan drew a small tube of blood from a prick in Billy's finger, carefully labeled it, and completed the required forms. The specimen and accompanying paperwork were sent to the state laboratory for analysis. Susan explained to Mrs. Benson that the state health department, following Centers for Disease Control and Prevention (CDC) recommendations, has outlined a course of action for children with elevated lead levels, and if Billy's serum lead levels are elevated, further testing may be necessary.

Environmental factors play an important role in the processes of human development, health, and disease. Historically, public health efforts have addressed measures to improve or ensure adequate and safe supplies of food and water, manage waste disposal and sewage, and control or eliminate vectorborne illnesses (U.S. Department of Health and Human Services [USDHHS], 2000). Nationally these efforts have been phenomenally successful and are largely responsible for the increase in life expectancy witnessed during the twentieth century (McKeown, 1995).

According to the environmental health report in *Healthy People 2010*, "human exposures to hazardous agents in the air, water, soil, and food and to physical hazards in the environment are major contributors to illness, disability and death worldwide…[and] poor environmental quality is estimated to be directly responsible for approximately 25% of all preventable ill health in the world" (USDHHS, 2000, p. 8.5). Population growth, urbanization, technology, industrialization, and modern agricultural methods have demonstrated unprecedented progress in many areas but have concurrently created a number of hazards to human health. Risks from synthetic chemicals, naturally occurring radiation, and biological contamination of food and water supplies remain potential threats to the health of U.S. citizens. In response to these potential threats to health, one priority area of *Healthy People 2010* is environmental health; consequently, a series of related objectives have been published. The *Healthy People 2010* box presents selected goals related to issues of environmental health.

Environmental threats to the health of individuals may come from various sources. Hall and colleagues (2007) categorize environmental health issues and concerns into nine areas, which are listed and defined in Table 7-1. Assessment and intervention strategies, along with general information for health education for each of these areas, with the exception of violence risks, are discussed briefly. Violence risks and related nursing interventions are included in the discussions of children's and women's health in Chapters 12 and 14.

HOUSING AND LIVING PATTERNS

Numerous actual and potential health threats related to housing and living patterns exist. Some common concerns include overcrowding, household chemical

healthy people **2010**

Selected Objectives for Environmental Health, Food Safety, and Occupational Health and Safety

OBJECTIVE	BASELINE (1997)	TARGET
8.1a: Reduce the proportion of persons exposed to air that does not meet the EPA's health-based standards for harmful air pollutants (ozone).	43%	0%
8.6: Reduce waterborne disease outbreaks arising from water intended for drinking among persons served by community water systems.	6 outbreaks per year	2 outbreaks per year
8.11: Eliminate elevated blood lead levels in children.	4.4% of children aged 1-5	0%
8.15: Increase recycling of municipal solid waste.	27%	38%
8.18: Increase the proportion of persons who live in homes tested for radon concentrations.	17%	20%
10.2b: Reduce outbreaks of infections caused by key foodborne bacteria (*Salmonella*).	44 outbreaks per year	22 outbreaks per year
10.5: Increase the proportion of consumers who follow key food safety practices.	72%	79%
15.7: Reduce nonfatal poisonings.	348.4 per 100,000	292 per 100,000
16.15: Reduce the occurrence of spina bifida and other neural tube defects.	6 per 10,000 live births	3 per 10,000 live births
20.1c: Reduce deaths from work-related injuries (construction).	14.6 per 100,000 workers	10.2 per 100,000 workers
20.10: Reduce occupational needle-stick injuries among health care workers.	600,000	420,000

Data from U.S. Department of Health and Human Services: *Healthy people 2010*, Conference ed, Washington, DC, 2000, Government Printing Office.

exposure, potential for poisoning, presence of firearms, and violence. Table 7-2 describes sources of home pollution. Several related issues (e.g., radon gas) are listed elsewhere in this chapter. This section discusses potential problems related to indoor air quality and lead exposure in housing and living conditions.

INDOOR AIR QUALITY

Indoor air quality in the home may significantly affect health. Concerns center on combustion pollutants (e.g., carbon monoxide [CO], secondhand smoke), particles (e.g., asbestos, animal dander, pollen), and living organisms (e.g., dust mites, molds, bacteria). Several of these concerns—secondhand smoke, carbon monoxide poisoning, and biological contamination—are addressed in detail.

Secondhand smoke refers to the combination of smoke given off by the burning of a cigarette, pipe, or cigar and the smoke exhaled from the lungs of smokers. Secondhand smoke has been classified by the Environmental Protection Agency (EPA) as a known carcinogen and is estimated to cause approximately 3400 lung cancer deaths in nonsmokers each year (CDC, 2006). Health threats from secondhand smoke that pose risks to infants and children include increased numbers of respiratory tract infections (e.g., pneumonia and bronchitis), decreased lung function, symptoms of chronic respiratory irritation, middle ear infections, and development and exacerbation of asthma. In adults secondhand smoke causes eye, nose, throat, and lung irritation and may affect the cardiovascular system. The

TABLE **7-1** Areas of Environmental Health

AREA	DEFINITION
Living patterns	The relationships among persons, communities, and their surrounding environments that depend on habits, interpersonal ties, cultural values, and customs
Work risks	The quality of the employment environment and the potential for injury or illness posed by working conditions
Atmospheric quality	The protectiveness of the atmospheric layers, the risks of severe weather, and the purity of the air available for breathing purposes
Water quality	The availability and volume of the water supply and the mineral content levels, pollution by toxic chemicals, and the presence of pathogenic microorganisms; consists of the balance between water contaminants and existing capabilities to purify water for human use and plant and wildlife sustenance
Housing	As an environmental health concern, refers to the availability, safety, structural strength, cleanliness, and location of shelter, including public facilities and individual or family dwellings
Food quality	The availability and relative costs of foods, their variety and safety, and the health of animal and plant food sources
Waste control	The management of waste materials resulting from industrial and municipal processes and human consumption and efforts to minimize waste production
Radiation risks	Health dangers posed by the various forms of ionizing radiation relative to barriers preventing exposure of humans and other life forms
Violence risks	The potential for victimization through the violence of particular individuals and the general level of aggression in psychosocial climates

From Hall JM, Robinson CH, Broyles TJ: Environmental health. In Nies M, McEwen M, editors: *Community/public health nursing: promoting the health of populations*, ed 4, St Louis, 2007, Saunders.

Health Teaching box "Reducing the Health Risks of Secondhand Smoking" presents the EPA's recommendations to reduce the health risks of passive smoking.

Pollution from indoor combustion comes from appliances such as space heaters, gas ranges and ovens, furnaces, gas water heaters, and wood- or coal-burning stoves and fireplaces. Potential problems from indoor combustion typically relate to ineffective or improper venting of the appliances, cracked heat exchangers, burning of green or treated wood, or use of the wrong fuel.

Carbon monoxide (CO) exposure is particularly important, because more than 500 deaths each year are caused by accidental CO poisoning (CDC, 2007). Symptoms of CO poisoning include severe headaches, dizziness, confusion, and nausea. If CO poisoning is suspected, the EPA suggests getting all affected persons into fresh air immediately. Doors and windows should be opened, all combustion appliances should be turned off, and everyone should leave the house. A trip to the emergency room may be needed, and the physician should be told that CO poisoning is a possibility.

To reduce exposure to combustion pollutants, it is essential that combustion appliances undergo proper selection, installation, inspection, and maintenance. Suggestions to reduce or eliminate exposure to CO and other combustion gases are discussed in the Health Teaching box "Prevent Carbon Monoxide Exposure."

Indoor biological contaminants that may be detrimental to health include bacteria, molds, mildew, viruses, animal dander, dust mites, cockroaches, and pollen. Contaminated central air and heating units can become breeding grounds for

TABLE **7-2** Sources of Home Pollution

POLLUTANT	DESCRIPTION AND SUGGESTIONS	SOURCE AND EXAMPLES OF SUBSTANCE IN HOME
Radon	Colorless, odorless, radioactive gas from the natural breakdown (radioactive decay) of uranium; it is estimated that radon causes up to 20,000 lung cancer deaths per year	Soil or rock under the home; well water; building materials
Asbestos	Mineral fiber used extensively in building materials for insulation and as a fire retardant; asbestos should be removed by a professional if it has deteriorated; exposure to asbestos fibers can cause irreversible and often fatal lung diseases, including cancer	Sprayed-on acoustical ceilings or textured paint; pipe and furnace insulation materials; floor tiles; automobile brakes and clutches
Biological contaminants	Include bacteria, mold and mildew, viruses, animal dander and saliva, dust mites, and pollen; these contaminants can cause infectious diseases or allergic reactions; moisture and dust levels in the home should be kept as low as possible	Mold and mildew; standing water or water-damaged materials; humidifiers; house plants; household pets; ventilation systems; household dust
Indoor combustion	Produces harmful gases (i.e., carbon monoxide, nitrogen dioxide), particles, and organic compounds (e.g., benzene); health effects range from irritation of eyes, nose, and throat to lung cancer; ventilation of gas appliances to the outdoors will minimize risks	Tobacco smoke; unvented kerosene or gas space heaters; unvented kitchen gas stoves; wood stoves or fireplaces; leaking exhaust flues from gas furnaces and clothes dryers; car exhaust from an attached garage
Household products	Can contain potentially harmful organic compounds; health effects vary greatly; the elimination of household chemicals through the use of nontoxic alternatives or by using only in well-ventilated rooms or outside minimizes risks	Cleaning products; paint supplies; stored fuels; hobby products; personal care products; mothballs; air fresheners; dry-cleaned clothes
Formaldehyde	Widely used chemical that is released to the air as a colorless gas; it can cause eye, nose, throat, and respiratory system irritation, headaches, nausea, and fatigue; may be a central nervous system depressant and has been shown to cause cancer in laboratory animals; remove sources of formaldehyde from the home if health effects occur	Particleboard, plywood, and fiberboard in cabinets, furniture, subflooring, and paneling; carpeting, durable-press drapes, other textiles; urea-formaldehyde insulation; glues and adhesives
Pesticides	Including insecticides, termiticides, rodenticides, and fungicides—all contain organic compounds; exposure to high levels of pesticides may cause damage to the liver and the central nervous system and increase cancer risks; when possible, nonchemical methods of pest control should be used; if the use of pesticides is unavoidable, they should be used strictly according to the manufacturer's directions	Contaminated soil or dust that is tracked in from outside; stored pesticide containers; residue if used inside

TABLE **7-2** Sources of Home Pollution—cont'd

POLLUTANT	DESCRIPTION AND SUGGESTIONS	SOURCE AND EXAMPLES OF SUBSTANCE IN HOME
Lead	A long-recognized harmful environmental pollutant; fetuses, infants, and children are more vulnerable to toxic effects; if the community health nurse suspects that a home has lead paint, it should be tested	Lead-based paint that is peeling, sanded, or burned; automobile exhaust; lead in drinking water; food contaminated by lead from lead-based ceramic cookware or pottery; lead-related hobbies or occupations

From Primomo J, Salazar MK: Environmental health risks: at home, at work and in the community. In Maurer FA, Smith CM, editors: Community/public health nursing: health for families and populations, ed 3, St Louis, 2005, Saunders.

---

health teaching

Reducing the Health Risks of Secondhand Smoking

- Do not smoke in the home, and do not permit others to do so.
- If a family member insists on smoking indoors, increase ventilation in the area.
- Do not smoke if children, particularly infants and toddlers, are present.
- Do not smoke in an automobile with the windows closed if passengers are present.
- Find out about the smoking policies of day care centers, schools, and other caregivers of children, and take measures to ensure that children are not exposed.
- Teach others about the risks associated with secondhand smoke.
- Encourage and support policies that enact and maintain smoke-free workplaces.
- Prohibit smoking indoors, or limit smoking to rooms that have been specially designed to prevent smoke from escaping to other areas of the work site.
- Encourage employer-supported smoking cessation programs.
- Locate designated outdoor smoking areas away from building entrances or building ventilation system air intakes.
- Know the local and state laws regarding smoking in public buildings.
- Support stringent smoking control ordinances in the community.

From the Environmental Protection Agency: *Secondhand smoke* (EPA Publication No. 402-F-93-004), Washington, DC, 1993, Government Printing Office.

---

health teaching

Prevent Carbon Monoxide Exposure

Do have your heating system, water heater and any other gas, oil, or coal-burning appliances serviced by a qualified technician every year.

Do install a battery-operated CO detector in your home and check or replace the battery when you change the time on your clocks each spring and fall. If the detector sounds, leave your home immediately and call 911.

Do seek prompt medical attention if you suspect CO poisoning and are feeling dizzy, light-headed, or nauseous.

Don't use a generator, charcoal grill, camp stove, or other gasoline or charcoal-burning device inside your home, basement, or garage or near a window.

Don't run a car or truck inside a garage attached to your house, even if you leave the door open.

Don't burn anything in a stove or fireplace that isn't vented.

Don't heat your house with a gas oven.

From Centers for Disease Control and Prevention (website): http://www.cdc.gov/co/guidelines.htm.

---

mold, mildew, and other sources of biological contaminants and can then distribute the contaminants throughout the home. Biological contaminates can trigger allergic reactions, including asthma, and spread infections and illnesses (i.e., colds, influenza, and chicken pox). Symptoms of health problems caused by biological pollutants include sneezing, watery eyes, coughing, shortness of breath, dizziness, lethargy, fever, and digestive problems. Children, elderly people, and people with respiratory problems and allergies are particularly susceptible to biological agents in the indoor air.

To reduce exposure to biological contaminants, a number of activities are recommended (EPA, 2007a). These are listed in the Health Teaching box "Reducing Exposure to Biological Contaminants."

LEAD EXPOSURE

According to *Healthy People 2010* (USDHHS, 2000), there has been significant success over the past decade in reducing childhood **lead poisoning** in the United States because of measures to decrease lead in gasoline, air, food, and industrial sources. Indeed, the fairly dramatic reduction is attributed to identification of those at risk, widespread screenings, and effective community efforts to clean up problem areas. More remains to be done, however, and the risk is disproportionately high in persons having low income and persons from racial and ethnic minorities. Therefore reduction of blood lead levels remains a national priority (CDC, 2005).

Despite successes, it is estimated that about 2.2% of American children younger than 6 years (about 435,000 children), particularly minority and poor children from inner cities, have blood lead levels high enough to adversely affect their intelligence,

---

health teaching

Reducing Exposure to Biological Contaminants

- Maintain a relative humidity of 30% to 60% in the home.
- Install and use exhaust fans that are vented to the outdoors in kitchens and bathrooms.
- Vent clothes dryers outdoors.
- Vent the attic and crawl spaces to prevent moisture buildup.
- Keep the house clean. Dust mites, pollens, animal dander, and other allergy-causing agents can be reduced through regular cleaning.
- If using cool mist or ultrasonic humidifiers, clean appliances according to manufacturer's instructions and refill with fresh water daily.
- Thoroughly clean and dry water-damaged carpets and building materials (within 24 hours if possible) or consider removal and replacement.
- Take steps to minimize biological pollutants in basements (clean and disinfect basement floor drains regularly; operate a dehumidifier in the basement if needed to keep humidity levels between 30% and 50%).

From the Environmental Protection Agency: *Biological pollutants in your home* (website): http://www.epa.gov/faq/pubs/bio_1.html.

---

behavior, and development (CDC, 2004). As a result the CDC has implemented a multilevel program to screen young children for elevated lead levels, identify possible sources of exposure, monitor the medical management of children with elevated blood lead levels, support community programs to eliminate childhood lead poisoning, and provide health professionals, policy makers, and the public with educational information on preventing lead poisoning. (See the Community Application box "Preventing Childhood Environmental Lead Exposure.")

Lead-based paint in homes and buildings built before 1960 has been identified as the major source of lead poisoning. Chipping or peeling lead-based paint is of concern because it can easily be ingested by children or inhaled through lead-contaminated dust. Anemia, central nervous system disorders, and renal involvement may result from lead exposure. Of particular concern is chronic central nervous system dysfunction, including irreversible deficits in intelligence, behavior, and school performance. The CDC (1997; 2000) identifies those at greatest risk for lead poisoning as being children who:

- Live in a house or regularly visit a day care center, preschool, babysitter's home, or other house built before 1960
- Live in or regularly visit a house built before 1960 with recent, ongoing, or planned renovation
- Have a brother, sister, or playmate being treated for lead poisoning
- Live with an adult whose job, hobby, or use of ethnic remedies involves lead
- Live near an active lead smelter, battery recycling plant, or other industry likely to release lead

Maximum permissible blood levels of lead have been revised downward from 30 mcg/dl in 1975. Currently levels greater than 10 mcg/dl are denoted as "action" or "intervention" levels (CDC, 1997; CDC, 2004). Federal, state, and local efforts to decrease lead exposure should be supported by all health professionals.

WORK RISKS

An estimated 4.2 million job-related injuries and illnesses occur each year, with about 1.2 million severe enough to result in time lost from work

COMMUNITY APPLICATION
Preventing Childhood Environmental Lead Exposure

PRIMARY PREVENTION
Individual/Family Interventions

- Encourage parents to keep children away from peeling or chipping paint.
- Encourage families to remove lead-based paint from older homes.
- Wet mop and wet wipe hard surfaces with a high-phosphate solution.
- Do not vacuum hard surfaces because this might scatter dust.
- Wash children's hands and faces before they eat.
- Wash toys and pacifiers frequently.
- If soil around the home is likely to be lead contaminated (if the house was built before 1960 or is near a major highway), plant bushes next to the house and plant grass or other groundcover to reduce dust
- During remodeling of older homes be certain children and pregnant women are not in the home until the process is completed; thoroughly clean the house before inhabitants return.
- Do not use pottery or ceramic ware that was inadequately fired or is meant for decorative use for food storage or service.
- Do not store drinks or food in lead crystal.
- Make sure children eat regular meals; lead is more readily absorbed on an empty stomach.

Community Interventions

- Provide education programs and opportunities to learn about lead poisoning and prevention.
- Encourage communities to remove lead-based paint from older homes, particularly in low-income housing.
- Support policymakers who encourage funding for programs to reduce lead exposure.

SECONDARY PREVENTION
Individual/Family Interventions

- Recommend screening of high-risk children at age 6 months and at least every year.
- Recommend screening of all children at 12 months and yearly thereafter.
- Identify the source of lead exposure for children with serum lead levels above 10 mcg/dl.
- Refer for treatment if needed: If blood lead levels are greater than 20 mcg/dl, the child should receive environmental evaluation and remediation and a medical evaluation; drug therapy may also be indicated. If blood lead levels are greater than 45 mcg/dl, medical and environmental intervention and chelation therapy are necessary.
- Refer families with identified lead poisoning to local or state-sponsored programs if assistance is needed to remove the source of exposure.

Community Interventions

- Encourage community-sponsored testing for lead-based paint for all homes built before 1950.
- Promote accessibility of screening services.
- Monitor incidence of heavy metal poisoning.
- Educate the public on signs and symptoms of lead poisoning.
- Support government-sponsored financing of lead paint abatement when individual homeowners cannot afford it.

TERTIARY PREVENTION
Individual/Family Interventions

- Monitor progress and effects of treatment.
- Provide assistance in dealing with long-term effects of lead poisoning (e.g., referral for special education programs).
- Advocate lead abatement programs in older residential areas.
- Educate the public on the hazards of lead.
- Promote access to social services needed to manage the effects of lead poisoning.

Data from Centers for Disease Control and Prevention: *Preventing lead poisoning in young children*, Atlanta, 1991, Centers for Disease Control and Prevention; and from U.S. Department of Health and Human Services: *Healthy people 2010*: *national health promotion and disease prevention objectives*, Washington, DC, 2000, Government Printing Office.

(U.S. Department of Labor, 2006a; U.S. Department of Labor, 2006b). Workers face a variety of job hazards. Use of heavy equipment; exposure to chemicals, biohazards, sunlight, heat, cold, and noise; and potential for assault or violence pose risks to workers. Heavy lifting, working at elevations, and performing repetitive tasks, for example, can lead to serious injuries such as sprains, fractures, and carpal tunnel syndrome. According to the Department of Labor (2006b), sprains and strains are by far the leading injury and illness category in every major industry, with back sprains being the most common injury. Importantly, nurses' aides and orderlies had very high rates of back sprains and lost days from work attributed to overexertion. Other occupations with relatively higher rates of injury include mining, logging, agriculture, construction, manufacturing, trucking, and warehousing.

The extent of illness and injuries directly attributable to occupational risk can be difficult to define because many illnesses may result from prolonged exposure to a noxious substance over decades or from a combination of factors. Occupational lung disease, occupational cancers, and noise-induced hearing loss, for example, may take many years to develop. Psychological disorders and cardiovascular changes associated with job stress may be suspected but are difficult to verify.

To improve occupational health and safety, a combination of federal and state regulations were implemented during the twentieth century. Probably the most far-reaching piece of legislation was the Occupational Health and Safety Act (1970). The Occupational Health and Safety Act was responsible for the development of the Occupational Safety and Health Administration (OSHA) and the National Institute for Occupational Safety and Health (NIOSH). These agencies have been instrumental in setting and enforcing standards to improve worker safety and health and in providing research to address various health issues. Over the last three decades, OSHA has issued hundreds of occupational health and safety standards covering a wide range of hazards, such as toxic chemicals, hazardous equipment, and working conditions. These standards require employers to use appropriate practices, means, methods, operations, or processes to protect employees from hazards on the job (Rogers, 2003).

Prevention of **occupational health risk** hazards includes engineering controls, improving work practices, using personal protective equipment, implementing health-promotion strategies (e.g., programs for smoking cessation or stress reduction), and monitoring the workplace for emerging hazards. Nurses in community-based practice should be aware of occupational risks and measures that may be taken to prevent or minimize these risks (see the Community Application box "Preventing Work-Related Illness and Injury").

ATMOSPHERIC QUALITY

Air pollution threatens the health of both humans and animals. It can harm crops and other vegetation; contributes to the erosion, decay, and economic devaluation of buildings and structures; may diminish the protective ozone layer; and contributes to major climatic changes through the greenhouse effect. Exposure to air pollutants is associated with increases in morbidity and mortality. Air pollution can cause serious problems to humans, including lung damage, inflammatory responses, impairment of defenses, and acute changes in lung function. Major air pollutants affecting **atmospheric quality** are listed in Table 7-3.

In the United States, efforts to detect, monitor, reduce, eliminate, and control air pollution have been in effect since the Clean Air Act was passed in 1963. This legislation set standards for "ambient air quality" (which applies to the air quality in a city or town) and industrial emissions standards. The Clean Air Act was amended most recently in November of 1990 (EPA, 2007b). Goals of the 1990 amendments are the following:

- Cut acid rain in half through implementation of systems to reduce sulfur dioxide emissions from power plants.
- Reduce smog and other pollutants through upgrading inspection and maintenance programs for motor vehicles, adoption of clean fuel programs, and limiting use of wood stoves and fireplaces.
- Reduce air toxins (emissions from chemical plants, steel mills, and other businesses) through employment of stringent regulations to reduce industrial emissions.
- Protect the ozone layer through the reduction or elimination of **chlorofluorocarbons (CFCs)** in automobile air conditioners and residential, commercial, and industrial cooling and refrigeration systems.

OZONE

Ozone occurs in two layers in the atmosphere. In the stratosphere ozone acts to shield the earth from harmful effects of ultraviolet radiation given off by the sun. But at ground level, high concentrations of ozone are a major health concern because ozone is one of the primary problem gases in air pollution (EPA, 2007c).

The EPA (2007b) explains that there is evidence the Earth's stratospheric ozone layer is being destroyed by CFCs and other ozone-depleting gases found in refrigerants, aerosols, and some solvent cleaning agents. Theoretically radiation from the

COMMUNITY APPLICATION
Preventing Work-Related Illness and Injury

PRIMARY PREVENTION: HEALTH PROMOTION

Providing health education—individual and group programs
    on a variety of topics
Promoting healthful nutrition
Encouraging exercise and fitness
Assisting with stress reduction and coping mechanisms
Providing prenatal monitoring for pregnant workers
Teaching parenting skills

PRIMARY PREVENTION: ILLNESS PREVENTION

Providing health risk appraisal
Assisting with modification of identified risk factors
Promoting smoking cessation
Encouraging weight control
Providing appropriate immunizations (e.g., hepatitis B for
    health workers)

PRIMARY PREVENTION: INJURY PREVENTION

Providing accident investigation
Promoting use of safety devices
Removing safety hazards
Teaching good body mechanics
Providing safety education
Providing instruction on and monitoring of safe handling
    of hazardous substances

SECONDARY PREVENTION: SCREENING

Providing preplacement and termination of physical examinations
Providing environmental and ergonomic screening
Providing periodic screening for workers at risk

**SECONDARY PREVENTION: MANAGEMENT OF EPISODIC
CONDITIONS**

Assisting client in seeking professional health care when needed
Serving as an advocate to correct a health problem
Monitoring recovery from minor illness or injury
Acting as a resource for information on illness, prevention, and
    treatment

SECONDARY PREVENTION: EMERGENCY RESPONSE

Providing first aid for minor injuries
Establishing and maintaining a triage system for injuries
Diagnosing and treating injuries.
Mobilizing the emergency medical system when appropriate

TERTIARY PREVENTION

Monitoring chronic illness
Preventing or minimizing complications of chronic conditions
Serving as case manager for clients with chronic conditions
Assisting the worker in seeking reimbursement of health costs
    from health insurers
Providing on-site therapy where possible

---

sun elicits a chemical reaction between the CFCs and ozone, resulting in thinning of the ozone layer. In the early 1980s a significant depletion of ozone in an area about the size of North America was first observed in the southern hemisphere. At that time it was estimated that between 50% and 90% depletion in the ozone layer had occurred, creating a hole over Antarctica. A similar thinning of the ozone layer has also been detected over the North Pole.

To reduce the threat posed by **ozone depletion**, part of the Clean Air Act Amendment of 1990 initiated the phase-out of CFCs (EPA, 2007c). The major concern from a drop in stratospheric ozone levels is the increase in ultraviolet-B light. Increased incidence of skin cancer and cataracts and alterations in the immune system are linked to ozone depletion. Skin cancer is of particular concern. An increase in melanoma and in basal and squamous cell carcinoma is expected. In addition to the harmful effects

on humans, there is concern over the effects of increased ultraviolet-B light on animals, plants, and marine ecosystems.

Ground-level ozone is also a serious problem. Ground-level ozone is formed when nitrogen oxides and other volatile organic compounds are emitted from motor vehicles, power plants, and other sources of combustion in the presence of heat and sunlight. This exchange most readily occurs during hot weather (EPA, 2007c).

When inhaled, ozone can cause acute respiratory problems, aggravate asthma, and cause inflammation of lung tissue. It also impairs the body's immune system, making people more susceptible to respiratory illnesses. Those most at risk from exposure to ozone include children and asthmatics. Excessive ground-level ozone can also harm the environment by making plants susceptible to disease, pests, and environmental stresses (EPA, 2007c). To combat air

TABLE **7-3** Major Air Pollutants

POLLUTANT	SOURCES	EFFECTS
OZONE		
A colorless gas that is the major constituent of photochemical smog at the earth's surface. In the upper atmosphere (stratosphere), however, ozone is beneficial, protecting us from the sun's harmful rays.	Ozone is formed in the lower atmosphere as a result of chemical reactions between oxygen, volatile organic compounds, and nitrogen oxides in the presence of sunlight, especially during hot weather. Sources of such harmful pollutants include vehicles, factories, landfills, industrial solvents, and numerous small sources, such as gas stations and farm and lawn equipment.	Ozone causes significant health and environmental problems at the earth's surface, where we live. It can irritate the respiratory tract, produce impaired lung function, such as inability to take a deep breath, and cause throat irritation, chest pain, cough, lung inflammation, and possible susceptibility to lung infection. Smog components may aggravate existing respiratory conditions such as asthma. Ozone can also reduce yield of agricultural crops and injure forests and other vegetation. Ozone is the most injurious pollutant to plant life.
CARBON MONOXIDE		
Odorless and colorless gas emitted in the exhaust of motor vehicles and other kinds of engines where incomplete fossil fuel combustion occurs.	Automobiles, buses, trucks, small engines, and some industrial processes. High concentrations can be found in confined spaces like parking garages, poorly ventilated tunnels, or along roadsides during periods of heavy traffic.	Reduces the ability of blood to deliver oxygen to vital tissues, affecting primarily the cardiovascular and nervous systems. Lower concentrations have been shown to adversely affect individuals with heart disease (e.g., angina) and to decrease maximal exercise performance in young, healthy men. Higher concentrations can cause symptoms such as dizziness, headaches, and fatigue.
NITROGEN DIOXIDE		
Light brown gas at lower concentrations; in higher concentrations it becomes an important component of unpleasant-looking brown urban haze.	Result of burning fuels in utilities, industrial boilers, cars, and trucks.	One of the major pollutants that causes smog and acid rain. Can harm humans and vegetation when concentrations are sufficiently high. In children, may cause increased respiratory illness, such as chest colds and coughing with phlegm. For asthmatics, can cause increased breathing difficulty.
PARTICULATE MATTER		
Solid matter or liquid droplets from smoke, dust, fly ash, and condensing vapors that can be suspended in the air for long periods.	Industrial processes, smelters, automobiles, burning industrial fuels, wood smoke, dust from paved and unpaved roads, construction, and agricultural ground breaking.	These microscopic particles can affect breathing and respiratory symptoms, causing increased respiratory disease and lung damage and possibly premature death. Children, the elderly, and people suffering from heart or lung disease (such as asthma) are especially at risk. Also damages paint, soils clothing, and reduces visibility.

TABLE **7-3** Major Air Pollutants—cont'd

POLLUTANT	SOURCES	EFFECTS
SULFUR DIOXIDE		
Colorless gas, odorless at low concentrations, but pungent at very high concentrations.	Emitted largely from industrial, institutional, utility, and apartment-house furnaces and boilers; also from petroleum refineries, smelters, paper mills, and chemical plants.	One of the major pollutants that causes smog. At high concentrations, can also affect human health, especially among asthmatics (who are particularly sensitive to repiratory tract problems and breathing difficulties that sulfur dioxide can induce). Can also harm vegetation and metals. The pollutants it produces can impair visibility and acidify lakes and streams.
LEAD		
Lead and lead compounds can adversely affect human health either through ingestion of lead-contaminated substances, such as soil, dust, and paint, or through direct inhalation. This is particularly a risk for young children, whose normal hand-to-mouth activities can result in greater ingestion of lead-contaminated soils and dusts.	Transportation sources using lead in their fuels, coal combustion, smelters, car battery plants, and combustion of garbage that contains lead products.	Elevated lead levels can adversely affect mental development and performance, kidney function, and blood chemistry. Young children are particularly at risk because of their greater chance of ingesting lead and the increased sensitivity to lead of young tissues and organs.
TOXIC AIR POLLUTANTS		
Includes pollutants such as arsenic, asbestos, and benzene.	Chemical plants, industrial processes, motor vehicle emissions and fuels, and building materials.	Known or suspected to cause cancer, respiratory effects, birth defects, and reproductive and other serious health effects. Some can cause injury if accidently released in large amounts.
STRATOSPHERIC OZONE DEPLETERS		
Chemicals such as chlorofluorocarbons (CFCs), halons, carbon tetrachloride, and methyl chloroform that are used in refrigerants and other industrial processes. These chemicals last a long time in the air, rising to the upper atmosphere, where they destroy the protective ozone layer that screens out harmful ultraviolet radiation before it reaches the earth's surface.	Industrial household refrigeration, cooling and cleaning processes, car and home air conditioners, some fire extinguishers, and plastic foam products.	Increased exposure to ultraviolet radiation could potentially cause an increase in skin cancer, increased cataract cases, suppression of the human immune system, and environmental damage.

Continued

TABLE **7-3** Major Air Pollutants—cont'd

POLLUTANT	SOURCES	EFFECTS
GREENHOUSE GASES		
Gases that build up in the atmosphere that may induce global climate change or the greenhouse effect. They include carbon dioxide, methane, and nitrous oxide.	The main human-made source of carbon dioxide emissions is fossil fuel combustion for energy use and transportation. Methane comes from landfills, cud-chewing livestock, coal mines, and rice paddies. Nitrous oxide results from industrial processes, such as nylon fabrication.	The extent of the effect of climate change on human health and the environment is still uncertain but could include increased severity and frequency of storms and other weather extremes, melting of the polar ice cap, and sea-level rise.

From Environmental Protection Agency: *What you can do to reduce air pollution* (EPA Publication No. 450-K-92-002), Washington, DC, 1992, Government Printing Office.

pollution the EPA (2007d) has made several suggestions, which are included in Box 7-1.

WATER QUALITY

The availability of clean, safe water is vitally important in maintaining a healthy environment. According to the USDHHS (2000), only 73% of community water systems meet safe drinking water standards established by the EPA. Sewage (containing human waste, detergents), industrial processes and wastes (producing heavy metals, detergents, salts, heat, petrochemicals), and agricultural chemicals (e.g., fertilizer, pesticides) are the main sources of water pollution. To ensure and promote water quality, federal legislation was passed in 1948 and has been amended several times (1972, 1974, 1977, 1986, 1987). The Clean Water Act(s) serves to safeguard the quality of the nation's water supply through setting water standards and maximum allowable water contaminant levels.

MICROBIAL CONTAMINATION

Although surface and groundwater treatment through disinfection and filtration dramatically reduced the incidence of waterborne diseases in the United States during the twentieth century, each year thousands of Americans become ill by drinking contaminated water. Indeed, the CDC (2006) reported that in 2003-2004, there were 36 waterborne disease outbreaks affecting at least 2700 persons, with 58 hospitalizations and one death.

Waterborne diseases are those diseases that result from ingestion of contaminated water, inhalation of water vapors, body contact through bathing or swimming, and accidental ingestion of water during recreational activities (e.g., swimming, water skiing). Because symptoms are usually mild and short lived, it is assumed that only a small fraction of waterborne illnesses are recognized, reported, and investigated. Bacteria, viruses, and protozoa are the microorganisms of primary concern in waterborne disease. Table 7-4 lists the most common waterborne diseases found in the United States.

Water treatment processes include filtration, disinfection, and treatment of organic and inorganic contaminants. Removal of solids and microorganisms (e.g., *Giardia* and *Cryptosporidium* species) is accomplished by filtration systems (e.g., sand, diatomaceous earth, membrane, or cartridge filtration). Disinfection techniques include use of chlorine, ozone, and chloramines. Granular or powdered activated carbon column aeration, diffused aeration, oxidation, reverse osmosis, and aeration are also used to remove organic contaminants from water supplies.

7-1 What You Can Do to Clean the Air

AT HOME

- Use compact fluorescent lights with energy-efficient lighting
- Turn off appliances and lights when you leave the room
- Use the microwave to cook small meals
- Plant deciduous trees in locations that will shade your home in summer but admit light in winter
- Recycle paper, plastic, glass bottles, cardboard, and aluminum cans
- Reuse materials like paper bags and boxes when you can
- Properly dispose of household paints, solvents, and pesticides
- Paint with a brush, not a sprayer
- Keep woodstoves and fireplaces well maintained
- Purchase "green power" for your home's electricity
- Have leaky air conditioining and refrigeration systems repaired; have air conditioning systems checked in the spring and heating systems checked in the fall
- Cut back on air conditioning and heating use
- Insulate your home, water heater, and pipes
- Check filters monthly

DRIVE WISE

- Drive less, especially during peak traffic periods or on hot days
- Use public transportation, walk, or ride a bike
- Shop by phone, mail, or internet
- Telecommute
- Combine errands into one trip
- Avoid revving or idling engines over 30 seconds
- Avoid waiting in long drive-thru lines; park your car and go in
- Accelerate gradually, maintain the speed limit, and use cruise control on the highway
- Follow your owner's manual on recommendations for maximum fuel efficiency
- Use an energy-conserving grade of motor oil
- Minimize use of air conditioning if you can
- Get regular engine tune-ups and car maintenance checks
- Use EPA-certified facilities for air conditioner repair
- Replace your car's air filter and oil regularly
- Keep your tires properly inflated and aligned
- Fill gas tank during cooler evening hours to cut down on evaporation; don't "top off" the tank
- Look for the most efficient, lowest-polluting model of vehicle

BE INFORMED

- Share what you know with your family and friends
- Contact your state or local air pollution agency about how to become involved in local air pollution control issues

From the Environmental Protection Agency: *What you can do to clean the air* (website): http://www.epa.gov/air/actions/. Accessed October 10, 2007

CHEMICAL AND METAL CONTAMINANTS

Chemical contaminants of surface and ground water include pesticides (e.g., insecticides, fungicides, herbicides), petrochemicals and other organic compounds (e.g., improperly disposed of motor oil, paint, antifreeze), and a variety of industrial wastes (e.g., suspended solids, radionuclides, asbestos). Metal contaminants include lead, mercury, copper, arsenic, and iron.

Lead contamination is of particular concern because a significant number of public water systems in the United States provide drinking water that contains lead levels exceeding the action level standard established by the EPA. Also, lead is particularly harmful to infants, young children, and developing fetuses. Lead contamination is largely caused by widespread use of lead in pipes, brass faucets or fittings, and lead solder and is of most concern in homes that are very old or very new. Plumbing installed before 1930 is likely to contain lead. In newer plumbing system construction, lead solder and brass faucets and fittings are often used and can leach lead during the first 5 years of use. Thus water in buildings less than 5 years old may have lead contamination (CDC, 2007).

Recommendations from the CDC (2007) to reduce lead in drinking water include the following:

- Before drinking or cooking, flush the water system by running cold water 1 to 2 minutes, particularly if the water has been in contact with plumbing for more than 6 hours (e.g., overnight or during a workday).
- Use only cold water for consumption. Use only water from the cold water tap for drinking, cooking, and, especially, for making baby formula because hot water is more likely to contain higher levels of lead (boiling water will not reduce the amount of lead in water).
- Have household water tested for the presence and amount of lead. This is particularly important for apartment dwellers.
- Consider the use of filtering devices. Filters may help in reducing lead levels if properly used (e.g., filters must be changed as specified by the manufacturer).
- Consider bottled water for consumption. Bottled water is regulated by the Food and Drug Administration (FDA) if sold in interstate commerce and is under state regulation if sold within a state.
- Ensure that repairs to copper pipes do not use lead solder.

TABLE **7-4** Waterborne Diseases of Concern in the United States

DISEASE	MICROBIAL AGENT	GENERAL SYMTOMS
Campylobacteriosis	Bacterium (*Campylobacter jejuni*)	Fever, abdominal pain, diarrhea
Cryptosporidiosis	Protozoan (*Cryptosporidium parvum*)	Diarrhea, abdominal discomfort
Giardiasis	Protozoan (*Giardia lamblia*)	Diarrhea, abdominal discomfort
Hepatitis	Virus (hepatitis A)	Fever, chills, abdominal discomfort, jaundice, dark urine
Shigellosis	Bacterium (*Shigella* species)	Fever, diarrhea, bloody stool
Viral gastroenteritis	Viruses (Norwalk, rotavirus, and other types)	Fever, headache, gastrointestinal discomfort, vomiting, diarrhea

From Centers for Disease Control and Prevention: *Selected diseases spread through drinking water (United States)* (website): http://www.cdc.gov/ncidod/diseases/water/drinking.htm. Accessed October 10, 2007; and from Craun MF, Craun GF, Calderon RL et al: Waterborne outbreaks reported in the United States, *J Water Health* 4(suppl 2):19, 2006.

COMMUNITY AND NURSING INTERVENTIONS

Research into improving water treatment and detecting, analyzing, and eliminating contamination is ongoing. Efforts to monitor and improve water quality should be supported by all health care providers and by concerned citizens. Improved public and professional appreciation of the risks of contaminated drinking water and increased willingness of the public to pay for improved drinking water quality are essential (USDHHS, 2000). Suggestions for improving water quality and ensuring safe water include the following:

- Be aware of the community's water source and supplier. How is the water supply treated and tested for contamination? Does the supplier adhere to guidelines and standards set by the EPA?
- Learn about potential contamination sources of ground water and surface water.
- Urge the community water supplier and state and local regulatory and health officials to ensure that the water supply complies with all standards.
- Support efforts to educate the public and elected officials about the need to protect and improve the quality of drinking water.
- Express willingness to pay higher water rates, if necessary, to finance improvements in water quality.
- Support local and state efforts to develop programs and strategies to protect surface and ground water and to develop programs to control contaminating sources and activities.

- Support ongoing research and training efforts to improve water quality.

FOOD QUALITY

The FDA and the Department of Agriculture are responsible for setting standards for food safety, inspection of many foods, regulation of restaurants and food sales, approval of food additives, and for oversight of other aspects of food safety. Although safety of food consumed by U.S. residents is taken for granted, outbreaks of food-related illnesses and threats to health occasionally occur. Food quality and safety concerns include potentially harmful intentional and unintentional additives and biological and chemical contaminants. A variety of other issues related to food, such as genetically engineered foods and misrepresentations of nutrient qualities and substandard inspection, should also be of concern to all nurses.

MICROBIOLOGICAL CONTAMINATION

The USDHHS (2000) estimates that each year some 76 million illnesses, 325,000 hospitalizations, and 5000 deaths are associated with microorganisms in food. Problems cited include emerging pathogens; improper food preparation, storage, and distribution practices; an increasingly global food supply; and an increase in the number of people at risk because of aging and compromised capacity to fight these diseases.

Several **foodborne pathogens** have been cited as being of primary concern with regard to foodborne illnesses. These include *Salmonella, Campylobacter, Escherichia coli* 0157:H7, and *Listeria monocytogenes* (Table 7-5). Campylobacteriosis and salmonellosis are the most frequently reported foodborne illnesses in the United States, but *E. coli* 0157:H7 and *L. monocytogenes* infections are more severe. The very young, elderly, and immunocompromised persons experience the most serious foodborne illnesses. Other high-risk populations include residents in nursing homes; hospitalized cancer and organ transplant patients; and individuals with AIDS, cirrhosis, or reduced stomach acid. Campaigns have been launched to reach all consumers on food safety. The "Seven Commandments of Food Safety" developed by the FDA will help prevent foodborne illnesses (see the Community Application box, "Seven Commandments of Food Safety").

INTENTIONAL FOOD ADDITIVES

Intentional food additives are those substances added to food during processing to enhance the nutritional content of foods (e.g., vitamins and minerals), improve flavor (e.g., monosodium glutamate, salt, sugars, "natural flavors"), enhance color (e.g., dyes), improve texture or consistency (e.g., leavening agents, gums, thickening agents), and/or increase the shelf life (e.g., various preservatives).

The FDA has regulated food additives to some degree since the passage of the Food, Drug, and Cosmetic Act in 1938. This law requires food manufacturers to list product ingredients on the food label. Subsequent amendments and legislation have resulted in allowing the FDA to establish and enforce standards for the processing of food, including food additives. The "Delaney clause," added in 1960, forbids the use of any additive shown to cause cancer in humans or animals. The Nutrition Labeling and Education Act was passed in 1990 to require listing of color additives by name and the listing of ingredients in standardized foods. The Dietary Supplement Act of 1992 set more stringent guidelines for health claims and nutrition content of foods to ensure that claims made about health and nutritional benefits are truthful.

Instruction on food additives should be a component of thorough nutrition counseling. Client education should include encouragement to read food labels and to choose foods appropriate for individual nutritional needs.

UNINTENTIONAL (INCIDENTAL) FOOD ADDITIVES

Unintentional food additives refer to those substances that enter and remain in food as a result of their use as pesticides or herbicides, after being added to animal food, from packaging material, or through chemical changes brought about by processing methods. Glass chips, insect fragments, mercury and other heavy metals in fish, and residual antibiotics and hormones in beef and milk products are examples of food contaminants that have been the source of concern (Foulke, 1994; Hall, Robinson, Broyles, 2007; Wagner, 1992).

To further reduce and virtually eliminate ingestion of pesticide residues, the FDA provides the following recommendations:
- Wash fruits and vegetables with large amounts of cold or warm water and scrub with a brush when appropriate (do not use soap).
- Throw away the outer leaves of leafy vegetables such as lettuce and cabbage.
- Peel and cook when appropriate, although some nutrients and fiber are lost when produce is peeled.
- Trim fat from meat and fat and skin from poultry and fish. Residues of some pesticides concentrate in animal fat.

OTHER ISSUES IN FOOD QUALITY

Other concerns and issues in food quality include genetically engineered foods; irradiation of foods; and ongoing development of substances, additives, and chemicals to change food. Recent scientific developments have advanced the production of foods with decreased caloric content, increased nutritive value, and improved shelf life. The Department of Agriculture and the FDA sets policy for foods produced from new plant varieties and plant breeding, and the FDA must approve new food additives before marketing. As a result of these efforts, clients should be reassured that efforts are being made to ensure food safety. However, clients should also be encouraged to stay informed on current developments regarding food quality.

WASTE CONTROL

There are two major concerns in the issue of waste control: (1) volume of solid wastes produced in the United States and (2) concerns over the disposal of

TABLE **7-5** Selected Foodborne Microorganisms

MICROORGANISM	ONSET, DURATION, AND FREQUENCY	ACUTE SYMPTOMS	ASSOCIATED FOODS	PREVENTION
Salmonella species	*Onset of symptoms:* 6-48 hours after ingestion. *Duration of symptoms:* 1-2 days. *Frequency:* 77 reported outbreaks in 1989 involving 2400 individuals. Most cases, however, go unreported, and the FDA estimates 2-4 million annual cases of salmonellosis in the United States.	Nausea, vomiting, abdominal cramps, diarrhea, fever, and headache.	Meats, poultry, eggs, milk and dairy products, fish, shrimp, frog legs, yeast, salad dressings and sauces, cream-filled desserts and toppings, peanut butter, cocoa, and chocolate.	Raw eggs and foods containing raw eggs (e.g., homemade ice cream, Caesar salad, mayonnaise) may cause salmonella infections. Eggs and all meats, particularly poultry, should be thoroughly cooked. Buy refrigerated eggs and keep refrigerated at temperatures less than 40° F. Wash hands, utensils, equipment, and work areas with hot soapy water before and after they come in contact with eggs and poultry. Buy only pasteurized milk and keep refrigerated.
Campylobacter jejuni	*Onset of symptoms:* 2-5 days after ingestion of contaminated food or water. *Duration of symptoms:* 7-10 days, with relapses in about 25% of cases. *Frequency:* C. jejuni is the leading cause of bacterial diarrhea in the United States. Estimates exceed 2-4 million cases per year.	Diarrhea—often bloody and may contain fecal leukocytes—fever, abdominal pain, nausea, headache, and muscle pain.	Raw chicken, raw milk, contaminated water, and raw clams.	Wash and thoroughly cook chicken. Wash hands and cooking utensils that come in contact with raw chicken with hot soapy water. Complete pasteurization of milk and chlorination of drinking water will kill C. jejuni.

Escherichia coli 0157:H7	*Onset of symptoms:* 6-48 hours after ingestion. *Duration of symptoms:* approximately 8 days. *Frequency:* appears to be uncommon; however, probably only the most severe cases are reported.	Severe cramping, abdominal pain, and diarrhea that initially is watery but becomes grossly bloody. Occasionally vomiting occurs. Fever is low-grade or absent.	Raw and undercooked hamburger meat (ground beef) is the primary source. Has also been traced to processed salami. Raw milk and other meats may contain *E. coli* 0157:H7.	Thoroughly cook all beef, particularly ground beef. Maintain cooked beef at appropriately hot or cold temperatures. Do not drink unpasteurized milk.
Listeria monocytogenes	*Onset of symptoms:* in general, 7-30 days after exposure, although may be 2-3 days after consumption of heavily contaminated foods. Symptoms in infants may appear hours or days after birth. *Frequency:* appears to be relatively rare—about 1600 cases per year.	Fever, headache, nausea, and vomiting; of particular concern to pregnant women and their unborn children because infection may lead to fetal death, premature labor, or infections in newborns. Major concern—mortality rate is almost 25%.	Dairy products, particularly soft cheeses; also found in some imported seafood (e.g., frozen crab meat, cooked shrimp, and cooked surimi).	Consume only pasteurized milk and dairy products made from pasteurized milk.

Adapted from the Food and Drug Administration: *Foodborne pathogenic microorganisms and natural toxins,* Washington, DC, 1992, Government Printing Office.

COMMUNITY APPLICATION
Seven Commandments of Food Safety

1. Wash hands before handling food.
2. Keep it safe—refrigerate.
3. Do not thaw food on the kitchen counter.
4. Wash hands, utensils, and surfaces after contact with raw meat and poultry.
5. Never leave perishable food out over 2 hours.
6. Thoroughly cook raw meat, poultry, and fish.
7. Freeze or refrigerate leftovers promptly.

Data from U.S. Department of Health and Human Services: *Healthy people 2010: national health promotion and disease prevention objectives*, Washington, DC, 2000, Government Printing Office.

toxic and hazardous wastes. Each is discussed briefly.

SOLID WASTE MANAGEMENT

The United States is the world's biggest producer of solid wastes. Burying wastes in landfills, incineration, and recycling are the current available options for management of solid wastes. It is estimated that U.S. residents throw away about 4.6 pounds of garbage per person per day (EPA, 2007e). Figure 7-1 depicts components of America's trash. Besides involving esthetic and practical concerns, effective solid waste management is essential in decreasing pathogen transmission through insect and rodent control and in eliminating potential exposure to toxic and infectious materials.

In response to this growing problem, the EPA has endorsed an "integrated waste management" strategy of source reduction, recycling, waste combustion and landfilling, and community response and activities to produce less waste. Box 7-2 outlines practical ways all citizens can work to manage solid waste more effectively.

TOXIC AND HAZARDOUS WASTE CONTROL

Hazardous materials make up approximately 10% of industrial wastes and include poisons, inflammable materials, infectious contaminants, explosives, and radionuclides. The EPA regulates **hazardous waste** under the Resource Conservation and Recovery Act and, together with the Agency for Toxic Substances and Disease Registry, is responsible for overseeing hazardous waste disposal and monitoring potential

and actual threats posed to health and safety. The EPA has identified 1450 sites as being on the "National Priorities List" designated for cleanup under the Comprehensive Environmental Response, Compensation, and Liability Act of 1980 (the Superfund law). This law requires industry to pay for cleaning up the worst hazardous wastes sites by taxing industries that produce these wastes.

Some of the most common contaminants include lead (e.g., from paint and glass manufacturing and smelting), mercury (e.g., from batteries, paints, pesticides), polychlorinated biphenyls (PCBs) (e.g., from electrical insulation); chromium (e.g., from copy machines, stainless steel manufacturing, chrome plating), trichlorolorethane or trichloroethylene (e.g., from dry-cleaning agents), and benzene (e.g., from chemical manufacturing). To regulate these and other hazardous wastes, the EPA has instituted a tracking system that monitors identified hazardous substances from the time the substance is produced until it reaches an approved site for disposal.

Medical waste is defined by the EPA as cultures and stocks of infectious agents, items contaminated with human blood and blood products, human pathological wastes, contaminated animal carcasses, wastes from clients isolated with highly communicable diseases, and all used sharps. Disposal of medical waste is largely regulated at the state level. Currently incineration is the method of disposal of choice for medical waste; approximately 90% of hospital waste is incinerated on site. The remainder is sterilized in autoclaves or transported off site for treatment (EPA, 2007).

Hazardous waste management consists of a combination of treatment to reduce toxicity (e.g., incineration, detoxification), storage, and/or disposal following prescribed methods. In addition, the EPA strongly encourages waste minimization to reduce the volume of hazardous wastes.

LANDFILLS

A landfill is a place where garbage is dumped and covered daily with a layer of soil. The soil cuts down on odor, flies, insects, and animals. Newer landfills, called *sanitary landfills*, are lined with clay and strong plastic sheets designed to keep the landfill from leaking into the environment—particularly from contaminating ground water. Although some 70% of

Food scraps, 11.9%

Glass, 5.2%

Wood, 5.7%

Metals, 7.6%

Plastics, 11.8%

Other, 3.4%
(e.g., rubber, leather, textiles, miscellaneous inorganic wastes)

Yard trimmings, 13.1%

Paper, 34.2%

Total weight = 246 million tons
(2005 figures)

Figure 7-1. Total waste generation in the United States. (From Environmental Protection Agency: *Municipal solid waste in the U.S.–2005 facts and figures*, 2007 [website]: http://www.epa.gov/epaoswer/non-hw/muncpl/msw99.htm. Accessed October 10, 2007.)

the garbage in a landfill is biodegradable, most garbage, including food and paper, remains intact for decades because lack of light, oxygen, and water prevents composting.

INCINERATION

Incineration as a method of solid and hazardous waste management is controversial. Incineration reduces the volume of waste by up to 90% and is effective in destroying most biological contaminants. However, increasing air pollution, particularly with toxic chemicals, and subsequent disposal processes for residual heavy metals are the primary concerns. Commercial waste incinerators are designed to control emissions into the air. A variety of methods and devices, including filters, "scrubbers," and electrostatic precipitators, are employed to collect particulates and neutralize exhausts. Following incineration, residual ash is tested for toxicity and disposed of accordingly. If no toxins are found, the residue is typically dumped into a regular landfill. If toxins are found, the residue is shipped to hazardous waste

BOX 7-2 Tips for Reducing Solid Waste

REDUCE
Reduce the amount of unnecessary packaging.

REUSE
Consider reusable products.
Reuse bags, containers, and other items.
Borrow, rent, or share items used infrequently.
Sell or donate goods instead of throwing them out.

RECYCLE
Choose recyclable products and containers, and recycle them.
Select products made from recycled materials.
Compost yard trimmings and some food scraps.

RESPOND
Educate others on source reduction and recycling practices.
Make preferences known to manufacturers, merchants, and community leaders.
Be creative—find new ways to reduce waste quantity and toxicity.

landfills. A positive byproduct of waste incineration now gaining attention is energy production. Capturing the energy (i.e., heat) that is produced and recycling it is commonplace in newer, state-of-the-art incineration plants.

RADIATION RISKS

Threats to health from ionizing radiation come from several sources. Figure 7-2 illustrates potential sources of exposure to radiation. Unless exposure is occupational in nature (e.g., for radiology technicians, dentists, nuclear plant employees), the most common and most potentially hazardous radiation risks come from two sources: (1) radon gas and (2) the sun.

RADON GAS

Radon, an odorless, invisible gas, is a byproduct of the decay of uranium and occurs nearly everywhere in very small amounts. Radon enters buildings through cracks in solid floors, construction joints, cracks in walls, gaps in suspended floors, gaps around service pipes, cavities inside walls, and the

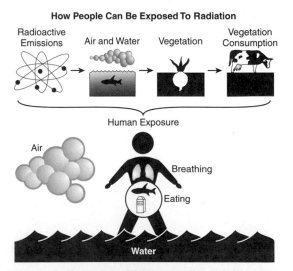

Figure 7-2. How people can be exposed to radiation. (From Centers for Disease Control and Prevention/National Center for Environmental Health: *Radiation studies*, Atlanta, 1993, U.S. Department of Health and Human Services, Centers for Disease Control and Prevention.)

water supply (EPA, 2007f). The amount of radon present varies greatly, and dangerously high levels can be found in many homes. Millions of homes have elevated radon levels, and most homes, particularly in high-incidence areas, should be tested for radon. When elevated levels are confirmed, the problems should be corrected.

Indoor radon gas is a national health problem contributing to an estimated 21,000 deaths each year. Indeed, about 10% of all lung cancer deaths are linked to radon, making radon the second leading cause of lung cancer in the United States (EPA, 2007f).

Radon is measured in units called *picocuries per liter* (pCi/L). The average radon level in most houses in the United States is approximately 1 pCi/L. The EPA has established a level of 4 pCi/L or less as desirable (EPA, 2005).

To measure radon levels, test kits can be purchased through the mail or from hardware stores and other retail outlets. Test kits should stipulate that they "meet EPA requirements" and should be designated "short term" (to remain in the home for 2 to 90 days) or "long term" (to remain in the home for 90 days or more). Because radon levels tend to vary from day to day, a short-term test is less likely to accurately detect radon. If one short-term test records a level of 4 pCi/L or greater, a second test should be conducted. The EPA recommendations following radon testing are discussed in Box 7-3.

The EPA recommends employing only trained contractors to perform repairs needed to lower home radon levels. Repair costs range from $800 to $2500, depending on the house and choice of radon reduction methods.

ULTRAVIOLET RADIATION AND SKIN CANCER

Skin cancer is the most common form of cancer in the United States, with more than 1 million new cases diagnosed each year, resulting in approximately 11,000 deaths (about 8000 from melanoma and about 2700 from non-melanoma skin cancer) (American Cancer Society [ACS], 2007a). Exposure to the sun is associated with three major types of skin cancer: (1) basal cell carcinoma (75% of all cases of skin cancer), (2) squamous cell carcinoma (20% of all cases of skin cancer), and (3) malignant melanoma (4.5% of all cases of skin cancer) (ACS, 2007b). Exposure to **ultraviolet radiation** from the sun is

BOX 7-3 Environmental Protection Agency Recommendations for Randon Testing

Step 1. Take a short-term test. If the result is 4 pCi/L or higher, take a follow-up test to be sure.

Step 2. Follow up with either a long-term test or a second short-term test:

For a better understanding of the year-round average radon level, take a long-term test.

If test results are needed quickly, take a second short-term test. (If the short-term test results are 10 pCi/L or

higher, a second short-term test should be conducted immediately.)

Step 3. If the second test was a long-term test: Home repairs are needed if long-term results are 4 pCi/L or greater.

If the second test was a short-term test: Home repairs are needed if the average of both tests is 4 pCi/L or greater.

Adapted from Environmental Protection Agency: *A citizen's guide to radon* (EPA Publication No. 402-K02-006), Washington, DC, 2005, Government Printing Office.

believed to cause most basal and squamous cell carcinomas. The correlation between melanoma and sun exposure is less certain.

Rates of skin cancer appear to be rising, and an estimated one in six people will develop skin cancer during his or her lifetime. At highest risk are those individuals with a fair complexion, who sunburn easily, and those who have blond or red hair and blue eyes. As stated, exposure to ultraviolet radiation, particularly during the early years of life, contributes to skin changes that eventually result in development of skin cancer.

Signs, Symptoms, and Detection of Skin Cancer

Basal and squamous cell carcinomas occur most frequently in older individuals, and although basal cell carcinoma rarely metastasizes, squamous cell carcinoma produces regional metastasis in approximately 5% of cases. Skin changes that may indicate basal or squamous cell carcinomas most often occur on the face, head, neck, and hands. The National Cancer Institute (NCI, 2005) recommends observation for any of the following conditions on the skin and examination by a health care provider of any lesions that last longer than 2 weeks:

1. A small, smooth, pale, shiny or waxy lump
2. A firm red lump
3. A sore or lump that bleeds or produces a crust
4. A flat, red spot that is rough, dry, or scaly and may become itchy or tender
5. A red or brown patch that is rough and scaly

Malignant melanoma is the most serious and potentially deadly form of skin cancer, developing in about 60,000 individuals and causing approximately 8100 deaths annually in the United States. Melanoma can occur at virtually any age; indeed, it is one of the most common cancers in people younger than 30 years of age (ACS, 2007b). It is about 10 times more common among whites than blacks and slightly more common among men than women (ACS, 2007a).

Melanoma develops from pigment-forming cells in the skin, most commonly from preexisting or newly developed nevi. Although melanoma can develop virtually anywhere on the body, intermittently sun-exposed areas, such as the back or calf, are the most common sites in whites. In people with very dark skin (e.g., blacks), the palms, soles, and under the nails are the most common sites (ACS, 2007b).

The ACS recommends a simple "ABCD" rule to observe for signs of melanoma in preexisting or new moles. These signs are listed in Box 7-4.

With early detection and prompt treatment, most skin cancers, including melanoma, can be treated. Treatment options include excisional surgery, chemotherapy, radiation therapy, and immunotherapy (ACS, 2007b). Recommendations for early detection include skin examination by a primary care provider every 1 to 3 years (depending on the client's age) and teaching and encouraging clients to perform monthly skin self-examination. See the Health Teaching box "Guidelines for Preventing Skin Cancer."

ENVIRONMENTAL HEALTH AND NURSING PRACTICE

Nurses, particularly those who work in community settings, must be knowledgeable about actual and potential environmental threats to health and should adapt their assessment and diagnostic skills to

BOX 7-4 ABCD Rule for Signs of Melanoma

A. Asymmetry: One half of a mole or birth mark does not match the other half.

B. Border: The edges are irregular, ragged, notched, or blurred.

C. Color: The color is not the same all over and may include shades of brown or black and sometimes patches of red, white, or blue.

D. Diameter: The spot is larger than 6 mm (about ¼ inch, the size of a pencil eraser) or is growing larger.

health teaching

Guidelines for Preventing Skin Cancer

- Limit the time spent in the sun. Ultraviolet radiation is most intense between 10:00 am and 3:00 pm and in the months of June to September. Limit outdoor activities during these times when possible.
- Use protective clothing. Long sleeves, long pants, and brimmed hats can protect against ultraviolet radiation.
- Use sunscreen. Sunscreen should be applied at least 30 minutes before exposure and should be reapplied every 2 to 3 hours. Waterproof products with an SPF (sun protection factor) rating of 15 or higher provide the best protection.
- Protect children from overexposure.
- Protect skin on hazy days and on sunny days. Clouds normally do not screen out ultraviolet rays.
- Be aware that certain foods, medications, and chemicals can worsen the effects of ultraviolet radiation on the skin. Medications such as some antihypertensive drugs, antibiotics, and antiinflammatory agents may produce photosensitivity. Some cosmetics, shampoos, and deodorants may also enhance photosensitivity.
- Avoid indoor tanning. Ultraviolet-A radiation is emitted by sun lamps and can increase the risk of skin cancer, eye injury, and skin aging.

include community environmental health issues. In nursing, environmental health has traditionally been limited to the immediate environment of the individual (e.g., hospitalized patient) or to the family home (e.g., home safety). It is essential, however, that all nurses be prepared to address a multitude of environmental health issues as described here. In taking a proactive role in health teaching, counseling, and advocacy regarding actual and potential environmental threats, nurses are indeed able to promote health and prevent illness and disability.

SUMMARY

A significant number of potential environmental health problems have been described in this chapter. They include threats related to housing and living patterns, air pollution, water pollution, food quality, radiation, and solid waste. Nurses like Susan, the pediatric nurse in the chapter-opening case study, must recognize the common environmental threats in their communities and work with other health care providers to identify and intervene in those areas and take steps to prevent environmental health problems.

By taking a proactive role in health teaching, counseling, and advocacy regarding actual and potential environmental threats, nurses are able to promote health and prevent illness and disability.

KEY POINTS

- Environmental factors have a great impact on human development, health, and disease. Public health efforts have been very successful in reducing threats to health through improving the safety

of food and water, managing waste disposal and sewage, and controlling or eliminating vector-borne illnesses. Contemporary environmental health threats come from toxic and ecological effects associated with the use of fossil fuels, synthetic chemicals, and other sources.

- Threats related to housing and living patterns include overcrowding, household chemical exposure, and violence. Indoor air quality may be affected by combustion pollutants (e.g., secondhand smoke, exhausts from space heaters), particles (e.g., asbestos, pollen), and living organisms. Lead may be present in peeling paint and in some water pipes.
- Millions of illnesses and injuries each year are related to workplace risks and hazards. Use of heavy equipment; exposure to chemicals and biohazards, sunlight, cold, and noise; and potential for assault or violence can threaten workers. The OSHA has been given the responsibility for protection of workers and has set and enforces standards to improve worker safety and health.
- Atmospheric quality is threatened by air pollutants that can cause lung damage, inflammatory

COMMUNITY APPLICATION
Prevention Interventions for Environmental Safety and Health

PRIMARY PREVENTION

- Advocate safer environmental design of products, automobiles, equipment, and buildings.
- Teach home safety related to falls and fire prevention, especially to families with children and elderly members.
- Counsel women of childbearing age regarding exposure to environmental hazards.
- Advocate vehicle protection systems, such as seat belts.
- Advocate use of protective devices, such as earplugs for noise.
- Immunize occupationally exposed workers for hepatitis B.
- Develop work site health and safety programs.
- Develop programs to prevent back injuries at work.
- Support the development of exposure standards for toxins.
- Support disclosure of radon and lead concentrations in homes at time of sale.
- Advocate for safe air and water.
- Teach avoidance of ultraviolet exposure and use of sunscreen.
- Advocate for reduced waste reduction and effective waste management.
- Support programs for waste reduction and recycling.

SECONDARY PREVENTION

- Assess homes, schools, work sites, and communities for environmental hazards.
- Routinely obtain occupational health histories for individuals, counsel about hazard reduction, and refer for diagnosis and treatment.
- Screen children from 6 months to 5 years for blood lead levels.
- Monitor workers for levels of chemical exposure.
- Screen at-risk workers for lung disease, cancer, and hearing loss.
- Participate in data collection regarding the incidence and prevalence of injury and disability in homes, schools, and work sites.

TERTIARY PREVENTION

- Encourage limitation of activity when air pollution is high.
- Support cleanup of toxic waste sites and removal of other hazards.
- Provide appropriate nursing care at work sites or in the home for persons with chronic lung diseases and injury-related disabilities.
- Refer homeowners to approved lead abatement resources.

From Smith C: Environmental health risks: at home, at work and in the community. In Maurer FA, Smith CM, editors: *Community/public health nursing: health for families and populations*, ed 3, St Louis, 2005, Saunders.

responses, and respiratory symptoms. Major air pollutants include ozone, carbon monoxide, nitrogen dioxide, particulates, sulfur dioxide, and lead. The burning of fossil fuels (i.e., gasoline, coal, oil) contributes greatly to air pollution.

- Ensurance of a safe, clean water supply is necessary to health. Sewage, industrial processes and wastes, and agricultural chemicals are the main sources of water pollution. Waterborne diseases can be caused by bacteria, viruses, and protozoa. Common chemical contaminants include pesticides, petrochemicals, lead, and other compounds.
- Food quality may be threatened by both intentional and unintentional food additives (e.g., biological and chemical contaminants). Microbiological contamination is usually caused by improper storage, handling, and/or preparation of food. Intentional food additives include substances added to food during processing to enhance the nutritional content, improve flavor, enhance color, improve consistency, or increase the shelf life.

Unintentional food additives are those substances that enter and remain in food as a result of being used as pesticides or added to animal food or from packaging.

- The volume of solid wastes and problems concerning the disposal of toxic and hazardous wastes present threats to the health and well-being of U.S. residents. Effective solid waste management is essential to decreasing pathogen transmission through insect and rodent control and eliminating potential exposure to toxic and infectious materials.
- Radiation threats to health come from several sources, most commonly radon gas and the sun. Radon is a colorless, odorless gas that causes thousands of deaths each year, most commonly from lung cancer. Radon enters buildings through cracks in solid floors, construction joints, and other ways, and dangerously high levels can be found in many homes. Skin cancer is the most common form of cancer in the United States, and

exposure to the sun is associated with all three major types of skin cancer.

Learning Activities & Application to Practice
In Class

1. With classmates, discuss each of the areas of environmental health presented. Give examples of health problems you have encountered related to each area. Discuss prevention efforts for each problem discussed, including primary, secondary, and tertiary interventions.

In Clinical

2. Observe for illnesses or health conditions or risks associated with environmental health threats encountered during clinical experiences. For example, in a clinic you might care for a toddler who is being screened for lead, an adult with carpal tunnel syndrome associated with using a computer, or an elder with skin cancer. Record these in a clinical log or diary and share with other students in the clinical group. How could the risk(s) be prevented or minimized?

3. Be prepared to teach clients about environmental threats to health and safety. Identify times when health education is appropriate (e.g., teaching a new mother not to use hot tap water to make formula, teaching the ABCDs of skin cancer and skin assessment to all adults, and teaching ways to reduce food contamination to high school students).

REFERENCES

American Cancer Society (2007a): *Cancer facts & figures–2007*, Atlanta, 2007, American Cancer Society.

American Cancer Society (2007b): *Skin cancer–melanoma* (website): http://www.cancer.org/docroot/CRI/CRI_2_3x.asp?dt=39. Accessed October 10, 2007. Blumenthal D: Red no. 3 and other colorful controversies, *FDA Consum*, May, 1990.

Centers for Disease Control and Prevention (2007a): *Carbon monoxide poisoning* (website): http://www.cdc.gov/co/guidelines.htm. Accessed October 10, 2007.

Centers for Disease Control and Prevention (2007b): *Selected diseases spread through drinking water (United States)* (website): http://www.cdc.gov/ncidod/diseases/water/drinking.htm. Accessed October 10, 2007.

Centers for Disease Control and Prevention (2007): *Lead in water: questions and answers* (website): http://www.cdc.gov/print.

do?url=http://www.cdc.gov/nceh/lead/faq/leadinwater.htm. Accessed October 11, 2007.

Centers for Disease Control and Prevention (2006a): *Secondhand smoke: fact sheet* (website): http://www.cdc.gov/tobacco/data_statistics/Factsheets/SecondhandSmoke.htm. Accessed October 10, 2007.

Centers for Disease Control and Prevention (2006b): Surveillance for waterborne disease and outbreaks associated with recreational water–United States 2003-2004; Surveillance for waterborne disease and outbreaks associated with drinking water and water not intended for drinking–United States 2003-2004, *MMWR Morb Mortal Wkly Rep* 55(SS-12):1, 2006.

Centers for Disease Control and Prevention (2005): *Preventing lead exposure in young children: a housing-based approach to primary prevention of lead poisoning* (website): http://www.cdc.gov/nceh/lead/publications/Primary%20Prevention%20Document.pdf. Accessed October 10, 2007.

Centers for Disease Control and Prevention: Recommendations for blood lead screening of young children enrolled in Medicaid, *MMWR Morb Mortal Wkly Rep* 49(RR-14):1, 2000.

Centers for Disease Control and Prevention: *Screening young children for lead poisoning: guide for state and offices*, Atlanta, 1997, Centers for Disease Control and Prevention.

Centers for Disease Control and Prevention: *Preventing lead poisoning in young children*, Atlanta, 1991, Centers for Disease Control and Prevention.

Craun MF, Craun GF, Calderon RL et al: Waterborne outbreaks reported in the United States, *J Water Health* 4(suppl 2):19, 2006.

Environmental Protection Agency (2007a): *An introduction to indoor air quality: biological pollutants* (website): http://www.epa.gov/iaq/biologic.html#Reducing%20Exposure%20to%20Biological%20Contaminants. Accessed October 11, 2007.

Environmental Protection Agency (2007b): *The plain English guide to The Clean Air Act* (website): http://www.epa.gov/air/caa/peg/. Accessed October 10, 2007.

Environmental Protection Agency (2007c): *Ozone* (website): http://www.epa.gov/ozone/. Accessed October 10, 2007.

Environmental Protection Agency (2007d): *What you can do to clean the air* (website): http://www.epa.gov/air/actions/.Accessed October 10, 2007.

Environmental Protection Agency (2007e): *Basic facts about waste* (website): http://www.epa.gov/epaoswer/osw/facts.htm. Accessed October 10, 2007.

Environmental Protection Agency (2007f): *Radon health risks* (website): http://www.epa.gov/iaq/radon/healthrisks.html. Accessed October 10, 2007.

Environmental Protection Agency (2007): *Basic information: medical waste* (website): http://www.epa.gov/epaoswer/other/medical/basic.htm#three. Accessed October 11, 2007.

Environmental Protection Agency: *A citizen's guide to radon* (EPA Publication No. 402-K02-006), Washington, DC, 2005, Government Printing Office.

Foulke JE: Mercury in fish: Cause for concern?, *FDA Consum* 28(7):1, 1994.

Hall JM, Robinson CH, Broyles TJ: Environmental health. In Neis M, McEwen M, editors: *Community/public health nursing: promoting the health of populations*, ed 4, St Louis, 2007, Saunders.

McKeown T: Determinants of health. In Lee PR, Estes CL, editors: The nation's health, ed 4, Boston, 1995, Jones and Bartlett.

National Cancer Institute (2005): *What you need to know about skin cancer* (website): http://www.cancer.gov/cancertopics/wyntk/skin. Accessed October 10, 2007.

Primomo J, Salazar MK: Environmental health risks: at home, at work and in the community. In Maurer FA, Smith CM, editors: *Community/public health nursing: health for families and populations*, ed 3, St Louis, 2005, Saunders.

Rogers B: *Occupational health nursing: concepts and practice*, ed 2, Philadelphia, 2003, W.B. Saunders.

U.S. Department of Health and Human Services: *Healthy people 2010. national health promotion and disease prevention objectives*, Washington, DC, 2000, Government Printing Office.

U.S. Department of Labor Bureau of Labor Statistics (2006a): *Workplace injuries and illnesses in 2005* (website): http://stats.bls.gov/iif/oshwc/osh/os/osnr0025.pdf. Accessed October 10, 2007.

U.S. Department of Labor Bureau of Labor Statistics (2006b): Nonfatal occupational injuries and illnesses requiring days from work–2005 (website): http://stats.bls.gov/iif/oshwc/osh/case/osnr0027.pdf. Accessed October 10, 2007.

Wagner B: FDA keeps antennae out for insect fragments, *FDA Consum*, November, 1992.

Cultural Influences on Health

objectives

objectives

Upon completion of this chapter, the reader will be able to:

1. Discuss the importance of providing culturally sensitive and culturally competent nursing care.

2. Differentiate among race, ethnicity, and culture, and describe characteristics of each.

3. Explain the relationships between socioeconomic status and culture and socioeconomic status and health.

4. Perform a cultural assessment.

5. Describe cultural variations related to diet, communication patterns, language, and religion.

6. Discuss variations in health patterns and common health problems among European Americans, Blacks, Hispanics, American Indians, and Asian/Pacific Islanders.

key terms

Culture	Subculture	
Ethnic group	Transcultural nursing	*See Glossary for definitions.*
Race		

case study

Trisha Thomas is a registered nurse working in a city-sponsored pediatric clinic in a large southwestern city. At the clinic Trisha primarily sees low-income clients, most of whom are eligible for Medicaid or have no personal health insurance. More than 75% of the clients seen in the clinic are from minority groups, and almost half are Hispanic. Other racial and ethnic groups seen include African-Americans, Southeast Asians (Vietnamese, Cambodian, and Laotian), and increasingly immigrants from Middle-Eastern and African countries (Iraqi Kurds and refugees from Somalia, Ethiopia, and Uganda).

Because Trisha has practiced nursing at the clinic for almost 4 years, she has learned to speak Spanish fairly well. She is able to perform assessments, take health histories, and teach effectively in that language. In addition, the clinic has interpreters for several of the most common languages heard at the clinic.

Continued

Trisha's experience working with people from many different cultures has given her an awareness of their health practices, beliefs, diet, and religions. This in turn has enabled her to conduct more thorough assessments and provide more effective teaching and anticipatory guidance than most of her colleagues.

On Thursday Trisha saw Carlos Sepulveda for his well-child visit. Carlos is 5 years old and will begin kindergarten this fall. Because Carlos' health care is financed through Medicaid, Trisha performed an Early and Periodic Screening, Diagnosis, and Treatment (EPSDT) examination (see Chapter 12), which includes a complete physical examination, developmental testing, height and weight measurements, and screenings for vision and hearing, lead, and anemia. Review of Carlos' immunization records showed that he was due for his second diphtheria-pertussis-tetanus and polio boosters and his second measles/mumps/rubella and varicella vaccinations.

Although Mrs. Sepulveda does not speak English, Trisha was able to gain information about Carlos' diet, sleeping habits, and activity. She learned that the family lives in a subsidized apartment in a safe area. The apartment has smoke detectors, and all medications and cleaning products are in cabinets with child-proof latches.

All of the findings from the physical assessment were normal. However, Carlos was small for his age (less than the twentieth percentile). Knowing that because of financial constraints and cultural preferences Carlos' diet might be deficient in protein, calcium, and some vitamins, Trisha directed her health teaching to his nutritional needs. After questioning Mrs. Sepulveda about his daily diet, Trisha gave her information on how to increase these nutrients and referred her to the Women, Infants, and Children (WIC) program (see Chapter 12) located in their building. Before Mrs. Sepulveda and Carlos left to see the WIC counselor, Trisha made an appointment for Carlos to return in 6 months for further evaluation.

The United States is becoming increasingly ethnically diverse. According to U.S. Department of Health and Human Services (USDHHS) reports, members of ethnic minority groups in the United States are disproportionately impoverished and have poorer health outcomes and fewer options for seeking health care (USDHHS, 2000). One of the two broad goals of *Healthy People 2010* is to "Reduce health disparities among Americans," and a number of objectives are specifically directed toward members of various racial and ethnic groups. The *Healthy People 2010* box provides examples of objectives that address the improvement of the health of members of minority groups.

Although the Americas have been a melting pot since colonization began in the 1600s, the makeup of the population is changing. Figures 8-1 and 8-2 depict year 2000 and estimated year 2020 population breakdowns by racial and ethnic groups. As these pie charts show, the percentage of whites is declining and the greatest growth is being seen in Hispanics and other immigrants, largely from Southeast Asia.

Many of the objectives from *Healthy People 2010* that address the disparity between people from various ethnic groups cite health problems that lead to differences in morbidity and mortality. For example, alcoholism is more common in American Indians, resulting in increases in liver disease and accidental injuries. Diabetes is much more prevalent in American Indians, Hispanics, and blacks, contributing to related complications and deaths in those groups. To further illustrate some of the differences between health problems found in racial and ethnic groups, Table 8-1 lists the ten leading causes of death for whites, Hispanics, blacks, American Indians, and Asians.

TRANSCULTURAL NURSING

Nurses who practice in community settings are often in a position to provide nursing care to clients from diverse racial and ethnic groups. To foster understanding and assist those individuals with nursing and health care needs, the Transcultural Nursing Society was established in 1973 by Madeline Leininger (Leininger, 2001a).

healthy
people 2010

Selected Objectives Addressing the Health of Racial and Ethnic Minorities

OBJECTIVE	BASELINE (1998)	TARGET
1.1: Increase the proportion of persons with health insurance (Hispanic or Latino)	70%	100%
1.8g: Increase nursing degrees awarded to underrepresented populations (black)	6.9%	13%
3.1: Reduce the overall cancer death rate (black)	262.1 per 100,000	158.7 per 100,000
5.3: Reduce the overall rate of diabetes that is clinically diagnosed (Hispanic)	61 per 1000	25 per 1000
8.11: Eliminate elevated blood lead levels in children (black)	11.5%	0%
9.7: Reduce pregnancies among adolescent females (black)	133 per 1000	42 per 1000
5.1: Reduce firearm-related deaths (black)	23.7 per 100,000	4.9 per 100,000
16.1h: Reduce deaths from SIDS (American Indian or Alaska Native)	1.56 per 1000	0.3 per 1000
18.1: Reduce suicide rate (American Indian or Alaska Native)	12.4 per 100,000	6 per 100,000
19.2: Reduce the proportion of adults who are obese (Hispanic)	29%	15%
27.1: Reduce cigarette smoking by adults (American Indian or Alaska Native)	34%	12%

SIDS, Sudden infant death syndrome.
Data from U.S. Department of Health and Human Services: *Healthy people 2010*, Conference ed, Washington, DC, 2000, Government Printing Office.

According to Herberg, "**Transcultural nursing** is concerned with the provision of nursing care in a manner that is sensitive to the needs of individuals, families and groups" where "a thorough assessment of the cultural aspect of a client's lifestyle, health beliefs and health practices will enhance the nurse's decision making and judgment when providing care" (1995, p. 3). Culturally sensitive nursing interventions show appreciation of and respect for differences and attempt to decrease the possibility of stress or conflict arising from cultural misunderstanding.

The American Academy of Nursing (1992) is commited to quality and "culturally competent" nursing care. Their recommendations include the following:

- Promotion of culturally competent care that is equitable and accessible
- Development and maintenance of a disciplinary knowledge base and expertise in culturally competent care

- Synthesis of existing theoretical and research knowledge regarding nursing care of different ethnic or minority, stigmatized, and disenfranchised populations
- Creation of an interdisciplinary knowledge base that reflects heterogeneous health care practices within various cultural groups
- Identification and examination of methods, theories, and frameworks appropriate for utilization in the development of knowledge related to health care of minority, stigmatized, and disenfranchised populations
- Establishment of ways to teach and guide faculty and nursing students to provide culture-specific care and to support the regulation of content reflecting diversity in nursing curricula

In accordance with these recommendations, nurses—particularly those working in community settings—should be knowledgeable of cultural

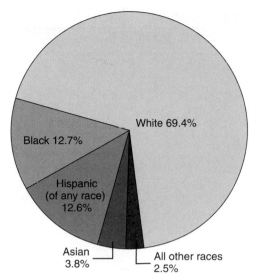

Figure 8-1. Population by race/Hispanic origin, 2000. (Data from: U.S. Bureau of the Census: *Projected population of the United States by race and Hispanic origin: 2000 to 2050* (website): http://www.census.gov/ipc/www/usinterimproj/natprojtab01a.pdf . Accessed August 28, 2007.

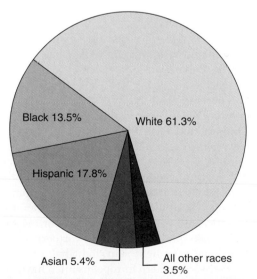

Figure 8-2. Population by race/Hispanic origin, 2020 (estimated). (Data from U.S. Bureau of the Census: Projected population of the United States by race and Hispanic origin: 2000 to 2050 (website): http://www.census.gov/ipc/www/usinterimproj/natprojtab01a.pdf. Accessed August 28, 2007.

differences and how those differences influence health and health practices. Nurses should be prepared to work within these differences to improve health. Nursing care and interventions to address problems related to cultural, hereditary, social, and other factors that contribute to differences in morbidity and mortality are described in this chapter.

CULTURE AND RELATED CONCEPTS

The terms *race*, *ethnic group*, and *culture* are frequently confused. They may be used interchangeably in error because they refer to different, although sometimes overlapping, concepts. Lack of recognition of the differences and subsequent misuse of the terms may incur confusion or misunderstanding.

RACE

Race refers to classification or grouping of humans primarily based on physical characteristics (e.g., skin color, hair color and texture, eye shape and color, height). Anthropologically, individuals from a given race have a common geographic ancestral origin. Early anthropologists recognized three races, based largely on skin color: (1) Caucasoid (white), (2) Mongoloid (yellow), and (3) Negroid (black). According to Garn (1965), research studies during the twentieth century led anthropologists to conclude that nine major geographical races exist, roughly based on continental divisions. These races are the following:

- African: A collection of related races in sub-Saharan Africa. Members have curly, tightly coiled hair, thick lips, and large amounts of melanin in the skin, hair, and gums. American blacks are mostly of African origin.
- American Indian: The earliest inhabitants of the Western Hemisphere, American Indians are related to Asians but have different blood groups. Skin color ranges from light to dark brown, and hair is black and straight.
- Asian: Populations are found in continental Asia (except South Asia and the Middle East), including Japan, Taiwan, the Philippines, and parts of Indonesia. Members have straight black hair, inner eyefolds, and pads of fat over their cheekbones. Most have light brown skin and are smaller in stature than Europeans.

TABLE **8-1** Ten Leading Causes of Death for Various Races (2004)

WHITE NON-HISPANICS	BLACKS	HISPANICS	AMERICAN INDIANS	ASIANS/PACIFIC ISLANDERS
Heart disease	Heart disease	Heart disease	Heart disease	Cancer
Cancer	Cancer	Cancer	Cancer	Heart disease
Stroke	Stroke	Injuries	Injuries	Stroke
COPD	Diabetes	Stroke	Diabetes	Injuries
Injuries	Injuries	Diabetes	Stroke	Diabetes
Alzheimer's disease	Homicide	Liver disease	Liver disease	Pneumonia/influenza
Diabetes	Kidney disease	Homicide	COPD	COPD
Pneumonia/ influenza	COPD	COPD	Suicide	Suicide
Kidney disease	AIDS	Pneumonia/influenza	Pneumonia/influenza	Kidney disease
Suicide	Septicemia	Perinatal conditions	Kidney disease	Alzheimer's disease

COPD, Chronic obstructive pulmonary disease.
From U.S. Department of Health and Human Services/ National Center for Health Statistics: *Health: United States–2006* (website): http://www.cdc.gov/nchs/data/hus/hus06.pdf#027. Accessed July 26, 2007.

- Australian (Australian Aborigine): These groups are native to Australia. Members have large teeth, narrow skulls, and very dark skin coloring; some have hair that is brown or red-gold in childhood.
- European: Comprises groups throughout Europe, the Middle East, and northern Africa. Group members have lighter skin than do other peoples. The "whites" of Australia, North and South America, and South Africa are members of the European race.
- Indian: Populations in South Asia from the Himalayas to the Indian Ocean. Skin color ranges from light in the north to dark in the south. Blood groups differ somewhat from those of Europeans.
- Melanesian-Papuan: Peoples of New Guinea and Solomon Islands. Melanesians resemble Africans in skin color and have hair that curls and frizzes but have different blood group frequencies than Africans.
- Micronesian: Comprises occupants of islands in the Pacific (e.g., Carolines, Gilberts, Marianas,

Marshalls). Micronesians are small and dark-skinned and have wavy or woolly hair. They resemble Polynesians somewhat in blood group frequencies.
- Polynesian: Far southern Pacific Islanders, Polynesians include people from Hawaii, New Zealand, and Easter Island. Members are tall, may be heavy, and have light to moderate skin color (Garn, 1965).

Although descendants of a given geographical race are similar, variations exist in people from different subgeographical areas, and they may differ quite noticeably from other members of the same race. For example, people from Northern Europe usually have very light skin, light hair, and blue eyes, whereas Southern Europeans often have olive skin, dark hair, and dark eyes. Likewise, Alaskan Inuits vary significantly from Southern American Indian tribes in height and other characteristics, and members of central and eastern African tribes may vary greatly from the Bushmen of South Africa. Race is largely unchanging, although intermarrying between races and subsequent mixing of races occurs frequently. This results in the lessening of some of the distinctive characteristics of each race.

ETHNIC GROUP

An **ethnic group** is a group of people who share common, distinctive characteristics such as race, ancestry, nationality, language, religion, food preferences, literature, and music and have a common history. According to Spector (2004), at least 106 ethnic groups are recognized in the United States, and more than 500 American Indian Nations exist.

Although members of ethnic groups share similar cultural patterns, values, beliefs, customs, behavior, and traditions, intraethnic variations usually exist. For example, in the United States, Hispanic-Americans represent a large ethnic group that varies significantly based on country or area of origin; this ethnic group contains Cuban-Americans, Puerto Ricans, Mexican-Americans, and people from Central America, among others. Likewise, African-Americans differ from Caribbean blacks or sub-Saharan Africans, and different tribal groups in Africa may vary greatly from each other.

CULTURE

In 1871 Sir Edward Tylor, an English anthropologist, defined **culture** as the "complex whole, including knowledge, beliefs, art, morals, law, customs and other capabilities and habits acquired by virtue of the fact that one is a member of a particular society" (Andrews, 2007, p. 210). Other definitions of culture include "nonphysical traits, such as values, beliefs, attitudes and customs that are shared by a group of people and passed from one generation to the next" (Spector, 2004, p. 310); "the totality of socially transmitted behavioral patterns, arts, beliefs, values, customs, life-ways...characteristics of a population of people that guide their worldview and decision making" (Purnell and Paulanka, 2003, p.3); and "a way of perceiving, behaving and evaluating the world...a guide for determining people's values, beliefs and practices" (Andrews, 1999a, p. 3). Culture, therefore, provides the organizational structure or basis for behavior within the group. Culture is not necessarily tied to race because members of a given culture may be

from different races. Culture, however, *is* a component of ethnicity.

To illustrate the differences in these concepts, a second-generation Cuban-American who lives in Miami and whose ancestors were African slaves might be classified as follows:

- Race: African/Black
- Ethnicity: Hispanic
- Cultural group: South Floridian/Cuban-American
  Another example would be an immigrant from Korea residing in Houston:
- Race: Asian
- Ethnicity: South Korean
- Cultural group: Korean-American/Texan
  Various terms are used in discussing race, ethnicity, and culture. To clarify some of the differences, Box 8-1 gives definitions of terms commonly used in reference to culture and cultural issues.

CHARACTERISTICS OF CULTURE

According to Allender and Spradley (2005), anthropologists and sociologists have identified a number of characteristics common to all cultures. Some characteristics that are particularly pertinent to the practice of nursing are listed in Box 8-2.

A **subculture** is a relatively large subsection of a cultural group; it has distinctive characteristics that set it apart from the group as a whole. Teenage gangs, professional football players, members of the military, and nursing students might be considered subcultures. Based on the characteristics described in Table 8-2 (p. 134), members of each of these groups must learn the cultural values, norms, practices, and other characteristics of the group. The soldier must learn terminology, skills, behaviors, and so forth to become a member of the group. In the same way the beliefs, values, and practices of professional football players are integrated into other aspects of their actions. Cultural values, beliefs, and practices of teenage gang members are shared. Nursing students (and other health care providers) do not need to explain thoughts, actions, and beliefs to other health care providers—rationale for actions is largely understood or implied. Finally, each of the subculture examples listed must remain adaptive and dynamic to subsist and grow.

To illustrate differences in subcultural groups, consider a white middle-class family from rural

BOX 8-1 Terms Used in Transcultural Nursing Care

CULTURE SHOCK

"Feelings of bewilderment, confusion, disorganization, frustration, and stupidity, and the inability to adapt to differences in language and word meanings, activities, time, and customs that are part of the new culture" (Murray, Zentner, Samiezade'-Yazd 2001, p. 46)

CULTURAL BLINDNESS

Failure to acknowledge or respect cultural differences and behaving as though the differences do not exist

DOMINANT VALUE ORIENTATION

The basic value orientation that is shared by the majority of the members of a cultural group as a result of early common experiences

DISCRIMINATION

The differential treatment of individuals because they belong to a minority group; denying equal opportunity by acting on a prejudice

ENCULTURATION (ACCULTURATION)

The process of becoming a member of a cultural group; adapting to another culture

ETHNICITY

A classification of individuals based on a shared culture or affiliation, values, perceptions, feelings, and assumptions

ETHNOCENTRISM

The belief that one's own group is superior to others

MINORITY GROUP

A segment of the population that differs from the majority based on physical or cultural characteristics

NORMS

The rules by which human behavior is governed that are the result of the cultural values held by a group

PREJUDICE

A hostile attitude toward individuals because they belong to a particular racial or ethnic group presumed to have objectionable qualities; generalized negative beliefs or preferences about a group that lead to prejudgment

RACISM

Excessive belief in the superiority of one's own racial group

STEREOTYPING

The belief or notion that all people from a given group are the same

VALUES

Personal perceptions of what is good or useful; desirable beliefs and standards

BOX 8-2 Characteristics of Culture

CULTURE IS LEARNED

- Cultural behaviors are acquired, not inherited; enculturation is learned through socialization and language acquisition.

CULTURE IS INTEGRATED

- The various components of a culture are simultaneously interrelated and independent; they are an integrated web of ideas, beliefs, and practices.

CULTURE IS SHARED

- Cultural values, beliefs, and practices are shared by the members of the culture and identify and stabilize the cultural group.

CULTURE IS MOSTLY TACIT

- Much of culture is outside of awareness; members of a culture know how to act and what to expect without need for discussion.

CULTURE IS DYNAMIC

- Every culture experiences constant change.

Data from Allender JA, Spradley BW: *Community health nursing: promoting and protecting the public's health*, ed 6, Philadelphia, 2005, Lippincott Williams & Wilkins.

Iowa and a white middle-class family from Los Angeles. In these two families, variations in values, language, dress, diet, leisure activities, expectations, and so on would exist. Similarly, a working-class Puerto Rican family living in New York City varies markedly from a Mexican family living in the Rio Grande valley.

CULTURAL ASSESSMENT

Nurses who work in community-based settings must recognize the impact of culture on health and health practices, and they should be familiar with the beliefs, values, and practices of the members of cultural groups they may care for. To gain an understanding, pertinent information should be assessed by the nurse; this may be accomplished by using all or part of one of several cultural assessment instruments. Excellent assessment guides for nurses have been developed by Andrews and Boyle (2003) and Giger and Davidhizar (2004) (see Appendix A). Some of the components to be considered in cultural assessment are values, socioeconomic status, communication patterns and language, nutrition and dietary habits, religion and religious practices, health beliefs and practices, and biocultural aspects of disease incidence. These are briefly addressed.

CULTURAL VALUES

Values are personal perceptions of what is good or useful and are a universal feature of all cultures. Among other purposes, values give meaning to life, provide self-esteem, serve as goals or motivators that direct behaviors, and form the foundation for the individual person on personal, professional, social, political, and philosophical issues.

Much of U.S. culture has been shaped by a dominant cultural group (white middle class) whose values include marriage and family, parental responsibility to children, work ethic, individuality, material wealth, comfort, humanitarianism, physical beauty, democracy, newness, cleanliness, education, science and technology, achievement, free enterprise, punctuality, rationality, independence, respectability, effort and progress, family unity and stability, pursuit of recreational activities, equality of people, future orientation, economic security for the present and future, sporting events, and cultural arts (Leininger, 2001b; Murray, Zentner, and Samiezade'-Yazd, 2001). Because these values are so entrenched in U.S. culture, often members of the dominant cultural group fail to recognize that these values are not universally shared or even understood by members of other cultural groups.

To assist nurses in understanding differences in values among various cultural groups, Leininger (2001a) and others have researched several different groups. Table 8-2 compares cultural values identified by the research of Leininger (2001b) for several of the most prevalent U.S. cultural groups.

SOCIOECONOMIC STATUS

In addition to variations based on racial or ethnic groups, cultural variations based on socioeconomic levels, or class, strongly influence health and health-seeking behaviors. Like other components of culture, socioeconomic class creates a set of values and role expectations regarding factors such as sex, marriage, parenting, birth, education, dress, housing, reading, occupation, and religion. In the United States health status is more closely linked to income level than to race or ethnicity (USDHHS, 2000). Indeed, poor people, regardless of race or ethnicity, are more likely to experience poor health and poor health care. Murray, Zentner, and Samiezade'-Yazd (2001) describe the following socioeconomic subcultures:

- Upper-upper level: This "affluent, or corporate level" is characterized by a small number of people who have money and power. Values include home, position, lineage, power and prestige, economic achievements, education, possession of art, and philanthropy.
- Lower-upper level: The "new rich" are persons who possess large incomes and lifestyles that flaunt their money. They have and value an abundance of possessions.
- Overclass: This is a new social class made up of professionals and managers who are upwardly mobile and have earned wealth through hard work. Many are urban singles and couples without children. They tend to be transnational, although many live on the coasts. Values include competitive achievement both on the job and in leisure.
- Upper-middle level: This level, which may be described as "well off," includes college-educated

TABLE **8-2** Comparison of the Values of Various Cultural Groups

CHARACTERISTIC	ANGLO-AMERICANS	AFRICAN AMERICANS	MEXICAN AMERICANS	AMERICAN INDIANS	ARAB-AMERICANS/ MUSLIMS	JAPANESE AMERICANS
Dependency	Value independence and freedom; focus on self-reliance	Interdependent with other blacks	Extended family valued; interdependent with kin and social activities	Stress harmony between land, people, and environment	Providing family care and support is a responsibility	Duty and obligation to kin and work group
Health and Healing	Value scientific/ medical facts and technology	May employ folk healing and home remedies	May use traditional folk care healers; may believe in hot-cold theory	Folk healers (e.g., Shamans) may be used	Obligation and responsibility to visit and help the sick	Attention to physical complaints; value personal cleanliness; may use folk therapies
Religion/ Spirituality	N/A	Religion valued (many are Baptists)	Religion valued (many are Catholic)	Maintain spiritual inspiration (spirit guidance)	Follow the teaching of the Koran; offering prayers (5 times each day)	N/A
Achievement/ Possessions	Value competition and achievement; materialism	Value technology (e.g., radio, car)	N/A	Value the practice of cultural rituals and taboos	Helping to "save face" and preserve cultural values is important	Ambitious and achievement oriented; maintain high educational standards
Hierarchical Structure/ Authority	Focus on the individual; less respect for authority and elders	Reliance on extended family networks	Patriarchy; respect for authority and elders	Authority of tribal elders; respect and value of children	Respect and protect different gender roles	Patriarchal obligations and respect elders; value; honor elders
Other	Value youth and beauty; leisure time important	Value music and physical activities	Value native foods; little concern for exact time	Pride in cultural heritage and "Nations"	Value knowing cultural taboos and norms	Futurists; politeness and ritual valued

N/A, not specifically addressed
Data from Leininger MM: *Culture care diversity and universality: a theory of nursing*, Boston, 2001, Jones and Bartlett.

professionals (e.g., doctors, dentists, engineers, lawyers). Children and family stability are highly valued. Education, hard work, career success, responsibility, honesty, security, materialism, various leisure activities, and travel are also valued.

- Middle level: Included in this level are people who have small or medium-sized businesses, skilled workers, office workers, teachers, and nurses. They are usually educated above the high school level. They live in middle-class neighborhoods and have two cars (often a van or SUV). Persons at this level are usually characterized by nuclear families and are child-oriented. Education, creativity, hard work, thrift, patience, planning ahead, and postponing immediate rewards are valued.
- Lower-middle level: Often referred to as the "working class," this level includes high school graduates with industrial or "blue-collar" jobs, clerical workers, technicians, semiskilled workers, and waitresses. Chances of advancement are minimal. Persons at this level live in small homes or apartments and possess one or two cars. Their values include patriotism, religion, authority, work ethic, honesty, neatness, respectability, self-reliance, independence, conformity, competition, achievement, education, and saving for the future. Adults are typically less educated and read less. Childrearing is taken for granted, and parents often rely heavily on the extended family for support.
- Upper-lower level: Included at this level are those who work at menial tasks (e.g., fast-food workers, domestics, gardeners, maintenance, garbage collectors) but are grateful for employment. Persons in this group often did not complete high school, were early parents with a rapid succession of children, and may have an early separation or divorce.
- Underclass: Comprises those in both acute and chronic poverty. Members of the underclass usually have a history of being unemployed or underemployed. Many of the underclass are children (about 45% of people living in poverty are children). Single-parent (usually matriarchal) families are very common. Other underclass groups are homeless people, migrant workers, immigrants and refugees and their families, and many elders. Low self-esteem, mistrust of others, anger, susceptibility to drug and alcohol abuse, teen pregnancy, and incarceration are not uncommon. Frequently the poor have not finished high school and are unskilled; they may be employed in temporary or seasonal jobs and/or rely on public assistance.

LANGUAGE AND COMMUNICATION

LANGUAGE
Language barriers are among the most commonly encountered problems in working with members of other cultural groups. Ideally the nurse speaks the client's language; in areas of high concentration of a minority group, many nurses are bilingual. For example, South Florida, Southern California, Arizona, New Mexico, and South Texas have a greater percentage of Spanish-speaking Hispanic and non-Hispanic nurses. In areas with many immigrants from China, Japan, and Southeast Asia (e.g., San Francisco), nurses who speak one or more Asian languages or dialects are often found. However, it is becoming increasingly common for the nurse and the client to be unable to speak the same language, and nurses need to be prepared and creative to adjust to this challenge. The Community Application boxes "Overcoming Language Barriers: Use of an Interpreter" and "Overcoming Language Barriers When No Interpreter Is Available" offer strategies for dealing with language barriers.

COMMUNICATION PATTERNS
When caring for clients from culturally diverse backgrounds, the nurse should recognize and identify variations in communication patterns. Communication is transmitted by body cues (e.g., touch, space, distance, position), paralinguistic cues (e.g., voice inflection, intonation, rhythm), and pronunciation and vocabulary (Giger and Davidhizar, 2004). Recognition of variations in communication patterns and familiarity with differences are important to delivering culturally appropriate care.

Nonverbal communication includes pitch, tone, and quality of the voice; use of silence; use of eye contact; posture; facial expression; gestures; object cues (e.g., clothes, jewelry, hair style); touch; and use of territorial space. Wide variations may exist in each of these, and nurses should recognize and interpret variations correctly and adapt practice accordingly.

COMMUNITY APPLICATION
Overcoming Language Barriers: Use of an Interpreter

- Before locating an interpreter, be sure you know what language the client speaks at home because it may be different from the language spoken publicly (e.g., French is sometimes spoken by aristocratic or well-educated people from certain Asian or Middle Eastern cultures).
- The nurse should avoid interpreters from a rival tribe, state, region, or nation (e.g., a Palestinian who knows Hebrew may not be the best interpreter for a Jewish client).
- The nurse should be aware of gender differences between the interpreter and client to avoid violation of cultural mores related to modesty.

- The nurse should be aware of age differences between interpreter and client.
- The nurse should be aware of socioeconomic differences between interpreter and client.
- The nurse should ask the interpreter to translate as closely to verbatim as possible.
- An interpreter who is not a relative may seek compensation for services rendered.

From Andrews MM: Cultural diversity and community health nursing. In Nies MA, McEwen M, editors: *Community/public health nursing: promoting the health of populations*, ed 4, Philadelphia, 2007, W.B. Saunders.

COMMUNITY APPLICATION
Overcoming Language Barriers When No Interpreter Is Available

- Be polite and formal.
- Greet the client using the last or complete name; gesture to yourself and say your name; offer a handshake or nod; smile.
- Proceed in an unhurried manner; pay attention to any effort by the client or family to communicate.
- Speak in a low, moderate voice. Avoid talking loudly, and remember that people tend to raise the volume and pitch of their voice when the listener appears not to understand; the listener may think that you are shouting or angry.
- Use any words known in the client's language. This indicates awareness of and respect for the client's culture.
- Use simple words, such as "pain" instead of "discomfort." Avoid medical jargon, idioms, and slang. Avoid using contractions such as "don't," "can't," and "won't." Use nouns repeatedly instead of pronouns. For example, say "Does Juan take medicine?" instead of "He has been taking his medicine, hasn't he?"
- Pantomime words and simple actions while verbalizing them.

- Give instructions in the proper sequence. For example, say "First wash the bottle; second, rinse the bottle," instead of "Before you rinse the bottle, sterilize it."
- Discuss one topic at a time, and avoid using conjunctions. For example, say "Are you cold (while pantomiming)?" and "Are you in pain?" instead of "Are you cold and in pain?"
- Validate whether the client understands by having the client repeat instructions, demonstrate the procedure, or act out the meaning.
- Write out several short sentences in English and determine the client's ability to read them.
- Try a third language. Many Indo-Chinese speak French. Europeans often know three or four languages. Try Latin words or phrases.
- Ask who among the client's family and friends could serve as an interpreter.
- Obtain phrase books from a library or bookstore, make or purchase flash cards, contact hospitals for a list of interpreters, and use both formal and informal networking to locate a suitable interpreter.

From Andrews MM: Cultural diversity and community health nursing. In Nies MA, McEwen M, editors: *Community/public health nursing: promoting the health of populations*, ed 4, Philadelphia, 2007, W.B. Saunders.

DIET AND NUTRITION

Diet is one of the most significant contributors to health and illness. It is widely known and accepted that excessive intake of certain nutrients (e.g., saturated fats and calories) or lack of nutrients (e.g., protein, vitamins, minerals) adversely affects health.

Heart disease, stroke, certain types of cancer, poor outcomes of pregnancy, growth retardation, and other health problems have been linked to diet.

Food preferences are usually developed during childhood and are reflective of cultural heritage, lifestyle, socioeconomic status, religion, education, and lifestyle. In addition, there may be dramatic regional variations in food consumption and preferences. In most cultures food is very important. Food brings people together, promotes common interests, and stimulates bonds with other people and society. Andrews (1999b, pp. 345-346) outlined the following cultural functions of food:

* Food enables people to maintain body functions and produce energy.
* Food is used to establish and maintain social and cultural relationships with relatives, friends, strangers, and others.
* Food functions to assess social relationships or interpersonal closeness or distance between people.
* Food helps in coping with emotional stresses, conflicts, and traumatic life events.
* Food is used to reward, punish, and influence the behavior of others.
* Food reflects the political and economic status of an individual or group.
* Food is used to assess, treat, and prevent illness or disabilities of people.

Nurses need to be aware of the dietary practices of members of the cultural groups with which they work to recognize potential threats to health and to attempt to modify them as appropriate. Reducing sodium intake for blacks with hypertension; encouraging overweight, middle-class whites with cardiac problems to eat more fruits and vegetables and reduce saturated fats in their diets; modifying the carbohydrate and fat content of food for diabetic Hispanics; and increasing protein intake in pregnant Asians are examples of frequently encountered dietary challenges.

RELIGION

Having at least a basic understanding of the religious beliefs and practices of clients is extremely important in delivering holistic nursing care. Increasingly, spiritual care is being recognized to be as important as caring for the biological and psychosocial needs of clients. This is particularly evident when working with clients who are very ill or elderly or who are at significant developmental stages (e.g., childbirth, puberty, death). Knowledge of religious prohibitions, practices, rules, and rituals can be extremely helpful. For example,

awareness of baptism rites, circumcision practices, prayer requirements, and an appropriate religious leader (e.g., priest, minister, rabbi) can assist the nurse in providing the most appropriate assistive care for both client and family.

Almost 56% of U.S. residents are Protestant Christians (e.g., Baptist, Methodist, Presbyterian, Lutheran, Episcopalian). Roman Catholics are the second most common religious group (27% of the general population) and make up the majority in some areas (e.g., South Louisiana and areas with large concentrations of Hispanics) (Spector, 2004). Other fairly commonly encountered religions, varying greatly by geographic area, include Islam, Judaism, Buddhism, and Hinduism. Table 8-3 describes general information that may affect health and health care for the more commonly encountered religions.

CULTURAL VARIATIONS IN HEALTH AND ILLNESS

When working with clients from a variety of ethnic and racial groups, nurses in community settings must also be familiar with biocultural variations in health and illness. All nurses should recognize these differences and plan care accordingly (e.g., provide anticipatory teaching on signs and symptoms of diabetes to clients in high-risk groups, such as Native Americans or Filipino-Americans). To assist in learning a little about differences in health and illness among different cultural groups, some important characteristics of several groups are described briefly.

AFRICAN-AMERICANS

In the United States, African-Americans account for about 12.7% of the total population (U.S. Census Bureau, 2004). The majority of black Americans are direct descendants of West African slaves brought to the United States during the seventeenth century (Spector, 2004). More recently black immigrants have come to the United States from Caribbean countries (predominately Haiti, the Dominican Republic, and Jamaica). Although blacks live throughout the country, greater percentages live in certain states (predominately the southern states) and urban areas (e.g., Washington, DC; Detroit; and Chicago). About 24% of blacks live below the poverty level (U.S. Census Bureau, 2007).

Text continued on page 142

TABLE **8-3** Selected Religious Beliefs and Practices and Nursing Implications

RELIGION	TITLE OF RELIGIOUS REPRESENTATIVE	BELIEFS AND PRACTICES	DIETARY PRACTICES	NURSING AND HEALTH CARE ISSUES	ISSUES RELATED TO DEATH AND DYING
Buddhism (Buddhist Churches of America)	Priest	Founded in sixth century BC in India by S. Gautama (Buddha). The goal of Buddhism is to attain "Nirvana," in which the mind has supreme tranquility, purity, and stability. Buddha means "enlightened one." Nirvana is attained through "right" views, intention, speech, action, livelihood, effort, mindfulness, and concentration.	No specified restrictions. Extremes of diet are discouraged.	Emphasis is on the person living now. Reproduction issues: Birth control is acceptable. Abortion may be acceptable under certain conditions.	Prolonging life: If there is hope for recovery and the continuation of the pursuit of enlightenment, all measures of support are encouraged; if the person cannot continue to seek enlightenment, conditions may permit euthanasia. Organ donation: If donation will help another seek enlightenment, it may be encouraged. Body disposal: Temple funeral with burial or cremation is common.
Catholicism	Priest	The Roman Catholic Church recognizes seven sacraments: Baptism, Reconciliation, Holy Communion (Eucharist), Confirmation, Matrimony, Holy Orders, and Anointing of the Sick (Extreme Unction).	Fasting and abstaining from meat and meat products may be condoned on certain Holy Days. Alcohol and tobacco may be used in moderation.	Reproduction issues: Only natural means of birth control (abstinence, rhythm method) are acceptable. The church teaches the sanctity of life and that abortion is morally wrong.	Prolonging life: Ordinary means of preserving life are obligated, but extraordinary means are not. Direct euthanasia is not permitted. Body disposal: The body is usually buried following a church service. Cremation may be acceptable in certain circumstances.
Christian (Protestant) Several different denominational groups with variations in beliefs and practices, based on denomination	Minister Pastor Priest Reverend	Salvation is through faith in the work of Jesus Christ, who was born about 4 BC and was crucified about 33 years later.	Usually no dietary restrictions/ Many denominations expect abstinence from alcohol and tobacco.	Reproduction issues: Birth control is usually permitted and decided on by the family. Abortion is prohibited by some denominations and based on individual decisions in others.	Prolonging life: Is based on individual decision Body disposal: Burial following a funeral service is typical. Cremation is usually permitted and based on individual decision.

Christian Scientist (Church of Christ, Scientist)	There are no clergy. Practitioners are lay members of the church.	Founded by Mary Baker Eddy in the 1800s. Christian Scientists believe that God heals through prayer, which results in drawing closer to God in thinking and living.	No dietary restrictions. Alcohol and tobacco are not used. Coffee and tea may also be declined.	Do not normally seek medical care or take medications. A surgeon may be employed to set a broken bone. They seek exemption from immunizations; will allow treatment for minor children if required by law. Reproduction issues: Birth control is left to individual judgement. An obstetrician or midwife may be used for delivery.	Prolonging life: A Christian Scientist family is unlikely to seek medical care to prolong life. Euthanasia is contrary to the teaching of Christian Science. Body disposal: Burial and burial service are decided on by the individual family.
Church of Jesus Christ of Latter-Day Saints (Mormonism)	Elder	Founded in the 1820s by Joseph Smith, whose writings included *The Pearl of Great Price and The Book of Mormon*, which were given to him by God through visions. There are two sects, the initial church based in Salt Lake City, Utah, and the reorganized church based in Independence, Missouri. Mormons believe salvation is based on faith in Christ, baptism by immersion, obedience to the teaching of the Mormon Church, good works, and keeping the commandments of God.	Abstinence from tobacco, alcohol, and beverages with caffeine (e.g., coffee, tea, colas) is required. Meat is permitted, but dietary intake of fruits, grains, and herbs is encouraged. Fasting one day per month is required.	Cleanliness is very important. A sacred undergarment may be worn at all times and should only be removed in emergencies. Reproduction issues: Procreation is one of the major purposes of life, and prevention of conception is contrary to teachings. Abortion is opposed except when the life of the mother is in danger.	Prolonging life: When possible, medicine and faith are used to reverse conditions that threaten life. If death is inevitable, efforts to promote peaceful and dignified death are encouraged.

Continued

TABLE 8-3 Selected Religious Beliefs and Practices and Nursing Implications—cont'd

RELIGION	TITLE OF RELIGIOUS REPRESENTATIVE	BELIEFS AND PRACTICES	DIETARY PRACTICES	NURSING AND HEALTH CARE ISSUES	ISSUES RELATED TO DEATH AND DYING
Islam	Imam	Monotheistic religion founded between 610 and 631 AD by Mohammed. Followers are Moslems or Muslims. Islam means subjection to the will of Allah (God). Good deeds will be rewarded at the last judgment, and evil deeds will be punished in hell. There are five essential practices: acknowledgement of Allah as the one God and Mohammed as his messenger; praying five times daily (dawn, noon, afternoon, sunset, and night) facing Mecca, Saudi Arabia; giving alms to the needy; fasting from dawn until sunset throughout Ramadan (the ninth month of the Islamic calendar); and making one pilgrimage to Mecca if able.	No pork is allowed. "Halal" (permissible) meats must be blessed and slaughtered in a directed manner (Zabihah). Alcohol is prohibited. All adults except pregnant women, nursing mothers, the elderly, and the ill are required to fast during Ramadan.	Reproductive issues: Contraception is permitted, but many conservative Muslims do not use it because it is viewed as interference in God's will. Abortion is objectionable although there is no official policy. The husband must sign consent forms regarding family planning. Women are very modest, and this should be respected during examination. Circumcision is practiced on male children at an early age. For adult converts, it is sometimes practiced, although not required.	Prolonging life: Any attempt to shorten a life or terminate it is prohibited. Body disposal: Donation of body parts or organs is not allowed. Burial of the dead is compulsory and follows a prescribed procedure consisting of ritually washing the body, wrapping the body in white cloth, special prayers for the dead, burial as soon as possible with the head facing Mecca. A fetus older than 130 days of gestation is treated as a human and buried in the same manner.
Jehovah's Witnesses	Religious titles are generally not used.	Founded by Charles Taze Russell during the 1870s and the 1880s in Pittsburgh, Pennsylvania. He began writing for the Watchtower Bible and Tract Society. Belief that 144,000 servants will rule with Jesus. Every Minister of the Watch Tower Bible and Tract Society devotes approximately 10 hours or more each month to proselytizing.	No dietary restrictions. Alcohol and tobacco are discouraged.	Blood transfusions violate God's laws and are not allowed. Some will accept alternatives to blood transfusions (e.g., nonblood plasma expanders, autologous transfusions, and autotransfusions) Reproduction issues: Birth control is a personal decision, although sterilization is prohibited. Abortion is opposed.	Prolonging life: Right to die is a matter of individual choice, but euthanasia is prohibited. Body disposal: Burial or cremation is permitted.

Judaism	Rabbi	Judaism is a monotheistic religion that dates to the time of the prophet Abraham around 1900 BC. The laws of God are contained in the Torah and explained in the Talmud and in oral tradition. There are several divisions (i.e., Orthodox, Conservative, Reform, and fundamentalist [Hasidic]). Each Sabbath (from sunset Friday to just after sunset Saturday) is a holy day, and there are a number of other holy days.	Dietary laws are very strict, but the degree to which they are observed depends on the sect. In general pork, predatory fowl, and milk with meat dishes are not eaten. Only fish with fins and scales are permissible (shellfish are prohibited). All animals should be ritually slaughtered to be kosher (properly prepared). Wine is part of many religious observances. Alcohol is permitted in moderation. Fasting is required during Yom Kippur.	Medical care is expected according to Jewish law. Circumcision is performed on all Jewish male children on the eighth day following birth. This may be done by a ritual circumciser, by the child's father, or by a pediatrician. Reproductive issues: Birth control is permissible, but having children is encouraged. Therapeutic abortion is permitted if the health of the mother is jeopardized.	Prolonging life: Death with dignity is a right; euthanasia is strictly prohibited. Jewish beliefs include the need to not be alone when the soul leaves the body, so family or friends should be allowed to stay with dying clients. Body disposal: Following death, the body should not be left alone and should not be touched by medical personnel. The body will be ritually washed (usually done at a funeral home). Human remains (including a fetus at any stage of gestation) are to be buried as soon as possible. Cremation is not in keeping with Jewish law.

Data from Andrews MM, Hanson PA: Religion, culture and nursing. In Andrews MM, Boyle JS, editors: *Transcultural concepts in nursing care*, ed 4, Philadelphia, 2003, J.B. Lippincott; Carson VB: *Spiritual dimensions of nursing practice*, Philadelphia, 1989, Saunders; Keegan L: Spirituality. In Black JM, Matassarin-Jacobs E, editors: *Luckmann and Sorensen's medical-surgical nursing: a psychophysiologic approach*, ed 4, Philadelphia, 1993, Saunders.

Common Health Problems

As mentioned previously, there is significant disparity between health indicators of blacks and other racial groups. For example, the life expectancy for blacks born in 2004 is 73.3 years, whereas for whites, it is 78.0 years. In addition, the difference in life expectancy between male and female whites and blacks is also significant. White women born in 2004 should expect to live 80.8 years, as opposed to 76.5 years for black women; and white men born in 2004 have a life expectancy of 75.7 years, compared with 69.8 years for black men (USDHHS/National Center for Health Statistics [NCHS], 2006).

Although coronary artery disease mortality rates are similar in black and white men, women's rates of heart disease are higher in blacks. Probably the most distinctive difference is in cerebrovascular disease, where stroke accounts for much of the excess mortality in blacks compared with whites. In part this may be related to the prevalence of hypertension in blacks, for whom high blood pressure develops at a younger age and tends to be more severe than in whites. Indeed, it is estimated that some 40% to 45% of blacks are hypertensive (USDHHS/NCHS, 2006).

Although the incidence of cancer is similar between the racial groups, the overall mortality rate for cancer is significantly higher in blacks (234.5 per 100,000 for blacks and 188.3 per 100,000 for whites) (ACS, 2006). In addition, the rates for some of the most common cancers are higher for blacks than for whites, as shown in Table 8-4. This may be the result of delayed diagnosis and treatment.

Several other significant differences are found in rates of morbidity and mortality. For example, diabetes is one third more common among blacks than among whites. Black babies are more than twice as likely as white babies to die in their first year of life. Homicide is the most frequent cause of death for black men 15 to 24 years of age, a rate several times greater than for white men in the same age group (USDHHS, 2000).

Acquired immunodeficiency syndrome (AIDS) is particularly devastating to blacks because they account for a larger proportion of AIDS cases than do whites. Indeed, although blacks make up less than 13% of the U.S. population, they account for about half (49%) of the people in the U.S. with AIDS. Further, 64% of women and 63% of children under the age of 13 who are diagnosed with HIV/AIDS are black (CDC, 2007).

AMERICAN INDIANS, INCLUDING ALEUTS AND INUITS

American Indians (including Aleuts and Inuits) make up less than 1% of the total U.S. population; they are the smallest minority group. Although

TABLE **8-4** Comparison of Cancer Death Rates Between Blacks and Whites (2001)

TYPE OF CANCER	DEATH RATES FOR BLACKS (PER 100,000)	DEATH RATES FOR WHITES (PER 100,000)
Lung cancer (males)	104.1	76.6
Lung cancer (females)	39.9	41.6
Prostate cancer (males)	70.4	28.8
Breast cancer (females)	35.4	26.4
Cervical cancer (females)	5.6	2.6
Colorectal cancer (males)	34.3	24.8
Colorectal cancer (females)	24.5	17.1
All cancers (male)	352.2	250.5
All cancers (female)	200.4	169.1

From American Cancer Society: *Cancer facts and figures for African Americans 2005-2006* (website): http://www.cancer.org/downloads/STT/CAFF2005AACorrPWSecured.pdf. Accessed July 26, 2007.

many American Indians (approximately one third) live on reservations, most live in urban areas. Income and educational levels tend to be low. Health problems of American Indians are often the result of poverty because slightly more than half live below the poverty level.

Common Health Problems

Alcohol abuse and obesity are the two major risk factors affecting American Indian populations. Alcohol abuse is a significant health problem that contributes to other health threats, including accidental death, homicide, and suicide. It has been observed that unintentional injuries are the leading cause of death for Native American men younger than 44 years, with 75% of the injuries being alcohol related (USDHHS, 2000). Alcohol also contributes to other health problems more commonly found among American Indians. For example, cirrhosis deaths are 2.5 times greater among American Indians than the total population, and fetal alcohol syndrome is 5 times greater among American Indians.

Diabetes is extremely prevalent among Native Americans. Overall the incidence rate of diabetes for American Indians is 8.7 per 1000 (compared with an overall incidence of 3.1 per 1000 among all Americans). In some tribal groups as many as 40% of adults are diabetic (USDHHS, 2000).

ASIANS AND PACIFIC ISLANDERS

A growing number of Americans have ancestors who immigrated from Korea, China, Japan, Vietnam, Cambodia, Laos, and other Asian countries. Asian and Pacific Islanders now account for slightly less than 4% of the total population (U.S. Census Bureau, 2004). In this group about 10% live below the poverty level (U.S. Census Bureau, 2007).

Because many Asians are recent immigrants and their health care customs are based on Eastern rather than Western practices, it is helpful to be aware of some of the basics of Eastern health care. Many Asian health practices are grounded in Chinese tradition. Chinese philosophy of health and illness is holistic in nature and integrated with the external environment. The onset, evolution, and change of diseases are considered in conjunction with geographical, social, and other environmental factors.

Yin and Yang

In Chinese philosophy the terms *yin* and *yang* refer to opposing but complementary powers that regulate the universe, with *yang* representing male, positive energy (which relates to light, warmth, and fullness) and *yin* representing female, negative energy (which relates to darkness, cold, and emptiness) (Spector, 2004). Yin and yang depict a "unity of opposites" and regulate themselves to promote normal activities of life and health. Illness is the result of a disharmony of yin and yang.

Acupuncture is an ancient Chinese practice of using needles inserted at specific points of the body to cure disease and relieve pain. The practice and principles of acupuncture are very complex. The basic treatment goal of acupuncture is to restore the balance of yin and yang through insertion of the needles into meridians (points on the skin corresponding to a network, or channel, of energy that runs longitudinally throughout the body) to treat the condition (Spector, 2004).

Herbology refers to the use of herbs to heal. The Chinese use many herbs and plants for medicinal and healing reasons. Herbal medicines are categorized according to their properties of yin or yang. Ginseng root is an example of an herb used to treat a number of health problems, including anemia, depression, indigestion, and impotence (Spector, 2004). Other herbal remedies include Jen Shen Lu Jung Wan, a general tonic used to improve health and improve digestion; tiger balm, a salve used for relief of minor aches and pains; and white flower, a liquid used to treat colds, influenza, headaches, and coughs (Spector, 1993).

Common Health Problems

Health problems of Asian-Americans vary greatly, based on nation of origin, socioeconomic status, and length of time in the United States. In general, however, Asian-Americans have some distinct health problems. For example, liver cancer among Southeast Asians is much higher than in whites. This is thought to be the result of endemic hepatitis B, which in chronic carriers predisposes to the development of hepatocellular carcinoma. Tuberculosis (TB) is still a leading cause of death in some Asian countries and is a significant threat in the United States, being much more commonly found in Asian-Americans than in white populations.

WHITES (AMERICANS OF EUROPEAN DESCENT)

Non-Hispanic whites make up around 69% of the U.S. population (U.S. Census Bureau, 2004). Members of this group are descendants of immigrants from Germany, Italy, England, Scotland, Ireland, France, Austria, Russia, and several other countries. About 8% live below the poverty level (U.S. Census Bureau, 2007).

Common Health Problems

The leading causes of deaths for whites are heart disease, cancer, stroke, and chronic obstructive pulmonary disease (COPD); these are for the most part diseases of aging. However, health habits and lifestyle choices contribute to morbidity and mortality. Diet and activity levels, in particular, and use of alcohol and tobacco products and unhealthy sex practices contribute to disease and death in whites.

HISPANIC, OR LATINO, AMERICANS (ALL RACES)

Hispanic Americans originate from Cuba (5%), Central and South America (14%), Mexico (60% +), Puerto Rico (11%), and other Spanish-speaking countries of the Caribbean (7.5%). They make up about 12.6% of the total U.S. population and represent the fastest-growing ethnic group. Although Hispanics live in all states, the greatest concentrations are found in southern border states (i.e., California, Arizona, New Mexico, Texas), Florida, and New York. As a rule the Hispanic population is very young and has a high birth rate. About 21% of Hispanics live below the poverty level (U.S. Census Bureau, 2007).

Balance of "Hot" and "Cold"

According to Stasiak (1991), Mexican-Americans consider health to be a state of well-being brought on by eating proper foods and maintaining a "hot/cold" balance in the foods eaten. Illness, to many Hispanic groups, is an imbalance in the body between "hot" and "cold" and "wet" and "dry." The belief is that a hot illness must be treated with a cold substance and vice versa.

Hot or cold does not refer to temperature but to the substance itself, and foods, beverages, illnesses, and people can be considered hot or cold. Examples of hot conditions are fever, infections, diarrhea, liver problems, and constipation. Cold conditions include cancer, pneumonia, menstrual period, earache, and stomach cramps. Examples of hot foods are chocolate, coffee, corn meal, cheese, eggs, onions, hard liquor, beef, and chili peppers. Cold foods include vegetables, fruits, dairy products, fish, chicken, and honey. Hot medicines and herbs include penicillin, tobacco, garlic, cinnamon, vitamins, and aspirin. Cold medicines and herbs include sage, milk of magnesia, and bicarbonate of soda (Gonzalez and Kuipers, 2004).

Traditional Illness Management and Healers

Although practices vary greatly depending on the ethnic group, traditional or folk healers and religious rituals are sometimes used by Hispanics to treat illness. The use of religious signs, symbols, rituals, and practices is common. The most popular forms of treatment combine Catholic rituals, such as offerings of money, penance, confession, lighting candles, and laying on of hands, with the medicinal use of teas and herbs (Spector, 2004). Examples of Hispanic folk healers are the curandero, the yerbero, and the partera.

A *curandero* (*curandera*) is a holistic healer, who may be "called" by God or be born with a "gift" of healing and/or may serve an apprenticeship (Spector, 2004). A curandero develops a very personal relationship with the client, and the goal of care is to restore harmony with the social, physical, and psychological parts of the person. A central focus of the treatment is relieving clients of their sins, which can cause an imbalance between God and people. Treatment, often provided in a room in the curandero's home that is decorated with religious paraphernalia, may include massage, diet, rest, practical advice, herbs, prayers, magic, and/or supernatural rituals (Gonzalez and Kuipers, 2004).

A *yerbero* is a folk healer who specializes in using herbs and spices (Gonzalez & Kuipers, 2004), and a *partera* is a Mexican-American midwife (Spector, 2004). Nurses should be aware of common folk treatments such as herbal teas and roots used by these traditional healers and question clients respectfully, not judgmentally. It should be noted that many traditional health practices have been shown to be beneficial (Stasiak, 1991).

Common Health Problems

Hispanics experience the greatest disparity in health and health problems among American minority groups. Infant mortality rates, for example, vary substantially between cultural groups—Puerto Ricans living in the United States have almost twice the infant mortality rate of Cuban-Americans. Hispanics have a very high birth rate (22.9 births per 1000 women, compared with 12.5 births per 1000 women in the total U.S. population) (NCHS, 2006). Unintentional injuries, AIDS, and homicide disproportionately affect Hispanics. Diabetes is also very prevalent among Mexican-Americans, as is obesity; this is particularly true for Mexican-American women.

PRINCIPLES FOR NURSING PRACTICE IN COMMUNITY SETTINGS

One of the barriers to providing culturally sensitive nursing care is failure to recognize and appreciate the impact of culture on health care providers themselves. Health care providers have been socialized into a given culture (usually the dominant cultural group of middle-class white) and then further socialized into the culture of their profession. "Professional socialization teaches the student a set of beliefs, practices, habits, likes, dislikes, norms and rituals…. [Therefore] health-care providers can be viewed as a foreign culture or ethnic group" (Spector, 2004, pp. 180). As a result it is very important that all nurses seek to realize the impact of their personal culture and the culture of health care providers on their own behavior, values, and practices.

Following recognition of their own cultural beliefs, values, and biases, nurses can learn to better recognize and appreciate the beliefs, values, and biases of others and use this information to improve nursing care. Allender and Spradley (2005) succinctly summarized cultural principles for practice for nurses who work in community settings. These principles are the following:
- Develop cultural self-awareness
- Cultivate cultural sensitivity
- Assess client group's culture
- Show respect and patience while learning about other cultures
- Examine culturally derived health practices.

Adherence to these principles promotes culturally competent nursing care.

SUMMARY

The population of the United States comprises people from many different cultural groups, and each of these groups has its own distinctive values, methods of communication, diet, and religious beliefs and practices, among other characteristics. In addition, members of different racial, ethnic, and cultural groups have health threats and risks associated with their particular biological, psychological, social, and lifestyle factors.

Like most nurses, Trisha, the nurse from the opening case study, works with clients from various cultures and realizes that culturally competent nursing care should be a priority of all nurses. In the community, however, a recognition of how culture impacts health behaviors, health beliefs, and health practices is particularly important. Thus to practice holistically, nurses should strive to learn about other cultures and to understand and use the information in providing nursing care.

KEY POINTS

- The United States is becoming increasingly ethnically diverse, and this affects health and health care delivery, particularly for nurses in community-based practice.
- Numerous nursing organizations have recognized the need to provide culturally sensitive and culturally competent nursing care; the Transcultural Nursing Society was established in 1973.
- *Race* refers to classification of humans based on physical characteristics, and there are nine recognized distinct races. An *ethnic group* is a group of people who share common distinctive characteristics, such as race, ancestry, nationality, language, religion, food preferences, literature, music, and a common history. There are more than 100 ethnic groups in the United States. *Culture* is closely tied to ethnicity and refers to values, beliefs, attitudes, and customs that provide the

organizational structure or basis for behavior within the group. A *subculture* is a relatively large subsection of a cultural group that has distinctive characteristics that set it apart from the group as a whole.

- Community-based nurses may need to perform a cultural assessment to help recognize the impact of culture on health and health practices. Identification of cultural values should be a component of a cultural assessment.
- Cultural variations based on socioeconomic levels or class can greatly influence health and health-seeking behaviors. Socioeconomic class creates a set of values and role expectations regarding sex, marriage, parenting, birth, education, dress, housing, occupation, and religion.
- Language barriers are frequently encountered when working with members of other cultural groups. Appropriate use of an interpreter and tips for communication without an interpreter can be helpful for nurses working in community-based settings. Familiarity with variations in communication patterns between various cultural groups can also be helpful.
- Cultural factors that also contribute significantly to health and illness include diet and nutrition and religion.
- Cultural variations occur in health, illness, and health practices. Nurses working with significant numbers of persons from a cultural group should be aware of these variations and practices.

Learning Activities & Application to Practice
In Class

1. Talk with classmates from racial or ethnic minorities. Share differences in values, norms, religion, and health beliefs, and discuss how these factors influence health practices and might affect health care delivery. Explore ways nurses can develop sensitivity to other cultural groups.
2. Review *Healthy People 2010* objectives that relate to minority health. Discuss interventions to address the objectives with classmates.
3. Complete a cultural self-assessment, and share findings with classmates.

In Clinical

4. Review census data from your area to identify the percentages of persons from non-European origin in the local community. If possible, compare with previous data (e.g., has the percentage increased since 1990? Since 2000?). What are projections for the future?
5. Identify an individual or family from a cultural minority, and perform a cultural assessment. Share findings with the clinical group.
6. Outline in a diary or log some health practices, health problems, and other observations uniquely related to race, culture, or ethnicity you might encounter in clinical practice. Share these with the clinical group. Were any assessments or interventions performed based on racial, ethnic, or cultural variations?

REFERENCES

Allender JA, Spradley BW: *Community health nursing: promoting and protecting the public's health*, ed 6, Philadelphia, 2005, Lippincott Williams & Wilkins.

American Academy of Nursing.: AAN expert panel report: culturally competent health care, *Nurs Outlook* 40(6):277, 1992.

American Cancer Society: *Cancer facts and figures for African Americans 2005-2006* (website): http://www.cancer.org/downloads/STT/CAFF2005AACorrPWSecured.pdf. Accessed July 26, 2007.

Andrews MM: Cultural perspectives on nursing in the 21st century, *J Prof Nurs* 8(1):1, 1992.

Andrews MM (1999a): Theoretical foundations of transcultural nursing. In Andrews MM, Boyle, JS, editors: *Transcultural concepts in nursing care*, ed 3, Philadelphia, 1999, J.B. Lippincott.

Andrews MM (1999b): Culture and nutrition. In Andrews MM, Boyle JS, editors: *Transcultural concepts in nursing care*, ed 3, Philadelphia, 1999, J.B. Lippincott.

Andrews MM: Cultural diversity and community health nursing. In Nies MA, McEwen M, editors: *Community/public health nursing: promoting the health of populations*, ed 4, Philadelphia, 2007, W.B. Saunders.

Andrews MM, Boyle JS: *Transcultural concepts in nursing care*, ed 4, Philadelphia, 2003, J.B. Lippincott.

Andrews MM, Herberg P: Transcultural nursing care. In Andrews MM, Boyle JS, editors, *Transcultural concepts in nursing care*, ed 3, Philadelphia, 1999, J.B. Lippincott.

Centers for Disease Control and Prevention: *HIV/AIDS and African Americans* (website): http://www.cdc.gov/hiv/topics/aa/index.htm. Accessed August 24, 2007.

Garn SM: *Human races*, ed 2, Springfield, Ill, 1965, Charles C. Thomas.

Giger JN, Davidhizar RE: *Transcultural nursing: assessment & intervention*, ed 4, St Louis, 2004, Mosby.

Gonzalez T, Kuipers J: Mexican Americans. In Giger JN, Davidhizar RE, editors: *Transcultural nursing: assessment and intervention*, ed 4, St Louis, 2004, Mosby.

Herberg P: Theoretical foundations of transcultural nursing. In Andrews MM, Boyle JS, editors: *Transcultural concepts in nursing care*, ed 2, Philadelphia, 1995, J.B. Lippincott.

Leininger MM (2001a): The theory of culture care diversity and universality. In Leininger MM, editor: *Culture care diversity & universality: a theory of nursing*, Boston, 2001, Jones and Bartlett.

Leininger MM (2001b): Selected culture care findings of diverse cultures using culture care theory and ethnomethods. In Leininger MM, editor: *Culture care diversity & universality: a theory of nursing*, Boston, 2001, Jones and Bartlett.

Murray RB, Zentner RMJ, Samiezade'-Yazd C: Sociocultural influences on the person and family. In Murray RB, Zentner JP, editors: *Nursing assessment and health promotion: strategies through the life span*, ed 7, Upper Saddle River, NJ, 2001, Prentice Hall.

National Center for Health Statistics: *Births: final data from 2004* (website): http://www.cdc.gov/nchs/data/nvsr/nvsr55/nvsr55_01.pdf. Accessed August 28, 2007.

Spector RE: Culture, ethnicity and nursing. In Potter PA, Perry AG, editors: *Fundamentals of nursing: concepts, process & practice*, St Louis, 1993, Mosby.

Spector RE: *Cultural diversity in health & illness*, ed 6, Upper Saddle River, NJ, 2004, Prentice Hall.

Stasiak DB: Culture care theory with Mexican-Americans in an urban context. In Leininger MM, editor: *Culture care diversity & universality: a theory of nursing*, Publication No. 15-2402, New York, 1991, National League for Nursing Press.

U.S. Bureau of the Census: *Projected population of the United States by race and Hispanic origin: 2000 to 2050* (website): http://www.census.gov/ipc/www/usinterimproj/natprojtab01a.pdf. Accessed August 28, 2007.

U.S. Bureau of the Census: *Income, poverty, and health insurance coverage in the United States: 2006* (website): http://www.census.gov/prod/2007pubs/p60-233.pdf. Accessed August 28, 2007.

U.S. Department of Health and Human Services: *Healthy people 2010*: Conference edition, Washington, DC, 2000, Government Printing Office.

U.S. Department of Health and Human Services/ National Center for Health Statistics: *Health: United States–2006* (website): http://www.cdc.gov/nchs/data/hus/hus06.pdf#027. Accessed July 26, 2007.

Natural and Manmade Disasters

objectives

Upon completion of this chapter, the reader will be able to:

1. Define the terms *disaster* and *emergency*, and give examples of each.

2. Identify potential internal and external emergencies and disasters that a community might experience.

3. Describe the essential elements of a plan to meet emergencies and disasters.

4. Recognize the role of the nurse in emergency preparedness.

5. Recognize community resources and their role in emergencies and disasters.

key terms

American Red Cross
Crisis
Disaster
Disaster triage
Direct victims
Emergency
External emergencies

Federal Emergency
  Management Agency
  (FEMA)
First responders
Hazards
Indirect victims
Internal emergencies

Mass-casualty incident
Mitigation
Multiple-casualty incident
NA-TECH disasters
Terrorism
Workplace violence
See Glossary for definitions.

case study

Hope Spencer is a school nurse at Cottonwood Elementary School in Promise, a community of 32,700 people located about 100 miles inland from the Atlantic Ocean. There are 835 children, 43 faculty and staff, and a number of volunteers, visitors, and parents present in the school on any given day. The recent reports of school shootings by students and the apparent increase in natural disasters in the area have raised Hope's concerns about the preparedness of Cottonwood School should an emergency or disaster occur. Hope has been told that the school district has a plan for what to do in case of a fire, but she has not reviewed the school's emergency plans and does not know whether they include policies and procedures for internal emergencies and other disasters.

Continued

Because Hope is new to the district, she asked some of the faculty if they knew what to do in the event of an incident or emergency. The findings from her short, anecdotal assessment were troubling, as only one faculty member seemed to have any idea of what to do in the event of on-campus violence. And although all knew what to do in case of fire, no one could respond with assurance about what to do if there were an onsite explosion or one nearby. Armed with that data, Hope reviewed the school's Policies and Procedures Manual and found that the only emergency policy in the book dealt with measures to take during a fire; no other internal or external emergencies or disasters were addressed.

Hope searched the Internet for information on emergency-preparedness policies and learned about procedures that should be in place in schools. Finding a significant amount of information, she realized that the input of many people would be necessary to address disaster preparedness at Cottonwood Elementary School. Hope presented her observations to her principal and discussed her research on the history of violent incidents and other disasters in schools, essential elements to include in a disaster plan, and supplies and information that would be needed in each classroom should the school be faced with an emergency or disaster event. She proposed that a committee be established to develop a plan, policies, and procedures for emergencies and disasters specific to Cottonwood Elementary School.

After reviewing Hope's findings, the principal selected a committee to develop the policies and appointed Hope chairperson. As a result of the committee's work, Cottonwood Elementary School will be better equipped to ensure the safety of its students, staff, faculty, volunteers, and visitors during emergencies or disasters.

Disasters happen every day. They may be natural calamities, accidents, terrorism, or war. Disasters can affect one family at a time and cause thousands of dollars in damage (a house fire) or they can kill thousands and have economic losses in the billions (the terrorist attacks on the World Trade Center and the Pentagon on September 11, 2001).

A **disaster** refers to any event that causes destruction and devastation that cannot be alleviated without assistance; the event need not cause injury or death. The American Public Health Association (2005) notes that disasters are emergencies "of such severity and magnitude that the resultant combination of deaths, injuries, illness, and property damage cannot be effectively managed with routine procedures or resources" (p.1).

TYPES OF DISASTERS

Disasters may be the result of natural or manmade occurrences (see Table 9-1). Natural disasters include climactic events such as hurricanes, tornados, floods, blizzards, typhoons, and droughts; topographical events such as earthquakes, avalanches, and volcanic eruptions; or communicable disease epidemics. Natural disasters can be extremely destructive in terms of human life. Indeed, it is estimated that approximately 3 million lives have been lost in the past 20 years as the result of earthquakes, volcanic eruptions, landslides, floods, tropical storms, droughts, and other natural disasters. Floods have been the most common type of natural disaster and account for more than one third of all disasters (Lundy and Butts, 2001). Manmade disasters include war, chemical and biological terrorism, civil disasters (riots and demonstrations), and accidents (transportation accidents, structural collapse, explosion, and chemical and biological contamination). Fire can be either manmade (accidental or arson) or naturally occurring (lightning strike) (Beachley, 2005; Summerlin, 2007).

Terrorist attacks are a special category of manmade disasters. Although the use of terrorist tactics is not new, terrorists attacks have increased dramatically over the last decade. **Terrorism** refers to the "unlawful use of force or violence against persons or property to intimidate or coerce a government or civilian population in the furtherance of political or social objectives" (Allender and Spradley, 2005, p. 462). Throughout the world, terrorism results in thousands of deaths and injuries and billions of dollars in property damage each year. In most cases,

TABLE **9-1** Types of Disasters

NATURAL DISASTERS	MANMADE DISASTERS
Avalanches	Terrorism
Blizzards	Civil unrest (riots)
Communicable disease epidemics	Explosions, bombings
Droughts, wildfires	Fires
Earthquakes, tsunamis	Structural collapse (bridges)
Floods, mudslides	Toxic or hazardous spills
Hailstorms	Mass transit accidents
Heat waves	Pollution
Hurricanes	Wars
Tornados, cyclones	
Volcanic eruptions	

Source: Summerlin E: Natural and man-made disasters. In Nies M, McEwen M, editors: *Community/public health nursing: promoting the health of populations*, ed 4, p. 582, St Louis, 2007, Saunders.

terrorists use explosives or incendiary devices against their targets, but there is growing concern over the potential for use of biologic organisms (e.g., anthrax, smallpox) or chemical agents (e.g., sarin gas, mustard gas) in a terrorist attack.

Disasters may also be termed *NA-TECH* (natural-technological); **NA-TECH disasters** are natural disaster incidents that cause a technological problem. For example, a hurricane may cause high winds, heavy rain, and flooding, which damage buildings and electrical power lines, resulting in fires. Similarly, an earthquake can destroy roads and crack natural gas pipelines, resulting in the potential for explosions. Disasters are a global problem and disproportionately affect persons from developing countries where poverty, urbanization, and overcrowding of cities have increased the danger of both natural and manmade disasters. For example, the earthquake and tsunami off the coast of Sumatra, Indonesia, in December 2004 resulted in the deaths

of more than 200,000 people and displaced thousands more (USAID, 2008).

Disasters can result in multiple or mass casualties. A **multiple-casualty incident** is one in which between 2 and 100 persons are injured. Multiple casualties generally strain, and may in some cases overwhelm, the available emergency medical services and resources. A **mass-casualty incident** is a situation with a large number of casualties (100 or greater) that significantly overwhelms available emergency services (Summerlin, 2007). When there are mass casualties (i.e., the September 11, 2001, terrorist attacks; Hurricane Katrina), a community or region usually requires assistance of emergency personnel and resources from surrounding communities or states. Table 9-2 lists recent multiple- and mass-casualty disasters in the United States.

EMERGENCIES

An **emergency** is an unforeseen event or condition requiring immediate action. Emergencies can occur internally or externally. **External emergencies** are those hazardous or harmful events that occur somewhere in the community, outside of a defined business, industrial complex, residence or other facility. External emergencies require immediate action, but are typically managed by **first responders**—fire, police, and ambulance services—to the scene. Examples of external emergencies are vehicular accidents, house fires, and shootings in various community settings; these emergencies may result in multiple casualties. **Internal emergencies** are events that initiate within a facility. These include industrial fires, explosions, hazardous material spills, and workplace violence.

Internal emergencies are often managed by the facility's resources initially, and the assistance of first responders follows as necessary. For example, in the event of a fire at a facility (e.g., a hospital), trained internal personnel will be called upon to try to control the fire, limit its spread, and perhaps evacuate people while the public fire department is en route. Similarly, if a bus accident injures several children at a school, the school nurse and other personnel will try to manage or stabilize the situation while waiting for the first responders. The emergency becomes a **crisis**, a turn for the worse, when the incident has gotten out of control, leading to multiple casualties, severe destruction, or both (Sternberg, 2003).

TABLE **9-2** Multiple and Mass Casualty Disasters—United States, 2000 to 2007

DATE	TYPE OF DISASTER AND LOCATION	NUMBER OF DEATHS
January 2000	Crash of Alaska Air 261 (California)	88
June 2001	Tropical storm Allison in southeast United States	41
Sept 11, 2001	Terrorist attacks, New York City, Washington DC, and Pennsylvania	2973
September 16, 2004	Hurricane Ivan (Florida, Alabama)	32
March 23, 2005	Chemical plant explosion (Texas City, Texas)	15
August 29, 2005	Hurricane Katrina (Louisiana, Mississippi, Texas, Alabama, Florida)	Approximately 1800
September 24, 2005	Hurricane Rita (Texas, Louisiana)	120 (7 actual; 113 attributed [e.g., transportation accidents])
April 16, 2007	Shootings—Virginia Tech University	32
Feb 5-6, 2008	Tornados (Tennessee, Kentucky, Arkansas, Alabama)	60 (approximately)
Feb 7, 2008	Sugar plant explosion (Port Wentworth, Georgia)	11

Workplace violence is a relatively common type of internal emergency and refers to "violent acts against a person at work or on duty, including physical assaults (rape and sexual assault and aggravated and simple assault) and robbery" (Warchol, 1998, p.1). There are four types of workplace violence: (1) violence committed by clients or patients, (2) violence associated with robbery or other crimes, (3) violence among co-workers or managers, and (4) domestic violence that spills over into the workplace (AFL-CIO, 2007). Although workplace violence is not a new threat, its incidence appears to be increasing (see the Research Highlight "Workplace Violence"), and the potential is present in almost any setting.

IMPACT OF A DISASTER

Casualties of disasters may be classified as *direct victims* or *indirect victims*. **Direct victims** are those who are immediately affected by the disaster; they may be injured, dead, an evacuee, or a refugee.

Indirect victims are the family and friends of the direct victim or the first responders to the scene. In addition to the impact a disaster has on individuals, families, and friends, health care facilities in communities are also affected (Hassmiller, 2004; Summerlin, 2007).

How disasters affect individuals, families, and communities varies greatly, depending on the disaster type, cause, location, magnitude, extent of damage, duration, and amount of warning. Individuals are affected when they must leave their homes to seek safety and escape the effects of the disaster. The community is affected when it must provide temporary food, housing, and other services to those who are displaced.

IMPACT OF A DISASTER ON INDIVIDUALS

Individual responses to disaster can include fear, panic, disbelief, and anger. There is often disorientation, difficulty in making decisions, and reluctance to abandon property. Emotional responses include insomnia, headaches, apathy and depression,

Research Highlight

Workplace Violence

The problem of failing to plan for internal emergencies was addressed in a longitudinal study of workplace violence. In his research, Chavez (2002) learned that fatal attacks at worksites have continued at a steady rate despite the increased awareness and more stringent security measures following the September 11 attacks. The study analyzed violence initiated by employees, former employees, clients, and other categories by examining 18 separate events that resulted in the deaths of 34 people and the wounding of 23 others.

Certain important characteristics were noted about this kind of violence. Chavez learned that perpetrators were mostly men (94.3%), and overwhelmingly they were between the ages of 35 and 45. Current employees made up 43.6% of the perpetrators, and former employees made up 22.5%. Domestic violence accounted for 21.4% of the incidents, and client-type relationships accounted for 12.5%. Most offenders had significant tenure on the job, and their purpose was to seek out selected individuals. After the violence 33.9% committed suicide, 7.1% died in confrontation with

police, and 15.4% surrendered peacefully to police immediately after the violent act.

The reason Chavez posited for continued incidents of workplace violence despite increased focus on prevention was lack of awareness of potential threats and failure to develop and implement effective policies. Factors that contribute to workplace violence are the following: a weak or nonexistent policy against all forms of violence; inadequate employee hiring, supervising and retaining practices; inadequate training of employees on how to prevent or respond to violent situations; failure to inform employees of policies; inability to adequately assess threats; a weak reporting mechanism; and failure to take immediate action against those who have threatened or committed acts of violence.

It was concluded that training on violence prevention should be provided to all employees to minimize workplace violence. The training should focus on how to recognize and deal with the threats and must show employees that their safety and well-being is important to the organization.

From Chavez LJ (2002): *18 workplace violence incidents since September 11th: for the workplace killer, it is business as usual (website):* http://www.workplaceviolence911.com/Articles/articles.jsp?listType=1015-63K. Accessed September 21, 2007.

moodiness, irritability, anxiety about the future, domestic violence, frustration, feeling of powerlessness, and guilt. Physical disturbances include gastrointestinal upsets, diarrhea, and nausea (Hassmiller, 2004) (Table 9-3).

In general, individuals experience disasters in relation to how significantly they are directly affected. An individual's perception of a disaster may change over time as the person begins to acknowledge the full impact of the disaster. Beachley (2005) pointed out that psychological reactions fall into three categories: (1) mild to severe, (2) normal to pathological, and (3) immediate to delayed. Within these designations, a reaction may be severe, normal, or mild and yet abnormal. A few people are so overwhelmed by the disaster that they immediately experience extreme psychological distress. Others may appear unaffected initially, using denial as a defense mechanism to handle their thoughts and feelings.

If survivors do not recognize and deal effectively with emotional and psychological consequences, they may suffer long-term problems such

as posttraumatic stress disorder. Most experts recommend that disaster victims and aid workers have critical stress debriefings and possible referral to a mental health care professional (Beachley, 2005; Young, 1998).

IMPACT OF A DISASTER ON THE COMMUNITY

During and immediately following a disaster, significant problems in a community can arise when public services personnel are being overworked. In some cases important services such as telephone systems, television and radio broadcasting, electricity, transportation, and water and sanitation services may be disrupted. Resources such as food and medical supplies may be depleted. Floods, tornados, earthquakes, and terrorist attacks may damage or destroy both public and private buildings.

Summerlin (2007) noted that there are four phases of a community's reaction to a disaster. First there is the *heroic phase*, in which there is large-scale community support, with an emotional emphasis on helping people survive and recover. The second phase is the *honeymoon phase*. People

TABLE **9-3** Common Reactions to an Emergency or Disaster

EMOTIONAL	COGNITIVE	PHYSICAL	INTERPERSONAL
Shock	Impaired concentration	Fatigue	Alienation
Anger	Impaired decision making	Insomnia	Social withdrawal
Despair	Memory impairment	Sleep disturbance	School impairment
Numbing	Disbelief	Hyper-arousal	Increased conflict
Terror	Confusion	Headaches	Vocational problems
Guilt	Distortion	Startle response	
Grief or sadness	Decreased self-esteem	Somatic complaints	
Irritability	Decreased self-efficacy	GI problems	
Helplessness	Self-blame	Decreased appetite	

Modified from Young BH et al: *Disaster mental health services: a guidebook for clinicians and administrators*, Menlo Park, Calif, 1998, Department of Veterans Affairs, National Center for PTSD.

who simultaneously experienced the catastrophic event draw together for support and sharing. This is followed by the *disillusionment phase*, in which feelings of disappointment surface because of delays or failures when promises of aid are not fulfilled. Often this happens because people seek help to solve their own problems rather than community problems. Finally, there is the *reconstruction phase*. In this phase, there is reaffirmation of belief in the community when new buildings are constructed or other measures are taken to bring about closure (e.g., building the memorial at the World Trade Center).

DISASTER MANAGEMENT

Historically Americans have prepared for emergencies only in times of national threat, such as during World War II and in the early 1960s, when there was concern over nuclear war with the Soviet Union. The recent spate of natural disasters such as hurricanes and earthquakes; the terrorist attacks at Oklahoma City, the World Trade Center, and the Pentagon; and concern over the potential for global pandemics (e.g., bird flu) have created concerns across the nation for preparedness to meet both natural and manmade disasters (Beachley, 2005).

Federal, state, and local governments bear the primary responsibility for designing and implementing disaster relief. Local and national voluntary agencies, in particular the American Red Cross, also play a large part.

DISASTER SERVICES PROVIDED BY GOVERNMENTAL AGENCIES

Local governments are responsible for the safety and welfare of their citizens. Local disaster response organizations should include local area government agencies (i.e., fire departments, police departments, public health departments, emergency services, and the local Red Cross (Summerlin, 2007). Emergency operations plans should be based on the likelihood of a particular disaster, and "mock disaster" exercises should be planned and conducted accordingly. For example, localities on the Gulf Coast should plan for hurricanes; certain locations on the West Coast should plan for earthquakes; midwestern and southern states should plan for tornados; and northern states should plan for blizzards.

State governments coordinate each state's Emergency Operations Plan and establish emergency management agencies to manage the state's response to a disaster. If the disaster involves more than one local jurisdiction, the state may coordinate response services. When a disaster happens, the governor opens the Emergency Operations Center, where some state agencies (i.e., state police, National Guard, and state health and social service agencies) work together to direct activities for disaster relief. If the state does not have the resources to respond to and manage the disaster, the governor can request federal disaster relief assistance (Summerlin, 2007).

The federal government enacts laws and provides funds to support state and local governments. The Public Disaster Act of 1974 (PL 93-288) provided consolidation of federal disaster relief activities and funding under a single agency. As a component of this Act, the **Federal Emergency Management Agency (FEMA)** was established in 1979. During reorganization of federal governmental agencies to better prepare for effective management, response, and recovery following the events of 9/11, in 2003 FEMA became part of the Department of Homeland Security (Summerlin, 2007).

As the federal agency charged with assessing and responding to disaster events in the United States, FEMA's responsibilities include emergency planning, preparedness, mitigation, response, and recovery. Working closely with state and local governments, FEMA funds emergency programs and provides technical guidance and training in all phases of disaster management (Beachley, 2005; Allender and Spradley, 2005). A great deal of information on preparation for disasters and how to respond is readily available on the Agency's website: www.fema.gov. The Community Application Box "Disaster Planning" is an example.

COMMUNITY APPLICATION
Disaster Planning

EMERGENCY SUPPLIES

Food

Store at least a 3-day supply of nonperishable food.
Have a manual can opener.
Keep disposable plates, cups, and utensils.

Clean Air

Store snugly fitting face masks.
Store plastic sheeting, duct tape, and scissors to seal off a room.

Water

Store at least a 3-day supply, 1 gallon per day per person.
Store water in clean plastic bottles.

Supply checklist

Basic supplies include flashlight, batteries, radio, garbage bags, map, moist towelettes, whistle, clothing, bedding, and tools.

First-Aid Kit

Basic supplies include sterile gloves, dressings, soap, antibiotic ointment, bandages, eye wash, and nonprescription medications (e.g., aspirin).

Special Needs Items

Have a supply of prescription medications, special items for infants (diapers, formula), elders, or persons with disabilities.

MAKE A PLAN

Create a Family Plan

Plan how to contact one another if the family is separated.
Review the plan for different situations.

At Work and Schools

Schools, daycare providers, workplaces, apartment buildings, and neighborhoods should have site-specific emergency plans.

In a High-Rise Building

Plan for the possibility that you may be in a high-rise building at the time of an attack.
Note the closest emergency exit.
Be sure you know another way out, in case your first choice is blocked.
Take cover against a desk or table if things are falling.
Face away from windows and glass.
Move away from exterior walls.
Do not use elevators.
Stay to the right when going down stairwells to allow emergency workers to come up.

In a Moving Vehicle

If the vehicle becomes difficult to control, pull over.
Avoid road hazards.
Obey barriers and signs.

Deciding to Stay or Go

Depending on your circumstances and the nature of the attack, the first important decision is whether to stay put or get away . You should understand and plan for both possibilities.

Source: Department of Homeland Security.

DISASTER SERVICES PROVIDED BY THE AMERICAN RED CROSS

The **American Red Cross** (ARC) is a voluntary support agency founded in 1881 by Clara Barton. The ARC operates across the United States and has chapters in many localities throughout the country and throughout the world. The Disaster Relief Acts of 1970 and 1974 give the ARC the authority to act as the primary voluntary national disaster relief agency for the American people and to be ready for immediate action in every part of the United States (Beachley, 2005). As a result, the ARC provides disaster relief services to people 24 hours a day, 7 days a week.

Each year the ARC responds to more than 70,000 disasters, including house or apartment fires (the majority of disaster responses), hurricanes, floods, earthquakes, and tornados among others. Chapters of the ARC have been set up in more than 1300 communities to respond to needs of victims (ARC, 2008). The ARC chapters participate in drills and exercises that enable volunteers to respond quickly and effectively. It has created five programs to meet human needs during a disaster (Table 9-4). In addition to providing volunteers and services in the event of a disaster, the ARC also provides information for what to do during an emergency. For example, they provide instruction on how to "shelter in place." (See the Community Application box "Shelter-In-Place Instructions.") Their website

(www.redcross.org) has a wealth of information on emergency preparedness.

DISASTER PLANNING

Whether considering the potential for external disasters/emergencies or internal emergencies, the key to effective disaster management is predisaster planning and preparation. To better prepare for the future, planning requires the ability to forecast events, engineering to reduce risks, public education about potential hazards, a coordinated emergency response, and a systematic assessment of the effects of a disaster. Responsibility for addressing disaster planning is shared by the local, state, federal, and voluntary agencies. Beachley (2005) lists eight principles for disaster management:

1. Prevent the occurrence of the disaster whenever possible. Many disasters, particularly manmade ones, may be preventable through such activities as enforcement of building codes, proper land and water management, equipment maintenance, and safety education.
2. Minimize the number of casualties if the disaster cannot be prevented. Early warning systems can help alert the public to the possibility of immediate danger and help reduce the impact of predictable disasters. In addition, information on an evacuation plan can be used to improve the chance of survival.

TABLE **9-4** Programs Provided by the American Red Cross During Disasters

PROGRAM	EXAMPLES OF ACTIVITIES
Damage Assessment	Gather information about the physical damage resulting from a disaster
Mass Care	Provide food, shelter, and supplies (e.g., hygienic articles, toilet articles, cleaning supplies) to victims and disaster workers
Health Services	Provide medical, nursing, and health care (e.g., blood and blood products, emergency medical supplies) to meet the emotional and medical needs of victims and disaster workers
Family Services	Emergency assistance to help families by providing food, clothing, shelter, medical needs, household furnishings, and occupational supplies and equipment
Disaster Welfare Inquiry Service	Gathers information about the disaster, including what and who are affected and individuals killed or injured; information is disseminated to concerned relatives

Adapted from Beachley M: Nursing in a disaster. In Maurer FA, Smith CM, editors: *Community/public health nursing: health for families and populations*, ed 3, St Louis, 2005, Saunders.

COMMUNITY APPLICATION
Shelter-in-Place Instructions

LOCATION	INSTRUCTIONS
Home	Close all windows, turn off all fans, go to above-ground room, take disaster supplies with you, and bring pets inside; go to room with a telephone, wet some towels and jam them in the space under the door.
School	Close the school, activate emergency plan, and keep visitors in the building; provide for telephone inquiries from concerned parents; if children have cell phones, allow them to call a parent; select interior rooms above the ground floor.
Work	Close the business, bring everyone into one room, shut and lock the doors, keep customers in the building, turn on call-forwarding, change the recording to indicate the business is closed; if danger of explosion, close the window shades, blinds, or curtains.
Vehicle	If close to home, office, or a public building, go there. If unable to get to a home or building, pull over to the safest place possible, turn off the engine, close windows and vents, listen to the radio regularly for updated advice, and follow directions from law enforcement officials.

Adapted from: American Red Cross (2003): *Fact sheet–shelter in place* (website): http://www.redcross.org/services/disaster/beprepared/shelterinplace.pdf. Accessed January 20, 2008.

3. Prevent further casualties from occurring after the initial impact of the disaster. Identify and lessen any unsafe conditions that occur after a disaster; these often affect disaster workers (i.e., police and firefighters).
4. Rescue the victims. Aid workers must locate and free trapped victims and then move them to a safe place.
5. Provide first aid to those injured.
6. Evacuate the injured to medical facilities. Aid workers must plan for transport vehicles and routes while considering current weather conditions, conditions of roads, and location of hospitals.
7. Provide medical care. All hospitals have disaster plans and hold disaster drills; how they are used during a disaster depends on the availability and location of medical care facilities and personnel.
8. Promote reconstruction of lives. Care should continue until recovery, and both victims and disaster workers should receive psychological counseling and emotional support.

All communities should have a disaster plan. In addition, many organizations and groups (i.e., fire-fighters, police, emergency personnel, public health officials, hospitals) that would be called upon during a disaster must have their own plans to integrate with the community plan. Elements of a disaster plan are listed in Box 9-1.

PREPARATION FOR INTERNAL EMERGENCIES

Most hospitals and many other businesses, industries, and organizations are required to have plans in place for emergencies and disasters. Oftentimes, however, clinics, schools, churches, and retail businesses are not always prepared for internal emergencies. In view of the fact that emergencies and disasters can occur anywhere, nurses need to do what they can to assure that organizations and facilities are able to manage an emergency or disaster.

Virtually all businesses, organizations, or facilities have some risk for experiencing emergencies (e.g., workplace violence, fire, weather-related emergencies). Incidents have occurred in schools, churches, clinics, daycare centers, occupational/work settings, businesses, and hospitals. These incidents may occur in any season of the year and may be confined or

BOX 9-1 Elements of a Disaster Plan

Chain of authority (person or agency responsible for issuing warnings and with authority for delegation)
Lines of communication
Equipment and supplies
Human resources (health professionals, disaster specialists, governmental officials, engineers)
Team coordinators (persons assigned to coordinate aspects of a disaster)
Modes of transportation
Documentation
Evacuation routes
Rescue personnel and equipment
Acute care (triage and first aid)
Supportive care for victims and families
Means for evaluation

Sources: Lundy KS, Butts JB: The role of the community health nurse in disasters. In Lundy KS, Janes S, editors: *Community health nursing: caring for the public's health*, p. 546, Boston, 2001, Jones and Bartlett; Allender JA, Spradley BW: Communities in crisis: disasters, group violence and terrorism. In Allender JA, Spradley BW, editors: *Community health nursing: promoting and protecting the public's health*, ed 6, Philadelphia, 2005, Lippincott Williams & Wilkins; Summerlin E: Natural and manmade disasters. In Nies M, McEwen M, editors: *Community/public health nursing: promoting the health of populations*, ed 4, St Louis, 2007, Saunders.

may cover a wide-ranging area. Since the 9/11 attacks, a great deal of attention has focused on precautions to take to be prepared for biological, chemical, and nuclear terrorist attacks, but measures to prepare for internal emergencies and disasters have been neglected (Chevez, 2002).

Regardless of the setting, nurses have a responsibility and role in an organization's or facility's emergency and disaster preparedness and response plans. To this end, nurses need to ask questions such as the following: What are the potential hazards for this facility? Does a disaster plan exist? Does the disaster plan include policies and procedures for emergencies and disasters that might occur within the facility? Does the disaster plan include procedures for community disasters? If a plan exists, when was it last reviewed and updated? Has the plan been tested by a drill? Nurses should be prepared to evaluate the completeness of a facility's planning for an unexpected emergency or disaster event and to act as a resource for

other agencies and organizations to help them do the same.

ROLE OF THE NURSE DURING DISASTERS

During a disaster, nurses and other emergency personnel are usually advised not to attempt to provide care until the situation has stabilized. Depending on the disaster, nurses may be involved in triage, in acute care/first aid for immediate treatment, or in shelters or other areas of support.

TRIAGE

During a disaster the first obligation of relief workers is to remove victims from danger. This job usually falls to first responders (e.g., firefighters and others trained in search and rescue), and nurses are rarely involved.

After victims have been removed from danger, if there are multiple severe casualties, disaster triage allows health care personnel to identify the most salvageable clients so that treatment can be initiated immediately. *Triage* is the sorting of casualties. **Disaster triage** is different from triage conducted in the emergency rooms of hospitals. The focus of disaster triage is to do as little as possible for the greatest number in the shortest period of time. Triage can determine where and how the victim is to be managed. In some circumstances the victim might be treated onsite; in others they might be removed to a hospital via ambulance, helicopter, or other type of transport. Nurses may be involved in several areas during triage. They may conduct the triage, monitor those persons waiting for care, or work on the logistics of transfer.

Once a decision has been made during triage regarding the individual's condition, a specific color-coded triage tag is placed on the person. A green tag is used for those with minor injuries who can wait for care. Yellow is for those who have serious systemic injuries that are not life threatening and can wait. A red tag is considered "top priority" and is used for those who need immediate treatment to address a life-threatening condition but who have a probability for survival. A black tag is reserved for the deceased or for those whose injuries are so extensive that nothing can be done to save them.

EMERGENCY CARE/FIRST AID

Following initial triage, disaster nurses may provide care onsite at emergency treatment stations, or they may work at local hospitals and clinics. At first-aid stations, nurses are needed to provide direct nursing care, evaluate health care needs, and arrange for transport once victims are stabilized. They may also be involved in managing the procurement, distribution, and replenishing of supplies and providing on-the-job training and supervision of volunteer staff and assigning them to appropriate duties. In some cases, nurses may be called on to arrange for psychological and spiritual care of victims; in other cases they may be asked to care for bodies and notify families (Allender and Spradley, 2005). They may also be involved in direct disaster counseling. The Community Application box "Disaster Counseling" offers suggestions for how to best provide emotional support to disaster victims.

SHELTER ASSISTANCE

Shelters are managed by trained volunteers and the ARC. In widespread disasters, such as hurricanes, shelters are opened in several areas to house the local residents and victims who have traveled to escape more immediate danger. Each shelter has a team manager, a nurse, people to keep records, and numerous volunteers. Activities include keeping records; coordinating meals; providing snacks, cots, blankets, and other essentials; and providing health care (Lundy and Butts, 2001).

COMMUNITY APPLICATION
Disaster Counseling

Disaster counseling involves both listening and guiding. Survivors typically benefit from talking about their disaster experiences and being assisted with problem solving and obtaining referrals to resources. These suggestions for disaster counselors are provided by the Center for Mental Health Services:

Establish Rapport: Survivors respond when workers offer caring eye contact and a calm presence. Rapport includes an attitude of interest and understanding and genuine concern. Conveying respect and being nonjudgmental are necessary for building rapport.

Active Listening: Workers listen most effectively when they take in information through their ears, eyes, and "extrasensory radar" to better understand the survivor's situation and needs. Some tips for listening are:

Allow silence: Silence gives the survivor time to reflect and become aware of feelings. Silence can prompt the survivor to elaborate. Simply "being with" the survivor and their experience is supportive.

Attend nonverbally: Eye contact, head nodding, caring facial expressions, and occasional "uh-huhs" let the survivor know that the worker is in tune with him or her.

Paraphrase: When the worker repeats portions of what the survivor has said, understanding, interest, and empathy are conveyed. Paraphrasing also checks for accuracy, clarifies misunderstandings, and lets the survivor know that he or she is being heard. Good lead-ins are: "So you are saying that . . . " or "I have heard you say that . . . "

Reflect feelings: The worker may notice that the survivor's tone of voice or nonverbal gestures suggests anger, sadness, or fear. Possible responses are, "You sound angry (scared, etc.), does that fit for you?" This helps the survivor identify and articulate his or her emotions.

Allow expression of emotions: Expressing intense emotions through tears or angry venting is an important part of healing; it often helps the survivor work through feelings so that he or she can better engage in constructive problem-solving. Workers should stay relaxed, breathe, and let the survivor know that it is OK to feel.

SOME DO'S AND DON'T'S

Do say:
- These are normal reactions to a disaster.
- It is understandable that you feel this way.
- You are not going crazy.
- It wasn't your fault; you did the best you could.
- Things may never be the same, but they will get better, and you will feel better.

Don't say:
- It could have been worse.
- You can always get another pet/car/house.
- It's best if you just stay busy.
- I know just how you feel.
- You need to get on with your life.

The human desire to try to fix the survivor's painful situation or make the survivor feel better often underlies the preceding "Don't say" list. However, as a result of receiving comments such as these, the survivor may feel discounted, not understood, or more alone. It is best when workers allow survivors to have their own experiences, feelings, and perspectives.

From Center for Mental Health Services (2008): *Disaster counseling* (website): http://mentalhealth.samhsa.gov/publications/allpubs/KEN-01-0096/default.asp. Accessed February 20, 2008.

In shelters, nurses consult with the shelter manager on the health status of residents and workers and identify potential problems and needs. They may also monitor those who are particularly vulnerable for poor outcomes or health problems (e.g., pregnant women, elders, small children, the ill or injured) and may refer clients for additional treatment or follow-up.

THE NURSE AND DISASTER PREPAREDNESS

Everyone should be encouraged to be prepared for a disaster. As health professionals, nurses in particular should be aware of potential dangers and prepare accordingly. In addition, nurses should know community resources that deal with disasters, and if interested should join a local disaster action team or act as a liaison with local hospitals. Hassmiller (2004) suggests three levels of preparedness for nurses: (1) personal preparedness, (2) professional preparedness, and (3) community preparedness.

Personal preparedness addresses personal and family preparation and includes recognizing what would be the most likely type of disaster that could happen to the family (i.e., Does the family live in an area that might be hit by a hurricane? An earthquake? A blizzard?). The family should review disaster plans at the workplace or school and create a disaster plan for the home. The family should maintain emergency supplies in case of a disaster. Supplies should include a 3-day supply of water (1 gallon per person per day); food that will not spoil; a change of clothing and blanket or sleeping bag for each person; a first-aid kit that includes prescription medications, emergency tools and supplies, and items needed for infants, elders, or disabled family members. For additional information, see the Health Teaching box "Family Disaster Plan."

Professional preparedness refers to the need for nurses to be aware of and understand the disaster plans in the community. Items for nurses preparing to help in a disaster include a copy of their professional license, personal equipment (e.g., stethoscope), flashlight and extra batteries, weather-appropriate clothing, materials to keep records, and pocket-size reference books. In addition, all workers should be trained in first aid and CPR.

---

health teaching

Family Disaster Plan

A home disaster plan should be focused on the most likely or logical type of disaster that might happen. The plan should include an evacuation plan/escape route, emergency telephone numbers, being sure that insurance coverage is adequate, having a fire extinguisher and knowing where it is kept and how to use it, installing smoke detectors on each level of the home, and identifying safe spots in the home for various types of disasters. The disaster plan should also include assembling emergency supplies and a first-aid kit. According to FEMA, the family disaster supplies kit should include the following:

- Water: a minimum 3-day supply of water for each person in the household (1 gallon of water per person per day)
- Food: a 3-day supply of nonperishable food. Foods should require no refrigeration, preparation or cooking, and little or no water. Include ready-to-eat canned meats, fruits and vegetables; canned juices; milk; soup; staples (e.g., sugar, salt, pepper); high-energy foods (e.g., peanut butter, jelly, crackers, granola bars); vitamins; foods for infants, elders, or persons on special diets; and comfort/stress foods (e.g., cookies, hard candy, cereals, instant coffee, tea bags)
- First-Aid Kit: sterile adhesive bandages in assorted sizes, sterile gauze pads, hypoallergenic adhesive tape, 2- and 3-inch sterile rolled bandages, scissors, tweezers, needle, moistened towelettes, antiseptic, thermometer, tongue blades, tube of petroleum jelly or other lubricant, assorted safety pins, cleansing agent/soap, latex gloves, sunscreen, and prescription and nonprescription drugs (pain reliever, antidiarrheal medication, antacid, syrup of Ipecac, laxative)
- Tools and Supplies: paper cups, plates, and plastic utensils; battery-operated radio and extra batteries; flashlight and extra batteries; cash or traveler's checks; a credit card; extra car keys; extra eyeglasses; manual can opener; fire extinguisher; pliers; tape; compass; candles and matches in a waterproof container; aluminum foil; plastic storage containers; signal flare; paper and pencil; needles and thread; wrench to turn off household gas and water; whistle; plastic sheeting; regional map; toilet paper; soap and liquid detergent; feminine supplies; plastic garbage bags; disinfectant; chlorine bleach
- Clothing and Bedding: sturdy shoes or work boots, rain gear, blankets or sleeping bags, hat and gloves, thermal underwear, sunglasses
- Special Items: for family members with special needs (infants, elders); include formula, diapers, medications, extra eyeglasses
- Important family documents (kept in a portable, waterproof container): wills, insurance policies, stocks and bonds, passports, Social Security cards, immunization records, bank account numbers, credit card account numbers, and an inventory of valuable household goods, important telephone numbers, and family records (birth, marriage, and death certificates).

From Federal Emergency Management Agency: *Your family disaster plan*, Jessup, Md, 2001, FEMA.

Community preparedness focuses on the community's ability to address a disaster. Some communities plan for disasters by having written disaster plans and participating in yearly disaster drills. Nurses can become a part of this process by becoming members of the disaster team at work or in the community.

EMERGENCY AND DISASTER MANAGEMENT

Emergency and disaster management involves prevention, preparation and planning, responding, and recovering from the emergency or disaster incident. Nurses and other staff members can respond more quickly if all the aspects of emergency or disaster management have been considered. Regardless of the setting, proactive measures need to be determined and taken so that everyone in a facility, community, or region is aware of what hazards are likely to happen both internally and externally and what procedures to follow should an emergency or disaster occur.

PREVENTION/MITIGATION

Measures taken before an emergency or disaster event are known as *prevention* or **mitigation**. The first step in prevention or mitigation is identifying the potential risk factors for a community or facility. **Hazards** are sources of danger that need to be identified, both within and outside the facility or community. Assessment for hazards, as well as identifying the direct and indirect effect each hazard presents, should be initial priorities. Assessment provides an opportunity to prevent or minimize some of the threats to safety (San Francisco Office of Emergency Services & Homeland Security, 2005). The characteristics of the emergency or disaster must also be considered before a plan to manage the danger is developed or revised. Characteristics to be considered are the frequency and the predictability of a hazard event occurring, the preventability of the hazard event, its imminence (how much warning the facility would have), how long the event might last, and the scope and number of potential casualties.

PREPARATION AND PLANNING

Once the hazards and their characteristics are identified, a well-written plan to manage the emergencies or disasters needs to be created. Box 9-2 lists items to include in a clinic or office disaster plan. The items suggested are broad and should fit any facility. A word of caution: a person should not be named to carry out responsibilities, but a position and an alternate should be identified. The specifics to be included under each of the suggested items are unique to each setting. FEMA, the ARC, Homeland Security, and the Internet have many fact sheets with suggestions about what to do to prepare for an emergency and what should be included or addressed in a plan. Once the plan is developed regular training and exercises to test the plan should be conducted. Review of an agency's or organization's plan should be included in any orientation for new staff and volunteers.

RESPONSE

In an internal disaster the role of the nurse may vary greatly, depending on the extent and type of emergency. The response stage of an emergency or disaster

---

BOX **9-2** Suggested Items to Include in a Clinic or Office Disaster Plan

GENERAL

Purpose of the disaster plan
Scope of the disaster plan
Plan activation
　Who can activate the plan
　Circumstances when the plan should be activated
Disaster plan mission statement
Leadership and succession of leadership
Delegation of authority
Supporting plans and resources
Legal authorities, codes, and policies

Plan administration (e.g., distribution, updates)
Staff activation and call down procedures
Mutual aid agreements
Communication procedures
Organizational chart
Job action sheets

SPECIFIC PLANS

Evacuation plan
Transportation plan
Medical management plan

Source: San Francisco Office of Emergency Services & Homeland Security (2005): *Clinic/office disaster & emergency planning* (website): http://www.sfgov.org/site/oes_index.asp. Accessed November 24, 2007.

starts immediately after the event occurs. The facility may close completely, go into a lockdown situation, institute shelter in place, evacuate the facility, conduct search and rescue, conduct emergency triage, provide direct care, or become a community shelter site. Policies and procedures should note roles and personnel responsible for different aspects of the plan. For example, if the facility closes, in what stages do the staff leave? Do any staff have to stay to secure the facility? If patients are present, what information should they receive, and who is responsible for informing them?

RECOVERY

Recovery begins when the danger or event is over, and the facility begins to resume its prior mission or service. Individuals have many reactions to an emergency or disaster event; this includes staff members of the facilities. Individuals will experience emotional, cognitive, physical, and interpersonal reactions as described previously. If the facility has a shelter role, many of these reactions will be present simultaneously. The nurse needs to know what the reactions may be and how to address them on a short-term basis and possibly a long-term basis. School nurses, parish nurses, occupational health nurses, clinic nurses, and public health nurses will all be involved in helping individuals who are experiencing reactions following an emergency or disaster. Nurses' role(s) during the recovery stage may include case finding, referring for treatment, providing counseling and support, case management, and direct patient care.

SUMMARY

Nurses have a very important role to play in the management of emergency or disaster incidents. In addition to assisting in the management of large-scale emergencies, they may be involved earlier in the process during the emergency-preparedness planning stage. Indeed, nurses should participate in the process of assessing potential emergency or disaster threats and advocating for both communities and facilities to take preventive/mitigation measures to minimize the effects.

As illustrated in the opening case study, educating administrators and community leaders about potential hazards and recognizing the effects of an emergency or disaster are extremely important.

Nurses have a personal and professional role to play in being prepared for any emergency. This should include seeking out additional training or education in disaster management; keeping credentials current; knowing what injuries, diseases, and reactions victims may experience; and knowing how to manage them. Care should also include recognizing individuals who are struggling to recover from an emergency or disaster event and providing counseling and support or referral when needed. Finally, all nurses can assist by: (1) partnering with others in their community or facility to develop emergency plans, (2) participating in drills to test the plans, and (3) evaluating the success of the plan in order to make revisions as needed.

KEY POINTS

- Sudden, unexpected emergency or disaster events occur everywhere, and no community, business, organization, or facility is exempt from experiencing them.
- Communities, businesses, organizations, and facilities should assess for potential hazards and take appropriate proactive measures to counter the hazards.
- Nurses need to be aware of potential threats or hazards as they approach planning phases and use governmental and professional guidelines for the essential elements to include in the plans for a particular community or facility (business, school, clinic, church).
- To ensure the safety of staff, clients, and visitors in their facility, nurses need to take an active role in facilitating or advocating for prevention, preparedness, planning, response, and recovery policies and procedures for managing emergencies and disasters.

Learning Activities & Application to Practice

1. Obtain a copy of an organization's, agency's, or business's disaster plan for analysis. Does it address hazards specific to the facility or only external disasters? What needs to be changed? Why?
2. Discuss with classmates how the role of the nurse would differ from setting to setting in different facilities. What nursing role is most important in each setting? What is the rationale for the decision?

3. In class, in groups of four to six, draft a personal and professional disaster plan for an emergency event occurring at your college/university while you are in class.

4. Interview a first responder in your community and ask for suggested safety issues for the following: home health agency, hospice care, parish nursing, nurse practitioner in a retail store. If possible, negotiate a "ride out" with the responder.

5. Research the history of emergencies or disasters that have occurred in two different settings in your community. What were the emergency or disaster events? Were the incidents from an internal hazard or external disaster? Who was involved in their management? Were changes made to the disaster plan(s) following the event?

REFERENCES

Allender JA, Spradley BW: Communities in crisis: disasters, group violence and terrorism. In Allender JA, Spradley BW, editors: *Community health nursing: promoting and protecting the public's health*, ed 6, Philadelphia, 2005, Lippincott Williams & Wilkins.

American Academy of Experts in Traumatic Stress: *A practical guide for crisis response in our schools*, Commack, NY, 2003, AAETS.

American Federation of Labor–Congress of Industrial Organizations: *Violence against women in the workplace* (website): http://www.aflcio.org/issues/jobseconomy/women/violence.cfm. Accessed November 14, 2007.

American Red Cross (2008): *Red Cross facts* (website): http://www.redcross.org/services/disaster/0,1082,0_562_,00.html. Accessed January 5, 2008.

American Public Health Association (2005): *Types of disasters and their consequences* (website): http://www.medscape.com/viewarticle/513258_print. Accessed October 6, 2007.

Beachley M: Nursing in a disaster. In Maurer FA, Smith CM, editors: *Community/public health nursing: health for families and populations*, ed 3, St Louis, 2005, Saunders.

Chavez LJ (2002): *18 workplace violence incidents since September 11th: for the workplace killer, it is business as usual* (website): http://www.workplaceviolence911.com/Articles/articles.jsp?listType=1015-63K. Accessed September 21, 2007.

Edwards TD, Young RA, Lowe AF: Caring for a surge of hurricane Katrina evacuees in primary care clinics, *Ann Fam Med* 5(2):170, 2007 (electronic version online): http://www.medscape.com/viewarticle/555951_print. Accessed September 13, 2007.

Hassmiller SB: Disaster management. In Stanhope M, Lancaster J, editors: *Community & public health nursing*, ed 6, St Louis, 2004, Mosby.

Lundy KS, Butts JB: The role of the community health nurse in disasters. In Lundy KS, Janes S, editors: *Community health nursing: caring for the public's health*, Boston, 2001, Jones and Bartlett.

MSNBC staff and news service reports (2007, December 9): *Gunmen, victim killed in Colo. church attack: police, four others wounded–no link to earlier Colorado shooting* (website): http://www.msnbc.msn.com/id/2217178. Accessed February 10, 2008.

San Francisco Office of Emergency Services & Homeland Security (2005): *Clinic/office disaster & emergency planning* (website): http://www.sfgov.org/site/oes_index.asp. Accessed November 24, 2007.

Sternberg E: Planning for resilience in hospital internal disaster, *Prehosp Disaster Med* 18:291, 2003.

Summerlin E: Natural and man-made disasters. In Nies M, McEwen M, editors: *Community/public health nursing: promoting the health of populations*, ed 4, St Louis, 2007, Saunders.

USAID (2008): *USAID rebuilds lives after the tsunami* (website): http://www.usaid.gov/locations/asia_near_east/tsunami/background.html. Accessed February 20, 2008.

U.S. Department of Labor/Occupational Safety and Health Administration: *Hospital hazards* (website): http://www.osha.gov/SLTC/healthcarefacilities/hazards.html. Accessed December 27, 2007.

Warchol G: *National crime victimization survey: workplace violence 1992-96*, Washington, DC, 1998, Department of Justice.

Young BH et al: *Disaster mental health services: a guidebook for clinicians and administrators*, Menlo Park, Calif, 1998, Department of Veterans Affairs, National Center for PTSD.

UNIT

Three

Settings for Community-Based Care

Nursing Care in Ambulatory Settings

objectives

Upon completion of this chapter, the reader will be able to:

1. Discuss specific aspects of nursing care in clinics, offices, schools, worksites, rural areas, parishes, and correctional facilities.

2. Discuss specific aspects of nursing care in ambulatory oncology centers, outpatient surgical centers, and public health departments.

3. Compare and contrast nursing practice in different ambulatory care settings.

4. Explain education and certification issues related to ambulatory nursing practice.

key terms

Ambulatory care
Ambulatory nursing practice
Ambulatory oncology
  nursing practice
Ambulatory surgery
Correctional nursing

Education for All
  Handicapped Children Act
  (PL 94-142)
Occupational health nursing
Occupational Safety and
  Health Act (PL 91-596)

Parish nursing
Public health nursing
Rural nursing
School nursing
Workers' compensation
See Glossary for definitions.

case study

Bill Barnett is a registered nurse (RN) working in a postanesthesia care (recovery) unit (PACU) in a day surgery center. The day surgery center is a freestanding facility located in a small city. The center houses six operating rooms and 30 to 40 surgical procedures are performed there daily.

    The various surgical procedures performed at the center involve virtually all surgical specialties. On a typical day, general surgery procedures (e.g., laparoscopic cholecystectomy, inguinal hernia repair), orthopedic procedures (e.g., arthroscopy), gynecological procedures (e.g., laparoscopy, cervical dilation, curettage), ophthalmic procedures (e.g., cataract extraction, radial keratotomy), plastic surgery (e.g., blepharoplasty, rhinoplasty), otolaryngology procedures (e.g., tonsillectomy, myringotomy/placement of pressure equalization [PE] tubes), and others are performed.

Continued

Bill is one of seven PACU RNs employed at the day surgery center, and he has worked there 5 years. During that time he has seen the caseload grow dramatically, with many of the procedures becoming increasingly complex. The first surgical cases are scheduled to begin at 07:30 and continue until about 15:00. The RNs work staggered shifts. Bill begins his day at 10:00 and is responsible for recovering patients from the later cases.

On a recent Thursday, Bill cared for Tony Mitchell, a 17-year-old high school football player who tore his left medial meniscus during practice. The surgeon performed arthroscopic surgery on Tony's left knee and shaved the torn part of the meniscus. The surgery was done under general anesthesia and lasted about an hour.

Tony was beginning to awaken from anesthesia when he was brought into the PACU by the anesthesiologist and the circulating nurse. His endotracheal tube had been removed in the operating room, but he still had an oral airway in place and was breathing without difficulty. Bill placed a blood pressure cuff on Tony's right arm and took his vital signs (blood pressure, 110/56; pulse, 88; respirations, 20; temperature, 97°F). His blood oxygen levels were monitored by a pulse oximeter and remained at 98.

When Bill called Tony's name and instructed him to open his eyes, Tony complied. He gagged slightly and reached toward his mouth to remove the oral airway. Bill assisted him and discarded the airway in a nearby container. Tony responded appropriately to questioning and stated that his left leg hurt a little. The left leg had been wrapped in a heavy dressing and Ace bandage in the operating room and then propped on two pillows. Bill assessed the foot and toes for swelling, color, and capillary refill. All were "normal." When asked, Tony moved his left toes without difficulty.

Bill received a report from the anesthesiologist and circulating nurse, both of whom stated that the procedure was uneventful. The anesthesiologist detailed the medications that had been used during the procedure and gave Bill the anesthesia records and operative report, and both left to prepare for their next cases.

Bill monitored Tony's vital signs and pulse oximeter every 5 minutes for about 20 minutes and then every 10 to 15 minutes for the next hour. By that time Tony was alert and requested something to drink. Within 2 hours after admittance to the PACU, Tony was sitting up in a recliner and drinking an iced soft drink; his intravenous line had been removed, and his parents were present. Bill used that time to reinforce the postoperative instructions that Tony and his parents had already been given. They repeated the instructions and stated that they would take Tony to the surgeon's office the next day for postoperative evaluation. They had already filled a prescription for pain medication given to them earlier and correctly verbalized the appropriate dosage. Tony was discharged from the day surgery center about an hour later and left on crutches with his parents.

The term **ambulatory care** refers to personal health care provided to an individual who is not a patient in a health care institution. Over the last several decades, ambulatory care has grown dramatically, and continued growth is anticipated indefinitely. Today approximately 60% of all surgical procedures are performed on an outpatient basis. Likewise, chemotherapy and other parenteral medications are delivered in homes and outpatient centers; diagnostic tests and procedures are performed in freestanding clinics and centers; and health promotion and health education services are provided in convenient settings such as home, work, church, and school. In most instances, ambulatory patients/clients engage in self-managed health activities or receive care from families (ANCC, 2007; Swan, Conway-Phillips, & Griffin, 2006).

It is not surprising that the growth in non-institution-based care has resulted in a concurrent growth in the number of nurses who are employed in these areas. Ambulatory care nursing includes "direct patient care, telehealth nursing practice, health maintenance and promotion, disease prevention and management, patient education and counseling, patient advocacy, case management and the coordination of care for patients throughout the health care system" (AAACN, 2007, p.10).

Many of the objectives of *Healthy People 2010* (U.S. Department of Health and Human Services [USDHHS], 2000) involve health teaching, symptom monitoring and management, and risk reduction activities that are most effectively delivered during primary care office visits, formal or informal health education classes, individual counseling sessions, or other health-promotion situations. The *Healthy People 2010* box lists some of the objectives that relate to ambulatory health care settings.

This chapter explores some of the numerous settings for community-based health care delivery and briefly describes nursing practice in those settings. The settings and descriptions of nursing practice are by no means all inclusive. Settings, clientele, and nursing practice vary greatly by geographical area, population needs, nursing practice guidelines and protocols, and a number of other factors. The purpose of this chapter is to give a general overview of practice opportunities for RNs apart from acute care, long-term care, and home health settings.

Included is nursing care in clinics and physicians' offices, schools, work sites, churches, and specialty practices such as oncology care, surgery, and public health.

NURSING PRACTICE IN SELECTED SETTINGS

Community-based nursing practice often involves being a member of a group or practice concerned with the provision of comprehensive, primary care for individuals or families in a geographically or institutionally defined area. In these instances nursing care is largely focused on health promotion, primary prevention, screening for early identification of disease, and assisting in treatment regimens for both acute and chronic illnesses (e.g., colds, influenza, ear infection, hypertension, diabetes).

Again, it is important to note that nursing roles and interventions may vary significantly in similar settings by organizational or institutional policy,

healthy people **2010**

Examples of Objectives Appropriate for Community-Based Settings (e.g., Clinics, Schools, Work Sites, Churches)

OBJECTIVE	BASELINE (1998)	TARGET
6.9: Increase the proportion of children and youth with disabilities who spend at least 80% of their time in regular education programs	45%	60%
7.1: Increase high school completion	85%	90%
7.4a: Increase the proportion of the nation's elementary, middle, junior high, and senior high schools that have a nurse-to-student ratio of at least 1:750	28%	50%
7.6: Increase the proportion of employees who participate in employer-sponsored health-promotion activities	28%	50%
14.23g: Maintain measles vaccination coverage levels for children in kindergarten through the first grade	96%	95%
15.39: Reduce weapon carrying by adolescents on school property	8.0%	6.0%
19.16: Increase the proportion of work sites that offer nutrition for weight-management classes or counseling	55%	85%
24.5: Reduce the number of school days missed by people with asthma from asthma	NA	NA

Data from U.S. Department of Health and Human Services: *Healthy people 2010*: Conference ed, Washington, DC, 2000, Government Printing Office.

state practice regulations or requirements, and other factors. For example, in one occupational setting, the nurse's practice may primarily be concerned with monitoring Occupational Safety and Health Association guidelines and workers' compensation cases and providing first aid to injured employees, whereas in another company the occupational health nurse's practice focuses on health promotion and illness-prevention activities, such as conducting screenings and health education classes and providing counseling. This section briefly describes nursing practice in selected settings.

HEALTH CARE PROVIDER OFFICE OR CLINIC

Probably the most familiar role of the nurse in community-based practice is that of the office or clinic nurse. Nurses working in physician-based practices, nurse-based practices, and health maintenance organizations collectively account for the largest group of nurses working outside hospitals. In the United States, approximately 11.5% of all RNs are employed in clinic or office settings (USDHHS/Division of Nursing [DON], 2006). The most common types of practice are the physician-based solo practice, group practice or partnership, and the health maintenance organization.

Nursing Practice in Ambulatory Clinics and Offices

As mentioned previously, the roles and responsibilities of the nurse vary greatly between clinics because the practice, focus, and clients are often very different. Physicians may be general or family practitioners who provide preventive care and diagnose and treat clients of all ages and for all types of health problems. Other general areas of practice include pediatrics, obstetrics and gynecology, and internal medicine. Practitioners in these areas provide "primary care" to more focused groups (i.e., children, women, and adults, respectively), but care is still comprehensive, covering multiple body systems. The many medical and surgical specialists (e.g., surgeons, cardiologists, dermatologists, ophthalmologists, psychiatrists, orthopedists) see clients with more specific health problems.

The roles and interventions that nurses practice in physicians' offices obviously are based on the type of care provided in that office or clinic. For example, a nurse working in a surgeon's office may assist with surgical procedures, provide follow-up through phone calls, remove sutures, and help with preprocedure and postprocedure assessments. A nurse working in a cardiologist's office might assist in monitoring stress tests and perform electrocardiograms and other tests, and a nurse working in a pediatric office may assist in physical and developmental assessment, collect specimens (e.g., finger sticks, strep cultures), teach parents about infant care, and administer immunizations.

The scope of **ambulatory nursing practice** includes such activities as measurement, specimen collection, client follow-up, assessment, health teaching, provision of comfort measures, coordination of services, and preparation of patients for surgical or nonsurgical procedures. Box 10-1 lists some of the roles and responsibilities in practice in ambulatory care clinics.

The American Academy of Ambulatory Care Nursing (AAACN) has published practice standards for ambulatory care nursing administration. The ten standards for practice outlined by the organization relate to structure and organization of ambulatory care nursing, staffing, competency, ambulatory nursing practice, continuity of care, ethics and patient's rights, environment, knowledge development, performance improvement and leadership (AAACN, 2007).

Education, Experience, and Certification Recommendations for Clinic Nurses

There are some specialized requirements for employment in physicians' offices and clinics. Skills and competencies needed include: knowledge of illness and symptom management; experience with triage; strong assessment and organizational skills; communication skills; and ability to collaborate as a member of a multidisciplinary team (Novotny, Lippman, Sanders & Fitzpatrick, 2003). Although some physicians or other providers prefer that the nurses they employ have at least 1 year of hospital experience, many hire new RNs. A baccalaureate degree is usually not required for nurse's positions in ambulatory settings. Certification for ambulatory care nurses is available through the American Nurses Credentialing Center (ANCC) (see www.nursecredentialing.org).

SCHOOLS

Documentation of efforts to promote student health through school health services began in New York City in the late 1800s. The distinguished public

BOX **10-1** Examples of Nursing Practice Roles and Interventions in Ambulatory Care

ENABLING OPERATIONS
- Maintaining safe work environment
- Setting up the room
- Ordering supplies
- Providing emotional support
- Taking vital signs

TECHNICAL PROCEDURES
- Preparing the client for procedures
- Assisting with procedures
- Chaperoning during procedures
- Informing the client about treatment
- Witnessing signing of consent forms
- Administering medications
- Collecting specimens

NURSING PROCESS
- Developing the nursing care plan
- Using nursing diagnosis
- Completing the client history
- Assessing client learning needs

- Evaluating client care outcomes
- Charting each client encounter

TELEPHONE COMMUNICATIONS
- Performing telephone triage
- Calling the pharmacy with prescription
- Calling the client with test results

ADVOCACY
- Making the clients aware of rights
- Acting as a client advocate
- Referring the client to an appropriate provider

TEACHING
- Instructing the client on medical/nursing regimen
- Instructing the client on home and self-care

CARE COORDINATION
- Acting as a resource person
- Coordinating client care
- Assessing needs and initiating referrals
- Finding resources in the community
- Instructing on health promotion

Adapted from Hackbarth DP, Haas SA, Kavanagh JA, Vlasses F: Dimensions of the staff nurse role in ambulatory care: part I–methodology and analysis of data on current staff nurse practice, *Nurs Econ* 13(2):89-98, p.92. 1995. Reprinted with permission of the publisher, Jannetti Publications, Inc.

health nurse Lillian Wald is credited with convincing New York City's school board to use a public health nurse to decrease absenteeism. As a result of her support, Lina Rogers was employed as the first school nurse in 1902. Reportedly Miss Rogers was so successful that 25 additional nurses were hired over the next several years, and the use of public health nurses in school-based practice spread rapidly to other cities, including Boston, Chicago, and Philadelphia (Kalisch & Kalisch, 2004; Pollitt, 1994). Currently, more than 78,000 school nurses practice in the United States, accounting for about 3.2% of all RNs (USDHHS/DON, 2006).

Early emphasis in school health programs was on control of communicable diseases such as tuberculosis, smallpox, diphtheria, whooping cough, pediculosis, scabies, and ringworm. As measures to control communicable diseases proved successful, attention moved toward sanitation, safety issues, and early detection and remediation of physical problems (e.g., vision and hearing deficits) that might impede learning. Throughout the next 40 to 50 years, school nursing roles and activities expanded to include assisting the physician with examination of students;

counseling of students, parents, and teachers; and developing and implementing health education programs. School nurses also made home visits, provided in-service education for teachers, and served as a resource for school administration.

The roles and practice of school nurses have continued to evolve. Most recently school health service programs have concentrated on the following components:
- Prevention of illness and disease transmission and early detection of possible disease
- Intervention in identified problems such as alcohol and drug use, sexually transmitted diseases (STDs), pregnancy, family violence, and the adaptation of children with special health needs to the school setting
- Promotion of healthy lifestyles
- Health education, both formal and informal

School health programs and the role of school nurses have strengthened and expanded during the past 2 decades. Currently, school-based teams are used nationwide in numerous ways, including caring for disabled children, investigating suspected child abuse, improving health education, promoting the safety of school children, implementation and management of school-based clinics, and research and evaluation of school health programs.

School Nursing Practice

The school nurse is responsible for maintaining the school health program. Pourciau and Vallette (2007) describe **school nursing** practice in the following terms:

- Prevention and control of communicable diseases/immunizations monitoring
- Care of ill or injured students
- Care of children with special health needs
- Health screening
- Health education
- Counseling and social services
- Providing a healthy school environment
- Health office management/ student records

Each of these components is discussed briefly in the following sections.

PREVENTION AND CONTROL OF COMMUNICABLE DISEASES/IMMUNIZATIONS MONITORING. Communicable disease control and prevention in school health programs typically involves monitoring immunization records to ensure student compliance with school district and state requirements, exclusion for communicable disease, and efforts for infection control (e.g., universal precautions for all individuals who contact body fluids, hand washing protocols for cafeteria workers, monitoring incidence of illness and absenteeism).

Although requirements differ, completion of a basic set of childhood immunizations is necessary for school attendance in all states. Exceptions to these requirements vary somewhat by state and may be made for philosophic, religious, or health reasons (e.g., having had a documented case of measles) (CDC, 2006; National Network for Immunization Information [NNII], 2004).

It is usually the responsibility of the school nurse to monitor the immunization records of each child to ensure compliance. When a deficiency is observed, the nurse follows school district guidelines to ensure remediation of the deficiency. In some districts this simply involves gaining parental permission and providing the vaccination at the school. In other settings the nurse sends a letter to the child's parent or guardian that explains which vaccinations are not current. Often this letter includes consequences (e.g.,

exclusion from school) if the immunization is not completed in a timely manner and information on where to go for low-cost or free immunizations.

Exclusion from school of those students who contract communicable diseases is based on school district policy and state laws. Therefore it is essential that the nurse be aware of these requirements and understand under what conditions a child is to be excluded from school and under what conditions he or she may return. For example, children with chicken pox are generally excluded from attending school until after 7 days from onset of the rash, and children with strep infections are excluded until 24 hours has passed following initiation of antibiotic therapy and fever has subsided.

CARE OF ILL OR INJURED STUDENTS. The school nurse is responsible for monitoring the health of students, providing first aid and emergency care when indicated, and administering treatments and medications when prescribed, following school district procedures and standard protocols. The nurse should maintain a file of basic information, health records, and emergency information for each student.

Providing simple first aid for minor injuries is common in school nursing practice. Normally, each school district develops a set of first aid protocols or instructions to follow when caring for simple problems such as scrapes, blisters, sprains, or stings. A first aid kit should be well stocked and readily available for treatment of minor injuries. When more serious emergencies occur, it is often the school nurse's responsibility to provide first aid, inform the parents, and make arrangements to transport the student to the emergency room or physician's office if necessary. School districts should also have guidelines for the nurse to follow in emergency situations.

For students with acute or chronic illnesses or conditions, administration of medication or treatments at school may be necessary. School districts maintain policies on who is to administer medications and treatments, the process to be followed, and guidelines for record keeping. Sometimes it is the responsibility of the nurse to perform these services, but often the nurse must train others to perform these tasks and monitor their care, per district policy.

CARE OF CHILDREN WITH SPECIAL HEALTH NEEDS. Congress enacted the **Education for All Handicapped Children Act (PL 94-142)** in 1975. Public Law 94-142 gives "all students, including those who are severely handicapped, the right to public education in the least restrictive environment possible, regardless of physical or mental disabilities" (Pourciau & Vallette, 2007, p. 613). The law was amended in 1986, expanding the eligible population to include preschool students. This amendment was added to reduce developmental delays, minimize institutionalization, and help families meet the special needs of children with disabilities. The Act was amended further in 2003 (The Individuals with Disabilities Education Act [IDEA]—PL 105-17) to provide special education and related services as well as assistive technology devices to "eligible" students. Conditions covered by IDEA are physical or mental impairments that substantially limit life activities. These include: physiological disorders, cosmetic disfigurement, or anatomical loss affecting the neurological, musculoskeletal, respiratory, digestive, genitourinary, hematological, endocrine or lymphatic systems, as well as impairments of the senses (auditory, vision). IDEA also covers serious psychological disorders such as mental retardation, organic brain syndrome, emotional or mental illness (e.g., depression), or specific learning disabilities (e.g., dyslexia) (Zimmerman, 2006).

Requirements of PL 94-142 and its amendments that specifically relate to school nursing are: (1) a provision that efforts must be made to screen or identify children in need of special education and related services, and (2) completion of an individualized education plan (IEP), which is developed by an interdisciplinary team and includes current educational level, goals, and specific services to be provided.

As part of the IEP, the school nurse will develop an individualized healthcare plan (IHP) by assessing the student and determining health needs. The IHP should specify coordination of care activities, educational needs, and instruction for assistive personnel. Within an IHP, school nurses and other designated individuals may be called on to monitor ventilator-dependent children, perform or supervise intermittent catheterization, and administer gastrostomy feedings. As with medication administration, performance of these procedures must be within the state's Nurse Practice Act, follow district policy, be authorized by parents, and be prescribed by a physician.

HEALTH SCREENING. Screening for actual and potential health problems and hindrances to education is a very important component of a school health program. State mandates, available staff, rate of incidence of certain conditions, resources, time, and facilities determine screening programs and procedures.

In most school health programs, screening includes vision, hearing, height and weight, and scoliosis. Screening for other health conditions (e.g., acanthosis nigricans, depression) may be required or provided by some states.

Although regulations and requirements vary across states (Selekman, 2006), the National Association of School Nurses (NASN, 2006) supports vision screening programs in schools. Such screenings may detect problems that can interfere with a student's ability to learn. Specifically the NASN recommends vision evaluation of young and never-screened children for near-, distance-, binocular-, and color visual function, and then periodic appraisal of the distance vision of older previously-screened children. Additional evaluation can be performed at the request or recommendation of the child's parents or teachers.

After identification of a suspected vision problem, the school nurse should make a referral following district protocol. As with all school referrals, a follow-up should be made within 4 weeks to ensure that the child has had further evaluation and treatment if indicated (Kimel, 2006; Selekman, 2006).

Hearing screening programs are conducted to promote a high level of hearing acuity for all students, minimize the number of students with hearing loss, and provide for individual education needs of students with permanent hearing impairment. As with vision screening, state requirements and regulations will vary somewhat regarding when school children are screened for auditory difficulties and who is responsible.

Hearing screening should be performed by nurses or other professionals (e.g., audiologists) trained in hearing screening and should include visual examination through an otoscope (to detect cerumen, foreign bodies, or a perforation of the tympanic membrane), audiometric testing or pure-tone screening (records the softest level at which a tone can be heard), and acoustic emittance testing (used to measure middle ear pressure). As with vision screening, a referral is made following identification of a possible problem.

Optimally height and weight of each child should be measured and recorded annually to detect potential problems. Students' Body Mass Index (BMI) should be calculated from height and weight information and compared to recommended norms. Recording of growth measurements should be completed and referrals made following district guidelines.

Although routine screening for scoliosis is no longer endorsed by the U.S. Preventative Services Task Force (2004), "postural screening" is required by most states to identify students who may have physical findings suggesting spinal deviations or curvature indicating scoliosis (Sekelman, 2006). As with vision and hearing screening, screening for scoliosis is largely dependent on school district and state mandates, and as with other screening programs, follow-up for suspected scoliosis is essential.

HEALTH EDUCATION. Promoting and encouraging positive health practices through health education is a central component of school nursing. Topics often covered by nurses in schools include nutrition education, dental health, developmental changes/sexuality, and prevention of substance abuse.

COUNSELING AND SOCIAL SERVICES. The school nurse should be available to perform health counseling for students, parents, staff, and others. Promotion of mental health and reduction or removal of threats to mental health are important nursing interventions (Pourciau & Vallette, 2007). School nurses help students learn to solve problems and assist them in identifying additional services or care as needed. For example, young girls who suspect pregnancy often call upon the school nurse for counseling, or if they have confirmed a pregnancy, they may seek assistance. Similarly, the school nurse will work with parents to help identify low-cost dental care, glasses, mental health services, or other needed care.

HEALTH OFFICE AND STUDENT RECORD MANAGEMENT. The school nurse's office should be amply equipped and supplied to allow for comprehensive and appropriate services. Minimally, the health offices should contain a desk and chair, locked filing cabinet for student files, locked cabinet for medications, cots for ill students, hot and cold running water, and private office space for conferences.

Student records should include immunization status, pertinent health concerns, results of screening and examinations, and IEPs/IHPs as appropriate. Finally, school nurses must be aware of and respect the confidentiality of health information requirements mandated by HIPAA.

Education and Experience Recommendations for School Nurses

A baccalaureate degree in nursing is recommended by the American Nurses' Association (ANA) and the NASN as the entry level for practice as a school nurse; many school districts require it. Throughout the United States, however, many diploma- or associate degree-prepared school nurses are currently practicing. Some school districts require a minimum of 1 year of experience, preferably in pediatrics, before employment.

OCCUPATIONAL HEALTH

Occupational health (industrial) nursing (OHN) in the United States began in the late 1800s. Reportedly a group of coal mining companies in Pennsylvania hired a nurse named Betty Moulder to care for miners and their families. At approximately the same time, Ada Mayo Stewart was hired as an "industrial health nurse" by the Vermont Marble Company. By 1912, 38 nurses were employed by businesses and industries, and that number had grown to 11,000 by 1943 (Rogers, 2003). There are currently more than 22,000 occupational health nurses practicing in the United States (USDHHS/DON, 2006).

Occupational Health Nursing Practice

The American Association of Occupational Health Nurses (AAOHN) has stated that OHN is an autonomous specialty in which nurses make independent nursing judgments in providing health care services. Further, OHN is "the specialty practice that focuses on promotion, prevention, and restoration of health within the context of a safe and healthy [work] environment. It includes the prevention of adverse health effects from occupational and environmental hazards. It provides for and delivers occupational and environmental health and safety programs and services to clients" (AAOHN, 2004, p. 270). The Research Highlight box "Occupational Health" provides details about deaths from injuries suffered in an occupational setting.

Occupational health nursing practice is a synthesis of knowledge from nursing, medicine, occupational health, epidemiology, environmental health, and social and behavioral sciences and includes business and economics concepts and principles, as well as legal and ethical principles (Rogers & Travers,

Research Highlight

Occupational Health

The CDC (2007) reported that during 2005, a total of 5702 individuals sustained work-related, fatal injuries (an average of almost 16 work-related deaths per day). Despite the relatively high number, there were some positive findings. For example, there was a 23% decline in the U.S. occupational fatality rate between 1992 and 2005. Additional findings included the following:

- Males accounted for 93% of all occupational injury deaths.
- Workers aged 25 to 34 accounted for the largest number of occupational injury deaths.
- Transportation incidents accounted for 43% of all deaths.
- "Contact with objects and equipment" (e.g. being struck by a falling object, being crushed during a cave-in) was the

second leading cause of occupational deaths (18%), followed by "assaults and violent acts" (14%), falls (13%), exposure to harmful substances or environments (e.g. heat stroke or hypothermia, poisoning though inhalation of harmful substances, insect stings, animal bites) (9%), and fires (3%).

- Industries with the largest number of deaths were construction (1186 deaths); transportation and warehousing (881 deaths); and agriculture/forestry/fishing/hunting (714 deaths).
- The highest death rates were for agriculture/forestry/fishing (32.5/100,000), mining (25.6/100,000), transportation (17.6/100,000), and construction (11.0/100,000).

Data from Centers for Disease Control and Prevention: Fatal occupational injuries–United States, 2005, *MMWR Morbid Mortal Wkly Rep* 56(13):297-300, 2007; and U.S. Department of Labor, Bureau of Labor Statistics, *Census of fatal occupational injuries, 2005* (website): http://www.bls.gov/news.release/cfoi.toc.htm. Accessed June 28, 2007.

2007). Occupational health nursing practice is directed by a combination of federal and state regulations, company policy and philosophy, the type of work or setting, worker input, nurse interest and expertise, and available resources.

The scope of practice of OHN includes the following (Rogers, 2003):

- Worker/workplace assessment and surveillance to identify potential problems and determine the state of health of the worker(s).
- Occupational health care and primary care to provide treatment, follow-up, referral for medical care, and emergency care.
- Case management to improve health care coordination for early intervention and to help foster the worker's return to work.
- Health promotion, health protection, and prevention for both individuals and groups of workers to enhance levels of health and move toward optimal health.
- Counseling to help employees clarify problems and make informed decisions and choices and giving positive reinforcement.
- Management and administration of the occupational health unit, which will contribute to the company's overall health goals.
- Community orientation, providing collaboration and partnerships with community agencies and groups, thereby enhancing available resources for employees and the company.

- Research and trend analysis to identify the relationship between the worker and elements in the work environment that might positively or negatively affect health.
- Legal/ethical management to ensure a safe and healthful work environment for all employees.
- Managing workers' compensation claims.
- Training for cardiopulmonary resuscitation (CPR) and first aid.

Legislation Affecting Occupational Health Nursing Practice

Much of the practice of the OHN is directed by or in response to federal legislation and state mandates. Several of the most significant laws affecting OHN practice are described here.

WORKERS' COMPENSATION ACTS (DATES VARY BY STATE). **Workers' compensation** is an insurance system operated by the states, with each state having its own law and program. The first workers' compensation law was passed in New York in 1910, and subsequently all 50 states and the District of Columbia have enacted workers' compensation laws (Rogers & Travers, 2007).

Workers' compensation insurance is "no fault" and benefits are provided through employer-carried insurance plans. Benefits are awarded to individuals who sustain physical or mental injuries from their employment, regardless of who or what caused the injury or illness. Although they vary by state, workers' compensation laws generally allow for ongoing payment of wages and benefits to the injured or disabled worker or dependent survivor for wages lost, medical care and related costs, funeral and burial costs, and some rehabilitation expenses.

OCCUPATIONAL SAFETY AND HEALTH ACT (1970). The **Occupational Safety and Health Act (PL 91-596)** is a comprehensive, multifaceted, and far-reaching piece of legislation. The purpose of the Occupational Safety and Health Act is to "assure so far as possible every working man and woman in the Nation safe and healthful working conditions and to preserve our human resources" (Public Law 01-596, 91st Congress, December 29, 1970; cited in Rogers, 2003, p. 531).

To accomplish the stated purpose, the Occupational Safety and Health Act did the following:

1. Formed the Occupational Safety and Health Administration (OSHA), which sets and enforces standards of occupational safety and health (Department of Labor).
2. Formed the National Institute for Occupational Safety and Health (NIOSH), which researches and recommends occupational safety and health standards to OSHA and funds educational centers for the training of occupational health professionals (USDHHS).
3. Established the National Advisory Council on Occupational Safety and Health, a consumer and professional council that makes occupational safety and health recommendations to OSHA and NIOSH.
4. Established federal occupational safety and health standards.
5. Established the Occupational Safety and Health Review Commission to advise OSHA and NIOSH regarding the legal implications of decisions or actions.
6. Created a mechanism for imposition of fines and other punitive measures for violation of federal occupational safety and health regulations.
7. Required employers to maintain records of work-related deaths, injuries, and illnesses (Rogers and Travers, 2007).

The party responsible for promulgating legally enforceable standards that employers must meet to be in compliance with the Occupational Safety and Health Act is OSHA. The responsibilities of OSHA are to perform the following:

- Develop and update mandatory occupational safety and health standards.
- Monitor and enforce regulations and standards.
- Require employers to keep accurate records on work-related injuries, illnesses, and hazardous exposures.
- Maintain an occupational safety and health statistics collection and analysis system (in collaboration with NIOSH).
- Supervise employer and worker education and training to identify and prevent unsafe or unhealthy working conditions (in collaboration with NIOSH).
- Provide grants to states to assist in compliance with the Occupational Safety and Health Act (Adams, 2001).

Education, Experience, and Certification Recommendations for Occupational Health Nurses

A baccalaureate degree is recommended for OHN practice. The AAOHN notes that OHNs usually have a baccalaureate degree in nursing and experience in community health, ambulatory care, critical care or emergency nursing (AAOHN, 2007). Certification in OHN is available through the American Board for Occupational Health Nurses (ABOHN). To be eligible for certification, RNs must have worked at least 4000 hours as an occupational nurse during the past 5 years, have completed 50 contact hours of continuing education in occupational health nursing-related areas during the past 5 years, and successfully pass a certification examination (ABOHN, 2006).

RURAL HEALTH

Like school nursing, early efforts to develop organized nursing practice in rural areas are traced to Lillian Wald. Miss Wald is credited for helping establish the Rural Nursing Service in 1912 (American Red Cross, 2007). A few years later, in 1925, Mary Breckinridge began the Frontier Nursing Service. These efforts focused on improving public health, primary health care, and midwifery services in rural areas (Frontier Nursing Service, 2007). Currently, approximately 4400 nurses are employed in rural health centers (USDHHS/ DON, 2006). Many other nurses practice in home health care and county or state public health agencies in rural areas.

The term *rural* is somewhat difficult to characterize. Typically, rural is defined based on geographic location and population density or in terms of distance or time needed to commute to an urban center. In general, rural areas are communities having less than 20,000 residents or fewer than 99 persons per square mile (Bushy, 2004).

About 20% of U.S. residents reside in rural areas, and in 13 states, more than 40% of the population are considered to be rural. The states with the lowest population density, therefore the most rural areas are: Alaska (1 person/square mile), Wyoming (5 people/square mile), Montana (6 people/square mile), North Dakota (9 people/square mile), South Dakota (10 people/square mile), and New Mexico (15 people/square mile) (U.S. Census Bureau, 2007). Although significant regional variations occur, several distinctive characteristics are common to rural populations in general that are important to nurses. For example, residents of rural areas are more likely to live in poverty. Bayne (2005) notes that of the poorest counties in the United States, 244 are rural; further, over 50% of the nation's poor live in rural areas (USDA, 2004). Other notable demographic characteristics of persons in rural areas include higher percentages of both children and elders, and lower levels of education. Box 10-2 compares characteristics of residents of rural and urban settings, illustrating how health threats and needs might be exacerbated in this population.

Issues in Rural Health Care

Distance, isolation, and sparse resources are inherent in rural areas, and these factors can negatively affect the health of rural residents. As with barriers to health care in other settings and populations, barriers to health care for individuals living in rural settings include availability and accessibility to health care providers and institutions, affordability of health care (because many residents are uninsured or underinsured), and acceptability. Lack of transportation, inequitable reimbursement policies for providers, weather conditions, lack of understanding of entitlements and services, and lower education levels also contribute to problems for rural residents in obtaining health care (Bushy, 2000; Bushy, 2007).

Rural Nursing Practice

Nurses practicing **rural nursing** most often practice in clinic settings, home health, or a combination. Skills needed by nurses in rural settings include technical and clinical competency; adaptability; flexibility; refined assessment skills; organizational abilities; independence; good decision-making skills; leadership ability; self-confidence; and skill in handling emergencies, teaching, and public relations. Box 10-3 presents characteristics of nursing practice in rural settings.

It is important that rural health nurses be willing to be cross-trained and educated to acquire competencies outside their primary specialty area. Rural nurses must also be able to remain current and competent in

---

BOX 10-2 Comparisons of Rural and Urban Americans

- A higher proportion of whites live in rural areas (82%) than in urban areas (62%) (however, this varies markedly by region).
- Rural communities have higher percentages of younger and older residents.
- Adults in rural areas have fewer years of formal education.
- Rural families tend to be poorer (more than 25% of rural Americans live in or near poverty and nearly 40% of all rural children are impoverished).
- Rural Americans are more likely to be uninsured or underinsured.

- Rural residents are more likely to have chronic illnesses (e.g., hypertension, arthritis, diabetes, cardiovascular disease, cancer).
- Rural residents have higher infant and maternal morbidity and mortality rates.
- Several health care risks are unique to rural occupations (e.g., machinery accidents, skin cancer from exposure to the sun, pulmonary and other problems related to exposure to chemicals and pesticides).
- Rural adults are less likely to have preventive health care (e.g., Pap smears, breast examinations, prostate specific antigen, cholesterol screenings).

Data from Bushy A: Community and public health nursing in rural and urban environments. In Stanhope M, Lancaster J, editors: *Community and public health nursing*, ed 6, St Louis, 2004, Mosby; Bushy A: Rural health. In Maurer FA, Smith CM, editors: *Community/public health nursing: health for families and populations*, ed 3, St Louis, 2005, Saunders.

BOX 10-3 Characteristics of Nursing Practice in Rural Environments

- Variety/diversity in clinical experiences
- Broader/expanding scope of practice
- Generalist skills
- Flexibility/creativity in delivering care
- Sparse resources (e.g., materials, professionals, equipment, fiscal)
- Professional/personal isolation
- Greater independence/autonomy
- Role overlap with other disciplines
- Slower pace
- Lack of anonymity

- Increased opportunity for informal interactions with clients/co-workers
- Opportunity for client follow-up upon discharge in informal community settings
- Discharge planning allowing for integration of formal and informal resources
- Care for clients across the life span
- Exposure to clients with a full range of conditions/ diagnoses
- Status in the community (viewed as prestigious)
- Viewed as a professional role model
- Opportunity for community involvement and informal health education

From Bushy A: Community and public health nursing in rural and urban environments. In Stanhope M, Lancaster J, editors: *Community and public health nursing*, ed 6, pp. 374-395, St Louis, 2004, Mosby.

practice in an environment characterized by sparse resources. Furthermore, it is recommended that all nurses in rural settings have training in trauma care and advanced life support, which may be required to assist in the stabilization of emergency cases. Finally, rural nurses need case management skills for transfer, referral, and coordination of care in areas characterized by the lack of specialized health care resources (Bushy, 2000; Bushy, 2007).

Education and Experience for Rural Nursing Practice

Nurses who practice in rural settings should have experience in a variety of areas, including rehabilitation, obstetrics, medical-surgical nursing, geriatrics, pediatrics, and emergency care. A knowledge of available resources and ability to coordinate formal and informal services is very important in rural health nursing (Bushy, 2000; 2004).

There are no specific educational recommendations for rural nursing practice. Educational preparation, however, should include public health principles, the process of community assessment, and content in health promotion and illness prevention, which historically has been a component of baccalaureate nursing education. Nursing authorities have recognized the need to consider changes in nursing education to develop curricula at each education level to address the unique needs of rural nursing (see the Research Highlight "Agricultural Health Nursing in the United States"). In particular, "schools and colleges of nursing which are situated in rural areas, or whose graduates tend to serve rural residents, have an obligation to structure their

programs to include rural content and clinical experiences in rural settings" (ANA, 1996, p. 24).

PARISH NURSING

Parish nursing is both a new and an old model of health care delivery. Indeed, the history of nursing is full of examples of religious orders or congregations providing care for the sick (Schank, Weis, and Matheus, 1996). The concept of modern-day parish nursing in the United States is attributed to a Lutheran chaplain, Granger Westberg, who reportedly advanced the role beginning in 1983 (Miskelly, 1995).

The philosophy of parish nursing is "to promote the health of a faith community (churches or synagogues) by working with the pastor and staff to integrate the theological, psychological, sociological, and physiological perspectives of health and healing into the work, sacrament and services of the congregation" (Solari-Twadell, Djupe, and McDermott, 1990, p. 51). Parish nursing programs are supported by many different denominations. There are thought to be at least 3000 parish nurses practicing in the United States (Siegrist, 2007).

The growing interest in parish nursing is attributed to several factors, including the following:
- Increasing focus on health promotion, disease prevention, and health and illness management.
- Problems of fragmentation of health care and the reemergence of the "wholeness" concept regarding health care.
- Increased emphasis on self-care and individual responsibility.
- Problems with access and cost.

Research Highlight

Agricultural Health in Nursing Curricula in the United States

Reed, Hoffman, and Westneat (2005) conducted a regional study of 185 nursing schools in the Southeastern part of the United States to assess both undergraduate and graduate nursing program curricula for emphasis on "agricultural health." The researchers discovered that of the responding programs, 84% did not include agricultural health issues at all or only mentioned it in passing. Indeed, only 15% of the programs noted that agricultural issues were covered in "20% or more of at least one class." Further, most faculty completing the surveys (49.5%) indicated that they were not aware of the need to teach nurses about agricultural health issues. It was determined that nursing faculty and students are interested in agricultural topics related to health and that more emphasis should be placed on exposing students to research and content in agricultural health and safety.

From Reed DB, Hoffman C, Westneat SC: Nurses' agricultural education in the southeastern United States, *J Nurs Educ* 44(6):271-276, 2005.

- Increasing numbers of people with chronic illness.
- Recognition of the need to identify and work with people in the community and in institutions (Schank, Weis, and Matheus, 1996).

Miskelly (1995) describes the following four models of parish nursing:

1. Institutional/paid model: The parish nurse is employed by a hospital, community agency, or long-term care facility that provides salary, benefits, support, and supervision and contracts with one or more churches to deliver care.
2. Institutional/volunteer model: A relationship exists between a church and an institution whereby the institution provides a stipend to the nurse or congregation and/or education and supervision; the nurses are volunteers.
3. Congregational/paid model: The nurse is employed by the congregation and receives benefits and supervision from the church itself.
4. Congregational/volunteer model: The parish health care program is supported by nurses volunteering their time.

Parish Nursing Practice

The goal of parish nursing is the enhancement of quality of life for all members of the congregation (Schank, Weis, and Matheus, 1996). Parish nurses coordinate and train volunteers. They organize and facilitate support groups, provide referrals to community resources, provide health education and counseling, and serve as a liaison within the health care system. In addition, parish nurses provide health education, advocacy, counseling, and screenings. Invasive nursing procedures and/or home health care are not usually components of parish nursing programs.

Through research, several health education needs appropriate for parish nursing care have been identified. These include stress management, development of a durable power of attorney and living wills, nutrition, grief support, cancer risk factors and prevention, CPR training, parenting skills, alcohol abuse, and infertility. Interventions include health counseling and screening (e.g., cholesterol, blood pressure, skin cancer, occult blood screening), support group facilitation (e.g., grief, parenting, caregiver), education (e.g., stress management, nutrition, exercise, CPR), and community resource referrals (e.g., weight control groups, infertility support groups, violence resources, alcohol abuse support groups). Provision and facilitation of information on health-related topics through use of a monthly newsletter and maintenance of a health section in the church library can be used to disseminate timely information on safety tips, home health care, health insurance, prevention of heart disease, and many other topics (Miskelly, 1995).

The parish nurse should develop the practice and program in response to the unique needs and priorities of the congregation and its members. Leadership, organizational, clinical, counseling, and teaching skills are essential.

Education and Experience for Parish Nursing Practice

A baccalaureate degree is recommended for parish nurses. Three to five years of experience in nursing practice, spiritual maturity, and ability to practice independently are important attributes for a parish nurse (Siegrist, 2007). It is recommended that all parish nurses complete a formal program of study.

These are typically offered in universities, hospitals, or established parish nursing programs and may be taken for college credit, continuing education, or postgraduate certification (Solari-Twadell and McDermott, 2006).

The curriculum for parish nursing courses should be comprehensive. Among others, topics for inclusion are an overview of the role of the church in health care, the history and philosophy of parish nursing, models of parish nursing, and roles and functions of the parish nurse (see the Community Application box). Other important issues and interventions for parish nurses are community assessment, health-promotion concepts, philosophy of self-care, legal and ethical issues (i.e., confidentiality, accountability, documentations, and end-of-life issues), how to be a part of a ministerial team, and how to start a parish nursing program.

CORRECTIONAL INSTITUTIONS

According to Droes, "the number of individuals incarcerated in the United States is the highest since data were first available in 1925" (1994, p. 201). In the United States the judicial system has mandated that correctional facilities have the responsibility to provide health care to all individuals confined to

their facilities (Hufft and Fawkes, 1994). In many cases, nurses are the primary health care providers in correctional facilities.

Issues in Caring for Persons in Correctional Facilities

In general, members of ethnic and racial minorities and people from lower socioeconomic groups are disproportionally represented in correctional facilities. In addition, residents of correctional institutions experience a higher rate of disease and disability than the general population. Infectious diseases (e.g., respiratory infections, influenza, gonorrhea, tuberculosis, hepatitis, and human immunodeficiency virus [HIV]), conditions related to the use and abuse of drugs and alcohol, seizure disorders, and acute mental health problems are particularly common. Trauma and chronic problems such as cirrhosis of the liver, gastritis, pancreatitis, and cardiac pathology are also prevalent (Snow, 2007).

One of the many distinctive characteristics of providing health care in correctional facilities is that clients usually have no choice in the selection of health care providers and may have no choice in the services provided. Likewise, a great deal of professionalism is needed for nursing practice in

---

COMMUNITY APPLICATION
Advocacy Roles for Parish/Congregational Nurses

Patterson (2007) notes that being an advocate is a critical component of parish nursing and discusses eight advocacy interventions appropriate for the practice. These are:

1. Help obtain access to care: Help locate health insurance programs or coverage options for those who cannot afford health insurance, or help find providers who will accept reduced fees.
2. Serve as a health navigator: Help those with insurance negotiate their way through the system by providing information about options for services and treatment.
3. Serve as an advocate in the healthcare system: Assist those who are patients in hospitals and nursing homes by monitoring care; encourage the patient and their family to speak up if they are concerned about the care the patient is receiving.
4. Work to acquire needed services in a community: Work with other local providers to give or coordinate free or

low-cost services (e.g., dental care) to poor/underserved community residents.
5. Mobilize for the health of neighbors: Support and assist programs that help meet needs of community members (e.g., providing classes on parenting and life skills management).
6. Raise awareness of legislative issues related to health: Educate members about health-related issues being addressed by lawmakers at all levels (local, state, national).
7. Advocate for environmental health concerns: Maintain awareness of environmental issues that might be harmful in the neighborhood/region; help educate others about environmental health concerns and what can be done to address them.
8. Work for those living in developing countries: Promote participation in outreach projects sponsored by the church to help manage or reduce health problems in developing countries.

From Patterson DL: 8 advocacy roles for parish nurses: what can a congregation do to address health issues that cry out for advocacy?, *J Christian Nurs* 24(1):33-35, 2007.

correctional facilities, in that providers in prison settings must have the ability to separate the action of the crime or offense of the individual inmate from his or her illness or health care needs (Hufft and Fawkes, 1994).

Nursing Practice in Correctional Facilities

Health services in correctional settings vary from health screening to full hospital services. In general, the main component of **correctional nursing** is the provision of primary care and emergency services for the inmates. Primary health care in these facilities typically includes screening activities, direct health care services, analysis of individual health behaviors, teaching and counseling, and assisting individuals in assuming responsibility for their own health (ANA, 1995).

Because of the situation and population encountered in this type of nursing practice, client needs and related nursing interventions in correctional facilities are quite unique. The ANA (1985) described the following specific interventions:

- Health education: Promotion of individual and group well-being through health education activities (e.g., health counseling, health teaching, and formal programs in health education).
- Suicide prevention: Ongoing assessment of suicide risk and planning and coordination of interventions that prevent suicidal behaviors.
- Communicable disease control: Promotion of a healthful environment to reduce the incidence of communicable disease within the correctional setting.
- Alcohol and drug rehabilitation: Collaboration with other members of the health care team to treat inmates who have substance abuse problems.
- Medication administration: Supervision of the administration of medications in accordance with state regulations and national standards.
- Psychosocial counseling: Provision of crisis intervention and episodic and ongoing psychosocial counseling.
- Emergency care: Initiation of emergency care as needed, according to community standards of care.
- Environmental health: Ongoing monitoring of the environment for conditions that would have a negative impact on health and safety within the facility and reporting of significant findings to the institution's management.

Nurses who work in correctional facilities must work toward the goal of preserving and promoting the health of the incarcerated individual within the institution's broader goal of security (see the Research Highlight "Caring in a Correctional Setting"). However, it is important to note that these nurses should provide *only* health care services; it is inappropriate for nurses to be involved in the security functions or disciplinary decisions of the setting (e.g., conducting body cavity or strip searches) (ANA, 1995). The institution should have a well-developed and periodically revised set of policies and procedures developed jointly by nurses, physicians, prisoners, and institution personnel (Stevens, 1993).

Education and Experience Recommendations for Nursing Practice in Correctional Facilities

Experience in mental health nursing is desirable for nurses who wish to practice in correctional facilities. Likewise, experience in emergency services, medical/surgical nursing, and community or public health nursing is also very beneficial. Educationally the ANA recommends a baccalaureate degree in nursing for the practice of nursing in correctional facilities (ANA, 1985). Finally, because of the unique characteristics described here, Stevens (1993) suggests that "nurses considering this practice setting

---

Research Highlight

Caring in a Correctional Setting

Weiskopf (2005) reported on a phenomenological study that examined the experience of caring for prisoners in a correctional setting. She discovered five themes associated with RNs' work with inmates: (1) negotiating the boundaries between custody and caring; (2) struggling to create a caring environment, (3) striving to turn a life around, (4) managing risky situations, and (5) staying vigilant. She explained how caring for inmate patients is complex, conflicting, and restrictive and that nurses had to confront risks to help inmates while being cautious and vigilant regarding safety. Other factors, such as manipulative patients, uncaring co-workers, and feelings of helplessness and stress for not meeting patient needs, were reported sources of stress among the nurses in the study group.

From Weiskopf CS: Nurses' experience of caring for inmate patients, *J Adv Nurs* 49(4):336-343, 2005.

should first observe a colleague who practices in the setting" (p. 6).

NURSING PRACTICE WITH SELECTED POPULATIONS

In contrast to the provision of care to individuals and families in geographical settings, organizations, clinics, or agencies, community-based nursing care often involves caring for individuals or families undergoing directed care to treat specified illnesses or to prevent certain illnesses or health threats. Practice in these settings is often limited to single encounters to provide treatment or preventative services (e.g., day surgery, immunizations, STD treatment) or multiple visits providing care for a chronic illness (e.g., ambulatory oncology, tuberculosis management, renal dialysis). This section describes nursing practice in specialized, community-based settings.

PUBLIC HEALTH DEPARTMENTS

Public health departments safeguard the health of the public and improve the health status of the community. Local health departments are given the authority by the state to protect the health and welfare of their residents and are funded through local taxes and fees and grants from their state and from federal sources.

Approximately 2900 local health departments exist in the United States. Of these, around 66% serve populations of less than 50,000 and half have fewer than 17 full-time employees. In addition, all local health departments employ RNs (either directly or through contracted services) (Maurer and Kelly, 2005). State, county, and local health departments combined employ approximately 48,000 RNs (about 2.3% of all RNs) (USDHHS/HRSA/BHP/DON, 2006).

The scope of services provided by public health departments varies considerably across the country. In general, health departments have traditionally been responsible for environmental sanitation, communicable disease surveillance and prevention, and other services to prevent illness and promote health. Public health efforts include a variety of services and interventions, such as regulation of water and air quality; solid waste disposal; supervision of restaurants, grocery stores, and other food processors and handlers; and control of vectors that might spread disease (e.g., mosquitoes, rats).

To control communicable diseases, health departments are required to monitor them (see Chapter 19) and are usually involved in their prevention as well. This often includes provision of immunizations; easily accessible (affordable) treatment for STDs; and screening, diagnosis, and treatment of certain communicable diseases such as tuberculosis, AIDS, and Hansen's disease. In addition to these programs, again varying greatly by area, many public health departments provide prenatal and family planning services, well-baby care, community mental health services, and home health care.

Public Health Nursing Practice

Nursing practice in public health departments varies greatly, depending on the nurse's assigned area. Much of **public health nursing** practice focusing on control of communicable disease is described in detail in Chapter 19. Home health, family planning, maternal child health, and community mental health are covered in Chapters 11, 14, and 18, respectively. See those chapters to learn more about public health nursing practice.

Education and Experience Recommendations for Public Health Nurses

Because public health theory and practice are included in baccalaureate nursing programs, a baccalaureate degree in nursing is preferred by most health departments. However, most nurses currently working in public health departments were educated in diploma or associate-degree programs.

One or more years of nursing experience is often required for employment in public health departments. Practical experience in maternal and child health, primary health care, mental health care, infection control, and management of clients with HIV and AIDS is particularly helpful in public health nursing.

AMBULATORY ONCOLOGY CARE

According to Buchsel and Glennon (2005), "It is estimated that 80 to 90% of care given to patients with cancer is delivered in the ambulatory care setting" (p. 1). Sites for delivery of care and some services offered for patients with cancer include the following:
- Physicians' offices: Services may include chemotherapy administration, procedures, laboratory and x-ray facilities, counseling, and educational programs.

- Outpatient clinics: Services performed include radiation therapy, chemotherapy, biotherapy, physician and psychosocial services, symptom control, bone marrow transplantation, and rehabilitation.
- Twenty-three-hour and 24-hour clinics and day hospitals: These provide urgent care and may include an emergency room for oncology patients, an outpatient procedure unit, observation, an investigational treatment area, an after-hours telephone triage center, and on-call physician support (Lamkin, 1994).

The following health care services are related to care of oncology patients:

- Prevention, screening, and detection
- Chemotherapy
- Radiation therapy
- Blood component therapy
- Patient and family education
- Discharge planning and referral
- Nutritional support
- Group or individual counseling
- Physical therapy and rehabilitation
- Outpatient surgery
- Prescription supply and procurement
- Survivor services
- Treatment planning
- Symptom management (Lamkin, 1994; Buchsel and Yarbro, 2005)

Nursing Practice in Ambulatory Oncology Settings

Nursing interventions in **ambulatory oncology nursing practice** include client counseling (e.g., client advocacy, emotional support during visitations and by telephone), health care maintenance (e.g., general assessment of health, assessment of compliance, measurement of physiological indices), primary care (e.g., triage in person or by telephone, obtaining client history, performing physical examination), client education (e.g., group educational programs, explanation of plan of care, reinforcement of physician instructions), therapeutic care (e.g., administration of treatments such as irrigations, dressing changes, specimen collection; administration of medications), normative care (e.g., preparing client for physician, assisting physician, providing follow-up appointment), complements to client-centered care (e.g., maintaining supplies and equipment, developing educational

materials and standards of care for staff, maintaining knowledge of new care practice), communication (e.g., providing information to other health care providers regarding client care issues), and documentation and planning (Buchsel and Yarbro, 2005; Cooley, Lin, and Hunter, 1994).

Ambulatory oncology nurses often provide telephone triage, which includes follow-up, symptom management, patient education, scheduling appointments and tests, and contacting physicians to discuss patient care issues. Well-defined assessment skills that incorporate physical, psychosocial, and financial aspects are essential for this specialized practice.

Client and family education is essential to accomplishing one important goal of outpatient oncology care: to prepare the client for self-care. Client education needs include treatment options, information about specific treatments and diagnostic tests, symptom management, nutrition, pharmacology, accessing social services, technical skills (e.g., caring for catheters, central lines, self-injection), and how and when to access assistance when needed (Lamkin, 1994).

Education, Certification, Experience, and Recommendations for Ambulatory Oncology Nurses

Nurses who practice in ambulatory oncology centers should have at least 1 year of clinical experience in oncology or chronic illness. They must have good clinical skills, be certified in CPR, and be able to handle emergency situations. Certification in oncology nursing is available at three different levels: (1) oncology certified nurse (ONC), (2) certification in pediatric oncology (CPON), and (3) advanced oncology certified nurse (AOCN) for those with graduate degrees (Oncology Nursing Certification Corporation, 2007).

AMBULATORY SURGERY

Ambulatory surgery refers to the process in which patients have surgery, recover, and are discharged home the same day. Ambulatory surgery is not a new concept (it reportedly dates back to ancient Egypt), but it has increased dramatically in recent years because of advances in anesthesia and surgical techniques and a desire for convenience and cost containment. Indeed, it is estimated that more than 31 million surgical procedures, or about 63% of all surgical procedures, are performed in ambulatory settings each year in the United States (Odom-Forren, 2004).

Cost containment is one of the primary reasons for the proliferation of same-day surgical procedures. Indeed, many third-party payers require that certain procedures be done on an outpatient basis unless documentation can be provided that this would be unsafe for the patient. To determine eligibility for having a surgical procedure performed on an ambulatory basis, considerations should include general health status (patients should be evaluated to determine possibility of complications during and after the surgical procedure), results of preoperative tests (e.g., laboratory tests, chest x-ray, electrocardiogram), willingness and acceptance by the patient and family (including provision for competent care at home), anticipated recovery period, and reimbursement sources (Phillips, 2007).

Several terms can be used to describe ambulatory surgical care facilities. These include outpatient surgery centers, same-day surgical units, one-day surgery centers, or ambulatory surgery centers. Several different organizational structures are available for ambulatory surgery facilities, including the following:

- Hospital-based dedicated unit: Patients are admitted to an autonomous, independent, self-contained unit within or attached to the hospital but physically separated from the inpatient operating room suite.
- Hospital-based integrated unit: Patients share the same operating room suite and other hospital facilities with inpatients but have a separate preoperative holding area.
- Hospital-affiliated satellite surgery center: Patients are cared for at an ambulatory surgery center that is owned and operated by the hospital but physically separated from it.
- Freestanding ambulatory surgery center: Patients are cared for at a totally independent facility that is privately owned and operated for the purpose of providing surgical care.
- Office-based center: Patients are seen at a physician's office that is equipped for surgery. Many general surgeons, dermatologists, plastic surgeons, periodontists, podiatrists, and others perform surgical procedures in their offices (Phillips, 2007).

Freestanding postsurgical recovery centers provide short nonhospital stays for less-intensive recovery and for less-complex surgical cases. These centers are designed for individuals who are otherwise well but may need monitoring or services that cannot be easily, safely, or economically provided in the home. For example, a patient who has undergone extensive plastic surgery may need to be monitored for a day or two and treated for pain and to prevent complications (e.g., infection) but may not require hospitalization. For this person a short stay in a recovery center would be appropriate. Likewise, if a day surgery patient has no one to provide care at home, an overnight stay in a recovery center might help avoid an otherwise unnecessary hospitalization.

Advantages of ambulatory surgery include decreased cost to the patient and institution, increased bed availability for seriously ill patients, decreased risk of acquiring a nosocomial infection, and less disruption to the patient's personal life. Disadvantages include increased anxiety of the patient and caregiver, complications (e.g., allergic responses to drugs and anesthetics, prolonged procedures, secondary diagnosis), and unrealistic patient expectations of physical capabilities postoperatively. Occasionally patients require hospitalization because of prolonged procedures, secondary diagnosis, surgical accident, or other complications (e.g., excessive pain, nausea and vomiting, bleeding, swelling) (Phillips, 2007). Contraindications to ambulatory surgery include patients who are physically unstable, morbidly obese, acute substance abusers, or individuals who do not have adequate support at home (Groah, 1996). Box 10-4 lists surgical procedures commonly performed on an outpatient basis.

Nursing Practice in Ambulatory Surgery

Nursing care during ambulatory surgery is typically provided in three phases: (1) preoperative care, (2) intraoperative care, and (3) postanesthesia care.

PREOPERATIVE CARE. In the preoperative phase, the patient is admitted to the facility, given preoperative instructions, and prepared for the procedure. Any tests that have been performed in preparation are reviewed, and other tests may be performed at that time. The nurse conducts a preoperative interview to verify information about past medical and surgical history, the pending procedure(s), current medications, drug allergies, and other pertinent information

10-4 Commonly Performed Outpatient Procedures

GYNECOLOGY
- Conization of cervix
- Dilation and curettage
- Salpingectomy
- Salpingogram
- Tubal ligation
- Bartholin cyst excision

ORTHOPEDIC SURGERY
- Arthroscopy
- Ligament repair
- Ganglion excision
- Ulnar nerve transplant
- Fracture reduction
- Bunionectomy
- Tendon repair

OPHTHALMOLOGY
- Cataract procedures
- Ptosis
- Tear duct probe
- Eyelid surgery
- Eye muscle surgery

THORACIC SURGERY
- Esophageal dilation
- Pacemaker battery replacement

NEUROSURGERY
- Carpal tunnel release
- Ulnar nerve transfer

DENTAL/ORAL SURGERY
- Dental extraction
- Intraoral biopsy

OTOLARYNGOLOGY
- Nasal septum repair
- Otoplasty
- Tonsillectomy
- Adenoidectomy
- Bronchoscopy and laryngoscopy

PLASTIC SURGERY
- Augmental mammoplasty
- Blepharoplasty

- Skin grafts
- Basal cell carcinoma excision
- Ganglionectomy
- Scar revision

GENERAL SURGERY
- Breast biopsy
- Laryngoscopy
- Esophagoscopy/gastroscopy
- Node biopsies
- Herniorrhaphy
- Bronchoscopy
- Debridement
- Hemorrhoidectomy
- Sigmoidoscopy/colonoscopy

UROLOGY
- Transurethral resection of the prostate
- Circumcision
- Vasectomy
- Cystoscopy
- Orchiectomy
- Testicular biopsy

Adapted from Katz R: Issues in outpatient surgery, *Seminars in Anesthesiology* 258, 1987; Fairchild SS: Topics and issues affecting practice. In Fairchild SS, editor: *Perioperative nursing: principles and practice*, ed 2, Boston, 1996, Little, Brown.

(e.g., whether the patient wears contact lenses or has dental work or any prostheses). The nurse confirms that any instructions regarding eating or drinking before admission have been followed.

The nurse then allows the patient to change into a gown and escorts him or her to the holding area, where baseline vital signs are taken (Figure 10-1). In the holding area the patient may be given preoperative medications and further prepared for the procedure (e.g., the operative site may be shaved or an intravenous line started). Agency protocol determines how the consent forms for surgery and other paperwork are completed and who is responsible. The nurse should ensure that all consent forms are complete and accurate.

INTRAOPERATIVE CARE. As with perioperative nursing care in the hospital, the intraoperative team usually consists of a circulating nurse, a scrub nurse, an anesthesiologist or certified registered nurse-anesthetist (CRNA), and the surgeon. Often the surgeon has an assistant. In most agencies it is the responsibility of the circulating nurse to ensure that the procedure runs smoothly. The circulating nurse typically retrieves the patient from preoperative holding when

the anesthesiologist or CRNA is ready. The circulating nurse assists the scrub nurse and the anesthesiologist or CRNA with their preparatory work while helping reduce the patient's anxiety.

Both the circulating nurse and the scrub nurse assist the surgeon throughout the procedure. At the end of the procedure, the circulating nurse attends the anesthesiologist or CRNA while the patient awakens if general anesthetic is used. The circulating nurse assists the patient to a stretcher (a wheelchair may be used for procedures done under local or regional anesthesia) and takes the patient to the postanesthesia care area.

POSTANESTHESIA CARE AND DISCHARGE. Following the procedure, the patient is taken to the designated PACU or recovery area for observation; for management of pain, nausea, and vomiting; and to ensure maintenance of fluid and electrolyte balance. In the PACU, the vital signs are taken periodically, and the patient is monitored for complications related to surgery, anesthesia, or the presenting health condition.

Discharge is based on the absence of indications of serious complications (e.g., bleeding, unusual pain), when the patient is alert and able to walk

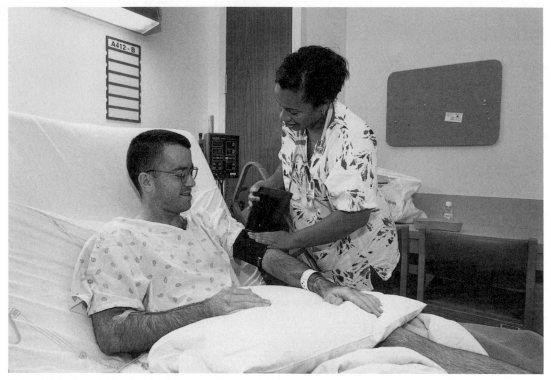

Figure 10-1. Nurse taking the blood pressure of a patient before surgery in an ambulatory surgical facility. (Courtesy Rick Brady, Photographer, Riva, Maryland.)

safely, and whether a responsible person is in attendance. Discharge criteria include the patient being alert and oriented and having stable vital signs; no respiratory distress; no hoarseness or cough following endotracheal intubation; a gag reflex; ability to swallow and cough; no dizziness, nausea, or vomiting; no bleeding and minimal swelling or drainage on dressings; ability to tolerate fluids and having been able to void; no excessive pain that will not be alleviated with oral medications at home; ability to ambulate (based on developmental age or physical limitations); capable of self-care or accompanied by a responsible adult and appropriate mode of transportation (Dark, 2004; Phillips, 2007).

The PACU nurse is usually responsible for reviewing postprocedure instructions with the patient and the caregiver(s). It is essential that they be aware of signs and symptoms of complications and when to call the surgeon or go to the hospital. Instructions should also include pain management, bathing instructions, wound care (if applicable), activity limitations, diet, and the importance of a follow-up appointment with the surgeon. Instructions should be written and explicit to ensure that they are easily understood (Dark, 2004; Groah, 1996).

Experience, Education, and Certification for Ambulatory Surgery Nursing Practice

There are no specific educational requirements for RNs practicing in ambulatory care surgery. However, many ambulatory surgery centers require a minimum of 1 year of experience in either the operating room or postanesthesia care.

Certification in operating room nursing care is definitely an advantage. The Association of Operating Room Nurses (AORN) grants certification through the Certification Board of Perioperative Nursing to qualifying operating room nurses and RN first assistants.

NURSING CARE IN OTHER AMBULATORY SETTINGS

Additional settings in which nurses are employed in community-based practice are nursing in poison control centers, ambulatory diagnostic centers (e.g., outpatient imaging and radiology services for diagnosis and treatment), community hotlines (e.g., suicide, AIDS, drug and alcohol abuse, family violence), summer camps, and migrant health centers. Nurses who desire to practice in nonacute care settings should be alert to the variety of opportunities.

SUMMARY

Most health care is provided to clients who are not inpatients in health care facilities. Indeed, the majority of care is provided in ambulatory settings. Increasingly, in addition to services such as health-promotion and illness-prevention interventions, which have traditionally been provided in community settings, many surgical procedures, chemotherapy, and diagnostic procedures are taking place in ambulatory settings. As a result many nurses, such as Bill, the PACU nurse from the case study, are needed to fill positions in these areas.

The type and practice of nurses in ambulatory settings are incredibly variable. Settings include health care offices or clinics, schools, occupational settings, rural health clinics, parish practices, correctional facilities, public health departments, ambulatory oncology centers, and many others. The practice and focus of the nurses in ambulatory settings is wide, and whatever their area of specialization or interest, nurse are encouraged to examine opportunities to work in ambulatory settings.

KEY POINTS

- *Ambulatory care* refers to personal health care or health services (e.g., outpatient surgery and chemotherapy, diagnostic tests and procedures) provided to noninstitutionalized patients.
- Ambulatory nursing care is largely focused on health promotion, primary prevention, screening for early identification of disease, and assisting in treatment regimens for both acute and chronic illnesses.

- About 11.5% of all RNs practice in a health care office or clinic (with a provider such as a physician, nurse practitioner, or physician assistant). Clinic or office nurses assist with assessments and procedures, provide education, collect specimens, and administer medications. Coordination of services and preparation of patients for procedures are other roles and responsibilities.
- Currently, about 3.2% of all RNs are school nurses. School nurses work to prevent illnesses, intervene in identified problems, promote healthy lifestyles, and provide health education. Caring for students with special health needs (e.g., urinary catheterization, tube feedings, tracheotomy care) is becoming increasingly common.
- Occupational health nurses provide health care services to workers, focusing on health promotion and protection from injury and illness within the context of a safe and healthy work environment. Occupational health nurses provide assessment of the environment for threats to health and safety, assessment of the health status of workers, nursing care for occupational and nonoccupational injuries and illnesses, counseling, and health education. Several laws directly affect the practice of the occupational health nurses. These include Workers' Compensation Acts and the Occupational Safety and Health Act.
- Delivery of nursing and health care to clients in rural areas has a number of distinctive characteristics and challenges. Distance, isolation, and sparse resources, combined with shortage of nurses and other health care providers in rural areas, are particular challenges. Rural nurses must be clinically competent in a very broad number of areas and are typically cross-trained to manage client needs in areas including trauma, routine obstetrical care, care of children and elders, and care of clients with mental health needs.
- Parish nurses seek to promote the health of a community (centered in a church or synagogue) by integration of theological, psychological, sociological, and physiological perspectives of health. Parish nurses work to enhance the quality of life for members of a congregation and often the surrounding neighborhood. Parish nursing interventions include organization of support

groups, provision of referrals to community resources, health education, counseling, and acting as a liaison within the larger health care system.

- The U.S. government requires health care services for all inmates in correctional facilities. As a result, approximately 9000 RNs work in jails, prisons, and juvenile detention facilities. The main component of nursing practice in correctional facilities is provision of primary care and emergency services for the inmates.

- Approximately 48,000 nurses practice in local, county, and state public health departments. Depending on mandates of the individual locality, health departments are responsible for diverse areas, including environmental sanitation, communicable disease surveillance and prevention, and maternal and child health.

- Ambulatory oncology care allows cancer patients to receive diagnosis and treatment as outpatients. Nurses may care for oncology clients in physicians' offices, outpatient clinics, and day hospitals. Health care services may include prevention, screening, chemotherapy, radiation therapy, education, discharge planning, nutritional support, counseling, and outpatient surgery.

- More than half of all surgical procedures can be performed on an ambulatory basis; thus nursing in outpatient surgical centers continues to grow. Nurses who work in outpatient surgical centers may provide preoperative care, intraoperative care, or postanesthesia care. Preoperative care involves giving the patient and family preoperative instructions and preparing them for the procedure. Intraoperative nursing consists of acting as circulating nurse; scrub nurse; or, in some cases, first assistant during the surgical procedure. During postanesthesia care, the nurse observes the patient for complications, manages complications and side effects (e.g., nausea, pain), and prepares him or her for discharge.

Learning Activities & Application to Practice
In Class
1. Interview a nurse who practices in an ambulatory setting. What roles and responsibilities does the nurse have? What are common interventions? Describe positive and negative aspects of practice. What are education and experience requirements?

What are employment opportunities, work hours, and salaries? Share findings with the class.

In Clinical
2. Spend one or more days in one or more of the ambulatory settings described. If possible, select an acute or chronic care setting (e.g., ambulatory surgery, oncology) and a primary care setting (e.g., physician office, school, parish nursing). In a log or journal, compare and contrast nursing practice in the two settings.

REFERENCES

Adams C: Promoting and protecting the health of adults and the working population. In Allender JA, Spradley BW, editors: *Community health nursing: concepts and practice*, ed 5, Philadelphia, 2001, Lippincott.

American Academy of Ambulatory Care Nursing: *Ambulatory care nursing administration and practice standards*, ed 7, Pitman, NJ, 2007, American Academy of Ambulatory Care Nursing.

American Academy of Ambulatory Care Nursing: *Ambulatory care nursing administration and practice standards*, Pitman, NJ, 2004, Author.

American Association of Occupational Health Nurses: *Fact sheet: occupational and environmental health nursing* (website): http://www.aaohn.org/press_room/fact_sheets/profession.cfm. Accessed June 27, 2007.

American Board for Occupational Health Nurses: *Certification criteria* (website): http://www.abohn.org/certif.htm. Accessed June 27, 2007.

American Nurses' Association: *Scope and standards of nursing practice in correctional facilities*, Washington, DC, 1995, American Nurses' Association.

American Nurses' Association: *Rural/frontier nursing: the challenge to grow*, Washington, DC, 1996, American Nurses' Association.

American Nurses' Credentialing Center: *Ambulatory care nursing certification fact sheet* (website): www.nursecredentialing.org. Accessed June 26, 2007.

American Red Cross: *The history and organization of the Red Cross Nursing Service* (website): http://www.redcross.org/services/nursing/0,1082,0_389_,00.html. Accessed June 27, 2007.

Bayne T: Rural health care. In Allender JA, Spradley BW, editors: Community health nursing: promoting and protecting the public's health, ed 6, Philadelphia, 2005, Lippincott.

Buchsel P, Glennon C: Ambulatory care administrative concepts: an overview. In Buchsel PC, Yarbro CH, editors: *Oncology nursing in the ambulatory setting: issues and models of care*, ed 2, Sudbury, Mass, 2005, Jones and Bartlett.

Buchsel PC, Yarbro CH: *Oncology nursing in the ambulatory setting: issues and models of care*, ed 2, Sudbury, Mass, 2005, Jones and Bartlett.

Bushy A: *Orientation to nursing in the rural community*, Thousand Oaks, Calif, 2000, Sage.

Bushy A: Community and public health nursing in rural and urban environments. In Stanhope M, Lancaster J, editors: *Community & public health nursing*, ed 6, St Louis, 2004, Mosby.

Bushy A: Rural health. In Maurer FA, Smith CM, editors: *Community/public health nursing: health for families and populations*, ed 3, St Louis, 2005, Saunders.

Bushy A: *Rural Nursing: practice and issues*, American Nurses Association Continuing Education Program (online): http://www.nursingworld.org/mods/mod700/rural.pdf. Accessed October 23, 2007.

Centers for Disease Control and Prevention (2006): *Child and school immunization requirements 2005-2006* (website): http://www.cdc.gov/vaccines/vac-gen/laws/downloads/izlaws05-06.pdf

Centers for Disease Control and Prevention (2001a): Fatal occupational injuries–United States, 1980-1997, *MMWR Morbid Mortal Wkly Rep* 50(16):317, 2001.

Centers for Disease Control and Prevention (2001b): Hepatitis B outbreak in a state correctional facility, 2000, *MMWR Morbid Mortal Wkly Rep* 50(25):529, 2001.

Chafey K, Hill WG, Burg GR: Rural and migrant health. In Nies M, McEwen M, editors: *Community/public health nursing: promoting the health of populations*, ed 4, St Louis, 2007, Saunders.

Cooley ME, Lin EM, Hunter SW: The ambulatory oncology nurse's role, *Semin Oncol Nurs* 10(4):245, 1994.

Dark PM: Patient discharge education in the phase II setting. In Quinn DMD, Schick L, editors: *Perianesthesia nursing core curriculum: preoperative, phase I and phase II PACU nursing*, St Louis, 2004, Saunders.

Droes NS: Correctional nursing practice, *J Community Health Nurs* 11(4):201, 1994.

Fairchild SS: Topics and issues affecting practice. In Fairchild SS, editor: *Perioperative nursing: principles and practice*, ed 2, Boston, 1996, Little, Brown.

Frontier Nursing Service: *A brief history of the frontier nursing service* (website): http://www.frontiernursing.org/History/HowFNSbegan.shtm. Accessed June 27, 2007.

Groah LK: Ambulatory surgery. In Groah LK: *Perioperative nursing*, ed 3, Stamford, Conn, 1996, Appleton & Lange.

Hackbarth DP, Haas SA, Kavanagh JA, Vlasses F: Dimensions of the staff nurse role in ambulatory care: part I–methodology and analysis of data on current staff nurse practice, *Nurs Econ* 13(2):89, 1995.

Hufft AG, Fawkes LS: Federal inmates: a unique psychiatric nursing challenge, *Nurs Clin North Am* 29(1):35, 1994.

Kalisch PA, Kalisch BJ: *American nursing: a history*, ed 4, Philadelphia, 2004, Lippincott.

Kimel LS: Lack of follow-up exams after failed school vision screenings: an investigation of contributing factors, *J Sch Nurs* 22(3):156, 2006.

Lamkin L: Outpatient oncology settings: a variety of services, *Sem Oncol Nurs* 10(4):229, 1994.

Maurer FA, Kelly G: State and local health departments. In Maurer FA, Smith CM, editors: *Community/public health nursing: health for families and populations*, ed 3, St Louis, 2005, Saunders.

McDermott MA, Solari-Twadell PA, Matheus R: Promoting quality education for the parish nurse and the parish nurse coordinator, *Nurs Health Care Persp* 19(1):4, 1998.

Miskelly S: A parish nursing model: applying the community health nursing process in a church community, *J Community Health Nurs* 12(1):1, 1995.

National Association of School Nurses: *Issue brief: school vision screening* (website): http://www.nasn.org/Portals/0/briefs/2006briefvision.pdf. Accessed June 26, 2007.

National Network for Immunization Information: *Common questions about school immunization laws* (website): http://www.immunizationinfo.org/assets/files/PDFs/4_SCH.pdf. Accessed June 22, 2007.

Novotny JM, Lippman DT, Sanders NK, Fitzpatrick JJ: *101 Careers in nursing*, New York, 2003, Springer.

Odom-Forren J: Evolution of perianesthesia care. In Quinn DMD, Schick L, editors: *Perianesthesia nursing core curriculum: preoperative, phase I and phase II PACU nursing*, St Louis, 2004, Saunders.

Oncology Nursing Certification Corporation: *Certification requirements for oncology nurses* (website): http://www.oncc.org/getcertified/TestInformation/certificationsavailable.shtml. Accessed October 21, 2007.

Phillips NF: *Berry & Kohn's operating room technique*, ed 11, St Louis, 2007, Mosby.

Pollitt P: Lina Rogers Struthers: the first school nurse, *J Sch Nurs* 10(1):34, 1994.

Pourciau CA, Vallette EC: School health. In Nies M, McEwen M, editors: *Community health nursing: promoting the health of populations*, ed 4, St Louis, 2007, Saunders.

Reed DB, Hoffman C, Westneat SC: Nurses' agricultural education in the southeastern United States, *J Nurs Educ* 44(6):271, 2005.

Rogers B: *Occupational and environmental health nursing: concepts and practice*, Philadelphia, 2003, Saunders.

Rogers B: *Occupational health nursing: concepts and practice*, Philadelphia, 1994, W.B. Saunders.

Rogers B, Travers PH: Occupational health. In Nies M, McEwen M, editors: *Community health nursing: promoting the health of populations*, St Louis, 2007, Saunders.

Schank MJ, Weis D, Matheus R: Parish nursing: ministry of healing, *Geriatr Nurs* 17(1):11, 1996.

Selekman J: Health promotion. In Selekman J, editor: *School nursing: a comprehensive text*, Philadelphia, 2006, F.A. Davis.

Siegrist BC: Parish health. In Nies M, McEwen M, editors: *Community health nursing: promoting the health of populations*, ed 4, St Louis, 2007, Saunders.

Snow A: Forensic and correctional nursing . In Nies M, McEwen M, editors: *Community health nursing: promoting the health of populations*, ed 4, St Louis, 2007, Saunders.

Solari-Twadell PA, McDermott MA: *Parish nursing: development, education and administration*, St Louis, 2006, Mosby.

Solari-Twadell P, Djupe A, McDermott M, editors: *Parish nursing: the developing practice*, Park Ridge, Ill, 1990, National Parish Nurse Resource Center.

Stevens R: When your clients are in jail, *Nurs Forum* 28(4):5, 1993.

Swan BA, Conway-Phillips R, Griffin KF: Demonstrating the value of the RN in ambulatory care, *Nurs Econ* 24(6):315, 2006.

U.S. Census Bureau: *American fact finder: population, housing, units, area and density, 2000* (website): http://factfinder. census.gov/servlet/GCTTable?_bm=n&_lang=en&mt_ name=DEC_2000_SF1_U_GCTPH1_US9&format=US9&_ box_head_nbr=GCTPH1&ds_name=DEC_2000_SF1_ U&geo_id=01000US. Accessed June 28, 2007.

U.S. Department of Agriculture: *Rural poverty at a glance* (Economic Research Service Research Report Number 100) (website): http://www.ers.usda.gov/publications/ rdrr100/rdrr100_lowres.pdf. Accessed June 28, 2007.

U.S. Department of Health and Human Services: *Healthy people 2010: National health promotion and disease prevention objectives,* Washington, DC, 2000, Government Printing Office.

U.S. Department of Health and Human Services/ Health Resources and Services Administration, Bureau of Health Professions/Division of Nursing: *The registered nurse population, March, 2004,* Rockville, MD, 2006, Government Printing Office.

U.S. Preventative Services Task Force: *Recommendation statement: screening for idiopathic scoliosis in adolescents* (website): http://www.ahrq.gov/clinic/3rduspstf/scoliosis/scoliors .htm. Accessed June 27, 2007.

U.S. Preventative Services Task Force: *Guide to clinical preventive services,* ed 2, Washington, DC, 1996, U.S. Department of Health and Human Services.

Zimmerman B: Student health and education plans. In J. Selekman J, editor: *School nursing: a comprehensive text,* Philadelphia, 2006, F.A. Davis.

Chapter 11

Home Health Care Nursing

objectives

Upon completion of this chapter, the reader will be able to:

1. Discuss home health care nursing and explain its relationship to other types of nursing practice.

2. Explain the impact of Medicare regulations on home health nursing.

3. Describe the importance of documentation in home health nursing.

4. Discuss skills and knowledge necessary for the home health nurse, including discharge planning, case management, coordination of community resources, and interdisciplinary collaboration.

5. Explain the three stages of a home visit.

6. Discuss different types of specialized home health nursing, including infusion therapy, chronic wound care, perinatal home care, psychiatric home care, and hospice care.

key terms

Case management
Conditions of Participation
Coordination of community resources
Discharge planning
Enterostomal care
Home health care

Home health nursing
Hospice care
Infusion therapy
Interdisciplinary collaboration
Perinatal home care
Psychiatric home health care

Qualifications for home care
Skilled nursing services

See Glossary for definitions.

case study

Penny Mitchell has been a home health nurse for 2 years and is employed by a hospital-based agency in a small city. Before taking this position, she worked for 5 years as a staff nurse—primarily in a coronary care unit.

Each day Penny sees four to six clients, mostly elderly, with a variety of health problems. One recent Thursday, she saw four clients: Mr. Carter, who has congestive heart failure, to monitor his blood pressure and weight and perform medication teaching; Mrs. Kirk, who is

Continued

homebound because of osteoporosis and receives monthly calcitonin injections; Mrs. Thomas, to change her Foley catheter, which her caregiver reported to be leaking; and Mr. Wilson, for admission to home care services following discharge from the hospital the day before and to initiate PRN dressing changes for a granulating abdominal wound.

Penny prepares for each day by calling her scheduled clients the night before to set up times, outline the services she will be providing, determine if she needs to bring any special supplies, and learn if there are any specific instructions regarding the client's care that she is not aware of. Because Mr. Wilson is a new client and Penny has never been to his home, she is careful to obtain driving directions from his wife. She confirms with Mrs. Kirk that her medication is at her home and that it is not necessary to stop at the pharmacy. She inventories her car stock of dressings, gloves, solutions, and other supplies to identify anything she might need that is not readily available. Finally, she determines what forms will be needed for documentation of each client's care and gathers educational materials that will be beneficial in client teaching.

Each visit consists of a general assessment followed by implementation of the prescribed skilled nursing services. The clients and their family members or caregivers are given instruction on their illness, treatment regimen, and self-care. Referrals for additional services are made as appropriate, and physicians and/or others involved in the care of each client are called to report findings, clarify orders, and request assistance. Also, the process of admitting new clients such as Mr. Wilson into agency service necessitates additional assessments (e.g., complete physical assessment; health history; and medication, functional, social needs) and explanation and completion of several documents related to home health services and Medicare reimbursement.

After she has seen each client and made necessary notifications and referrals, Penny carefully completes documentation of all findings and services. Her orientation to the agency, 2 years of experience, and several related training sessions have taught her the importance of precise and thorough documentation. Therefore she painstakingly completes and reviews all documentation and organizes each case folder to return to the agency. Finally, she contacts the agency to give a brief report on each client and receive her assignment for the following day.

With reforms in health care financing and delivery over the last two decades, hospital occupancy rates have declined dramatically, outpatient surgery has markedly increased, and clients are being discharged "sicker and quicker." This, in turn, has resulted in a significant increase in home health care. Indeed, home care is one of the fastest growing specialty areas of nursing. According to the Health Resources and Service Administration's Division of Nursing, between 1980 and 2004, the number of nurses working in Community Health settings, including home health care, increased by 128.8% (U.S. Department of Health and Human Services [USDHHS], 2006). The growth in home health care is also demonstrated by the rapidly increasing number of Medicare-certified agencies, clients, and visits over the past decade. The growth in home care peaked in 1997 at more than 10,000, but because of changes in Medicare reimbursement, it has declined somewhat over the past few years.

Table 11-1 illustrates the changes in home health care since 1967.

HISTORY OF HOME HEALTH CARE DELIVERY AND FINANCING

Until the early 1900s, care for the ill and injured was provided almost exclusively in the home by family members, friends, or trained health care providers. In the United States organized home health nursing services began when the first visiting nurse associations (VNAs) were established in Buffalo, Boston, and Philadelphia during the mid-1880s. The early VNAs were established to care for the poor and disenfranchised suffering from illness or injury. The renowned public health nurse, Lillian Wald, is credited with starting a visiting nursing service for New York City in 1893 and persuading the Metropolitan Life Insurance Company to furnish home

TABLE **11-1** Growth in Medicare-Certified Home Health Care

YEAR	NUMBER OF HOME HEALTH AGENCIES	MEDICARE EXPENDITURES (MILLIONS)	NUMBER OF CLIENTS (THOUSANDS)	NUMBER OF VISITS
1967	1753	$46	N/A	N/A
1980	2924	$662	957	22,428
1992	6004	$7878	2565	135,012
1998	8080	$10,446	3062	154,992
2006	8838	$12,885	3228	95,534

Data from National Association for Home Care & Hospice: *Basic statistics about home care*, Updated 2007. Washington, DC, 2007, National Association for Home Care and Hospice.

nursing services for policyholders in 1908 (Rice, 2006). Provision of home health nursing services for insured clients became increasingly common during the following decades. Public health departments, the Red Cross, and philanthropic efforts funded many of the earliest home health agencies.

Initially, home health nursing services and interventions were determined by the nurse. Teaching on hygiene and infant care; instituting measures to control communicable disease; assistance with self-care; performance of activities of daily living for persons with serious or chronic illnesses; and caring for elderly, ill, and dying patients were among the services provided.

Passage of Medicare in 1965, however, dramatically changed home health care. In the early years, home health care was directed and delivered virtually exclusively by nurses; physician guidance and oversight were not required. With Medicare, the payment source, client eligibility, purpose of home care, and provision of home care changed. Medicare developed very stringent requirements for eligibility, services, and physician oversight. Physician-prescribed and directed care became a necessity, guidelines for services were defined, and requirements for eligibility were predetermined. The independent practice of nurses providing care to individuals and families in their homes was greatly altered, and home health care services came under physician directives.

Until recently **home health care** in the United States was largely provided by "official" agencies (governmental or public) or voluntary agencies (private, nonprofit agencies such as VNAs funded by fees-for-service, united community funds, grants, and other sources). As Table 11-2 shows, however, the majority of home health agencies now are proprietary or hospital-based. This trend also reflects the changes in the health care system. As care moved from acute care institutions, largely because of the advent of diagnoses-related group reimbursement policies, both proprietary and nonprofit hospitals and providers have recognized the need for home care services and the potential for revenue generation.

DEFINITIONS RELATED TO HOME HEALTH CARE

Home health care has been defined as "that component of a continuum of comprehensive health care whereby health services are provided to individuals and families in their places of residence for the purpose of promoting, maintaining, or restoring health, or maximizing the level of independence, while minimizing the effects of disability and illness, including terminal illness" (Warhola, 1980, p. 9). Emphasis is placed on the premise that "health care" (not medical care) should be "comprehensive" and designed to promote, maintain or restore health, with the objective being to "maximize independence."

Home health nursing combines aspects of community health nursing with selected technical skills from other specialty nursing practices and delivers care for individuals in collaboration with the family and/or designated caregivers. **Home health nursing** refers to "nursing practice applied to patients of

TABLE **11-2** Medicare-Certified Home Health Agencies by Sponsor: 1967, 1990, and 2005

SPONSOR	1967		1990		2005	
	NUMBER	PERCENTAGE	NUMBER	PERCENTAGE	NUMBER	PERCENTAGE
Visiting Nurse Association (VNA)	642	36.6	521	9.1	459	5.2
Public	939	53.6	985	17.3	1132	13.0
Proprietary	0	0	1884	33.1	4919	56.5
Private (nonprofit)	0	0	710	12.5	562	6.5
Hospital-based	133	7.6	1486	26.1	1547	17.8
Other	39	2.2	109	2.0	85	1.0
Totals	1753	100	5695	100	8704	100

Data from National Association for Home Care & Hospice: *Basic statistics about home care*, Updated 2007. Washington, DC, 2007, National Association for Home Care and Hospice.

all ages in the patients' residences, which may include a private home, assisted living, or personal care facility" (American Nurses' Association [ANA], 2007, p. 9).

The home health nurse's role involves coordinating and directing all involved disciplines and caregivers to optimize client outcomes. This is accomplished through sharing information of community health resources with the client and caregivers. In addition, a comprehensive knowledge base incorporating aspects of the specialty areas within nursing is required to deliver holistic care in the home.

Unlike many other types of nursing practice, home health care nursing is not limited to a particular age group or diagnosis. Depending on the specific client's needs, care may be episodic or continuous and may be primary, secondary, and/or tertiary in nature. Home health nursing should be holistic and focused on the individual client, integrating family/caregiver, environmental, and community resources to promote optimal well-being for the client. The goal of care is to maintain or improve patients' quality of life or support them and their family/caregivers at the end of life.

Similar to other nursing practice standards, the Home Health Nursing standards endorsed by the ANA follow the steps of the nursing process, addressing assessment, diagnosis, outcome identification, planning, implementation, and evaluation. In addition, standards of professional performance relate to quality of care, performance appraisal, education (i.e., knowledge and competency), collegiality, ethics, collaboration, research, and resource utilization (ANA, 2007).

HOME HEALTH CARE REIMBURSEMENT AND DOCUMENTATION

Public sources (Medicare and Medicaid) financed more than 70% of home health services in 2005 (Center for Medicare and Medicaid Services, 2007); therefore the discussion related to financing and documentation is directed toward meeting Medicare requirements. To be reimbursed by Medicare for services rendered to clients, home health agencies must be Medicare certified. Medicare certification is awarded only to those agencies that have successfully demonstrated that they meet Medicare's **"Conditions of Participation"** for home health agencies. These conditions are regulations that consist of explicit rules, standards, and requirements established at the federal government level and are therefore consistent within all states. These regulations outline requirements for virtually all aspects of home health care and detail such areas as personnel qualifications, notifying clients of their rights, acceptance of clients, plan of care, medical supervision, types of services that are offered by the agency, and the duties of each service provider (e.g., skilled nursing, various therapies, home health aide) (CMS, 2004).

To process Medicare claims, the Centers for Medicare & Medicaid Services (CMS) contracts with regional insurance companies, or fiscal intermediaries. The home health agency sends the fiscal intermediary a bill for services each month, accompanied by the required documentation. These materials are reviewed by the intermediary and if all documentation is included and appropriately meets the coverage criteria for home care, the bill is paid. Often there are questions regarding client eligibility or appropriateness of services (Milone-Nuzzo, 2005).

For eligibility for coverage under Medicare guidelines, the following **qualifications for home care** must be met (CMS, 2004):

- The person to whom the services are provided must be eligible for Medicare.
- The client's care must require intermittent skilled nursing care, physical therapy, or speech therapy.
- The client must be homebound.
- The client must be under the care of a physician who develops and monitors a home health plan.
- The home health agency must be certified to participate in Medicare.

Each home health professional service (e.g., nursing, physical therapy, speech therapy) has guidelines on what Medicare defines as *covered services.* For a service to be covered by Medicare the RN makes the initial evaluation visit, regularly reevaluates the client's nursing needs, initiates the plan of care, plans necessary revisions, provides services requiring specialized nursing skills, initiates appropriate preventive and rehabilitative nursing procedures, prepares clinical and progress notes, coordinates services, informs the physician and other personnel of changes in the client's condition, counsels the client and family, and supervises and teaches other nursing personnel. Examples of **skilled nursing services** that are reimbursable under defined circumstances are listed in Box 11-1.

HOME HEALTH CARE DOCUMENTATION

When asked what they like most about home health care, nurses often cite the autonomy, being able to spend more time caring for clients, or the hours. When asked what they like least about home health care, nurses almost always mention the paperwork. Completion of all required documentation has several purposes:

- Recording services rendered
- Describing the client's condition and response to care
- Promoting continuity of care
- Validating reimbursement claims
- Forestalling legal actions

For reimbursement by Medicare, documentation of all services and care given must be meticulously completed. Individual agencies design forms for documentation that best meet the needs of their particular clientele and nurses' preferences. Documentation of a thorough nursing assessment, including physical, psychosocial, functional, nutritional, and safety components, and gathering information on all medications, is necessary.

Orientation of nurses new to home health care practice or to a new agency demands in-depth instruction on documentation requirements, including specifics on how to complete all forms thoroughly

BOX 11-1 Medicare-Reimbursable Skilled Nursing Services

- Observation and assessment of a client's condition
- Management and evaluation of a client care plan
- Teaching and training activities for the client and the client's family or caregivers
- Tube feedings
- Tracheotomy aspiration
- Insertion and irrigation and replacement of catheters in selected clients
- Wound care
- Ostomy care
- Heat treatments
- Administration of medical gasses
- Rehabilitation care
- Venipuncture
- Psychiatric evaluation, therapy, and teaching (by a psychiatrically trained nurse)

and accurately. Table 11-3 presents information to guide home health nurses in documentation of home health care services.

ELEMENTS OF HOME CARE NURSING PRACTICE

Home health care nursing practice requires unique skills and knowledge. Home health care nursing responsibilities are varied and numerous. A few basic and essential activities home health care nursing comprises are described in the following sections.

DISCHARGE PLANNING

Discharge planning is the process of determining and planning to meet client needs following release from a health care facility. The discharge planning process allows client and family needs to be identified and evaluated, with responsibility for meeting those needs being transferred to the client, the client's caregiver or significant others, or other health care providers. The purposes of discharge planning include promoting continuity of care to improve client health status and coordinating the client's needs with available resour-ces. Reduction in average length of service, lower cost, efficient use of resources, fewer requests for additional services, improved communication, and better information on client needs are benefits attributable to discharge planning.

Ideally the discharge planning process should begin before the client is hospitalized, with anticipation of the client's needs during recovery. When the course of recovery is predicted to be difficult for any of several reasons and follow-up care through a home health agency is anticipated or requested comprehensive discharge planning is beneficial. Discharge planning as a service is performed by different health professionals, including nurses, social workers, physicians, and chaplains. Many institutions employ professionals—usually nurses or social workers—for this position. These individuals are responsible for identifying clients in need of ongoing care following discharge, consulting with caregivers (both in the institution and when the client is discharged), educating staff regarding discharge plans, and coordinating activities. Many health care

TABLE **11-3** Guidelines for Medicare Documentation to Validate the Need for Home Care Services

AVOID THE FOLLOWING WORDS	USE INSTEAD
Monitor, supervise. Denotes a stable client.	**Assess, evaluate.** "Monitor" may be used when managed care is ordered and the skilled nurse is supervising paraprofessionals to ensure safe delivery of the therapeutic regimen.
Healing well. Suggests that visits are unnecessary and supports client discharge from home health services.	Objectively describe the wound in terms of size, depth, drainage, color, and odor.
Discussed. Does not require the skills of a professional; anyone can discuss.	Teach, educate, instruct, demonstrate.
Prevent/prevention. Not covered. Must be done incidental to a skilled service such as assessment teaching and treatment.	Focus on **restorative, rehabilitative, and/or palliative** (hospice) interventions.
Stable, independent. Negates medical necessity and supports client discharge from home health services.	Document response to treatment.
Feeling better. Subjective and supports functional ability, client discharge from health services.	Focus on the client's physical assessment, functional ability, and problems/needs.

AVOID THE FOLLOWING WORDS	USE INSTEAD
Noncompliant/uncooperative.	Document specific problems with coping or refusal to follow the plan of care as a source of referral to a psychiatric home health nurse or social worker. Document refusal to follow the plan of care as a justification for a learning contract or, per home health agency policy, client discharge.
Went to the market/going to church, etc. Negates homebound status.	Document equipment, manual assistance, and number of people required for client to leave home. Verify homebound status each visit. If the client leaves the home, explain why trips were taken as related to lifestyle or medical necessity.
Client not at home.	**Not available for visit or no answer to locked door.** Document on next visit why client was not available for visit.
Continue care plan.	Describe what your next visit plans are based on (e.g., assess cardiopulmonary status of client with congestive heart failure).
Maintenance. Never use this word because it negates the necessity of visits and supports client discharge from home health services.	Document response to the plan of care of case-management needs.
Confused.	Describe disorientation to person, place, or time. Describe ability to follow commands and short- and long-term recall.
Chronic condition. Is indicative of a stable condition.	Describe exacerbation of the chronic condition that requires the services of a skilled nurse.
Reinforce, reinstruct. Repetitive instruction will not be covered unless learning difficulties are documented.	Document comprehension difficulties, attention deficit, or other problems that hamper ability to learn and necessitate repeating instructions. Use words such as **demonstrate, teach, instruct, or educate**.
Observed. Anyone can observe.	Use **assess or evaluate**. Skilled observation may be used as a component of client education to document client/caregiver return demonstration.

From Rice R: *Manual of home health nursing procedures*, ed 2, St Louis, 2000, Mosby.

institutions utilize assessment instruments to identify clients who need more.

CASE MANAGEMENT

Case management has been defined as "a collaborative process of assessment, planning, facilitation and advocacy for options and services to meet an individual's health needs through communication and available resources to promote quality cost-effective outcomes" (Clark, 2008 p. 277). According to Lyon (2007), case management "assists the client through a complex, fragmented, and often confusing health care delivery system and achieves specific client-centered goals" (p. 137).

The case manager's role is comprehensive and includes assessment of the client's needs and resources, outlining a plan of care to meet the identified needs, arranging for the most cost-effective complement of services and providers to meet the identified needs, and coordinating the activities of various health care providers (Clark, 2008). In home health care nursing, *case management* generally refers to the comprehensive supervision of the care given to each client. The case manager, usually the RN, functions as the team leader who provides or arranges primary care, supervises paraprofessionals, and collaborates with other health professionals (e.g., a physical or occupational therapist or medical social worker). The case manager is responsible for maintaining communication between the disciplines and with the client and monitoring and evaluating client goals. More detailed information on case management is provided in Chapter 4.

COORDINATION OF COMMUNITY RESOURCES

Coordination of community resources requires the nurse to be knowledgeable about services offered by his or her agency and any resources available in the community that would benefit clients. In addition to being aware of resources, the home health nurse must understand the referral process.

During the referral process, a client is directed to appropriate agencies or organizations for information or assistance with care. To make effective and appropriate referrals, the nurse must do the following:

- Be aware of community services available for needs related to home health nursing practice.
- Determine if the client is eligible for the services offered by the agency or organization.
- Have an understanding of how to refer a client for a particular service and who may refer a client (e.g., some services or service providers require a referral from a physician only).
- Know the costs of services and the payment mechanism.
- Be aware of the location, telephone number, hours of operation, and contact person.

Often the nurse provides the client or caregiver with the necessary information for the referral and allows them to make initial contact. At other times it may be appropriate for the nurse to call the individual, agency, or organization directly.

To identify sources for community referrals, the home health nurse may use a directory of community services, which is available in many cities and towns. In addition, home health agencies often provide nurses with a list of available community resources. Experienced home health nurses usually develop a personal listing of service providers that have been helpful for clients in the past. Names of agencies, contact persons, and their telephone numbers are essential. Examples of commonly utilized community resources are various government programs (e.g., Medicaid; Veteran's Affairs; Women, Infants, and Children [WIC] program); Meals on Wheels; adult day care providers; area hospices, if not provided by the nurse's agency; organizations that assist with financial obligations; and transportation providers for the handicapped or elderly.

INTERDISCIPLINARY COLLABORATION

Home health nursing practice requires the nurse to initiate and maintain a collegial and collaborative relationship with all health care providers working with the client. In health care, especially in matters of the plan of care, *collaboration* implies joint decision making with all professionals involved with the client's care. **Interdisciplinary collaboration** is integrated within the roles and functions of the home health nurse discussed here and is vitally important in the process of discharge planning and case management. To comply with Medicare requirements and to best direct client care, the nurse must work with the physician to receive orders and outline the plan of care. As the case manager the nurse must share the plan of care with all involved in the client's care and make recommendations and modifications based on their input. Case conferences should be held regularly, particularly for clients with complicated or prolonged care, to share information among the providers and discuss the client's response to the treatment plan. In addition, the nurse may oversee, evaluate, or supervise the care of others. Professionals involved in home health care planning and delivery are described in Box 11-2.

THE PROCESS OF HOME HEALTH NURSING

Home health nursing may be specialized or generalized and is always detail intensive. Orientation, education, and training of nurses in home health

BOX 11-2 Professionals Involved in Home Health Care Planning and Delivery

Nurses: Registered nurses have been the traditional providers of health care in the home. Nurses provide skilled nursing services, coordinate care as case managers and referral agents, and act as client advocates.

Physicians: Most clients are referred for home care services by physicians, and physician oversight of the plan of care is required for Medicare reimbursement and for payment from other insurers.

Physical therapists: Most home care agencies employ physical therapists to assess a client's needs for assistive devices that will support rehabilitation and safety, evaluate neuromuscular and functional ability, prescribe and administer therapy procedures to meet client needs, and teach the client or caregivers to perform these therapies and related activities.

Occupational therapists: Whereas physical therapists usually concentrate on gross motor skills and rehabilitation, occupational therapists assist the client in restoration of small motor coordination and improving physical tasks related to activities of daily living. The goal of occupational therapy is reaching the highest level of functioning possible.

Speech therapists/speech pathologists: Speech therapists work to treat, manage, or alleviate problems associated with limitations in communication related to speech, language, hearing, and swallowing difficulties.

Social workers: Social workers assist clients with social, emotional, and financial needs. In addition, social workers often serve as advocates and refer clients to available community resources.

Registered dietitians/nutritionists: Dietitians provide direct counseling and teaching for clients with special dietary needs and problems. In addition, they may act as consultants or resource persons for nurses and other health care providers.

Home health aides: Home health aides are paraprofessionals who assist in the home with the client's personal care, basic nursing (e.g., vital signs, assistance with self-administered medication), light housekeeping, and related tasks (e.g., shopping, meal preparation). For Medicare reimbursement, home health aides must be supervised by an RN.

Other providers: Other professionals and paraprofessionals that occasionally provide care to clients in the home or might assist home health nurses include pharmacists, phlebotomists, laboratory technicians, respiratory therapists, enterostomal therapists, chaplains, and massage therapists.

---

nursing practice should be comprehensive and specific and include significant time spent with preceptors. This section focuses on the process of the home health nursing visit and gives specific instructions on how to conduct a home visit and what may be expected and required of the provider.

The process of the home health nursing visit can be divided into three stages: (1) the previsit/planning stage; (2) the visit, or implementation, stage; and (3) the postvisit stage. Each of these stages and the home health nurse's activities are described in the following sections.

PLANNING FOR THE HOME HEALTH NURSING VISIT

To be efficient, safe, and productive, home health care nursing requires a significant amount of previsit planning. Previsit planning involves determining which clients are to be seen during the day and prioritization of the scheduled visits based on a number of factors. For example, one client needs a blood sugar drawn before breakfast, another client needs dressing changes twice a day, and the caregiver of a third client will only be present in the morning to let the nurse into the residence. Other factors to be considered in scheduling include distance between visits, the need to take specimens to the laboratory, the need to coordinate the visit with other health professionals, and the need to work with physicians. In addition to scheduling, the nurse must be aware of supplies, equipment, medications, teaching materials, and anything else that might be needed and make arrangements for obtaining materials that are not immediately at hand.

The previsit/planning phase consists of those activities that prepare the nurse to accomplish the required tasks of the home visits scheduled. This phase requires several considerations as the nurse plans care for all clients to be seen each day. These considerations and activities are outlined.

Caseload Scheduling

Assignments and scheduling guidelines for home health clients differ among agencies. The plan of care developed by the admitting nurse and/or case manager in collaboration with the physician determines how often the client will be seen and what services are to be provided during each visit. Often agencies assign home health nurses a caseload of clients, and each nurse determines which clients to see on which days. In other agencies all assignments are made from the central office, based on individual client needs and available personnel. Typically the agency assigns nurses based on geographical or distance considerations (e.g., one nurse sees clients in a given area) or based on specialized needs of the client or abilities of the nurse (e.g., infusion therapy or wound care).

Home health nurses generally see four to six clients each day, although this may vary somewhat, based on client acuity and prescribed services (e.g., an intravenous infusion may take 2 hours or more) or distances that must be traveled (e.g., in rural areas, the nurse may drive 100 miles or more to see one client). When planning the day's schedule, the nurse begins with a list of all clients that will be seen that day. This list should include the following:

- A synopsis of the client's diagnosis(es)
- What services need to be provided during the day's visit
- Any supplies, equipment, or medications needed in the home that are not at hand
- General directions regarding location of each residence (e.g., map coordinates)

From this list the nurse can begin the process of scheduling client visits. This is typically accomplished during the afternoon or evening before the day's visit.

Telephone Contact

After the day's preliminary schedule is determined, each client is contacted to inform him or her of the anticipated time for the nursing visit and to briefly explain the purpose of the visit. In addition, the nurse should get specific directions to the residence if this is the first visit and determine if any special additional instructions, requests, or information regarding each client may be needed; for example, scheduling around the presence of a caregiver or the need to bring additional supplies.

Occasionally it is impossible to contact the client to schedule the visit. For example, the client may not have a telephone, may not be able to answer it, or may not speak English. In these cases contacting a relative, neighbor, or other caregiver to establish the time and purpose of the visit should be attempted.

Each agency has guidelines on what to do if telephone scheduling is not possible. If no problems (e.g., the client has a physician's appointment or requests an earlier or later time to avoid a conflict) are encountered with the preliminary schedule, the nurse uses this schedule when seeing the day's caseload.

Review of the Client's Chart

Following scheduling, the home health nurse should become familiar with the client's plan of care. Chart or case review is a very important step in the care of the home health client. However, this may not be a simple process. Many providers from the home health agency may see the same client. Depending on agency protocols, the client's comprehensive chart may be at the agency or in the possession of the case manager. In many instances other providers see the client without seeing the master chart and need as much information as possible regarding that client, the condition, and the plan of care. Each agency uses different methods to deliver this information. Voice mail or other recorded reports, faxed information, e-mail downloads, and charts and data left in the home are methods used to manage information about each client and deliver it to health care team members.

The nurse scheduling the visit should review all available information before seeing the client. If anything is unclear, or if the nurse has any questions regarding the care plan, the case manager (if someone other than the scheduled nurse), the physician, the nurse's supervisor, or other appropriate individual should be contacted to answer questions or clarify information, plans, or procedures before the nurse sees the client. This enables the nurse to be prepared for and better expedite each visit and ensures that all concerns and questions regarding the client's care are addressed.

Assessment of Personal Supplies and Equipment

Another important step in previsit planning involves daily inventory of the nurse's bag and routine periodic inventory of the car stock of supplies. The accompanying Community Application boxes ("Suggested Contents of a Home Health Nurse's Bag" and "Suggested Contents of a Home Health Nurse's Car Stock") detail what should be included

COMMUNITY APPLICATION
Suggested Contents of a Home Health Nurse's Bag

- Large shoulder bag with multiple compartments and zippered closure
- Laptop computer
- Cell phone

MEDICAL EQUIPMENT/SUPPLIES

- Antimicrobial soap (preferably liquid) and paper towels; alcohol foam
- Stethoscope
- Sphygmomanometer
- Thermometer (oral and tympanic) and appropriate covers
- Penlight or flashlight
- Tape measure and/or small ruler
- Alcohol wipes
- Nonsterile gloves (dozen pairs)
- Nonsterile disposable gown or apron
- Nonsterile waterproof pads (chux)
- Disposable masks
- Goggles
- Sterile gloves (three or four pairs)
- Dressing supplies (4-inch gauze squares [4 × 4s], 2-inch gauze squares [2 × 2s]), 3-inch and 4-inch dressing gauze,

sterile applicators, silk and paper tape, sterile saline, adhesive bandages)
- Venipuncture supplies (e.g., assortment of vacutainer needles, tubes, syringes, tourniquet)
- Glucometer and strips
- Sterile specimen cup, culture tubes
- Bandage scissors
- Forceps
- Biohazard containers and bags

OTHER MATERIALS

- Map
- Agency and Medicare required forms and charting materials and information
- Laboratory forms and plastic pouches for transporting laboratory specimens
- Teaching materials
- Pocket medication reference book
- Pocket nursing interventions reference book
- Plastic trash bags
- Bathroom scale

---

in each one. Based on agency guidelines and variations in the nurse's practice (e.g., if he or she is a member of the intravenous team or is a wound specialist), these supplies may vary. The car stock should be checked periodically for expired supplies and to ensure that no supplies are damaged; it should be replenished as necessary. The bag should be inventoried and replenished daily.

Safety Concerns and Previsit Planning

It is important to note that several safety concerns apply to home health care nurses. Typically home health nurses work alone. They may go into questionably safe neighborhoods, drive many miles in adverse weather conditions, and some may encounter threatening situations. To enhance communication between the nurse and the agency and to promote safety, most agencies supply nurses with cellular telephones and pagers. To assist in minimizing threats, the Community Application box "Safety Tips for Home Health Nurses" provides general information on safety in home health.

The final aspect of previsit planning should include notifying the agency of the nurse's anticipated sched-

ule. This allows the agency to trace or monitor the movement of the nurse and, with the use of the pager or cellular telephone, make contact if necessary.

THE HOME VISIT ACTIVITIES

Smith (2005) divides the home health visit into three phases: (1) initiation, (2) implementation, and (3) termination. Specific activities for each are described in the following sections.

Initiation Phase

The initiation phase begins when the nurse knocks on the door and gains entrance into the residence. The nurse should identify herself or himself and the agency and briefly review the purpose of the visit. For example, the nurse might say "Good morning Mrs. Johnson. I'm Mary Smith from the Visiting Nurse Association, and I am here to change Mr. Johnson's dressing." The nurse should greet all in attendance and determine who is the primary caregiver for the client if appropriate. (Often the client lives alone.)

There may a brief social phase that can be used to begin assessments and establish rapport. A standard

COMMUNITY APPLICATION
Suggested Contents of a Home Health Nurse's Car Stock

DRESSING SUPPLIES

- Two or three dozen packages of sterile 2 × 2s and 4 × 4s
- 3-inch and 4-inch gauze dressings (6 to 12 packages of each)
- Sterile abdominal dressing (ABD) pads (box)
- Hypertonic dressing gauze
- Nonstick dressing gauze (e.g., telfa, adaptic)
- Hydrocolloid dressings (several boxes in a variety of sizes)
- Adhesive bandages (one box of assorted sizes; "spots" for venipunctures)
- Alcohol wipes (one box)
- Sterile gloves (one or two boxes)
- Nonsterile gloves (one or two boxes)
- Assortment of tapes
- Sterile scissors (two or three pairs)
- Sterile forceps (two or three pairs)
- Staple remover (one or two)
- Suture removal kit(s)
- Steri strips (several sizes)
- Sterile saline (several containers)
- Hydrogen peroxide (two or three bottles)
- Other dressings, ointments, solutions, and supplies based on factors such as client needs and physician preferences

CATHETERS AND RELATED EQUIPMENT AND SUPPLIES

- Adult briefs (variety of sizes)
- Catheter insertion kits (two)
- Indwelling catheters (variety of sizes)
- Red rubber catheters (variety of sizes)

- Catheter drainage bags (two)
- Catheter irrigation kit (two)
- Sterile water for irrigation (three or four bottles)
- Catheter leg bag (two)
- Underpads (waterproof pads—chux) (two packages)
- Urine specimen containers (sterile; three or four)

MISCELLANEOUS EQUIPMENT AND SUPPLIES FOR ROUTINE VISITS

- Variety of needles and syringes
- Lancets and chemstrips for glucometer (if used)
- Restraints
- Lubricating jelly
- Levine tube (two)
- Trash bags (one box)
- Pill boxes (two)
- Disposable masks and aprons or gowns (several of each)

MISCELLANEOUS EQUIPMENT AND SUPPLIES FOR SPECIALIZED HOME CARE (WHEN APPLICABLE)

- Enterostomal therapy supplies (e.g., colostomy, ileostomy bags, stomahesive)
- Infusion therapy supplies (e.g., variety of administration sets, syringes, injectable solutions)
- Respiratory therapy or tracheotomy supplies (e.g., suction tubes, suction tips and catheters, tracheotomy care trays)
- Gastrointestinal feeding supplies (e.g., variety of bags, tubings)

COMMUNITY APPLICATION
Safety Tips for Home Health Nurses

- Maintain car; keep gas tank at least half full
- Ensure cell phone is charged and readily accessible
- Lock all car doors at all times; keep windows rolled up
- Park as close to the entrance to the client's residence as possible
- Use a map or global positioning system (GPS) device; know where clients live; get directions
- Keep purse in the car trunk; carry change and identification in a pocket
- Dress appropriately, conservatively, professionally (according to agency guidelines); wear comfortable shoes, minimal jewelry, and name tag
- Pay attention to uncomfortable, intuitive "feelings"; if the setting or situation seems unsafe, leave at once

- Avoid walking by groups of individuals loitering near building entrances and/or isolated places
- Never walk into a home uninvited; always knock and wait at the door to be let in either physically or verbally
- If pets are annoying or threatening, request that they be removed to another room before entering the home
- Know the agency's policy regarding safety; some agencies will provide a security guard, assistant, or escort to accompany providers in questionably safe areas
- Visit only during scheduled hours; if exceptions must be made, notify supervisor

greeting, such as "How are you doing this morning," allows the nurse to begin collecting data on the client's physical, psychological, and social well-being (Figure 11-1). A brief discussion about the weather, holidays, or news events allows the nurse to assess cognitive status. Talking for a few minutes with the caregiver(s) can convey caring, assist with assessment of the family situation, and assist with the concerns, abilities, and understanding level of the caregiver. At this point and throughout the visit, the nurse should continually assess the surroundings to determine potential threats to the client's condition or safety.

During this brief social phase, the nurse should review the chart or records left in the home. If this is the initial visit, the nurse should make sure that permissions are signed or should obtain them. At this time the nurse may open the medical supplies bag and begin removing needed equipment, such as a blood pressure cuff and stethoscope. The nurse should also remove the soap and paper towels from the bag and ask to use the bathroom or kitchen to wash hands. The nurse is now ready to begin the physical assessment and implement the plan of care.

Implementation Phase

The implementation phase is the working component of home health care provision. During this phase assessments are conducted, skilled nursing care is provided, and teaching is accomplished.

ASSESSMENT. Assessment in home health nursing involves several different areas. In addition to thorough physical assessment, assessment of psychosocial needs, functional abilities, medication, nutrition, safety issues, and the client's environment is essential. Home health agencies often develop their own assessment tools and provide the requisite forms for documentation of assessment in each of these areas.

Typically a thorough database is completed during the initial admission visit. From this database the plan of care is developed to address identified needs and appropriate skilled nursing interventions and other therapies (e.g., physical therapy, occupational therapy) and ancillary assistance (e.g., home health aide assistance with activities of daily living) that will be administered as appropriate. During subsequent visits less comprehensive, more directed assessments are conducted. After hand washing, at each visit the nurse takes vital signs and performs a

Figure 11-1. A nurse visits with an elderly client in her home. (Courtesy Rick Brady, Photographer, Riva, Maryland.)

routine head-to-toe assessment, including assessment of the following:

- Respiratory system (e.g., listening to breath sounds, quality of respirations, assessing presence or absence of cough)
- Cardiovascular system (e.g., rate, rhythm, heart sounds, presence or absence of chest pain, peripheral pulses, capillary refill, edema)
- Neurological system (e.g., whether the client is alert and oriented, reactivity of pupils, ability to move extremities, and equal strength of same)
- Gastrointestinal system (e.g., abdomen; bowel sounds; any distention, masses, or tenderness; nausea, vomiting, or diarrhea; last bowel movement; and appetite)
- Urinary system (e.g., frequency of urination, any burning, unusual odor)
- Skin integrity (e.g., turgor, temperature, color, any redness, open areas or wounds)

Particular attention is given to those areas related to identified problems or potential problems. For example, if the client has diabetes, the nurse should very carefully assess the feet for adequate circulation and evidence of skin breakdown. If the client has been diagnosed with congestive heart failure, careful attention to cardiovascular and respiratory function, including monitoring of weight and signs of peripheral edema, is essential.

An individual routine is usually established, wherein the nurse develops a pattern to ensure that all systems and areas are covered during the assessment. Most nurses usually begin by taking and charting vital signs. Comparison with previous readings and notation of significant changes may dictate unplanned actions or interventions (e.g., if the client has developed an elevated temperature since yesterday or if the blood pressure is unusually high, the physician may need to be called immediately). While taking the vital signs, and throughout the physical assessment, the nurse can take the opportunity to question the client to obtain additional information (e.g., "When did you last have a bowel movement?" "What did you eat for breakfast?" "Have you noticed any dizziness or pain?"). Follow-up questions to the client's responses of change or identification of possible problems allows the nurse to obtain more information (e.g., "When did you first notice burning when you urinate?" "I see your ankles are a little swollen—have you been up quite

a lot?" "Your blood pressure is a little higher than it has been—did you take your medication this morning?"). Any problems should be noted in the visit record and discussed with the physician or case manager as appropriate.

Following the initial visit, much less documentation is required. A revisit summary outlining the routine assessment and all findings should be included. This should be followed by narrative description of the purpose of the visit and details of the skilled nursing care given.

PROVISION OF SKILLED NURSING CARE. As described earlier, skilled observation and assessment are essential services for Medicare reimbursement. Other covered services include wound care, venipuncture, administration of medications, tracheotomy and catheter care, and teaching clients and caregivers various skills and services. During each visit, the nurse performs the identified and assigned interventions and documents them according to agency guidelines.

Often the nursing care performed requires the nurse to use materials carried in his or her bag (e.g., drawing blood, removing sutures or staples) or supplies left in the home (e.g., changing dressings, performing tracheotomy care, administering intravenous medications). As in the acute care setting, the nurse must treat the bag and stock of supplies as clean and carefully avoid contamination and cross-contamination. It is important to remember to remove the supplies and equipment from the bag or stock before beginning the procedures and not to return to the bag without washing hands or removing contaminated gloves. In addition, the nurse should be careful to place the bag on a clean surface (not the floor) and to ensure that children or pets cannot reach it. When leaving equipment and supplies in the home, the same guidelines and procedures should apply, and manufacturer's recommendations regarding storage should be carefully maintained. Dressing supplies, for example, should be placed in a clean cupboard or on a shelf away from the reach of pets and children and away from moisture or extreme heat. Likewise, medications, formulas, and solutions should be stored according to guidelines. If the nurse is unsure of the ability of the client to store supplies properly, he or she should make other arrangements. For example, occasionally a family may not have reliable electricity or a working refrigerator and cannot properly store solutions for total parenteral nutrition (TPN). In such a case, the nurse may need to arrange to pick up the prescribed solutions at a pharmacy and bring them with him or her or to store them at a neighbor's residence.

When performing sterile procedures (e.g., dressing changes, insertion of catheters, hanging solutions), it is as important that meticulous technique be followed in the home as in the hospital. In addition, the nurse should ensure that all contaminated materials and waste be disposed of properly. The client and the caregivers should be taught proper management of infectious wastes and the rationale behind such management. Containers for handling "sharps" should be provided, and methods for appropriate disposal should be taught to the client and the caregiver.

TEACHING. In home health care, teaching is one of the most important functions of the nurse. The nurse teaches the client and the caregivers general information about the client's illness or condition, care or treatment regimen, medications, and identification and reporting of symptoms or complications. In addition, clients and their caregivers may be given specific instructions on a variety of health-related topics, such as self-administration of insulin or other injectable medications, management of an American Diabetic Association diet, self-catheterization, administration of gastrostomy tube feedings, tracheotomy care, bowel training, wound care, or colostomy or ileostomy care.

As discussed in Chapter 3, it is very important to realize that health teaching goes beyond information dissemination. In home health care the nurse must assess the readiness and ability of the client or caregiver to perform the necessary tasks; present the information in a manner that is understandable to the learner; possibly use several methods, tools, and materials in the instruction process; and carefully, accurately, and thoroughly evaluate the level of understanding and response to the teaching. Observation of the client during a sterile dressing change, use of return demonstration in drawing up insulin, and verbalization of principles of infection control are evaluation techniques that the nurse may use to determine how well the client understands the instructions.

Many agencies provide and encourage the use of written materials to assist their nurses in teaching clients and caregivers in home settings. Written instructions are particularly helpful for clients who will be required to perform procedures without the presence of the nurse. Step-by-step guides can be reviewed and discussed with the client and often prove to be very helpful tools. Providing written instruction on areas such as the steps in monitoring blood sugar and self-administration of insulin, the signs and symptoms of complications of anticoagulant therapy and when to notify the physician, the signs and symptoms of urinary tract infection for the client with an indwelling catheter, and the management of congestive heart failure can assist in enhancing the client's understanding of his or her health problems; in treating or alleviating symptoms; and in preventing, identifying, or recognizing changes or complications to the condition.

Termination Phase

Following completion of the skilled nursing interventions and teaching, the home health nurse evaluates the client's response to care and briefly summarizes the continuing plan of care with the client and caregiver. If care is to be ongoing, the nurse can set up a time for the next home visit. During this phase, the nurse should be careful to gather all equipment and supplies that he or she will take. If any specimens have been collected, these should be placed in appropriate containers and requisite paperwork should be completed.

At this point, the nurse should also review potential health emergencies and appropriate actions to take. For example, the nurse might say, "Mrs. Cooper, if you experience any chest pain or shortness of breath or if you gain more than 2 pounds when you weigh yourself in the morning, call your doctor immediately." The nurse should ensure that contact information for the doctor, the home health agency, and other providers is readily available.

Before departure, the nurse should ask the client and caregiver if they have any questions and clarify once more when he or she will return and the purpose of the next visit (e.g., "Good-bye for now, Mrs. Charles. Another nurse will see you this evening, but I will be back about the same time tomorrow to change your dressing." "Mrs. McClure, I will call your doctor today to report on your laboratory findings. If there are no changes in your Coumadin schedule, I will be back in 2 or 3 weeks to check your clotting times again. I will call you and let you know.").

POSTVISIT ACTIVITIES

After each visit, several activities must be completed to fulfill the responsibilities of the home health care nurse. These activities include communication of findings to other health care providers (reporting and referral) and documentation (completion of all forms and charting).

Communication

Reporting important assessment and evaluation findings to all appropriate personnel or referral to other providers for follow-up of identified concerns is a very important component of home health care practice. If the nurse seeing the client is the case manager, findings or significant changes in the client's condition are typically reported to the physician. Other providers may also be contacted to refer or initiate services (e.g., occupational therapy, speech therapy). Also, current care providers may be contacted to discuss their assessment of the client (e.g., the nurse might call Mrs. Thornton's physical therapist to discuss whether additional visits for more in-depth teaching of range-of-motion exercises might be appropriate).

The home health care nurse should keep the physician informed of the client's condition. Any changes in health status and any significant findings should be reported immediately. If the home health nurse seeing the client is not the case manager, a report to the case manager needs to be made following agency guidelines.

Referrals to nonagency providers (e.g., Meals on Wheels, adult day care centers) should be made as appropriate following agency guidelines. As nurses gain experience in home health care practice, they may maintain a list or booklet of community resources to share with their clients.

Documentation

The importance of complete, concise, and accurate documentation in home health nursing cannot be overstated. All forms and documents must be completed according to Medicare or other third-party payer guidelines and the home health care agency's requirements. An experienced home health nurse may be able to complete most of the paperwork while in the client's home or immediately thereafter. However, the nurse should comprehensively review each client's chart at the end of the day.

Documentation should include date and time of reporting to the physician and/or case manager described previously and any actions resulting from that report. For example, "Mrs. Cooper's BP 160/94; Dr. Black notified @ 13:00; he stated that no changes be made in medication at present, requests that pt's BP be reevaluated in 2 days. Plan: SNV on Thursday to reevaluate" or "Dr. Brown contacted @ 09:30 and informed that wound edges were reddened, drainage malodorous, and pt reports increased pain. M.D. requested wound C & S be performed and client seen again tomorrow. C & S to lab at 10:30; results available in 24 hrs. Plan: contact lab tomorrow a.m. and schedule p.m. SNV." Often home health agencies periodically review home care nurses' documentation to ensure comprehensiveness.

SPECIALIZED HOME HEALTH CARE

Related to changes in the health care system, specialized home health services have been added and expanded over the past decade. For example, **infusion therapy**, which includes TPN, chemotherapy, and administration of other pharmacotherapeutics, has become increasingly common. Other areas of specialized care now being provided in the home include care of ventilator-dependent clients, high-risk prenatal clients, routine postpartum clients, clients with chronic mental health problems, and clients with chronic wounds. Hospice, or care of the terminally ill, is also becoming more commonplace. Basic components of each of these areas are described in this section.

INFUSION THERAPY

Home infusion therapy is a very significant component of home health care. With shortened hospital stays, many patients are discharged needing additional or prolonged parenteral medication. Home health care agencies have responded by adding home infusion nurses or teams or incorporating home infusion therapy into specialized orientation or training for their regular home care nurses. In addition, many home health agencies that specialize in infusion therapy have developed.

The growth in home infusion or intravenous therapy programs has been phenomenal since the 1980s. Reasons cited for the growth include the following:
- Patient population (high patient acuity and increased complexity of cases)
- Technology (e.g., portable infusion pumps, flexible silicone catheters)
- Cost (decreasing inpatient hospitalization)
- Consumer awareness (clients and their families are more willing to participate in the recovery process) (Adams and Rice, 2006)

Types of Home Infusion Therapy

Several types of infusion therapy are routinely delivered in homes. Antibiotics, pain medication, TPN, hydration, and chemotherapy are the most routinely administered home intravenous therapies. Blood products, cardiac agents (dobutamine), medications to treat premature uterine contractions in high-risk pregnancies, chelation therapy, steriods (e.g. for multiple sclerosis and organ rejection following transplant), and human growth homone are other agents sometimes administered in the home (Adams & Rice, 2006). Table 11-4 lists common diagnoses for home intravenous therapy.

Home Infusion Therapy Management

Home infusion therapy is nursing-intensive and can be very complex. Orientation of new nurses to home infusion services should be comprehensive and cover specific procedures for each type of care (e.g., TPN, chemotherapy, antibiotic therapy). Resources for assistance, supervision, and consultation should be available at all times, and procedures for complications must be reviewed routinely and followed painstakingly.

In addition to delivering the prescribed medications, the nurse must evaluate the client for complications (e.g., medication reactions or infection) related to the illness or the treatment regimen.

TABLE **11-4** Home Infusion Therapy

TYPE OF INFUSION THERAPY	EXAMPLES OF MEDICAL DIAGNOSES
Antibiotic therapy	AIDS-related infections Bacterial endocarditis Cystic fibrosis Osteomyelitis Pneumonia
Parenteral nutrition	AIDS-related enteropathy Colitis Crohn's disease Pancreatitis Various cancers (e.g., colon, liver, stomach)
Chemotherapy	Leukemias Lymphomas Sarcomas Various carcinomas (e.g., breast, lung, pancreas)
Pain management	Chronic intractable pain (secondary to cancer) Various AIDS-related diagnoses
Hydration therapy	Gastroenteritis Hyperemesis gravidarum Intractable diarrhea

Adapted from Humphrey CJ, Milone-Nuzzo P: *Home care nursing: an orientation to practice*, New York, 1991, Appleton & Lange.

Management of the plan of care requires consideration of the drug therapy schedule, presence or absence of other caregivers who may be needed to assist, additional or preliminary medications or therapies, availability or source of the medication; preparation of the medication, use of an infusion pump if prescribed, and assessment and maintenance of the administration port.

Pain Management

In home health care, pain medications, including narcotics, are used to manage severe pain usually caused by cancer, acquired immunodeficiency syndrome (AIDS), or neurological or orthopedic conditions. Narcotics may be administered intravenously, intramuscularly, subcutaneously, intrathecally, or epidurally when oral or rectal drug administration is no longer adequate. In home care, use of client-controlled analgesia pumps is becoming common. Pain management is discussed in more detail later in this chapter in the section on hospice care.

Total Parenteral Nutrition

Use of TPN may be indicated when oral nutrition is not sufficient. The TPN requires a physician's order specifying the type of solution, frequency of administration, frequency of vital sign assessment, and periodic serum chemistry assessment. The TPN solutions are prepared in a pharmacy and must be refrigerated. An infusion pump is always used to ensure constant flow rates.

Enteral Nutrition Therapy

Enteral nutrition therapy is indicated for those clients who cannot receive sufficient oral nutrition. Enteral nutrition is the treatment of choice for clients with a functioning lower gastrointestinal tract but for whom food intake is not possible, is not adequate, or is too difficult. Home-based enteral nutrition is most commonly seen when providing care to clients with conditions such as pharyngeal or esophageal strictures or neurological disorders resulting in dysphagia, anorexia, and coma.

The client's diagnosis, condition, long-term needs, and prognosis determine the type of feeding tube and placement. In acute care facilities, nasogastric or orogastric tubes are often used to insert nutrients directly into the stomach. Surgically implanted feeding tubes (gastrostomy or jejunostomy

tubes) are used for clients with long-term nutrition assistance and/or conditions that necessitate bypassing portions of the gastrointestinal system. In home care, as in institutional settings, the feeding regimen is determined and prescribed by the physician or an interdisciplinary team including a nutritionist, a physician, and possibly a pharmacist. Choice of feeding solutions or formulas requires consideration of the metabolic needs of the client, financial limitations, learning ability of the client or caregivers, and other necessary therapies. Instruction for enteral therapy should include the specific supplements, amount, time, route, and procedure. Feedings may be prescribed as continuous, intermittent, or bolus. As in other areas of home health care, much of the nurse's responsibility lies in teaching the client or caregiver procedures for home nutrition therapy and supporting and monitoring the care.

WOUND MANAGEMENT

Wound care is one of the most common services provided by home health nurses. In the home, nurses typically work with wounds that are difficult to heal, usually because of underlying disease processes (e.g., diabetes, peripheral vascular disease), anemia, poor nutrition, wound contamination, chemical irritants, neglect, medications, age, and other factors (Rice, Wiersema-Bryant & Bangert, 2006). When wounds do not respond to care or when providing care to a client with an ostomy, nurses with special training or experience may be used.

Chronic Wound Care

Basic wound care, including frequency of dressing change, type of dressing used, cleaning solutions, and topical medications, is generally determined by the physician. Nurses who specialize in wound care, however, often have latitude to make decisions based on their expertise. Goals for wound treatment and management include prevention of further tissue destruction by reducing or controlling predisposing causes of tissue destruction, prevention of infection, and planning treatments as appropriate based on the type of wound (pressure, venous, or surgical) and condition and size of the wound (stage, amount of drainage, and related factors).

In addition to changing dressings, nursing interventions in wound care include assessment of the wound and evaluation of the efficacy of treatment, cleansing and debridement, obtaining cultures when indicated, teaching the client and/or caregiver how to change the dressing using sterile technique, and teaching caregivers signs and symptoms of infection and how to prevent further tissue breakdown.

A number of wound care products are available and used by home care nurses to treat and prevent wounds. These include transparent dressings, hydrocolloid dressings, nonadherent dressings, and hypertonic saline gauze. The nurse may assist in securing specialized equipment or supplies to prevent pressure sores. Gel pads, foam mattresses, and air support mattresses, for example, may be helpful.

Enterostomal Care

Many home care agencies employ enterostomal nurses, or enterostomal therapists (ET), to assist clients with a colostomy, an ileostomy, or a urostomy. Client and caregiver education and support and monitoring for complications or side effects are primary functions of **enterostomal care**.

In addition to providing client education for ostomy care, enterostomal nurses are often specialists in wound care and management. Typically enterostomal nurses case-manage clients with ostomies and act as resources for other home health nurses. Often the enterostomal nurse is consulted to assist in preventing skin breakdown for high-risk clients (e.g., those who are bed bound, very frail, paraplegic, or quadriplegic) or if a wound is not healing as anticipated.

CARE OF VENTILATOR-DEPENDENT CLIENTS

As with other areas of specialized care, home health care for ventilator-dependent clients is growing. Individuals who are ventilator-dependent or need ventilator assistance are sometimes discharged from acute care or long-term institutions into the home with conditions such as severe chronic obstructive pulmonary disease or other chronic lung problems (e.g., cystic fibrosis or complex pneumonia) or spinal cord injuries or defects. Home health nurses who work with ventilator-dependent clients must have intensive training and consistent agency support. When providing care to ventilator-dependent clients, the home health nurse must work closely with the physician, respiratory therapist, and family members. The nurse's role in the care of ventilator-dependent clients is largely supportive and includes the following:

- Assessing the home situation for the availability of 24-hour caregivers who are properly trained, competent, and able to perform cardiopulmonary resuscitation.
- Working with the physician and respiratory therapist to outline guidelines for concern (e.g., complications such as infection or respiratory difficulty) and appropriate interventions to teach the caregivers.
- Implementing and periodically reviewing emergency plans with the care providers.
- Coordinating referrals with social workers, physical or occupational therapists, respite caregivers, support groups, or others as appropriate.
- Teaching and monitoring tracheostomy care and suctioning.
- Providing skilled nursing care for other needs of the client.
- Assisting in monitoring blood gas levels and acid-base balance as ordered or needed.

Ventilator-dependent clients are at risk for problems and complications such as infection, fluid volume overload, impaired skin integrity, and injury (e.g., tracheostomal trauma from suctioning, overinflation of the tracheostomy tube cuff, tissue adhesions and stricture) (Rice, 2001). Agency policy and physician orders dictate care for these clients. In general, the stoma should be cleaned daily, with the skin being assessed for signs of infection. Needed suctioning using disposable or properly cleaned catheters should be performed using aseptic technique, and tracheostomy tubes should be changed at least monthly. Knowledge of commonly used equipment and supplies is essential for nurses who work with ventilator-dependent clients.

PERINATAL HOME CARE

Home care for pregnant and postpartum clients has increased dramatically during the past few years. Technologically advanced care for high-risk pregnancies and for neonates with identified breathing difficulties is now delivered in the home under certain conditions. In addition, postpartum care for clients, particularly following shortened hospital stays, is becoming increasingly common and even mandated in some locations. High-tech perinatal home care, apnea monitoring for high-risk infants, and postpartum home care are discussed briefly.

Home Care of High-Risk Perinatal Clients

One of the newest areas for home health nursing involves the care of high-risk perinatal clients. Until recent years, high-risk maternity clients were hospitalized for extended periods for monitoring or treatment. In many cases they are now being cared for in the home. **Perinatal home care** services include the following components:

- Uterine monitoring: A portable monitor may be used to assess contractions. The monitor may then be taken back to the provider, agency, or institution for evaluation or the information may be transmitted to a receiving center via telephone lines.
- Fetal monitoring: A portable fetal monitor may be used to perform a nonstress test to assess fetal development and condition. Like the uterine monitor, the fetal monitor produces a printed strip that can be transmitted via phone lines to the institution or agency for interpretation.
- Ultrasound: A portable ultrasound machine is used to perform a biophysical profile to evaluate fetal movement, fetal heart rate, muscle tone, and fluid volume.
- Infusion pump treatment: Subcutaneous infusion therapy utilizes a microinfusion pump to deliver continuous or intermittent low doses of a prescribed medication. For example, a medication such as terbutaline can be administered to control uterine contractions associated with preterm labor; an insulin pump may be used to administer insulin subcutaneously for an uncontrolled, brittle diabetic; or heparin may be administered via pump for a pregnant woman prone to developing blood clots.
- Infusion therapy: Antibiotics may be needed for severe infection; hydration therapy and TPN may be administered for hyperemesis.
- Hypertension monitoring: The nurse can teach the client or family to monitor blood pressure and report findings. As with uterine or fetal monitors, remote blood pressure monitors enable the client to transmit findings to a center or provider for interpretation (Dahlberg, Blazek, Wikoff, Tuckwell, and Koloroutis, 1995).

Postpartum Home Care

Increasingly, shortened postpartum hospital stays, attributable to health care reform and cost containment, have led to steady growth in postpartum home care. The average length of stay (LOS) for all deliveries in the United States is 2.6 days; typically insurers will reimburse a minimum LOS of 48 hours for a vaginal birth and 96 hours for a cesarean birth (Dasing, Ryberg and Keller, 2006). Benefits attributed to early discharge are quicker reestablishment of family routines, decreased separation from the family, decreased costs, decreased risk of nosocomial infection, emotional and psychological benefits from familiar surroundings, and increased confidence in learning to care for the neonate in the home setting. Disadvantages include decreased educational opportunities, need for increased help at home to provide meals and other home maintenance services, lack of rest for the mother, lack of nursing guidance for breastfeeding and neonatal care, and potential for undiagnosed complications, such as neonatal hyperbilirubinemia, low neonatal temperature, maternal hemorrhage, and excessive maternal pain.

Postpartum nursing care, whether in the hospital or home, includes monitoring the physical and emotional well-being of family members, identification of potential or developing complications, and bridging the gap between discharge and ambulatory follow-up for mothers and infants (Dasing, Ryberg and Keller, 2006). To meet the educational, physiological, and supportive needs of the childbearing family, several different models of postpartum home health care have been developed. In general, postpartum home care services include health promotion and health education activities that have been within the traditional scope and functions of postpartum inpatient care. Postpartum home care services generally include follow-up telephone calls 1 to 3 days after discharge, home visits 1 to 3 days after discharge, new parent information telephone lines staffed by a nurse and available 24 hours a day, lactation consultation to assist with problems encountered with breastfeeding, and organized support groups and outpatient clinics that encourage the first visit 3 to 4 days postdischarge to assess both mother and infant and provide relevant teaching and interventions.

During postpartum home visitation, the most common concerns of the mother are pain associated with episiotomy or cesarean incision, breast engorgement, backache, and uterine cramping. In addition, teaching regarding nutritional needs and avoidance of infection and constipation is also warranted. Infant concerns and questions are typically related to nutrition—particularly ineffective breastfeeding and bottle-feeding problems—and hyperbilirubinemia.

Apnea Monitoring

Apnea monitoring is most often indicated for premature infants with apnea, infants who have experienced or are at risk for experiencing a life-threatening event, and infants at risk for sudden infant death syndrome. In home care the primary role of the nurse is in educating the parents or caregivers about normal infant breathing patterns, recognition of and response to apnea episodes, infant cardiopulmonary resuscitation, and use and maintenance of the apnea monitor. In addition, the home care nurse should review the infant's cardiopulmonary status, review teaching, evaluate the parents' level of understanding, and assess the parents' stress. Referral for social services or respite care may be appropriate.

PSYCHIATRIC HOME CARE

Although psychiatric home health care was first recognized as a reimbursable treatment alternative eligible for Medicare reimbursement in 1979, it has only relatively recently become widely available. Psychiatric home care is appropriate for individuals with diagnosed or suspected mental illness who need psychiatric services but cannot use traditional outpatient mental health services. For example, psychiatric home care can prevent or shorten psychiatric hospitalization, particularly for acutely depressed individuals and those diagnosed as schizophrenic. The goals of **psychiatric home health care** are the following:
- Reduce the need for hospitalization or rehospitalization of clients in psychological crisis.
- Promote the client's adjustment to the community and home.
- Monitor medication compliance, effectiveness, and side effects.

- Provide assistance with problem solving to families.
- Reinforce predischarge therapy and treatment.
- Provide education to clients and their families regarding issues such as disease process, medication, diet, and community resources.
- Provide in-home respite services to the client's family (Gilkison and Neathery, 1995).

Client conditions or diagnoses in which home care might be beneficial, or even preferable to traditional outpatient or inpatient care, include confusion or disorientation, severe depression, altered perception or cognition, risk for self-harm, vulnerability in the community, requirement of 24-hour supervision, excessive fear or anxiety, agoraphobia, need for assistive devices for mobility, or inability to leave home independently (Carson, 1996). (See the Community Application box "Nursing Interventions and Services in Psychiatric Home Health Care.")

HOSPICE CARE: HOME CARE OF THE TERMINALLY ILL

The hospice movement in the United States is relatively recent, beginning in the 1970s (Wallace, 2002). **Hospice care** is intended to provide palliative care to the terminally ill. Most hospice patients have a diagnosis of cancer, but other diagnoses commonly seen in hospice care include AIDS, severe chronic obstructive pulmonary disease, terminal heart conditions, and neurological conditions such as amyotrophic lateral sclerosis or multiple sclerosis.

Hospice programs may be located either at a client's place of residence or in an inpatient facility. Models for hospice care include hospice-based programs within a hospital or within an extended care facility, a free-standing hospice, or home care hospice programs.

Although hospice care is frequently delivered to clients and their families in the home, there are distinctive differences between hospice care and traditional home health care. For example, in hospice nursing the primary focus is on quality of life and palliation, whereas in conventional home health the primary focus is on rehabilitation and restoration. In hospice, the nurse sees the client intermittently, with visits intensifying in frequency until death. In conventional home health, the nurse sees the client

COMMUNITY APPLICATION
Nursing Interventions and Services in Psychiatric Home Health Care

- Individual psychotherapy, as appropriate, to improve self-concept, decrease fear or anxiety, decrease hopelessness, increase motivation, increase spiritual well-being, improve eating patterns, improve sleep patterns, increase social interaction, and promote diversional activities
- Ongoing assessment and monitoring of psychiatric and emotional status
- Medication administration and management (including injection of medications such as haloperidol or fluphenazine decanoate) and assessment for medication effectiveness, compliance, and side effects
- Teaching about medication regimens, disease process, communication skills, and signs and symptoms of exacerbation of illness

- Crisis and symptom management
- Laboratory services (e.g., medication blood levels, white blood counts for clozapine)
- Case management to link clients and caregivers to community resources
- Assessment of family and community support systems and their effectiveness
- 24-hour on-call nursing support
- Development, implementation, and evaluation of a nursing care plan
- Coordination with other home care services, such as pharmacy, support, therapy, social service, and home care aide services

Data from Carson VB: The journey through home mental health care. In Carson VB, Arnold EN, editors: *Mental health nursing: the nurse-patient journey*, Philadelphia, 1996, W.B. Saunders; Dittbrenner H: Psychiatric home care: an overview, *Caring* June:26-30, 1994; Hauk DO: The mental health patient. In Rice R, editor: *Home health nursing: concepts and application*, ed 2, St Louis, 1996, Mosby; Lima B: In-home psychiatric nursing: the at-home mental health program, *Caring*, July:14-20, 1995.

intermittently, with the number of visits decreasing in frequency until the client is medically stable. Finally, hospice care requires expertise in managing terminal symptoms with active efforts to try alternative comforting approaches, in contrast to treating acute or chronic illnesses.

Hospice care focuses on the client and the family. According to the ANA (2002), hospice care emphasizes the following:

1. Assistance in dealing with emotional, spiritual, and medical problems
2. Support of the family
3. Keeping the client in his or her home for as long as feasible while making what remains of life as comfortable and meaningful as possible
4. Coordinated home care; inpatient, acute, and respite care; and bereavement services
5. Coordinated professional services and volunteer services appropriate to the individual client
6. Palliative care focusing on pain management

Eligibility for Hospice Care

Medicare Part A reimburses providers for hospice care. To be eligible for hospice benefits, clients must have life expectancy of 6 months or less, according to a physician's estimate, and they must not be undergoing or contemplating active treatment for their disease. In addition, they must have decided to forgo resuscitative measures at the time of death (Rice, 2006).

Caregiver Support

Caregiver support involves teaching about the course and progression of the disease and pain and symptom management. In addition, reassurance and provision of respite care or relief for the caregivers is very important. The hospice nurse can assist by referring the caregiver to providers of respite care or by instructing other family members or intermediate caregivers how to care for the client. Reassurance that the care is appropriate and that they are "doing the right thing" is emotionally beneficial. Common reactions seen in caregivers of the dying include grief, loneliness, isolation, feelings of uselessness or helplessness, anxiety, anger, depression, and fatigue. The hospice nurse can anticipate these and be prepared to intervene (Kemp, 1999).

Symptom Management

Control of symptoms is one of the primary goals in caring for hospice clients. Symptoms encountered can be the result of treatment and palliative measures taken (e.g., constipation from pain medications or nausea from radiation therapy) or the disease process and progression. Among the most frequently encountered problems are anorexia, weakness, fatigue, constipation, edema, urinary problems, dyspnea, skin problems, insomnia, dry mouth, dysphasia, coughing, and confusion and agitation (Rice, 2006). The nurse should anticipate these problems and take preventative measures whenever possible. Teaching the caregivers symptom prevention and/or management is essential.

Pain Management

According to Kemp (1999), pain is the most problematic and feared symptom in terminal care. Effective pain management includes accurate assessment of the pain and establishment of an effective individualized pain management plan. Thorough assessment of a client's pain should include information regarding each of the following elements:
- Location of the pain
- Extension or radiation
- Onset and pattern
- Duration
- Character or quality
- Precipitating, aggravating, or alleviating factors
- Intensity
- Associated symptoms
- Effect on activities of daily living
- Methods of pain relief

Often pain treatment is inadequate and inconsistent because of failure to routinely assess pain and pain relief; lack of knowledge among nurses and physicians of pain management; social or cultural fears; persistent myths (e.g., that pain is inevitable or use of opioids will result in loss of control or addiction); fear of respiratory depression; social or legal impediments to using opioids; communication problems among clients, caregivers, and professional staff; disease characteristics; and client characteristics (Kemp, 1999). To assist in development of a pain management plan, Box 11-3 contains basic principles for pain management.

Nurses who care for hospice clients should be very knowledgeable about pain management in general and about pharmacological management in particular. Utilization of appropriate drugs, dosages, and combinations requires experience and may require experimentation (e.g., some drugs or combinations of drugs or routes of administration work better for different clients or for different diagnoses). Hospice nurses must be well informed of the different types of pain medications and adjuvant medications and appropriate dosages and combinations. It is important to note that dosages and schedules may vary dramatically for terminally ill clients, and opioid doses may seem very high to nurses who do not routinely work with clients with severe pain. To assist in understanding the uses of different pain medications, Figure 11-2 presents the World Health Organization's three-step program to manage cancer pain.

Psychological and Spiritual Support of the Dying Client

Addressing the psychological and spiritual needs of the dying client can be extremely difficult for the nurse and the caregiver. Review of Kubler-Ross's

BOX 11-3 Principles of Effective Pain Management

- Use medications or techniques appropriate to the severity and specific type of pain.
- Give medications in amounts sufficient to control the pain and at intervals appropriate to the medication's duration of action.
- Use oral medications when possible.
- Give medications around the clock at regular intervals (prophylactically) to achieve a constant titer.
- Use adjuvant medications (e.g., nonsteroidal antiinflammatory drugs, corticosteroids, anticonvulsants, antidepressants, phenothiazines).

- Assess and treat side effects or complications.
- Anticipate side effects (e.g., constipation from narcotics, nausea).
- Assess for tolerance.
- Assess for and intervene in psychosocial and spiritual issues related to pain.
- Approach each patient as an individual and assess unique beliefs, strengths, and weaknesses.
- Teach the client and family principles of pain management.

From Kemp CE: *Terminal illness: a guide to nursing care*, ed 2, Philadelphia, 1999, J.B. Lippincott.

Figure 11-2. World Health Organization three-step analgesic ladder. Step 1: Nonopioid ± adjuvant. When pain persists or increases, proceed to Step 2. Step 2: Opioid for mild-to-moderate pain ± nonopioid ± adjuvant. When pain persists or increases, proceed to Step 3. Step 3: Opioid for moderate to severe pain ± nonopioid ± adjuvant. (Reproduced with permission from the World Health Organization: *Cancer pain relief*, ed 2, Geneva, 1996, World Health Organization.)

(1969) stages of death and dying (denial, anger, bargaining, depression, and acceptance) can be helpful. Recognition of these stages in the client and the family can assist in determining appropriate interventions. When observing a dying client, the nurse can expect feelings of loss and grief, loneliness, uselessness, anger, anxiety, fear, and depression.

Spiritual care involves understanding the client's spiritual beliefs and recognizing spiritual needs. Interventions can include listening to fears and concerns, exploring the client's understanding of the meaning of death, praying with the client if requested, reading aloud from the Bible or other appropriate religious literature if requested, expressing hope and comfort, and affirming the validity of spiritual concerns at the end of life. Referral to a minister, priest, rabbi, or other spiritual care provider may be respectfully offered .

Kemp (1999) describes personal qualities the nurse can demonstrate that are helpful in providing spiritual care at the end of life: realism (e.g., death is the end of a life on earth), hopefulness (i.e., includes hope of a better life in the present and in the future), truthfulness, faith, resourcefulness (i.e., ability to use the available resources), advocacy, sensitivity (e.g., acceptance of the client's uniqueness), and openness to the client's needs. Presence, or simply being near the client, can also be very comforting.

Interventions at Death

Infection, organ failure, lung or heart infarction, electrolyte imbalance, and hemorrhage are the most common causes of death in terminally ill clients (Kemp, 1999). Teaching the family what to expect as death nears and what to do following death are very important functions of the hospice nurse. Common signs of impending death include progressive anorexia, refusal of fluids, dreams and visions of persons who have died previously, withdrawal, changes in symptoms (e.g., increase or decrease in pain), respiratory symptoms (e.g., increasingly shallow and/or labored respirations, with periods of apnea, dyspnea, increased secretions), increased pulse rate, and changes in consciousness (e.g., drowsiness, unresponsiveness, confusion, agitation) (Kemp, 1999). The client's skin may become progressively cyanotic, cool, and mottled. The nurse should reassure the family that these signs are expected and manage them appropriately with comfort measures.

As death nears, families are instructed to call the primary hospice nurse or agency and not to call any emergency services. Depending on community or state requirements and agency policy, the nurse usually calls the physician, religious leader, funeral home, or others who have been identified in advance. Following the client's death, the nurse may bathe the client, remove all tubes and equipment, cover the body, and stay with the family until all arrangements have been made. It is appropriate for the nurse to cry or express grief with the family if he or she needs to do so. Frequently hospice nurses attend the client's wake, mass, funeral, or memorial service.

SUMMARY

Home health care is a dynamic, growing field for nursing practice that can be fun, autonomous, flexible, and very rewarding. Like Penny, the nurse in the opening case study, RNs who desire to work in home health care should be experienced and must be well trained and supported by agency management. A comprehensive orientation and ongoing assistance and supervisory support enhance the transition into home health practice and promote high quality nursing care.

As health care delivery continues to evolve and become increasingly community based, more and different types of care will be provided in the home. Emerging technology will allow for greater use of telecommunications, which in turn may dramatically change the types of care delivered in homes. Other factors, such as the aging of the population and the increasing numbers of clients with chronic diseases, will dictate an increased need for more home health agencies and providers. In particular, those that offer specialized care as described here will be in demand.

Because the knowledge base and information necessary for the practice of home health care nursing is vast, only a small portion has been discussed here; many issues and topics are beyond the scope of this book.

KEY POINTS

- Home health nursing integrates medical/surgical, community health, parent-child, gerontological, and psychiatric-mental health nursing into home health care practice. It refers to comprehensive nursing care provided to individuals and families in their place of residence, focusing on the environmental, psychosocial, economic, cultural, and personal health factors affecting health status.
- With the passage of Medicare in 1965, the practice of home health care nursing changed dramatically. Until recently home health care was largely provided by official (governmental or public) or voluntary (private, nonprofit) agencies. This has changed in the past decade, and the majority of home health agencies are now proprietary or hospital-based.

- Public sources (Medicare and Medicaid) finance about 70% of home health services. To be reimbursed by Medicare, home health agencies must be Medicare certified, follow Medicare's conditions of participation (explicit rules, standards, and requirements), and be certified by an accreditation organization.
- To qualify for coverage under Medicare, services must be "reasonable and necessary"; the client's care must require intermittent skilled nursing care, physical therapy, or speech therapy; the client must be homebound and under the care of a physician who develops a home health plan; and the agency must be certified to participate in Medicare.
- Thorough and accurate documentation is essential in home health nursing to record services, describe the client's condition and response to care, promote continuity of care, validate reimbursement claims, and forestall legal action. Completion of the required Medicare forms is necessary for payment.
- Home health care nursing requires unique skills and knowledge. Basic and essential activities include discharge planning (the process of determining the planning to meet client needs following release from a health care facility), case management (the process of ensuring that the services provided are appropriate for the client's needs), coordination of community resources, and interdisciplinary collaboration.
- Previsit planning involves determining which clients are to be seen and prioritization of the scheduled visits. Planning includes caseload scheduling, making contact by telephone or another method if necessary, review of the client's chart, assessment of supplies and equipment needed and what is on hand, and consideration of safety concerns.
- During the implementation stage, the scheduled plan of care is completed; it includes a comprehensive assessment, provision of skilled nursing care, health teaching as necessary, and other interventions. Following completion of the skilled nursing interventions and teaching, the nurse evaluates the response of the client to care, summarizes the continuing plan of care with the client and caregiver, and may set up a time for the next visit.

- Postvisit activities include communication of findings to other health care providers and completing requisite documentation.
- Home infusion therapy is a very significant component of home health care and includes delivery of antibiotics, pain medication, TPN, hydration, and chemotherapy.
- Home-based care of clients with chronic wounds is an important component of home health care. Nursing interventions in wound care typically include assessment of the wound and evaluation of the efficacy of treatment, cleaning and debridement, obtaining cultures, and teaching the client and/or caregiver how to change the dressing using sterile techniques.
- Enterostomal nurses are specialists in wound care and management, and they provide specialized care for clients with a colostomy, an ileostomy, or a urostomy.
- Home care of ventilator-dependent clients may be necessary for persons with severe chronic obstructive pulmonary disease or other chronic lung problems, spinal cord injuries, or other defects who have been discharged from acute care or long-term institutions into the home.
- Home care for pregnant and postpartum clients has increased dramatically during the past few years. Technologically advanced care for high-risk pregnancies (e.g., uterine monitoring, fetal monitoring, ultrasound, infusion pump treatment, and infusion therapy and hypertension monitoring) and care for neonates with complications (e.g., apnea monitoring) are becoming fairly routine. Postpartum care for uncomplicated clients following shortened hospital stays is also growing.
- Psychiatric home care is appropriate for individuals with diagnoses of suspected mental illnesses who need psychiatric services but cannot use traditional outpatient mental health services. Psychiatric home care can prevent hospitalization for clients with diagnoses such as severe depression, schizophrenia, and Alzheimer's disease.
- Hospice care provides palliative care to the terminally ill and is frequently provided in the home. Hospice care focuses on the family and the client and provides assistance in dealing with emotional, spiritual, and medical problems;

coordinates professional and volunteer services; and makes the client as comfortable as possible through pain and symptom management.

Learning Activities & Application to Practice
In Class
1. With classmates, practice conducting a home visit. One student can act as the client, one or two can act as caregivers, and one or two can act as the nurses. Practice each stage of the home visit and critique each other.
2. Talk with a nurse who routinely works in one of the specialized home health care areas examined in the chapter. Encourage the nurse to describe the types of clients seen, sources of reimbursement, changes in home health care in recent years, and anticipated changes. What professional experience is necessary for this type of practice? What strategies must be used to assist in teaching caregivers to provide the necessary care?
3. Box 11-4 lists a sample daily caseload for a home health nurse. Study the caseload and set a tentative schedule for ordering the visits. You will need to anticipate the amount of time needed for each visit and allow time for travel. Discuss the schedule with classmates.

In Clinical
4. Work with a practicing home health care nurse for a minimum of 6 days. Keep a log or a diary recording the types of clients seen. What skilled nursing interventions were performed? What practical experiences and skills are helpful for nurses considering home health practice? Describe the process of documentation.
5. In a log or diary, list the activities that were accomplished for one home visit within the three stages of a home visit described. Outline what preparations were made during the planning stage, what skilled nursing interventions and teaching were provided during the implementation stage, and describe postvisit activities. If possible, include the rationale chosen for scheduling of the caseload (i.e., what factors were considered in ordering the schedule?).
6. Work with a home health nurse who provides "specialty" care as described in this chapter.

BOX 11-4 Sample Home Health Nursing Daily Caseload

Mrs. E. Cooper: Map Coordinates, 37G; Admit Visit; dx—CHF, HTN

Assess: VS, C/P status, weight, edema—lower extremities, nutrition status, medication compliance
Teaching: HTN, low-Na diet, medication regimen
Special considerations: Daughter to be in the home 09:00-12:00—requests SNV when she is present

Mr. C. McClure: Map Coordinates, 38D; Return Visit; dx—postCVA (Anticoagulant Therapy)

Assess: VS, C/P status, neuro status, weight, nutrition status, medication compliance
Teaching: Anticoagulant therapy (s/sx of complications, medication regimen, safety)
Special considerations: Lab draw—protime—specimen to lab within 30 minutes; call MD with results before 14:00.

Mr. T. Johnson: Map coordinates, 23A; Return Visit; dx—Diabetes

Assess: VS, C/P status, weight, nutrition/diet, blood sugar (fasting), medication compliance
Teaching: IDDM (review materials left in home), observe DFS and self-administration of insulin, ADA diet

Special considerations: Requests SNV around 7:30 to allow breakfast by 8:30

Mrs. M. Charles: Map Coordinates, 38M; Return Visit; dx—Wound Right Foot—BID Dressing Changes (Early a.m. and Late Afternoon)

Assess: VS, C/P status, neuro status, nutrition status, medication compliance, wound—right foot
Wound care: Location—right foot; wet-to-dry dressing—cleanse with NS, pack with 2 4 × 4s and secure with 4" gauze
Teaching: s/sx of infection, safety
Special considerations: Pt had 99.8 temp yesterday—MD notified—requests to be called following visit regardless of findings; needs 1 week supply of gauze, NS, sterile gloves, and 4 × 4s

Mrs. G. Grace: Map Coordinates, 36A; Return Visit; dx—Urinary Incontinence—Indwelling Catheter

Assess: VS, C/P status, elimination status, neuro status, nutrition status, skin integrity
Teaching: s/sx of infection, monitoring fluid intake, catheter care
Special considerations: c/g reports catheter leaking—requests change

ADA, American Diabetes Association; *BID,* twice a day; *c/g,* caregiver; *CHF,* congestive heart failure; *C/P,* cardiopulmonary; *CVA,* cerebrovascular accident; *DFS,* diabetic finger stick; *dx,* diagnosis; *HTN,* hypertension; *IDDM,* insulin-dependent diabetes mellitus; *lab,* laboratory; *MD,* physician; *Na,* sodium; *neuro,* neurological; *NS,* normal saline; *pt,* patient; *s/sx,* signs and symptoms; *SNV,* skilled nursing visit; *VS,* vital signs.

REFERENCES

Adams SC, Rice R: The patient receiving home infusion therapies. In Rice R, editor: *Home care nursing practice: concepts & application,* ed 4, St Louis, 2006, Mosby.

American Nurses Association: *Standards for hospice nursing practice,* Kansas City, Mo, 2002, American Nurses Association.

American Nurses Association: *The scope and standards of home health nursing practice,* Washington, DC, 2007, American Nurses Association.

Carson VB: The journey through home mental health care. In Carson VB, Arnold EN, editors: *Mental health nursing: the nurse-patient journey,* Philadelphia, 1996, Saunders.

Center for Medicare and Medicaid Services: *National health expenditure projections 2006-2016* (website): http://www.cms.hhs.gov/NationalHealthExpendData/downloads/proj2006.pdf. Accessed September 4, 2007.

Center for Medicare and Medicaid Services: *Medicare and home health care* (website): http://www.medicare.gov/Publications/Pubs/pdf/10969.pdf. Accessed September 13, 2007.

Clark MJ: *Community Health Nursing: advocacy for population health,* ed 5, Upper Saddle River, NJ, 2008, Prentice Hall.

Dahlberg NLF, Blazek D, Wikoff B et al: High-tech, high-touch perinatal home care, *Caring* May:36-39, 1995.

Dasing L, Ryberg J, Keller T: Maternal-child nursing: postpartum home care. In Rice R, editor: *Home health nursing: concepts and application,* ed 4, St Louis, 2006, Mosby.

Dittbrenner H: Psychiatric home care: an overview, *Caring* June:26-30, 1994.

Gilkison JR, Neathery MB: Mental health in the home and community. In Antia-Otong D, editor: *Psychiatric nursing: biological and behavioral concepts,* Philadelphia, 1995, Saunders.

Freed PE: The mental health patient. In Rice R, editor: *Home care nursing practice: concepts and application,* ed 4, St Louis, 2006, Mosby.

Humphrey CJ, Milone-Nuzzo P: *Home care nursing: an orientation to practice,* Norwalk, Conn, 1991, Appleton & Lange.

Kemp CE: *Terminal illness: a guide to nursing care,* ed 2, Philadelphia, 1999, J.B. Lippincott.

Kubler-Ross E: *On death and dying,* New York, 1969, Macmillan.

Lima B: In-home psychiatric nursing: the at-home mental health program, *Caring* July:14-20, 1995.

Matassarin-Jacobs E: Pain assessment and intervention. In Black JM, Matassarin-Jacobs E, editors: *Luckmann and Sorensen's medical-surgical nursing: a psychophysiologic approach,* ed 4, Philadelphia, 1993, Saunders.

Milone-Nuzzo P: Home health care. In Maurer FA, Smith CM, editors: *Community/public health nursing practice: health for families and populations,* ed 3, St Louis, 2005, Saunders.

National Association for Home Care: *Basic statistics about home care,* Washington, DC, 2007, National Association for Home Care and Hospice. http://www.nahc.org/facts/07HC_Stats.pdf. Accessed March 23, 200.

Nichols G, Rice R: The hospice patient. In Rice R., editor: *Home health nursing: concepts and application*, ed 3, St Louis, 2001, Mosby.

Rice R: *Manual of home health nursing practice*, ed 2, St Louis, 2000, Mosby.

Rice R: The ventilator-dependent patient. In Rice R, editor: *Home health nursing practice: concepts & application*, ed 3, St Louis, 2001, Mosby.

Rice R: Home care nursing practice: historical perspectives and philosophy of care. In Rice R, editor: *Home care nursing practice: concepts & application*, ed 4, St Louis, 2006, Mosby.

Rice R, Wiersema-Bryant L, Bangert JB: The patient with chronic wounds. In Rice R, editor: *Home care nursing practice: concepts & application*, ed 4, St Louis, 2006, Mosby.

Smith CM: The home visit: opening the doors. In Maurer FA, Smith CM, editors: *Community/public health nursing practice: health for families and populations*, ed 3, St Louis, 2005, Saunders.

U.S. Department of Health and Human Services, Division of Nursing, Bureau of Health Professions: *The registered nurse population: findings for the national sample survey of registered nurses, March, 2004*, Washington, DC, 2006, Government Printing Office (online): ftp://ftp.hrsa.gov/bhpr/workforce/0306rnss.pdf. Accessed August 31, 2007.

Wallace DC: Clients with long-term care needs. In Clemen-Stone S, McGuire SL, Eigsti DG, editors: *Comprehensive community health nursing*, ed 6, St Louis, 2002, Mosby.

Warhola C: *Planning for home health services: a resource handbook* (DHHS Publication No. [HRA] 80-14017), Washington, DC, 1980, U.S. Department of Health and Human Services.

World Health Organization: *Cancer pain relief*, ed 2, Geneva, 1996, World Health Organization.

Four

Community-Based Nursing Care Across the Life Span

Health Promotion and Illness Prevention for Infants, Children, and Adolescents

objectives

Upon completion of this chapter, the reader will be able to:

1. Discuss the leading causes of morbidity and mortality for infants, small children, school-aged children, and adolescents.

2. Identify federal- and state-sponsored health programs and services for children, and explain eligibility requirements and referral processes.

3. Describe recommendations for screening and education for major causes of morbidity and mortality for infants, children, and adolescents.

4. Describe health promotion interventions for infants, children, and adolescents, including nutrition, physical activities, sleep and rest, dental health, and maturation and puberty.

5. Describe prevention interventions for infants, children, and adolescents, focusing on prevention of substance abuse, use of tobacco, and safety issues.

6. Discuss detection, prevention, and management of child abuse.

key terms

Anemia screening
Body Mass Index (BMI)
Bottle mouth syndrome
Child abuse
Child safety
Developmental screening

Early and Periodic Screening, Diagnosis, and Treatment (EPSDT) program
Head Start
Hearing screening
Newborn screenings

State Children's Health Insurance Program (SCHIP)
Vision screening
Women, Infants, and Children (WIC)

See Glossary for definitions.

case study

Bonnie Dalton is a registered nurse working in a private pediatric office in a small city. In her position, Bonnie assists the pediatrician and pediatric nurse practitioner (PNP) by taking health histories, weighing and measuring the children, performing health teaching for the children and parents, administering medications, and assisting with some diagnostic and screening procedures (e.g., strep cultures, fingersticks), and performing many other interventions.

Continued

Last Monday Bonnie saw Sally Benson for her 6-month wellness checkup. Sally was brought to the clinic by her mother. Bonnie observed that Sally was appropriately dressed, smiling, and responsive. Bonnie asked Mrs. Benson to remove Sally's clothes. While this was being completed, Bonnie asked her about Sally's eating and sleeping patterns and general health. She learned that Sally is breastfed and nurses six to eight times per day. Currently she is being given only supplemental apple juice and an occasional bottle of formula when Mrs. Benson leaves her with a babysitter. Sally sleeps 10 to 11 hours at night, occasionally waking, and naps twice daily for 1 to 2 hours.

Bonnie weighed and measured Sally and plotted the findings on a graphic chart kept in Sally's file. She noted that Sally weighed 17 pounds and measured 27 inches—a gain of 3 pounds and an increase of 1.5 inches since her 4-month visit. According to the chart, Sally's height and weight placed her within the seventy-fifth percentile for girls of her age.

When questioned, Mrs. Benson reported that Sally always rode in her car seat; outlet plugs were on all electrical outlets; and harmful substances and medications were in childproof, latched cabinets. Other safety issues discussed included smoke detectors near the bedrooms and hot water heater temperature.

Bonnie assisted the PNP with a head-to-toe physical examination and Denver II Screening Test. All findings from both the physical and developmental examinations were considered normal for Sally's age.

The PNP instructed Mrs. Benson on how to gradually introduce solid foods to Sally's diet, and Bonnie gave her several pamphlets and instruction guides kept in the clinic. The nurses also discussed several other safety issues, including poison control. Mrs. Benson was counseled to buy syrup of ipecac and to keep the phone number of the local poison control center near her telephone.

Routine neonatal screening tests (phenylketonuria, thyroid function, hemoglobin) had been performed shortly after Sally was born, and all results were normal. She was up to date on her immunizations and was scheduled to get her third vaccinations for pneumococcal infections, hepatitis B, diphtheria/tetanus/pertussis, polio, and *Haemophilus influenzae* B. Mrs. Benson reported that the only problem from previous immunizations was a slight fever during the afternoon and evening of the injections, which responded to administration of acetaminophen. Mrs. Benson was counseled again concerning possible side effects of immunizations and how to manage them.

Bonnie gave Sally the immunizations. Sally cried a little but was consoled by her mother and stopped crying quickly. Mrs. Benson was encouraged to give Sally acetaminophen and to call the office if she developed a temperature higher than 103°F or was crying inconsolably. Finally, Mrs. Benson was instructed to bring Sally back for her next wellness checkup when she was 12 to 15 months old.

THE HEALTH OF INFANTS, CHILDREN, AND ADOLESCENTS

Preventive health care for infants and children has had a profound effect on morbidity and mortality. In 1900 87% of infants lived to age 1 year, and only 77% survived to age 20 years. In comparison, in 2005 99.3% of infants survived until their first birthdays and 98.6% could expect to live to age 20 (National Center for Health Statistics [NCHS], 2007a). This increase has been attributed to several factors. Improved prenatal and intrapartum care has reduced infant mortality dramatically. Infant mortality declined from approximately 165 per 1000 births in 1900 to 47 per 1000 in 1940 to 29.2 per 1000 in 1950 to 6.8 per 1000 in 2004 (Kovner and Knickman, 2005; NCHS, 2004). In addition, clean water, improved quality and quantity of food, and immunization against communicable diseases have contributed dramatically to infants and children reaching adulthood.

CAUSES OF MORTALITY

As discussed in previous chapters, the overall leading causes of death among adults in the United States are heart disease, cancer, and stroke. However, these statistics are much different for infants, children, and adolescents, as is shown in Table 12-1. Indeed, for infants, congenital anomalies are the leading cause of death, and problems related to birth constitute the four leading causes of infant mortality. This trend

TABLE **12-1** Leading Causes of Death and Percentages for Infants, Children, and Adolescents (2004)

INFANTS (LESS THAN 1 YR)	CHILDREN (1-4 YR)	CHILDREN (5-14 YR)	ADOLESCENTS AND YOUNG ADULTS (15-24 YR)
Congenital anomalies (20.1%)	Accidents (34.3%)	Accidents (39.0%)	Accidents (46.2%)
Short gestation and low birth weight (16.6%)	Congenital anomalies (11.9%)	Cancer (14.9%)	Homicide (15.2%)
SIDS and respiratory distress syndrome (8.0%)	Cancer (8.3%)	Congenital anomalies (5.7%)	Suicide (12.9%)
Perinatal complications (6.1%)	Homicide (7.9%)	Homicide (4.8%)	Cancer (5.1%)

SIDS, Sudden infant death syndrome.
From the National Center for Health Statistics: *Health United States, 2006* (website): http://www.cdc.gov/nchs/hus.htm. Accessed October 23, 2007.

changes dramatically after the first year of life, with accidents claiming the most lives of children and adolescents. Strikingly, homicide and cancer rank high as causes of child and adolescent mortality, and congenital anomalies still contribute to many deaths.

CAUSES OF MORBIDITY

The leading causes of acute illness in children are respiratory conditions (i.e., colds, influenza, acute respiratory infections), other infective and parasitic diseases (e.g., viral infections, intestinal parasites), acute ear infections, and injuries. The most common chronic complaints in children are respiratory conditions (e.g., asthma, allergic rhinitis, chronic sinusitis, chronic bronchitis) and skin conditions (e.g., chronic dermatitis and acne). Musculoskeletal conditions (e.g., club foot, hip dysplasia, scoliosis) and vision, speech, and hearing impairments are identified in many children (NCHS, 2006).

Respiratory conditions contribute to the most time lost from school, accounting for more than 50% of days absent. Common childhood diseases (e.g., viral infections) are responsible for almost 22% of school absences. Other common acute complaints that cause school absenteeism include ear infections, injuries (e.g., fractures, sprains), and digestive complaints (e.g., nausea, vomiting).

Children younger than 1 year of age see physicians more often than any other age group younger than 65. From birth to age 1, infants average 6.7 physician contacts each year. In contrast, children and adolescents 5 to 14 years of age have 1.9 physician

office visits per year (NCHS, 2006). Major reasons for hospitalization of children include respiratory conditions (e.g., asthma, bronchitis, pneumonia), injury and poisoning, digestive disorders (e.g., gastroenteritis, diarrhea), infectious and parasitic diseases, mental disorders, chemotherapy, and unspecified viral illnesses (AHRQ, 2004).

OTHER INDICATORS OF HEALTH

To prevent, detect, and minimize disease, disability, and death in infants and children, a number of indicators of health and well-being should be assessed, and appropriate interventions should be developed and implemented when problems or potential problems are identified. Health indicators to be assessed should include growth and development, vision, and hearing. General strategies for health promotion (e.g., good nutrition, exercise and fitness, dental care) should be taught and encouraged. Finally, identified threats or risk factors, such as threats to safety or substance use (e.g., tobacco, alcohol, drugs), must be addressed.

A number of *Healthy People 2010* (USDHHS, 2000) objectives specifically target health-promotion and risk-reduction strategies for infants, children, and adolescents. The *Healthy People 2010* box lists some of these objectives. This chapter describes recommendations for primary health care, health promotion, and illness prevention activities and interventions appropriate for nurses caring for infants, children, and adolescents in community-based settings. Identification and management of common

healthy people 2010

Examples of Health-Promotion Objectives for Children and Adolescents

OBJECTIVE	BASELINE (1998)	TARGET
1.4b: Increase the proportion of children and youth aged 17 years and under who have a specific source of ongoing care	93%	96%
8.11: Eliminate elevated blood levels in children	4.5% of children aged 1 to 5 years	0%
9.7: Reduce pregnancies among adolescent females	72 per 1000 females aged 15 to 17 years	46 per 1000 females aged 15 to 17 years
14.4: Reduce bacterial meningitis in young children	13.0 per 100,000	8.6 per 100,000
15.20: Increase use of child restraints	92%	100%
16.1a: Reduce fetal and infant deaths during the perinatal period (i.e., 28 weeks of gestation to 7 days or more after birth)	7.5 per 1000	4.5 per 1000
16.15: Reduce the occurrence of spina bifida and other NTDs	6 per 10,000 live births	3 per 10,000 live births
18.2: Reduce the rate of suicide attempts by adolescents	2.6% per year	1% per year
19.3a: Reduce the proportion of children aged 6 to 11 years who are overweight or obese	11%	5%
24.2a: Reduce hospitalizations for asthma in children under age 5 years	60.9 per 10,000	25 per 10,000
27.2a: Reduce tobacco use by adolescents in grades 9 to 12	43%	21%

NTDs, Neural tube defects.
Data from U.S. Department of Health and Human Services: *Healthy people 2010*: conference ed, Washington, DC, 2000, Government Printing Office.

acute and chronic illness and conditions are also described.

SPECIAL HEALTH PROGRAMS AND SERVICES FOR CHILDREN

To meet the health care needs of disadvantaged, underserved, and disabled children, a number of federally sponsored programs have been developed over the past three decades. Nurses who practice in community settings, particularly those who care for underserved children, should be aware of services provided by these programs,

have an understanding of eligibility requirements, and know how to refer clients. Several of the most commonly encountered programs and services are briefly discussed in the following sections.

MEDICAID AND THE EARLY AND PERIODIC SCREENING, DIAGNOSIS, AND TREATMENT PROGRAM

Children are overrepresented among those with no health insurance or those covered by public insurance (e.g., Medicaid). Indeed, health care is financed by public sources for 26% of all persons 18 years and younger, and almost 27% of Medicaid dollars cover children. An additional 12% of all children have no health care insurance (Feldstein, 2003; HRSA/MCHB, 2003).

Most children without health insurance are the dependents of full-time workers whose employers provide no health insurance. Lack of health insurance has a significant effect on children's health because they are less likely to have a usual source of care, and their parents resort to the use of emergency rooms, hospital outpatient departments, or school health centers to substitute for a primary health care provider. As a result, children without health insurance are much less likely to receive preventive health care and are more likely to receive health care after illnesses are advanced and care is more expensive.

Medicaid is a welfare-assistance health program jointly sponsored by the federal government and each state. Children with Medicaid coverage are nearly as likely as children with private health insurance to have a usual source of care. This is very important for primary prevention, health education, and early identification and treatment of medical or developmental problems.

The Early and Periodic Screening, Diagnosis, and Treatment (EPSDT) program began in 1967 to identify and treat children's health problems before they became complex and costly. The EPSDT has evolved into a comprehensive preventive health care program for Medicaid-eligible individuals up to age 21 (HRSA, 2007). The program's services may be provided by a public health clinic, community health center, school health program, Head Start program, qualified independent practitioners, and others. Under federal guidelines, all eligible children and their families must be informed about EPSDT services and where to obtain them. Assistance with scheduling and transportation and assistance in using health resources effectively are components of EPSDT.

STATE CHILDREN'S HEALTH INSURANCE PROGRAM

The **State Children's Health Insurance Program (SCHIP)** was created in 1997 as part of the Balanced Budget Act of 1997 to provide health insurance coverage for uninsured children. Most children covered by SCHIP are from working families with incomes too high to qualify for Medicaid but too low to afford private health insurance. Like Medicaid, SCHIP is a partnership between the federal and state governments. Most states provide SCHIP coverage for children of families at or above 200% of the poverty level.

States have flexibility in organization of each SCHIP, which may be an expansion of the existing Medicaid program or a separate entity. Mandated covered services include inpatient and outpatient hospital care, physician's surgical and medical care, laboratory and x-ray services, and well baby/child care, including immunizations. Other components that may be offered include prescription drugs, mental health services, vision care, and hearing-related care (CMS, 2007).

WOMEN, INFANTS, AND CHILDREN PROGRAM

The Special Supplemental Nutrition Program for **Women, Infants, and Children (WIC)** provides food, nutrition counseling, and access to health services for low-income women, infants, and children. The WIC program is a federally funded program established in 1972 that is administered by each state. Pregnant or postpartum women, infants, and children up to age 5 who meet income guidelines and residency requirements and who are considered to be at nutritional risk are eligible. All persons receiving Aid to Families with Dependent Children, food stamps, or Medicaid are automatically eligible.

Most WIC programs provide vouchers that participants use at authorized stores to purchase nutritious foods. The foods included are high in protein, calcium, iron, and vitamins A and C. Typical WIC foods include iron-fortified infant formula and infant cereal, iron-fortified adult cereal, vitamin C-rich fruit or vegetable juice, eggs, milk, cheese, peanut butter, and dried beans. Special infant formulas are provided if prescribed. Participation in WIC has been shown to be effective in increasing gestation periods, raising birth weights, and reducing infant mortality. An estimated 2 million babies born in the United States are served by WIC (U.S. Department of Agriculture/Food and Consumer Service, 2006).

HEAD START

Head Start is a federally funded, comprehensive preschool program for children who are at risk for academic problems associated with poverty and lack of sufficient social stimulation. Head Start was begun in 1965 to incorporate health, nutrition, parent involvement, and children's learning into a comprehensive program for the disadvantaged. Low-income children 3 to 5 years of age are eligible for Head Start programs. Although programs vary by area, health care is often a component of Head Start programs.

EDUCATION FOR ALL HANDICAPPED CHILDREN ACT

In response to a lack of services for handicapped children, the Education for All Handicapped Children Act (Public Law [PL] 94-142) was passed in 1975. The PL 94-142 is important and encompassing because it mandates a free public education in the least restrictive environment for all handicapped children. In essence, this law requires public school districts to provide an educational environment that can meet the demands of any child with a disability, including children with physical impairments, learning disabilities, and mental and emotional disabilities.

To encourage early intervention, a 1986 amendment to PL 99-457 extended coverage for handicapped children from birth until age 21 years. These Acts, PL 94-142 and PL 99-457, are now known collectively as the *Individuals with Disabilities Education Act*. Services mandated by the Individuals with Disabilities Education Act include necessary physical or occupational therapy, speech therapy, transportation to and from school, and counseling or psychiatric services. Periodic health or medical procedures (e.g., intermittent catheterization, tube feeding, tracheostomy suctioning) may be provided in some areas. "Mainstreaming" or normalization (integration of special needs children with other children of the same age in a regular classroom) is encouraged whenever possible (Pourciau and Vallette, 2007).

PRIMARY HEALTH CARE RECOMMENDATIONS: U.S. PREVENTIVE SERVICES TASK FORCE

The U.S. Preventive Services Task Force (Agency for Healthcare Research and Quality [AHRQ], 2007) has developed guidelines to direct health care services for health promotion and illness prevention for individuals in all age groups. These recommendations include frequency of visits, screenings that should be performed (e.g., history, physical examination, laboratory or diagnostic procedures), appropriate parent or client counseling and health teaching, immunization recommendations, and specific guidelines for individuals in high-risk categories. Examples of specific assessment tools, health teaching information, and provider guidelines that address the specific recommendations are included throughout this chapter.

SCREENING RECOMMENDATIONS AND GUIDELINES

Various Federal and State Agencies, as well as private organizations, have published recommendations for screening for a number of genetic, congenital, developmental, maturational, and pathological problems and conditions. Guidelines and examples of tools and teaching tips are described briefly.

Newborn Screenings

Although there is considerable variation between states, all states require that all newborns be tested for congenital diseases. Testing for hypothyroidism and phenylketonuria, for example, is required by all states, and screening for galactosemia and hemoglobinopathies (e.g., sickle cell disease, thalassemia) is required by a majority of states. In addition, many states require newborn screening for maple syrup urine disease, congenital adrenal hyperplasia, cystic fibrosis, and other conditions. Recently a task force reviewed newborn screening practices and identified 29 specific conditions for which screening should be mandated (including the conditions mentioned above, as well as numerous others) and determined that reporting procedures should be standardized across states (HRSA/MCHB, 2005). Nurses who care for newborns in community settings must know the newborn screenings required by their state so they can offer effective preventive care for their clients.

Newborn screenings are usually accomplished by collecting drops of blood onto specially designed filter paper. An amount of blood sufficient to conduct testing must be placed on a specific area of the filter paper. This procedure can be difficult to accomplish and requires substantial practice to gain proficiency. The blood spot specimens should be obtained from every neonate before discharge or transfer from the hospital nursery or birthing suite, regardless of the status of the infant's feeding or age. For full-term well infants, the specimen should be obtained as close as possible to discharge and no later than 7 days of age. If the initial specimen is obtained earlier than 24 hours after birth, a second specimen should be obtained at 1 to 2 weeks of age. Premature infants, infants receiving parenteral feeding, and infants receiving treatment for illness should have a specimen obtained for screening at or near the seventh day of life (if it has not been done before that time), regardless of feeding status.

Nurses who work in community settings such as pediatric clinics and health maintenance organizations are frequently in a position to perform repeat testing, follow up on positive or inconclusive results, and offer referal and support services as needed. They may also be in a position to identify those at risk for not being screened (e.g., premature infants, infants undergoing adoption, infants born at home, children of homeless families, infants born outside the United States) (USDHHS/ODPHP, 1998).

All abnormal results from infant screening tests require confirmatory testing and a thorough physical examination. Counseling should be provided to all parents of children with abnormal results and should include information about the significance of the results, the need for retesting, implications for the child's health, treatment, associated symptoms and complications to watch for, and genetic counseling for future childbearing.

Body Measurement

Significant childhood conditions, such as growth retardation, malnutrition, eating disorders, and obesity, may be identified by regularly scheduled measurement of height and weight throughout infancy and childhood. In addition, head circumference should be measured at birth; at 2 to 4 weeks; and at 1, 2, 4, 6, 9, 12, 15, 18, and 24 months of age to identify potential abnormalities (e.g., hydrocephalus). General guidelines for body measurement are described here.

HEIGHT. For children younger than 2 years, height should be obtained by measuring recumbent length. A measuring board with a stationary headboard and sliding vertical foot piece can be used. If one is not available, a stationary vertical surface (e.g., the wall bordering the examining table) and a yardstick or tape measure may be used. In general the infant or child should lie flat against the center of the board, with the head held against the headboard and the legs extended. The foot piece, tape measure, or yardstick is positioned to the child's heels, and the height should be read to the nearest one-eighth inch.

For children 2 years and older, standing height is measured with a stadiometer or a graduated ruler or tape attached to a wall, with a flat surface placed horizontally on top of the head. The child should wear only socks or be barefoot, with the knees straight and feet flat on the floor. While the child looks straight ahead, the flat surface or moveable headboard should be placed on the top of the head, compressing the hair, and the height read and recorded. If height-measuring devices attached to weight scales are used, they should be checked frequently for accuracy.

WEIGHT. To improve accuracy, a balance beam or electronic scale should be used to obtain weights. The scale should be checked to ensure that it reads "0" before each use and should be checked periodically. Infants and small children should be weighed wearing only a dry diaper or light underpants. If possible the same scale should be used for each measurement.

HEAD CIRCUMFERENCE. The circumference of the head should be measured by extending a measuring tape around the most prominent part of the occiput to the middle of the forehead and lightly tightening to compress the hair. Head circumference is usually read to the nearest quarter inch or centimeter. A plastic or disposable paper tape is preferable to a cloth tape because the latter may stretch.

GENERAL   INSTRUCTIONS. All   measurements should be plotted on age- and gender-specific growth charts for comparison with reference standards. The CDC provides growth charts for comparisons with the National Health and Nutrition Examination Survey (NHANES) reference values. Recording serial measurements over time is recommended to detail an accurate growth record. Further, measurements should be interpreted within the context of the individual child's family and growth history (Figure 12-1). The child's **Body Mass Index (BMI)** should be calculated from the height and weight data at each visit. The BMI is a

Figure 12-1. These children of identical age (8 years) are markedly different in size. The child on the left, of Asian descent, is at the fifth percentile for height and weight. The child on the right is above the ninety-fifth percentile for height and weight. However, both children demonstrate normal growth patterns. (From Wong D: *Whaley & Wong's nursing care of infants and children*, ed 7, St Louis, 2007, Mosby.)

reliable indicator of body fat and correlates well with direct measures of body fat, such as underwater weighing. The BMI number should be plotted on a BMI growth chart appropriate for the child's age and gender. Plotting the child's BMI on a chart allows for comparision of the child's BMI to the BMI of children of the same age and gender from the NHANES reference group. Table 12-2 details the percentile ranges for childhood BMI, indicating which BMIs would be considered underweight, healthy weight, "at risk," and overweight.

If a child's measurements fall below the 5th percentile or above the 85th percentile, the clinician should assess past growth patterns and genetic and environmental factors to determine if follow-up is necessary (see Table 12-2). The rate of overweight among children has quadrupled in the past 10 years, leading to great concern about the future health of many children (CDC, 2006). Special growth charts are available for infants born prematurely.

Developmental Screening

Developmental screening is monitoring the progression of infants, children, and adolescents through evaluation of developmental tasks. It is a crucial component of comprehensive health care. Assessment of developmental level can be accomplished by using screening tools, a thorough history, physical assessment, and/or directed observation. To help nurses recognize appropriate developmental tasks, Table 12-3 outlines some common physical, psychosocial, and cognitive developmental tasks.

The Denver II is a revision of the classic tool, the Denver Developmental Screening Test. The Denver II is a screening tool used to assess the overall developmental status of children from birth to age 6 and to alert the health care professional to potential developmental difficulties. Areas covered in the Denver II are personal-social tasks (e.g., getting along with people and caring for personal needs), fine motor-adaptive tasks (e.g., hand-eye coordination, manipulation of small objects), language (e.g., hearing, understanding, using language), and gross motor abilities (e.g., sitting, walking, jumping) (Frankenburg and Dodds, 1990). All persons using this test are urged to participate in a training program to learn to administer and interpret the test correctly. Additional information can be obtained from the Denver Developmental Materials website (http://www.denverii.com/).

TABLE **12-2** BMI Weight Categories

WEIGHT STATUS CATEGORY	PERCENTILE RANGE
Underweight	Less than the 5th percentile
Healthy weight	5th percentile to less than the 85th percentile
At risk of overweight	85th to less than the 95th percentile
Overweight	Equal to or greater than the 95th percentile

TABLE **12-3** Developmental Tasks for Infants and Children (Includes Physical, Psychosocial, and Cognitive)

AGE	TASK
INFANCY	
3 mo	Experiences decrease in primitive reflexes, except protective and postural reflexes Develops social smile (indicates development of memory traces)
4 mo	Laughs
5 mo	Birth weight doubles When prone, can push up on arms Rolls over
6 mo	Begins teething Sits with support Exhibits "stranger anxiety" (is wary of strangers and clings to mother)
8 mo	Sits alone Crawls
9 mo	Can use pincer grasp Holds own bottle
10 mo	Stands with support
12 mo	Birth weight triples Takes first steps alone Develops trust Speaks five words Claps hands; waves "bye-bye"
TODDLERHOOD	
13 mo-2.5 yr	Masters walking Climbs stairs Feeds self (autonomy) Uses language (increases to 400 words and two- to three-word phrases) Masters toilet training/bowel and bladder control Has separation anxiety (screams when the mother leaves)
PRESCHOOL	
2.5-4 yr	Increases vocabulary; uses sentences Alternates feet on steps Copies circles and lines Builds a tower of blocks Begins to have concepts of causality, time, and numbers Develops body image Role plays Begins enculturation Begins development of conscience Has fears of loss of body integrity

Continued

TABLE **12-3** Developmental Tasks for Infants and Children (Includes Physical, Psychosocial, and Cognitive)—cont'd

AGE	TASK
SCHOOL AGE	
5-12 yr	Vision matures by age 6 yr
	Loses first baby tooth at age 6 yr; gets all permanent teeth except final molars by age 12 yr
	Develops peer relationships
	Enjoys activities/groups/teams
	Develops morality
	Has cognitive development: concepts of time/space, reversibility, conservation, parts/whole
	Can classify objects in more than one way
	Develops reading/spelling and math concepts
	Begins puberty: age 9 yr for girls; age 11 yr for boys
	Gains sense of industry
ADOLESCENCE	
13-19 yr+	Develops secondary sex characteristics
	Attains adult growth
	Adjusts to body changes
	Begins menses (girls)
	Develops abstract thought
	Develops an identity
	Fantasizes role in different situations
	Has increased heterosexual interests
	Has increased peer influences

From Selekman J: *Pediatric nursing*, Springhouse, Pa, 1993, Springhouse.

Vision Screening

Vision screening is used to assess children for problems with sight. Refractive errors (myopia, hyperopia, astigmatism) are the most common vision disorders in children, occurring in about 5% to 10% of children. Other visual disorders (affecting 2% to 5% of all children) include amblyopia (lazy eye), strabismus (ocular misalignment; cross eyes), and anisometropia (difference between the two eyes in nearsightedness, farsightedness, and astigmatism). These conditions typically develop between infancy and 5 to 7 years of age. Congenital cataracts, congenital glaucoma, retinoblastoma, and retinopathy of prematurity are other less commonly observed eye conditions occurring in infancy and childhood (USDHHS/ODPHP, 1998).

Normal vision is important for development, and failure to treat amblyopia, anisometropia, and strabismus before school age may result in irreversible visual deficits, permanent amblyopia, loss of depth perception and binocularity, cosmetic defects, and

educational and occupational restrictions. There are several reliable methods for screening children of all ages and developmental levels. Nurses working in schools, public health clinics, and specialized pediatric practices are encouraged to attend training classes to learn how to use screening equipment to properly screen children. Indicators of possible visual impairment are:

- holding objects very close to the face
- covering one eye or tilting the head
- squinting
- complaints of difficulty seeing
- difficulties with school work
- headaches

Early detection and treatment of vision disorders is essential for normal eye development. A careful history, thorough examination, vision testing, and referral of abnormal or asymmetrical results for further testing and treatment promote normal vision development. Guidelines for vision screening in children are available at http://www.aafp.org/afp/980901ap/broderic.html.

Hearing Screening

Hearing impairment affects all aspects of an individual's life, including developmental, educational, cognitive, emotional, and social components, so **hearing screening** is an essential component of a child's health assessment. An estimated 1% to 2% of children in the United States have some degree of hearing impairment. Hearing loss may be congenital or acquired during infancy or childhood. Temporary hearing loss associated with otitis media is fairly common among school-aged children, occurring in 5% to 7% of all children (USDHHS/ODPHP, 1998).

Infants at greatest risk for hearing loss include those with low birth weight, congenital infection (e.g., rubella, toxoplasmosis, syphilis, cytomegalovirus, herpes), craniofacial anomalies, hyperbilirubinemia requiring exchange transfusion, Apgar scores of 0 to 3 at 5 minutes, mechanical ventilation for cardiopulmonary disease for 2 days or more, and neonatal intracranial hemorrhage, prematurity, and hospitalization in the intensive care nursery. Indicators and risk factors for hearing loss in children younger than 2 years include parental concern that a hearing, speech, language, or developmental delay is present; bacterial meningitis; head trauma (particularly in the temporal bone area); infectious diseases known to be associated with sensorineural hearing loss (e.g., mumps, measles); a neurodegenerative disorder associated with hearing loss; and/or ototoxic medications used for more than 5 days (USDHHS/ODPHP, 1998).

Prevention, early detection, and intervention—particularly in infants—are critical in reducing functional limitation and disability from hearing impairment. Some congenital hearing impairments and some acquired during infancy are preventable. Hearing loss from otitis media and other diseases can be reduced through appropriate primary care. In addition, steps to minimize or manage hearing deficits through employment of assistive devices (e.g., hearing aids and special equipment) should be instituted as soon as possible to minimize developmental delays.

Lead Screening

The threat of childhood exposure to lead is discussed in Chapter 7. A few key points are repeated here and expanded to include guidelines for screening and treatment.

High blood lead levels have been identified as a very serious threat to children in the United States. This condition disproportionately affects minority and poor children in inner cities, where an estimated 3 million children younger than 6 years (about 4.4% of all children in this age group) have blood lead levels high enough to adversely affect their intelligence, behavior, and development (USDHHS/ODPHP, 1998).

At greatest risk for lead poisoning are the following:

1. Children who live in a house or regularly visit a day care center, preschool, babysitter's, or other house built before 1960
2. Children who live in or regularly visit a house built before 1960 with recent, ongoing, or planned renovation
3. Children who have a brother, sister, or playmate being treated for lead poisoning
4. Children who live with an adult whose job, hobby, or use of ethnic remedies involves lead
5. Children who live near an active lead smelter, battery recycling plant, or other industry likely to release lead

General guidelines for lead screening include initiation of risk assessment and counseling from prenatal visits until the child is 6 years of age. Disagreement exists among pediatric health care authorities, but in general, recommendations are that children with any risk factors listed here should be tested for lead exposure. Screening should be done at about 6 to 12 months of age and again at about 24 months. Infants at high risk should be initially screened at 6 months and every 6 months thereafter. After two consecutive measurements of less than 10 mg/dl, the child should be retested in 1 year. Rescreening should occur at any time when history suggests that exposure has increased, up to about age 6 years, unless otherwise indicated (USDHHS/ODPHP, 1998).

Anemia Screening

Iron deficiency anemia is the most common nutritional disorder in the United States, affecting an estimated 14% of children. The prevalence of anemia is higher among low-income children, breastfed infants, overweight children, and children from households where smoking is present and where occupants watch TV for 2 or more hours per day. Due in part to programs such as WIC and improved parental nutritional education, the prevalence of anemia in children has fallen substantially from 31% of preschool children in 1973 to 15.9% in 1995 (CDC, 2005a).

In infants and children, anemia is associated with fatigue, pallor, apathy, growth and development impairment, and decreased resistance to infection. Risk of anemia is related to low socioeconomic status, consumption of cow's milk before 6 months of age, consumption of formula not fortified with iron, and low birth weight. Native American and black children and immigrants from developing countries are also at risk. General recommendations are that the hemoglobin or hematocrit levels be checked during infancy (6 to 9 months) and early childhood. **Anemia screening** for adolescent females is also recommended (CDC, 2005a).

Therapeutic management of iron deficiency anemia focuses on increasing the amount of iron the child receives. Dietary supplementation includes the use of iron-fortified formulas and cereal for infants and limiting the intake of cow's milk, which decreases iron absorption. Oral supplements may be recommended and the child retested in 3 to 4 months if anemia is fairly significant. Oral iron is the preferred treatment for uncomplicated anemia. In children with iron malabsorption or those who do not tolerate oral iron, parenteral iron may be used (Linton & Kaplan, 2007). Prevention of iron deficiency anemia is described later in this chapter.

HEALTH PROMOTION

Health promotion refers to those activities related to individual lifestyle choices that can influence health. Physical activity and fitness, nutrition, and dental health are components of health promotion for infants and children that are of particular importance to nurses who practice in community settings. Basic information for assessment, health teaching, and counseling is presented in the following sections.

Nutrition

Good nutrition is essential for life, health, and well-being. Conversely, poor nutrition can be harmful because dietary factors are associated with 5 of the 10 leading causes of death (i.e., heart disease, some types of cancer, stroke, diabetes, atherosclerosis) (USDHHS, 2000). Malnutrition in the United States is rarely the result of a lack of a sufficient quantity of

food but is more often caused by deficiencies of certain nutrients (e.g., iron, calcium, protein, some vitamins) and excesses of others (e.g., calories, fats, simple sugars).

Food preferences and dietary habits are established early in childhood, and the importance of good nutritional habits should be taught from an early age. In general, good nutrition for children includes three healthy meals per day and two healthy snacks. Juice should be limited to 4 ounces per day because it is high in calories and may replace the calories that should come from more nutritious foods. Because of an increasing prevalence of peanut allergy, parents should be encouraged to withhold all foods containing peanuts until after age 3 (Mills & Woodring, 2007).

Children enjoy learning about food and are capable of learning basic nutrition concepts beginning in early elementary school. Providing nutrition education for children from preschool through high school should be encouraged to engage children in making wise food choices.

INFANT NUTRITION. As discussed previously, iron deficiency anemia is the most common nutritional disorder in infants and children. To prevent anemia the American Academy of Pediatrics recommends use of breast milk or commercial infant formula, or a combination of the two, for the first year of life. Other interventions include the use of iron supplementation (e.g., iron-fortified commercial formula or iron-fortified cereal for breast fed babies) to provide 1 mg/kg/day of iron by 4 to 6 months of age; use of iron (ferrous sulfate) drops (from 2 to 3 mg/kg/day to 15 mg/kg/day) to breastfed preterm infants after 2 months of age; use of iron-fortified infant cereal when solid foods are introduced; and limiting the amount of formula to no more than 1 L/day to encourage the intake of iron-rich solid foods (Vincent, 2007).

Addition of solid foods into the infant's diet should be done gradually from 4 to 6 months of age. Introduction of solid foods before this time may contribute to development of food allergies, overweight, and choking. Commercially prepared single-grain infant cereal (e.g., rice, barley, oatmeal) is usually introduced first. Rice cereal is often suggested because of its easy digestibility and low allergic potential. The nurse should stress that cereal be fed with a spoon, not added to the bottle. The practice of adding cereal to the bottle is common and contributes to overweight. Most often, strained fruits are introduced initially, followed by vegetables and then meats. Crackers or zwieback are offered at about 6 months of age. Small amounts of raw fruits and vegetables can be added gradually. General guidelines for the addition of solid foods is another important consideration in nutrition counseling. Most clinics and physicians' offices have pamphlets and brochures to provide parents more detailed information on these topics; the nurse can use these materials to supplement health teaching.

NUTRITIONAL NEEDS OF CHILDREN. Adequate caloric and nutrient intake is critical for supporting growth and development of children. In general, recommended nutrition intake for children includes 2 to 3 servings (2 to 3 ounces) per day of meat or meat substitutes (e.g., beans, lentils); 2 to 4 cups of milk or milk equivalent servings, depending on age and size; 5 or more servings of vegetables and fruits (including a dark green or deep yellow vegetable for vitamin A and fruits or vegetables that contain vitamin C); and 4 or more servings of breads and cereals. Fats, oils, and sweets should be eaten sparingly (Murray and Zentner, 2001).

NUTRITIONAL NEEDS OF ADOLESCENTS. In general, adolescents should consume more total nutrients than they did as young children. Accelerated physical and emotional development works to increase the metabolic rate and nutritional needs. Maximal growth takes place in girls between ages 10 and 12 and approximately 2 years later in boys. Protein, calcium, and calorie needs are higher during this time. In the United States, adolescent girls typically begin menstruating at 12.5 years, increasing the need for iron.

Meal skipping, frequent snacking, eating fast foods, and drinking soft drinks contribute to imbalances in the diet of adolescents. In general, adolescents between 12 and 18 years of age should consume 4 servings of dairy products (low-fat milk is preferred), 2 to 3 servings of meat and meat alternatives, 4 to 5 servings of fruits and vegetables, and 6 to 11 servings of breads and cereals. As with children, fats, oils, and sweets should be used sparingly.

Eating disorders (e.g., anorexia nervosa and bulimia) most often occur in adolescent girls. Teaching adolescents the importance of good nutrition should include discussion of the consequences of eating disorders and how to recognize them. More information on nutrition for children and adolescents is available online at http://www.mypyramid.gov

Physical Activity and Exercise

Exercise and physical activity are necessary for muscular development and refinement of coordination and balance, gaining strength, and enhancing other functions, such as circulation and elimination. Toddlers and small children usually have an abundance of energy and rarely need encouragement to promote physical activity. Many school-aged children and adolescents, however, often need to be encouraged to exercise. Several goals of *Healthy People 2010* (USDHHS, 2000) address the importance of physical activity in children 6 years of age through adolescence. In general, all children should engage in light to moderate physical activity for at least 30 minutes each day to develop and maintain cardiorespiratory fitness and improve overall physical fitness. In addition to exercises that improve heart and lung functioning, physical activities that enhance and maintain muscular strength, muscular endurance, and flexibility are recommended.

School-based physical education programs and non-school-related activities such as sports (e.g., soccer, baseball, basketball, hockey) and recreational activities (e.g., skating, swimming, bicycling) can be good sources of exercise. The use of appropriate safety equipment (e.g., helmets, pads, mouth protectors), however, must be stressed. Activities that can be easily incorporated into a child's daily routine and enjoyed all year should be encouraged because activity levels tend to decrease in the winter.

Childhood Overweight

The prevalence of overweight among children between the ages of 6 and 11 has quadrupled since 1970, increasing from 4% in 1970 to 16% in 2002 (NIDDKD, 2005). Ten percent of the world's school-age children are estimated to be overweight, putting them at increased risk for developing chronic disease. A quarter of these overweight children have a significant likelihood of having multiple risk factors for Type II diabetes and heart disease before or during early adulthood (Lobstein, Baur, Uauy, 2004). Complications of overweight include sleep apnea, slipped capital epiphyses, pseudotumor cerebri, gall bladder disease, nonalcoholic fatty liver disease, and metabolic syndrome, a constellation of traits including hyperinsulinemia, obesity, hypertension, and hyperlipidemia. An estimated 30% to 50% of overweight children have metabolic syndrome (Daniels, Arnett, Eckel, Gidding, Hayman, Kumanyika, et al., 2005). Hypertension and prehypertension have become significant health issues in children's health because of the strong association of high blood pressure with overweight and the increase in the prevalence of overweight among children. Overweight children tend to become overweight adults, raising doubts that this generation of children will have the quality of life or life expectancies of their parents (Olshansky, Passaro, Hershow, Layden, Carnes, Brody, et al., 2005). Overweight children often face social isolation. Stigmatization of overweight children is common and has a negative psychological impact on its victims.

There are many reasons why children become overweight:

- Genetic factors—certain genetic factors may lead to overweight, but for these factors to culminate in overweight, the environment must also be favorable.
- Diet—snacking on high calorie foods, such as soft drinks and candy, and eating meals away from home are associated with weight gain among children. Meals served in restaurants are larger than those served at home and contribute to overeating.
- Physical activity—the amount of time spent in physical education, recess, and outdoor play has decreased signficantly over the last two decades. As a result, children are spending more time engaged in sedentary activities such as watching television, playing video games, and using the computer. In addition, chilen also tend to snack in front of the TV, further increasing their intake (CDC, 2007a).

The U.S. Surgeon General recommends the following actions to decrease overweight and obesity:

- Change the perception of overweight and obesity at all ages, stressing health over appearance.
- Educate childbearing families about breast feeding. Breastfed babies are less likely to be overweight as they get older.
- Provide culturally appropriate education in schools and communities about healthy eating and physical activity.

- Ensure daily physical education in all school grades.
- Reduce time spent watching TV and other sedentary behaviors.
- Build physical activity into daily routines for children and their families. Children should aim for 60 minutes of moderate physical activity per day.
- Promote healthier food choices, including 5 servings of fruits and vegetables each day, and teach appropriate portion sizes.
- Ensure that schools provide healthful foods and beverages on campus and at school events.

(USDHHS, 2007)

Sleep and Rest

In addition to diet and exercise, sleep and rest are essential to good health. Sleep needs vary dramatically with age, ranging from 20 hours or more per day for neonates to 8 hours per day for older teenagers. Sleep patterns are affected by individual temperment, the environment, and bedtime routine.

The positioning of infants for sleep is very important because sleeping in a prone position has been associated with sudden infant death syndrome (SIDS). In 1992 the American Academy of Pediatrics recommended that almost all infants up to 6 months of age sleep on their sides or backs (exceptions are infants with gastroesophageal reflux and some infants with upper airway problems) (Vincent, 2007). Placing the infant on a firm mattress, rather than a pillow or soft bedding, is also suggested. Widespread adherence to these recommendations has resulted in a decline in SIDS deaths by more than 50% since 1990 (CDC, 2007b). All parents should be informed of these recommendations and taught to position infants on their backs, rather than prone, and to avoid overly soft bedding.

Dental Health

Although preventable, dental carries remains the most common chronic childhood disease. Indeed, tooth decay is 5 times more common than asthma (CDC, 2005a). In recent years, however, the oral health of children in the United States has improved dramatically, largely because of community water fluoridation, use of preventive services (e.g., sealants, topical fluoride treatment), and appropriate tooth care (e.g., brushing, flossing). Despite these improvements in oral health, more than half of all children have caries by the second grade, and about 80% have caries by the time they finish high school. *Healthy People 2010* objectives to promote oral health include increasing the percentage of communities with fluoridated water, encouraging the use of dental sealants, and increasing the use of topical or systemic fluorides (e.g., toothpastes, mouth rinses, fluoride drops) (USDHHS, 2000). Prevention of baby bottle tooth decay and screening of all preschool children for tooth decay are also encouraged.

It has been observed that community water fluoridation is the most effective and efficient means of preventing dental caries in children. Furthermore, widespread exposure to fluorides through drinking water and dental products has led to a 68% decline in the amount of decayed, missing, or filled teeth in the U.S. population (Centers for Disease Control and Prevention [CDC], 1999).

According to Ripa (1993), approximately 62% of U.S. residents have drinking water containing optimal levels of fluoride, with the highest levels (73%) being in Midwest states (i.e., Minnesota, Michigan, Wisconsin, Iowa, Missouri, Illinois, Indiana, Ohio) and the lowest (17.9%) in the Pacific states (i.e., Washington, Oregon, California).

Dental care of infants and young children may include fluoride supplementation. If the infant is fed with formula concentrate or powdered formula prepared with fluoridated water, supplements are not necessary. If the community does not have fluoridated water, supplemental fluoride drops should be used, with the amount of supplementation based on the amount of fluoride in the drinking water. For older children, dentists often recommend using fluoride tablets, fluoride application in the dental office, or use of fluoride toothpaste or mouthwash (ADA, 2005). Parents should be encouraged to purchase a toothbrush with soft bristles and the appropriate size head for their child. Children should brush twice daily with a flouridated toothpaste.

Dental sealants are thin plastic coatings painted on the chewing surfaces of the back teeth and are applied in the dentist's office, community clinic, or school. The process is simple, painless, and effective in preventing tooth decay. The process lasts up to 10 years and is fairly inexpensive. All parents should be encouraged to discuss dental sealants with their child's dentist.

Bottle mouth syndrome, or baby bottle tooth decay, occurs in older infants and toddlers who are allowed to fall asleep with a bottle of formula, milk, or another sweetened fluid in their mouths. These fluids pool in the mouth, particularly around the upper front teeth. Bacteria normally present in the mouth consume the carbohydrates from the milk or juice and (as a byproduct) produce metabolic acids. These acids decalcify tooth enamel, resulting in destruction of the tooth. All parents should be taught to prevent baby bottle tooth decay by using only plain water in naptime and bedtime bottles.

The primary teeth (deciduous teeth or baby teeth) begin erupting at about 6 months of age and continue until 2 years of age; they start shedding at about 6 years of age. The permanent teeth begin erupting at about 6 to 7 years of age and continue into adulthood. Figure 12-2 depicts normal tooth formation.

To promote oral health, the ADA (2005) offers the following recommendations:
- Take children to the dentist regularly, beginning within 6 months of the eruption of the first tooth, but no later than the child's first birthday.
- Encourage children to drink from a cup by their first birthday.
- Begin brushing the child's teeth with water as soon as the first tooth appears.
- Start flossing when two of the child's teeth begin to touch.
- Brush and floss the child's teeth daily until the child can be taught to do it alone; then encourage the child to brush and floss.
- Ensure that children get adequate fluoride for decay-resistant teeth (this varies based on the community—consult a dentist).
- Ask the dentist about dental sealants.

Thumb sucking or use of a pacifier generally does not cause permanent dental problems for children younger than 4 years of age. However, alignment problems in the permanent teeth may develop if thumb sucking persists beyond age 5 years. Observation of thumb sucking or use of pacifiers in small children should alert the nurse to inform the parents of potential problems. If thumb sucking persists, the child should be referred to a dentist.

Oral injuries are common during childhood. Children should be encouraged to wear mouth protectors or mouthguards when participating in activities

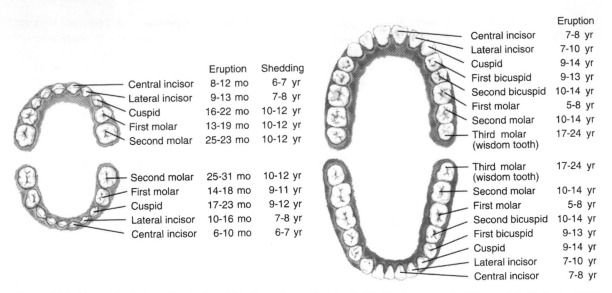

Figure 12-2. Normal tooth formation in the child. (From James S, Ashwill JW: *Nursing care of children*, ed 3, St. Louis, 2007, Saunders.)

that may involve falls, head contact, tooth clenching, or flying equipment (e.g., gymnastics, football, skateboarding, soccer, basketball). In addition to protecting teeth, mouthguards also prevent injury to lips, cheeks, and tongue and may reduce the severity and incidence of concussions (ADA, 2007). Mouth protectors are available at sporting goods stores or may be custom-made by the dentist.

If a dental injury occurs, the child should be taken to the dentist immediately. If a permanent tooth is knocked out, it should be rinsed gently with cool water without removing any attached tissue and immediately reinserted into the socket. If that is not possible, the tooth should be placed in cool water or milk, and the child should see a dentist as soon as possible, bringing the tooth along.

When working in community settings, nurses can dramatically affect the health of infants, children, and adolescents through measures to prevent illness and protect health and safety. Illness prevention and health protection strategies for children include prevention of communicable diseases; prevention of initiation of tobacco, alcohol, and drug use; promoting safety; and prevention and detection of child abuse. Prevention of communicable diseases, including vitally important pediatric immunizations, is discussed in Chapter 19. Interventions to

improve safety; prevent alcohol, tobacco, and drug use; and detect and prevent child abuse are described in the following sections.

Prevention of Substance Use

DRUGS AND ALCOHOL. Alcohol use contributes dramatically to the three leading causes of adolescent deaths. As stated earlier, injuries are the leading cause of death in adolescents, and an estimated 40% of injury deaths in this age group are related to the use of alcohol. Alcohol use also contributes significantly to adolescent homicide and suicide (the second and third leading causes of death in this age group). School-based alcohol and drug education programs have been somewhat successful; alcohol and marijuana use among adolescents (aged 12 to 17 years) decreased from 50% in 1999 to 43% in 2005 (CDC, 2006). To assist in reducing alcohol and drug use, health care providers are encouraged to screen and counsel adolescents for alcohol and other drug use. Components of alcohol and drug abuse counseling suggested by the USDHHS/ ODPHP (1998) include the following:

• Begin education on alcohol and drug use during the preteen years. All children and adolescents should be informed of the dangers of alcohol and other drugs, emphasizing associated dangers of human immunodeficiency virus (HIV) exposure and motor vehicle accidents while under the influence of alcohol and other drugs.

- Ask parents about their own use of alcohol and other drugs and whether they discuss the use of alcohol and drugs with their children. Assessment for a family history of alcoholism or drug use should be made.
- Establish a caring and confidential relationship with adolescents; however, the adolescent must be informed of the limits of confidentiality.
- As nonthreateningly as possible, question children and adolescents about drug and alcohol use in their environment (e.g., home, school, work). Suggested questions to be asked include "Do most of your friends drink alcohol or smoke marijuana at parties?" "Have you ever tried alcohol, marijuana, or other drugs?" "Do your parents know that you've used alcohol or drugs?" "Have you ever been drunk or stoned and driven a car?"
- If alcohol or drug use is determined, assess the type of drugs used and the quantity, frequency, and setting of use.
- Evaluate the extent to which alcohol or other drugs are affecting the adolescent's life (e.g., school performance, peer relationships, family relationships, work).
- Be aware of signs and symptoms of dependence, addiction, and withdrawal and teach them to parents and adolescents.
- Refer for evaluation and treatment if evidence of significant psychosocial impairment or physiological dependence is present. Familiarity with available treatment options in the community is essential.

TOBACCO. Use of tobacco products is the leading preventable cause of death in the United States, accounting for more than 440,000 deaths each year (about one out of every five deaths) (CDC, 2007c). Initiation of smoking occurs almost entirely during adolescence, and surveys have indicated that 82% of those who have ever smoked started by the twelfth grade. Approximately 23% of high school students report smoking cigarettes daily, and the average age of initial cigarette use is 12 years. White males have the highest prevalence of cigarette use among youth, and of the 23% of youth who report current cigarette use, 54.6% had tried to quit (CDC, 2006).

In addition to the direct health problems associated with tobacco use, concern arises because cigarettes are considered to be a gateway drug, and their use often leads to abuse of alcohol and illicit drugs. Indeed, teens who smoke are significantly more likely than nonsmokers to use alcohol, marijuana, and cocaine (Pourciau & Vallette, 2007). Because of the health problems associated with tobacco use, reduction of the initiation of cigarette smoking by teenagers has been termed a national priority. Strategies to prevent tobacco use among children and teenagers include enforcement of youth access laws, establishment of tobacco-free environments, and ongoing prevention programs in schools and the community.

Surveillance and enforcement of retail restriction of sale of tobacco to nonadults is essential to reduce the prevalence of smoking among teenagers. Most states have a minimum age of 18 years for purchasing cigarettes; however, 15% of youth who smoke report purchasing their own cigarettes at a store, with 48.5% of those who tried to buy tobacco in a store saying that they were not asked to show proof of age. Smokeless tobacco also represents a health risk to youth. Nationwide, 8% of students report having used smokeless tobacco, with white males having the highest prevalence of smokeless tobacco use. Youth also report smoking cigars. Nationwide, 14% of students report having smoked cigars, with black males having the highest prevalence of cigar use (CDC, 2006b).

The establishment of tobacco-free environments and tobacco use prevention education programs is an important component in decreasing the initiation of tobacco use among youth. The Pro-Children Act of 1994 requires that federally funded facilities that provide services to children (e.g., schools and libraries) be smoke free. Increasingly, state and city ordinances and laws are being enacted that prohibit smoking in public places. These efforts should be supported by all health care workers.

Health education and counseling strategies to encourage teenagers to prevent initiation of or to stop tobacco use include the following:

- Maintain a smoke-free environment in the health care office or clinic; do not permit smoking by staff, clients, or their parents. Post no-smoking signs and provide literature about the importance of smoking cessation and avoiding tobacco use.

- If parents or other family members smoke, stress the importance of stopping; emphasize the negative health consequences for children.
- Provide counseling or referral to those who want to quit smoking.
- Begin in elementary school to discuss tobacco use and its negative effects; emphasize the unattractive cosmetic consequences of tobacco use (i.e., stained teeth, oral sores, bad breath) and negative athletic consequences of tobacco use. Also emphasize the negative social consequences (e.g., disapproval by peers) because this is generally more effective with children and adolescents than discussing the long-term health consequences.
- Elicit information in a nonthreatening manner; have parents leave the room or ask adolescents to complete a previsit questionnaire discussing tobacco use and other sensitive issues.

Safety

In the United States, injuries are the leading cause of mortality in children and adolescents, with half of the fatal accidents involving motor vehicle crashes. In addition to motor vehicle accidents, significant risks are associated with other sources. Homicide accounts for about 11% of injury deaths; suicide, 9%; drowning, 21%; fire or burns, 14%; and "other" (e.g., choking, falls, poisoning, sports, accidents involving firearms), 14% (NCIPC, 2007a).

Interventions for childhood injury prevention are discussed in each of the following subsections.

VEHICLE SAFETY. As mentioned, motor vehicles are involved in almost half of all injury deaths and contribute to numerous hospitalizations of children and adolescents. More than 46,000 people are killed annually in motor vehicle accidents (NCHS, 2004a), including those who are occupants in a vehicle and those struck while riding bicycles or as pedestrians. Motorcycle (11% of total), bicycle (4.5% of total), and pedestrian (14.5% of total) casualties account for almost 30% of motor vehicle deaths each year (NCIPC, 2007a; NCIPC, 2007b).

Motor vehicle safety begins with the ride home from the hospital. Although some variation exists in specific regulations, all states require the use of child safety seats. Other interventions that have been suggested include adoption and enforcement of seat belt laws and ordinances, enforcement of strict penalties for operating a vehicle under the influence of drugs or alcohol, adoption and enforcement of laws and ordinances requiring motorcyclists and bicyclists to wear helmets, enforcement of speed limits, enforcement of minimum drinking age laws, and enforcement of laws and ordinances requiring child safety seat use and the extension of these laws and ordinances to cover all passengers sitting in all vehicles. Equipping vehicles with both driver and passenger airbags, improving vehicle designs to better protect both occupants (e.g., side impact protection, improved door design, roof crush resistance, and restraint system), and developing community-based pedestrian and bicycle safety programs are other safety measures (see the Health Teaching box "Basic Safety Counseling").

POISONING. In 2006, 77,346 children between the ages of 0-14 were victims of poisoning (NCIPC, 2007a). Most poisoning accidents take place in the home and involve children younger than 5 years. Any nonfood item is a potential poison, and many children die or are injured from swallowing medicines, polishes, insecticides, antifreeze, drain cleaners, and other household products. Parents of small children should be given information on how to protect their children from potential poisoning. In addition, instruction on emergency actions to be taken in the event of accidental poisoning should be a priority.

HEAD INJURY. Head injuries are the most common severe disabling injuries in the United States, with an estimated half million new cases occurring annually. The most common causes of head injury include motor vehicle (including bicycles and motorcycles) crashes, falls, diving and other water-related accidents, and violence. Recently efforts to prevent head injuries in children have targeted laws and ordinances requiring bicycle helmets.

Each year nearly 1000 bicyclists are killed in the United States, and more than 500,000 persons are treated in emergency departments for bicycle-related injuries. A very high prevalence of bicyclist fatalities occurs in males, and more than one third occur in boys between the ages of 5 and 15 years (CDC, 1995). The majority of bicycle fatalities are caused by bicyclist error (e.g., failure to yield right of way, improper crossing of an intersection or road, failure to obey traffic signs and lights), and alcohol is involved in many bicycle fatalities.

Head injury accounts for 62% of bicycle-related deaths and 67% of bicycle-related hospital admis-

Basic Safety Counseling

GENERAL INFORMATION

- Encourage parents and others to learn basic life-saving skills (e.g., CPR).
- Teach children to dial 911 and other local emergency numbers.
- Encourage parents and others to teach children how to manage peer pressure that might result in risk-taking behavior that may interfere with making good safety decisions.
- Encourage parents to be good role models for safe behavior (i.e., avoid drinking alcohol before driving, always wear a seat belt and bicycle helmet, drive within the posted speed limit).
- Be aware of community resources and programs related to safety.

CHOKING AND SUFFOCATION

- Advise parents and other caregivers to keep objects that can cause suffocation (e.g., plastic bags) and choking (e.g., coins, small toy parts, and certain foods such as grapes, gum, peanuts, hot dogs) away from small children.

DROWNING

- Never leave infants and small children in the bathtub without supervision.
- Do not allow children to swim alone.
- Advise that fences around swimming pools/spas should be at least 4 feet high with completely self-closing gates.

ELECTRICAL SAFETY

- Keep unused electrical outlets covered with plastic guards or install breaker outlets.
- Ground fault interrupter circuits should be used in bathrooms and other areas where water is likely to touch bare skin.

FALL PREVENTION

- Those caring for small children should use safety gates on both top and bottom of stairways, install window guards above the first floor, and move furniture away from upper-story windows so children cannot climb onto the window sill.
- Baby walkers should be used under supervision, particularly to avoid falls down stairs.

FIRE AND BURN PREVENTION

- To avoid scalding burns, reduce the temperature setting on the water heater to 49° C (120° F) or install antiscald devices on bathroom and kitchen faucets.
- Smoke alarms should be installed properly in sleeping areas and in the kitchen; batteries should be changed at least twice yearly. The family should have a fire escape plan and practice fire drills.

FIREARMS

- Parents and other caregivers should be advised about the dangers of keeping a firearm in the home. If a gun is kept in the home, it should be unloaded and locked up separately from the ammunition.

MOTOR VEHICLE SAFETY

- Use car seats for all children, based on state laws. Child safety seats should be in the rear seat of the car and should be used every time the children ride. Safety seats should face backward until child weighs at least 20 pounds or reaches 1 year of age.
- Booster seats should be used until children grow tall enough so the lap belt stays low on their hips. Children should never ride in the cargo areas of pickup trucks, vans, or station wagons. Infants and children should never be placed in the front seat of a vehicle equipped with a passenger-side air bag. If a vehicle does not have a rear seat, children riding in the front seat should be positioned as far back as possible from the air bag.

From U.S. Department of Health and Human Services/Public Health Service: *Clinician's handbook of preventive service*, ed 2, McLean, Va, 1999, International Medical Publishing.

sions. Based on evidence that 74% to 85% of the risk of head injury can be reduced by the use of bicycle helmets, the CDC (1995) has recommended that state and local agencies and organizations develop programs to increase their use. These recommendations are as follows:

- Bicycle helmets should be worn by all persons (i.e., bicycle operators and passengers) at any age when bicycling.
- Bicycle riders should wear helmets whenever and wherever they ride a bicycle (Figure 12-3).
- Bicycle helmets should meet the standards of the American National Standards Institute, the Snell Memorial Foundation, or the American Society for Testing and Material.
- To effectively increase helmet use rates, states and communities must implement programs that include legislation, education and promotion, enforcement, and program evaluation.

Other measures to improve bicycle safety include education and training to improve knowledge of and adherence to traffic laws, use of appropriate

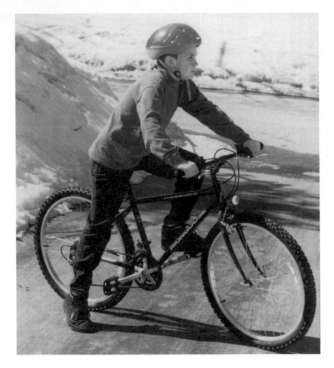

Figure 12-3. The right-size bike is important; the child should be able to sit on the bike and place the balls of both feet on the ground. The foot should comfortably reach and manipulate the pedal in the down position. Wearing a protective helmet is mandatory for safe cycling. The helmet should sit on top of the head in a level position and should not rock back and forth or from side to side. The strap should always be fastened securely under the chin. (From Wong DL: *Whaley & Wong's nursing care of infants and children*, ed 7, St Louis, 2007, Mosby.)

clothing (light colored and marked with reflective materials) when riding at night, and bicycle maintenance. Bicycle safety programs are available in most communities.

Head injury is also the most commonly recorded cause of deaths for motorcycle drivers and passengers who die in crashes. Nonhelmeted riders are two and a half times more likely than helmeted riders to sustain a fatal head injury. Further, helmet use is the single most important factor in preventing death and head injuries (Advocates for Highway and Auto Safety, 2005). All motorcycle riders should be informed of these statistics, and helmet laws should be encouraged in those states where they do not exist and strongly enforced in all other states. Nurses and other health care providers should consistently encourage parents, adolescents, and children to use protective helmets whenever using a bicycle or motorcycle.

FIRE AND BURNS. Fire and burns are the fifth leading cause of childhood deaths from injury, but they are the second leading cause of deaths from injury in children 1 to 9 years of age. In 2004 there were 461 deaths among children aged 0 to 9 years in the United States (NCIPC, 2007b). Although the death rate from residential fires has declined over the past several decades, many fire-related deaths are preventable and remain a major public health problem.

According to the USDHHS (2000), those who live in substandard housing without smoke detectors are at the highest risk for fire death. Improved public awareness of home fire safety, including use of functional smoke detectors in all sleeping areas and establishment of home evacuation plans, can help reduce home fire deaths and disabilities. The most common sources of fire and burns are wood stoves, space heaters, cooking equipment, cigarettes, matches, and lighters.

Many fire deaths and injuries are caused by smoke and gases because the victims inhale smoke that occurs ahead of the flames. Early warning and having an escape plan can dramatically diminish injury and death. General recommendations for fire safety include the following:

- Read the manufacturer's instructions on installation and location of fire detectors.
- Install smoke detectors on each floor of the house, near all sleeping areas, and in the kitchen.
- Follow the manufacturer's instructions for cleaning and maintenance; replace the battery annually or when a chirping sound is heard.

- Develop an escape plan and an alternate escape plan for the family and practice the escape routes periodically. The escape plan should include choosing a place outside the house where the family will meet to be sure that everyone got out safely.
- Ensure that there are at least two exits from each part of the house.

VIOLENT BEHAVIOR. Violence in the United States is pervasive and claims many lives and threatens the health and well-being of many more. On an average day in the United States, 53 people die from homicide, and at least 18,000 others survive interpersonal assaults. In addition, 84 people commit suicide each day, and 3000 others attempt suicide (USDHHS, 2000). Homicide was the cause of death of almost 20,000 Americans in 2004 (NCIPC, 2007b). It is the second leading cause of death for young persons 15 to 24 and the leading cause of death for blacks in this age group. Indeed, the homicide rate in the United States is 10 times higher than in Canada, 15 times higher than in Australia, and 28 times higher than in France or Germany (USDHHS, 2000).

Homicide most often affects men, teenagers, and minority group members—particularly blacks and Hispanics. To assist in the detection and prevention of violence, Box 12-1 lists sociological, developmental, and familial risk factors for violence.

Firearms, particularly handguns, have been implicated in an alarming number of homicides and suicides. Firearms accounted for 75% of the suicide/homicide deaths for the 15- to 24-year-old age group and 66% of deaths in those 10 to 14 years of age. All parents, children, and adolescents should receive information and counseling to prevent violence. Information on the danger of guns is particularly important.

OTHER SAFETY HAZARDS. Additional hazards threaten the safety of infants, children, and adolescents. These include participation in hazardous sports and recreational activities, choking or aspiration, suffocation, and other concerns.

To prevent injuries from sports and recreational activities, all children should be taught to wear appropriate protective gear at all times when participating. For example, batting helmets, and catcher's gear and athletic supporters and protective cups for all boys should be required when playing baseball; helmets, wrist guards, knee pads, and elbow pads should be worn for in-line skating and skateboarding; and hockey and football players should wear the full complement of pads, helmets, and mouthguards whenever they play. Parents should be counseled to ensure that children are properly supervised when engaging in activities that are associated with injury risk. Finally, many organized athletic organizations require a yearly physical examination by a health care professional before participation. A physical examination may identify undetected problems that might threaten health (e.g., asthma, heart problems, musculoskeletal problems).

Each year many children suffer serious injury or death through inappropriate use of objects or toys (e.g., beanbags, plastic bags, balloons), misuse of equipment (e.g., highchairs, baby walkers), and lack

---

BOX 12-1 Factors Associated with Risk of Violence

SOCIOLOGIC

Low socioeconomic status
Involvement with gangs
Drug dealing
Access to guns
Media exposure to violence
Community exposure to violence

DEVELOPMENTAL/PSYCHOLOGICAL

Alcohol or drug abuse
Rigid sex role expectations
Peer pressure, especially for adolescents

Poor impulse control
History of mental health problems
High individual stress level
Manual laborer, unemployed, or employed part time
Younger than 30 years

FAMILY

History of intergenerational abuse
Social isolation
Parents verbally threaten children
High levels of family stress
Two or more children

From Langford DR: Violence: a social and family problem. In Maurer FA, Smith CM, editors: *Community/public health nursing: health for families and populations*, ed 3, pp. 517-544, St Louis, 2005, Saunders.

of close supervision or precautions (e.g., leaving the side rail down on the crib, giving a toddler food that might cause choking, not covering electric outlets). Box 12-2 presents general guidelines for **child safety** that are essential components of health teaching for all parents.

Child Abuse: Detection and Prevention

Child abuse and neglect refers to any physical or mental injury, sexual abuse or exploitation, negligent treatment, or maltreatment of a child by a person who is responsible for the child's welfare. The

---

BOX 12-2 Child Safety Home Checklist

SAFETY: FIRE, ELECTRICAL, BURNS

- Guards in front of or around any heating appliance, fireplace, or furnace (including floor furnace)*
- Electrical wires hidden or out of reach*
- No frayed or broken wires; no overloaded sockets
- Plastic guards or caps over electrical outlets; furniture in front of outlets*
- Hanging tablecloths out of reach, away from open fires*
- Smoke detectors tested and operating properly
- Kitchen matches stored out of child's reach*
- Large, deep ashtrays throughout house (if used)
- Small stoves, heaters, and other hot objects (e.g., cigarettes, candles, coffee pots, slow cookers) placed where they cannot be tipped over or reached by children
- Hot water heater set at 49°C (120°F) or lower
- Pot handles turned toward back of stove, center of table
- No loose clothing worn near stove
- No cooking or eating hot foods or liquids with child standing nearby or sitting in lap
- All small appliances, such as iron, turned off, disconnected, and placed out of reach when not in use
- Cool, not hot, mist vaporizer used
- Fire extinguisher available on each floor and checked periodically
- Electrical fuse box and gas outlet accessible
- Family escape plan in case of a fire practiced periodically; fire escape ladder available on upper-level floors
- Telephone number of fire or rescue squad and address of home with nearest cross-street posted near phone

SAFETY: SUFFOCATION AND ASPIRATION

- Small objects stored out of reach*
- Toys inspected for small removable parts or long strings*
- Hanging crib toys and mobiles placed out of reach
- Plastic bags stored away from young child's reach, large plastic garment bags discarded after tying in knots*
- Mattress or pillow not covered with plastic or in manner accessible to child*
- Crib design according to federal regulations with snug-fitting mattress*†
- Crib positioned away from other furniture or windows*
- Portable playpen gates up at all times while in use*
- Accordion-style gates not used*
- Bathroom doors kept closed and toilet seats down*
- Faucets turned off firmly*
- Pool fenced with locked gate
- Proper safety equipment at poolside
- Electric garage door openers stored safely, and garage door adjusted to rise when door strikes object
- Doors of ovens, trunks, dishwashers, refrigerators, and front-loading clothes washers and dryers kept closed*

- Unused appliance, such as a refrigerator, securely closed with lock or doors removed*
- Food served in small noncylindric pieces*
- Toy chests without lids or with lids that securely lock in open position*
- Buckets and wading pools kept empty when not in use*
- Clothesline above head level
- At least one member of household trained in basic life support (cardiopulmonary resuscitation [CPR]), including first aid for choking‡

SAFETY: POISONING

- Toxic substances, including batteries, placed on a high shelf, preferably in locked cabinet
- Toxic plants hung or placed out of reach*
- Excess quantities of cleaning fluids, paints, pesticides, drugs, and other toxic substances not stored in home
- Used containers of poisonous substances discarded where child cannot obtain access
- Telephone number of local poison control center and address of home with nearest cross-street posted near phone
- Syrup of ipecac (containing two doses per child) in home
- Medicines clearly labeled in childproof containers and stored out of reach
- Household cleaners, disinfectants, and insecticides kept in their original containers, separate from food and out of reach
- Smoking in areas away from children

SAFETY: FALLS

- Nonskid mats, strips, or surfaces in tubs and showers
- Exits, halls, and passageways in rooms kept clear of toys, furniture, boxes, or other items that could be obstructive
- Stairs and halls well lighted, with switches at both top and bottom
- Sturdy handrails for all steps and stairways
- Nothing stored on stairways
- Treads, risers, and carpeting in good repair
- Glass doors and walls marked with decals
- Safety glass used in doors, windows, and walls
- Gates on top and bottom of staircases and elevated areas, such as porch or fire escape*
- Guardrails on upstairs windows with locks that limit height of window opening and access to areas such as fire escape*
- Crib side rails raised to full height; mattress lowered as child grows*
- Restraints used in high chairs, walkers, or other baby furniture; preferably walkers not used*
- Scatter rugs secured in place or used with nonskid back
- Walks, patios, and driveways in good repair

BOX 12-2 Child Safety Home Checklist—cont'd

SAFETY: BODILY INJURY

- Knives, power tools, and unloaded firearms stored safely or placed in locked cabinet
- Garden tools returned to storage racks after use
- Pets properly restrained and immunized for rabies

- Swings, slides, and other outdoor play equipment kept in safe condition
- Yard free of broken glass, nail-studded boards, other litter
- Cement birdbaths placed where young child cannot tip them over*

From Hockenberry MJ, Wilson D: *Wong's nursing care of infants and children*, ed 8, p. 559, St Louis, 2007, Mosby.
*Safety measures are specific for homes with young children. All safety measures should be implemented in homes where children reside and visit frequently, such as those of grandparents or babysitters.
†Federal regulations are available from U.S. Consumer Product Safety Commission, 1-800-638-CPSC.
‡Home care instructions for infant CPR and infant/child choking are available in Wong and Whaley's *Clinical Manual of Pediatric Nursing*.

incidence of child abuse appears to be rising. In 2002, 906,000 children were abused, with 1500 dying from this abuse. Among children who were abused, 61% experienced neglect, 19% were physically abused, 10% were sexually abused, and 5% suffered emotional or psychological abuse. Finally, shaken-baby syndrome affects an estimated 1200 to 1600 children per year (CDC, 2005).

Child abuse and neglect cases cross all age, race, education, and socioeconomic lines. Cases tend to be reported more frequently, however, among individuals who are poor, are young, and have little education (Maurer, 2005). It is important to realize that reported data may be biased, and observation

for and reporting of suspected cases should consider suspicious cases from any social class, race, or age.

Nurses who practice in community settings are sometimes in a position to recognize and intervene in cases of suspected child abuse. To assist in recognizing individuals at risk to be abusive parents, Box 12-3 lists characteristics of abusive parents and Table 12-4 details physical and behavioral indicators of child abuse and neglect.

Child abuse and neglect are crimes in all 50 states, and nurses have a legal responsibility to report suspected or actual cases of child abuse. Most institutions providing care to children have a written policy regarding the reporting of suspected

BOX 12-3 Characteristics and Behaviors of Abusive Parents/Child Care Providers

CHARACTERISTICS

- At or below poverty level
- History of abuse or neglect as a child
- Poor parenting skills
- Poor coping skills
- Involved in a crisis situation (e.g., unemployment, divorce, financial difficulties)
- Does not understand normal growth and development patterns
- Unrealistic expectations of their child's behavior
- Looking to child for satisfaction of needs of love, support, and reassurance
- Poor impulse control
- Low tolerance for frustration
- Poor or inadequate role models
- Socially isolated from support systems

- Women more frequently physically abuse children
- Men more frequently sexually abuse children
- Stepfathers are 5 to 8 times more likely to engage in sexual abuse of their children than are birth fathers

BEHAVIORS

- Frequent use of harsh punishment
- Projection of blame onto the child
- History of drug or alcohol abuse
- Delay getting medical attention for child
- Respond inappropriately to child during treatment (e.g., ignore, show no concern, or overinvolved with attention)
- Use different facilities for treatment of child
- Blame siblings, babysitters, or others without substantiation or place blame on child's clumsiness
- Tell contradictory stories to explain injury
- Vague about cause of the injury

Data from Langford DR: Violence: a social and family problem. In Maurer FA, Smith, CM, editors: *Community/public health nursing: health for families and populations*, ed 3, St Louis, 2005, Saunders; Stevenson L, Pappas A: Violence in the community. In Nies MA, McEwen M, editors: *Community/public health nursing: promoting the health of populations*, ed 4, St Louis, 2007, Saunders; Carson VB, Smith-DiJulio K: Family violence. In Varcarolis EM, Carson VB, Shoemaker NC, editors: *Foundations of psychiatric mental health nursing*, ed 5, St Louis, 2006, Saunders.

TABLE **12-4** Physical and Behavioral Indicators of Child Abuse and Neglect

PHYSICAL INDICATORS	BEHAVIORAL INDICATORS
Physical Abuse	
Unexplained bruises and welts in various stages of healing that may form patterns	Wariness of adult contacts
Unexplained burns by cigars or cigarettes or immersion burns (e.g., socklike, glovelike, or on buttocks or genitalia)	Apprehensive when other children cry
	Constantly on the alert
	Exhibiting extremes of behavior; aggressiveness or passive and withdrawn or overly friendly to strangers
Rope burns	Frightened of parents
Unexplained lacerations or abrasions	Afraid to go home
Unexplained fractures in various stages of healing; multiple or spiral fractures	Reporting injury by parents
Unexplained injuries to mouth, lips, gums, eyes, or external genitalia	
Physical Neglect	
Hunger	Begging or stealing food
Poor hygiene	Alone at inappropriate times or for prolonged periods
Poor or inappropriate dress	Delinquent
Lack of supervision for prolonged periods	Stealing
Lack of medical or dental care	Arriving early to and departing late from school
Constant fatigue, listlessness, or falling asleep in class	Reporting having no caretaker
Sexual Abuse	
Difficulty in walking or sitting	Exhibiting negative self-esteem
Torn, stained, or bloody underwear	Exhibiting inability to trust and function in intimate relationships
Genital pain or itching	Exhibiting cognitive and motor dysfunctions
Bruises or bleeding from the external genitalia, vaginal, or anal areas	Exhibiting deficits in personal and social skills
Sexually transmitted disease	Exhibiting bizarre, sophisticated, or unusual sexual behavior or knowledge
Drug and alcohol abuse	Delinquency or a runaway
Developmental delays	Exhibiting suicide ideation
	Reporting sexual assault
Emotional Maltreatment	
Failure to thrive	Exhibiting behavior extremes from passivity to aggression
Lags in physical development	Exhibiting habit and conduct disorders (e.g., antisocial behavior and destructiveness)
Speech disorders	Exhibiting neurotic traits
Developmental delays	Attempting suicide

From Stevenson L, Pappas A: Violence. In Nies MA, McEwen M, editors: *Community/public health nursing: promoting the health of populations*, ed 4, pp. 555-578, St Louis, 2007, Saunders.

child abuse. These policies need to be reviewed periodically. Finally, to assist in the reduction of family violence, see the Community Application box "Components of a Comprehensive Program to Reduce Family Violence."

NURSING CARE FOR COMMON HEALTH PROBLEMS

Nurses who care for infants and children in community settings should be aware of common illnesses and conditions. Table 12-5 describes some of the more frequently encountered acute and episodic illnesses and chronic conditions in infants and children, including prevention strategies, identification, and treatment.

SUMMARY

Nurses who practice in community settings are uniquely able to affect the health and well-being of children through appropriate assessment, counseling, health teaching, and providing other interventions as needed. Early detection of congenital, developmental, or acquired health problems and referral for treatment can dramatically influence the child's health and development.

Pediatric nurses like Bonnie from the opening case study recognize that preventive measures, such as encouraging appropriate, consistent use of safety devices (e.g., car seats, helmets, smoke detectors) and advance preparation (e.g., keeping poisons and

---

COMMUNITY APPLICATION
Components of a Comprehensive Program to Reduce Family Violence

PRIMARY PREVENTION—GOAL: PROMOTION OF OPTIMAL PARENTING AND FAMILY WELLNESS

Individuals

Family-life education in schools, churches, and communities
Education of children on methods of conflict resolution
Birth control services for sexually active teens
Child care education for teenagers who babysit
Preventive mental health services for adults and children
Training for professionals in early detection of violence

Family

Parenting classes in hospitals, schools, and other community agencies
Provision of bonding opportunities for new parents
Referral of new families to community health nurses after early discharge from the hospital for follow-up services
Social services for families

Community

Community education concerning family violence
Reduction of media violence
Development of community services such as crisis lines, respite placement for children, respite care for families with dependent older adult members, shelters for battered women and their children, and development and enforcement of anti-stalking measures including cyber-stalking
Handgun control

SECONDARY PREVENTION—GOAL: DIAGNOSIS OF AND SERVICE FOR FAMILIES IN STRESS

Individuals

Nursing assessment for evidence of family violence in all health care settings
A well-thought-out safety plan for victims
Knowledge of legal options to help ensure safety
Shelter or foster home placement for victims

Family

Social services for individuals or families
Referral to self-help groups in the community
Referral to community agencies that provide services for victims

Community

All health professionals skilled in assessment of violence and equipped with protocols for dealing with the victims to help ensure their safety
Hospital emergency rooms and trauma centers with 24-hour reporting, response, case intake, coordination with legal and medical authorities, coordination with voluntary agencies that have services, coordination with social services departments for provision of services
Death review teams to review deaths from injury, especially for infants and children
Public authority involvement by police, district attorneys, and courts
Epidemiological tracking and evaluation of violence
Handgun control

TERTIARY PREVENTION—GOAL: REEDUCATION AND REHABILITATION OF VIOLENT FAMILIES

Individuals

Empowerment strategies for battered women
Professional counseling services for individuals

Family

Parenting reeducation (i.e., formal training in child rearing)
Professional counseling services for families
Self-help groups

Community

Foster homes, shelters, and care for older adults
Public authority involvement
Follow-up care for known cases of abuse
Gun control

From Stevenson L, Pappas A: Violence. In Nies MA, McEwen M, editors: *Community/public health nursing: promoting the health of populations*, ed 4, pp. 555-578, St Louis, 2007, Saunders.

TABLE **12-5** Common Health Problems in Infants and Children

DISEASE/CONDITION	DEFINITION/ETIOLOGY	PREVENTION STRATEGIES	SIGNS AND SYMPTOMS/ COMPLICATIONS	MANAGEMENT/TREATMENT
Acute Respiratory/Ear, Nose, and Throat Conditions				
Viral infection (e.g., cold, influenza)	*Cold:* caused by up to 200 virus strains. *Incubation:* 1-7 days (usually 2-3 days). Children have 6-10 colds/year, decreasing with age.	Avoid exposure. Wash hands carefully; avoid touching nose or eyes with contaminated fingers. Influenza may be prevented or lessened with vaccination. Those in high-risk groups should be immunized yearly. Amantidine and remantadine may be used prophylactically in high-risk groups and during epidemics of influenza A.	*Cold:* nasal stiffness, sneezing, scratchy throat, coughing, malaise, headache, slight fever. *Influenza:* sudden onset of moderate-to-high fever (102° or higher), chills, headache, anorexia, malaise, muscle aches, cough, runny nose, sore throat, cervical lymphadenopathy, hoarseness, possible abdominal pain, vomiting, nausea, diarrhea. *Complications:* otitis media, pneumonia, bronchitis, and sinusitis are most common.	*Medications:* analgesics and antipyetics (avoid aspirini), decongestants, antitussives. *Symptom management:* bed rest, oral hydration. Observe for complications.
Bacterial pharyngitis (e.g., strep throat, tonsillitis)	*Strep throat:* caused by group A betahemolytic streptococci bacteria. Greatest incidence in children 5-18 years of age.	Avoid contact with respiratory secretions. Children should not return to school until after 24 hours of antibiotic therapy.	Sore throat, reddened throat, enlarged tonsils, soft palate petechiae, cervical adenopathy, fever (moderate-to-high), anorexia, chills, malaise, headache. Abdominal pain and vomiting may occur. *Complications:* Scarlet fever (red, papular rash beginning in the axilla and chest, spreading to the abdomen and extremities.) *Progressive complications:* rheumatic fever, glomerulonephritis, myocarditis.	Throat culture for suspected infection. For streptococcal pharyngitis, a 10-day course of penicillin is the standard. Erythromycin or cephalexin may be used for penicillin-allergic children. Teach parents the importance of completing the 10-day course of therapy. Monitor for complications.

Otitis media	Inflammation of the middle ear, usually bacterial. Almost 93% of children have one or more cases of the otitis media by age 7 years; 36% of children have six or more cases of otitis. Peak incidence is at 6-12 months; declines after age 7 years.	*Risk factors:* upper respiratory infection, smoking in household, family history of middle ear infections	Ear pain, decreased hearing, may have accompanying nasal discharge and cough, fever. *Infants:* irritability, may have slight fever. Otoscopic examination reveals decreased eardrum mobility, bulging eardrum redness. *Complications:* perforation of eardrum, hearing loss, scarring of eardrum, mastoiditis.	*Medications:* Amoxicillin, cephalosporin, Antihistamines and decongestants may be used but are not always effective. Referral for tympanostomy tubes and adenoidectomy for multiple infections, middle ear fluid that persists for 4-6 months, and/or hearing loss.
Respiratory infections: *bronchitis and pneumonia*	Inflammation and infection of the respiratory tract, usually as a secondary infection. May be caused by a virus or bacteria.	Vaccine is now recommended for all children to protect against bacterial pneumonia Monitor colds and influenza for complications and secondary infection.	Coughing—may be dry and hacking; nonproductive cough is common in bronchitis. Fever (may be mild to severe), chills, dyspnea, pulmonary rales and rhonchi, altered breath sounds, pleurisy, friction rub, headache. Tachypnea, malaise, wheezing.	Medications: antibiotics for bacterial bronchitis or pneumonia. Analgesics, antipyretics, cough suppressant.
Chronic Respiratory Diseases				
Asthma	Reversible airway disease characterized by bronchial constriction, mucosal edema, and increased mucous production.	*Avoidance of triggers:* allergens (e.g., pollens, molds, dust mites, animal dander), smoke and other pollutants, viral infections.	Abnormal pulmonary function tests, wheezing, cough, prolonged expiration, hyperresonance, decreased breath sounds, nocturnal dyspnea, cyanosis, use of accessory respiratory muscles.	*Medication:* steroids, beta-agonists, anticholinergics, theophylline; monitoring of peak expiratory flow rates (PEFR); Identify and eliminate irritants.

Continued

TABLE **12-5** Common Health Problems in Infants and Children—cont'd

DISEASE/CONDITION	DEFINITION/ETIOLOGY	PREVENTION STRATEGIES	SIGNS AND SYMPTOMS/COMPLICATIONS	MANAGEMENT/TREATMENT
Vaccine-Preventable Diseases				
Measles (rubeola)	Highly contagious, acute viral infection; incubation 8-12 days postexposure. Contagious from 1-2 days before symptoms to 4 days after onset of rash.	Vaccine-preventable. Postexposure prophylaxis-vaccine is protective if given within 72 hours postexposure; immune globulin prevents/modifies illness if given within 6 days postexposure.	*Prodromal phase:* fever and cold-like symptoms, conjunctivitis, photophobia, nasal congestion, cough, Koplik spots (small white spots circumscribed in red, opposite lower molars). *Acute phase:* rash begins as fever peaks; dark red, maculopapular rash begins behind ears and at hairline and spreads from head to feet and lasts 10-15 days. Rash turns brown and scaly after 5-6 days. *Complications:* otitis media, bronchitis, and pneumonia are most common.	Bed rest, antitussives, antipyretics (avoid aspirin). *Notify Health Department.*
Mumps	Acute viral infection presenting with unilateral or bilateral parotitis. Incubation period 14-24 days; 85% of cases occur before age 15 years.	Vaccine-preventable.	Parotid pain and swelling in one or both glands. Swelling peaks in 1-3 days and lasts 3-7 days. Mild-to-moderate fever.	Analgesics for pain (avoid aspirin). Liquid or soft diet, warm or cold compresses for swelling. *Complications:* orchitis or epididymitis are fairly common in postpubertal boys. *Less common:* meningoencephalitis, nephritis, pancreatitis, and oophoritis.
Chicken pox	Highly contagious infections caused by the varicella zoster virus. Most commonly affects children 5-9 years of	Vaccine-preventable. Postexposure varicella zoster immune globulin may be given to high-risk children. Avoidance of exposure (communicability—1 day	*Prodromal stage:* slight fever, malaise, mild headache, and anorexia for first 24 hours. Rash begins on the trunk, spreads to face and then extremities.	Isolate child in home until vesicles have dried (usually 1 week after onset); decrease itching with antipruritic agent (e.g., calamine lotion),

Condition	Description	Prevention	Clinical Manifestations	Management
	age but can develop in any age. *Incubation period:* 13-17 days postexposure.	before eruption of lesions until all vesicles have crusted).	Lesions may develop on oral and vaginal mucous membranes. Lesions begin as macules and rapidly progress to papule, then vesicle and present in varying degrees at one time	antihistamines, and oatmeal baths. Use mild antipyretics for fever but *avoid aspirin.*
Genitourinary Conditions				
Urinary tract infection (UTI)	Inflammation or infection of the urethra, bladder, or kidney. In neonates, UTIs are more common in boys; by 4 months, they are much more common in girls, and this continues throughout childhood. *Escherichia coli* causes 75%-90% of UTIs in children.	Good toileting hygiene (e.g., teaching girls to wipe from front to back); encourage frequent emptying of bladder; use cotton underpants. Avoid bubble baths.	Urinary urgency and frequency, burning, lower abdominal pain and cramping, hematuria, foul-smelling urine, fever. High fever and flank pain may indicate kidney infection. Recurrent infections may indicate renal anomalies and referral for diagnostic evaluation is very important.	*Medications:* antibiotics based on culture/sensitivity. A 7- to 10-day course of trimethoprim-sulfamethoxazole (TMP/SMZ) or amoxicillin is usually given. Stress the importance of completing all medications.
Gastrointestinal Problems				
Colic	Excessive crying seen in young infants who are otherwise well. Believed to be caused by paroxysmal abdominal cramping. Colic affects 10%-25% of infants age 3 weeks to 3 months.	Milk allergy may contribute to some cases	Inconsolable crying, often more than 3 hours per day; fist clenching, arching back, and drawing up of legs; excessive flatus.	Use of a pacifier, gentle rhythmic motions (e.g., rocking, car rides), music. Usually subsides by 3 months of age. Changing the baby's formula or removing dairy products from the diet of the lactating mother may help. Give smaller, frequent feedings; burp during and after feedings; place infant upright after feeding; place prone over a warm towel, hot water bottle, re-covered heating pad. Emotional support and respite care for the primary caregiver is very important.

Continued

TABLE **12-5** Common Health Problems in Infants and Children—cont'd

DISEASE/CONDITION	DEFINITION/ETIOLOGY	PREVENTION STRATEGIES	SIGNS AND SYMPTOMS/ COMPLICATIONS	MANAGEMENT/TREATMENT
Gastroenteritis/ stomach flu	In the United States, most cases of nausea, vomiting, and diarrhea are caused by viruses (rotavirus, parvovirus, adenovirus, and coronavirus). Symptoms usually occur 1-2 days after exposure.	Good handwashing, avoidance of exposure.	Nausea, vomiting, diarrhea, abdominal pain and distention, anorexia, malaise. Usually self-limiting, lasting 1-3 days. Dehydration in infants and small children may occur rapidly, however, and parents need to observe for fever, increasing thirst; decreasing urine production, sunken eyes or fontanel, diminished skin turgor, lethargy, cool extremities.	Replacement of fluids and electrolytes by encouraging consumption of clear liquids, such as uncaffeinated beverages, broth, flavored gelatin, water, or rehydration fluids (e.g., Pedialyte, Gatorade). As nausea and diarrhea decrease, slowly add mild foods, such as saltines, dry toast, rice, baked potato; avoid dairy products, most fruits, vegetables, meats. Hospitalization for intravenous rehydration may be necessary in severe cases.
Hepatitis A	Hepatitis A (infectious hepatitis) is the most common form of acute viral hepatitis. The virus is spread through the fecal-oral route directly or indirectly through ingestion of contaminated food or water. The highest incidence occurs among preschool and school-aged children. Incubation is approximately 4 weeks	Vaccine is available. Immune globulin for postexposure (given 1-2 weeks after exposure prevents illness in 80%-90% of individuals). Use proper handwashing.	Usually rapid onset of fever, malaise, nausea, anorexia, jaundice, dark urine, abdominal pain. *Complications:* rare.	Supportive/Symptomatic care: children should not return to school until jaundice has resolved and serum enzyme levels are no more than twice normal. Household contacts should be given immune globulin.
Pinworms (*Enterobium vermicularis*)	The most common helminthic infection in the United States, infecting about one third of all U.S. children at any one time.	Prevention of reinfection involudes treating all family members with 2 doses of medication 2 weeks apart. Washing all sleeping garments and bed linen in hot water and vacuuming	Intense perianal itching, particularly nocturnal, poor sleep, restlessness, enuresis, and distractibility.	*Tape test:* to diagnose, parents must press transparent tape firmly against the child's perianal area as soon as the child awakens in the morning. The tape is placed in a container and taken to a clinic

	Description/Cause	Prevention/Teaching	Signs and Symptoms	Treatment/Medication
	Predominant age is 5-14 years, with girls being more frequently infected than boys. More common in warm climates and crowded living conditions.	around the beds may be helpful. Careful, thorough handwashing after toileting and before eating and daily showering may also help.		for microscopic examination. *Medication:* Mebendazole (Vermox) is used to treat all family members (not recommended for children under 2 years or pregnant women).
Infectious diarrhea	Diarrhea and related symptoms are frequently caused by bacteria or parasites, in addition to viral gastrointestinal conditions described above. *Bacteria include E. coli; Staphylococcus, Salmonella,* and *Shigella* species; *Campylobacter jejuni; Vibrio cholerae;* and *Yersinia enterocolitica.* Parasitic organisms include *Giardia* species, *Cryptosporidium* species.	Source is typically contaminated food or water. Symptoms usually occur within a few hours of exposure. See Chapter 7 for information on food preparation and clean water. Good handwashing (particularly following toileting and changing diapers) is essential.	Symptoms vary somewhat based on causative organism. Severe, watery diarrhea; abdominal cramps, nausea, vomiting; headache; anorexia, malaise. Stools may contain blood or mucus. With *Giardia* species, pale greasy stools; fatigue; and weight loss are seen. Observe for signs and symptoms of dehydration (see above).	*Medication:* antibiotics appropriate for the organism. Symptomatic treatment (see above).
Constipation	Stool is passed infrequently or consists of hard, small masses. Cause is usually dietary, such as too much milk or insufficient fluids or bulk-forming foods. More common in boys 1-5 years of age, although not uncommon in infants.	Good dietary practices, including recommended servings of fruits, vegetables, and grain products. Prunes or prune juice may help infants and small children who have hard stools. Encourage drinking noncaffeinated, noncarbonated fluid and good elimination patterns.	Infrequent hard stools, pain or difficulty during defecation. Chronic constipation may be caused by underlying conditions (e.g., anorectal malformation, Hirschprung's disease, endocrine disorder or side effect of medication [e.g., iron]). Referral for evaluation may be indicated.	Occasional constipation in infants may be treated with glycerin suppositories, but caution parents not to overuse. Stool softener, such as docusate sodium (Colace), may be prescribed. Laxatives and cathartics are generally not recommended. Promote good toileting and dietary changes.

Continued

TABLE **12-5** Common Health Problems in Infants and Children—cont'd

DISEASE/CONDITION	DEFINITION/ETIOLOGY	PREVENTION STRATEGIES	SIGNS AND SYMPTOMS/ COMPLICATIONS	MANAGEMENT/TREATMENT
		Dermatologic Disorders		
Diaper dermatitis	Caused by irritation in the diaper area.	Change diapers frequently; use of ointments and periodically exposing the diaper area to air may help prevent. Wash cloth diapers in mild soap and rinse thoroughly. Avoid commercial wipes.	Redness and irritation in the diaper area.	
Impetigo	A superficial skin infection usually caused by *Staphylococcus aureus* or group A streptococci. Most common bacterial skin infection in children. Predominate age, 2-5 years. Most often occurring in hot, humid climates.	Good hygiene. Discourage children from scratching scabs or insect bites. Keep fingernails short and clean.	Begins as an erythematous papule, which progesses to a vesicle and crusts over. Pustules most frequently occur on face (around mouth or nose) or at a site of skin breakage (scratch or insect bite). Often multiple sites or satellite lesions occur. May be a complication of scabies, chicken pox, pediculosis, or eczema.	*Medication:* erythromycin cephalosporins, topical antibiotic ointments. Encourage cleanliness; wash areas two or three times per day with diluted antibacterial soap; wash linens and clothing separately from other family members' (this may need to be done daily until lesions have resolved). Exclude from school or day care until after antibiotics have been administered for 24 hours. Monitor for signs of spread.
Pediculosis	Infestation of lice—*Pediculus humanus capitis* (head lice) is the most common type of lice found in children. Whites, Asians, Hispanics, and Native Americans are most commonly affected, and girls are more commonly affected than boys.	Lice are transmitted by close personal contact. Encourage children to avoid sharing objects such as combs, brushes, hats, and clothing with other children. May also be transmitted through bed linen and upholstered chairs.	Nits (egg cases) are white spheres on the hair shaft. Nits are found most often on the back of the head and neck and behind the ears and are "glued" to the shaft and thus cannot be moved (distinguishing them from dandruff). Adult lice are small black specks that move and jump on the scalp and hair. Itching is very common. Eyelashes may be involved.	*Medication:* Lindane (Kwell) or permethrin (Nix) shampoo. Treat entire family. After treatment, remove nits with a nit comb. Wash all linens, brushes, combs, and hats in hot water. (Infants and pregnant women should not use Lindane.) Exclude from school or day care until treated.

	Description	Prevention	Clinical	Medication
Scabies	Skin infestation by the mite *Sarcoptes scabiei.* Most common in children and young adults.	Good general hygiene.	Generalized itching, which is often worse at night. Burrows are commonly found in finger webs, wrists, hands, feet, penis, scrotum, buttocks, and waistline. Vesicles and pustules may be evident if infection occurs.	*Medication:* Permethrin (Elimite cream), Lindane (Kwell), or Crotamiton (Eurax) cream or lotions are applied into the skin from the head to the soles of feet and left on for 8-14 hours, then thoroughly washed off. A second application 48 hours later is usually recommended. Treat all family members. Wash clothing, bed linen, and towels.
Ringworm (fungal infections of the skin)	Refers to several re-lated fungi infections. Comonly infected are the scalp (*Tinea capitis*), body (*Tinea pedis*), and groin (*Tinea cruris*—jock itch)	Associated with confined living quarters, poor hygiene. May become epidemic in schools and day care centers. Good personal hygiene and avoidance of sharing clothing, shoes, brushes, and combs can stop the spread. Identification and treatment of infected individuals and household pets are important.	Although some variation occurs depending on the site, lesions usually appear as round, raised, rough patches. May spread. Itching is very common.	*Medications:* Topical administration of antifungal agents. Encourage good hygenic pratices.
Acne	The most common skin disorder, acne is an inflammatory disorder of the sebaceous glands resulting in progression of comedones (white-heads, blackheads), to papules, inflammatory pustules. Scarring occasionally occurs. Acne most commonly affects adolescents during early to later puberty.	Diet probably has little effect on acne. Good nutrition and adequate sleep and exercise are beneficial.	Presence of comedones (whitehead and black-heads). Inflammatory lesions, including papules, pustules, and nodules occur. Most often affected are the face, upper chest, and upper back.	*Medications:* Topical medications such as benzoyl peroxide and topical erythromycin are helpful for milder cases. Low-dose oral tetracycline, erythromycin, and oral contraceptives can be effective in more severe acne. Isotretinoin (Accutane) may also help. Good skin care should always include daily washing with a mild soap.

Data from Hockenberry MJ, Wilson D: *Wong's nursing care of infants and children,* ed 8, St Louis, 2007, Mosby; Dambro MR: *Griffith's 5-minute clinical consult,* Philadelphia, 2006, Lippincott Williams & Wilkins; James SW, Ashwill JW: *Child health nursing: principles and practice,* ed 3, St Louis, 2007, Saunders.

matches away from children, having ipecac available), can be life saving. Furthermore, they understand that establishing healthy habits (e.g., good nutrition, dental hygiene, regular exercise) and failing to establish poor habits (e.g., smoking, drug and alcohol use) while in childhood can improve the quality and length of the individual's life.

This chapter has presented a great deal of information regarding health promotion and illness prevention for infants, children, and adolescents.

KEY POINTS

- The leading causes of mortality for infants are congenital anomalies, low birth weight, SIDS, and respiratory distress syndrome. After 1 year of age and through adolescence, the leading causes of death are unintentional injury, cancer, and homicide. In teenagers, suicide is added to the list.
- The leading causes of acute illness in children are respiratory conditions (e.g., colds, influenza, respiratory infections), other infections (e.g., viral infections, intestinal virus), acute ear infection, and injuries. Major chronic conditions are respiratory conditions (e.g., allergic rhinitis, asthma, chronic bronchitis); skin conditions (e.g., acne, dermatitis); musculoskeletal conditions; and vision, speech, and hearing impairment.
- Several federal- and state-sponsored health programs and services are available for disadvantaged, underserved, and disabled children. These include Medicaid, EPSDT, SCHIP, WIC, Head Start, and PL 94-142 (Education for All Handicapped Children Act).
- Screening guidelines and recommendations are available for infants and children to test for genetic, congenital, developmental, and pathological problems and conditions. These include routine infant screenings (e.g., testing of newborns for phenylketonuria, congenital hypothyroidism), body measurement (height, weight, and head circumference), developmental screening, vision screening, hearing screening, lead screening, and screening for anemia.
- Health-promotion activities for infants, children, and adolescents include nutrition education and counseling on nutrition, physical activity, and

exercise; sleep and rest patterns; dental health; and maturation and puberty.

- Illness prevention should include information on prevention of substance (drugs and alcohol) use and abuse, prevention of use of tobacco products, and safety issues (e.g., vehicle safety, poisoning, head injury prevention, drowning prevention, and prevention of fire and burns).
- Detection and prevention of child abuse are very important in community-based nursing practice, and nurses should be knowledgeable about patterns of abuse, how to identify suspected abuse, and how and when to intervene.

Learning Activities & Application to Practice
In Class
1. Discuss the *Healthy People 2010* objectives for infants, preschool children, school-aged children, and adolescents. What can nurses in communities do to help meet the objectives?

In Clinical
2. Observe and assist in completion of an EPSDT screening.
3. Observe and assist in collecting blood samples for routine infant screenings. Ensure that agency protocols are carefully followed.
4. Complete a developmental screening, such as the Denver II, on two or three children of differing ages. Share results with the clinical group.
5. Complete a "child safety home checklist" for a family encountered during clinical or for a neighbor or friend. Share findings and suggestions or recommendations for change with the clinical group.

REFERENCES

Advocates for Highway and Auto Safety (2005): *Motorcycle helmets: fact sheet* (website): http://www.saferoads.org/issues/fs-helmets.htm. Accessed October 26, 2007.

Agency for Healthcare Research and Quality (2004): *Care of children and adolescents in U.S. hospitals: HCUP fact book No 4* (online): http://www.ahrq.gov/data/hcup/factbk4/factbk4.htm. Accessed October 22, 2007.

Agency for Healthcare Research and Quality: *Guide to clinical preventive services,* 2007. recommendations from the U.S. Preventive Services Task Force (online): http://www.ahrq.gov/clinic/pocketgd.htm. Accessed October 26, 2007.

American Dental Association (2007): *Mouthguards* (website): http://www.ada.org/public/topics/mouthguards.asp. Accessed October 25, 2007.

American Dental Association (2005): *Flouride and fluoridation* (website): http://www.ada.org/public/topics/fluoride/index.asp. Accessed October 12, 2007.

American Dental Association (2005): *Baby's first teeth* (website): http://www.ada.org/prof/resources/pubs/jada/patient/patient_11.pdf. Accessed October 12, 2007.

Ashwill JW, Droske SC: *Nursing care of children*, Philadelphia, 1997, Saunders.

Carson VB, Smith-DiJulio K: Family violence. In Varcarolis EM, Carson VB, Shoemaker NC, editors: *Foundations of psychiatric mental health nursing*, ed 5, St Louis, 2006, Saunders.

Centers for Disease Control and Prevention: Injury-control recommendations: bicycle helmets, *MMWR Morb Mortal Wkly Rep* 44(RR-1):1, 1995.

Centers for Disease Control and Prevention: Achievements in public health, 1900-1999: fluoridation of drinking water to prevent dental caries, *MMWR Morb Mortal Wkly Rep* 48(41):933, 1999.

Centers for Disease Control and Prevention (2005a): *Pediatric nutrition surveillance* (website): http://www.cdc.gov/pednss/pednss_tables/pdf/national_table18.pdf. Accessed October 9, 2007.

Centers for Disease Control and Prevention/U.S. Department of Health and Human Services (2005b): *Preventing dental caries* (website): http://www.cdc.gov/nccdphp/publications/factsheets/Prevention/pdf/oh.pdf. Accessed October 12, 2007.

Centers for Disease Control and Prevention (2005c): *Child maltreatment: fact sheet* (website): http://www.cdc.gov/ncipc/factsheets/cmfacts.htm. Accessed October 15, 2007.

Centers for Disease Control and Prevention (2006a): *About BMI for children and teens* (website): http://www.cdc.gov/nccdphp/dnpa/bmi/childrens_BMI/about_childrens_BMI.htm. Accessed October 9, 2007.

Centers for Disease Control and Prevention (2006b): Youth risk behavior surveillance–2005, *MMWR Morb Mortal Wkly Rep* 55(SS-5):1-112, 2006.

Centers for Disease Control and Prevention (2007a): *Overweight and obesity* (website): http://www.cdc.gov/nccdphp/dnpa/obesity/childhood/. Accessed October 12, 2007.

Centers for Disease Control and Prevention (2007b): *Sudden infant death syndrome* (website): http://www.cdc.gov/SIDS/. Accessed October 12, 2007.

Centers for Disease Control and Prevention (2007c): *Smoking and tobacco use* (website): http://www.cdc.gov/tobacco/data_statistics/Factsheets/youth_tobacco.htm. Accessed October 14, 2007.

Center for Medicare and Medicaid Services (2007): *State children's health program* (website): http://www.cms.hhs.gov/home/schip.asp. Accessed October 21, 2007.

Dambro MR: *Griffith's 5-minute clinical consult*, ed 7, Philadelphia, 2006, Lippincott Williams & Wilkins.

Daniels SR, Arnett DK, Eckel RH, et al: Overweight in children and adolescents: pathophysiology, consequences, prevention, and treatment, *Circulation* 111:1999, 2005.

Feldstein PJ: *Health policy issues: an economic perspective*, ed 3, Chicago, 2003, Health Administration Press.

Frankenburg WK, Dodds JB: *DENVER II: Training manual*, Denver, 1990, Denver Developmental Materials, Inc.

Health Resources and Services Administration (2007): *EPSDT and Title V collaboration to improve child health* (website): http://www.hrsa.gov/epsdt/default.htm. Accessed October 22, 2007.

Health Resources and Services Administration/Maternal Child Health Bureau (2005): *Newborn screening: toward a uniform screening panel and system*; executive summary (website): http://mchb.hrsa.gov/screening/summary.htm. Accessed October 22, 2007.

Health Resources and Services Administration/ Maternal Child Health Bureau (2003): *Child health USA: 2003* (website): http://www.mchb.hrsa.gov/chusa03/index.htm. Accessed October 25, 2007.

Hockenberry MJ, Wilson D: *Wong's nursing care of infants and children*, ed 8, St Louis, 2007, Mosby.

Kovner AR, Knickman JR: *Jonas and Kovner's health care delivery in the United States*, ed 8, New York, 2005, Springer.

Langford DR: Violence: A social and family problem. In Maurer FA, Smith CM, editors: *Community/public health nursing: health for families and populations*, ed 3, St Louis, 2005, Saunders.

Linton CP, Kaplan NS: Hematological alterations. In Potts NL, Mandleco BL, editors: *Pediatric nursing: caring for children and their families*, ed 2, Scarborough, Ontario, Canada, 2007, Delmar.

Lobstein T, Baur L, Uauy R: Obesity in children and young people: a crisis in public health, electronic *Obes Rev* 5(Suppl. 1):4, 2004.

Mills DA, Woodring BC: Growth and development of the toddler. In Potts NL, Mandleco BL, editors: *Pediatric nursing: caring for children and their families*, ed 2, Scarborough, Ontario, Canada, 2006, Delmar.

Murray RB, Zentner JP: *Nursing assessment and health promotion: strategies through the life span*, ed 7, Norwalk, Conn, 2001, Appleton & Lange.

National Center for Health Statistics (2004a): *Deaths: preliminary data for 2004* (website): http://www.cdc.gov/nchs/data/nvsr/nvsr54/nvsr54_19.pdf. Accessed October 15, 2007.

National Center for Health Statistics (2004b): *Infant health* (website): http://www.cdc.gov/nchs/fastats/infant_health.htm. Accessed October 9, 2007.

National Center for Health Statistics (2006): *National ambulatory medical care survey: 2004 summary* (website): http://www.cdc.gov/nchs/data/ad/ad374.pdf. Accessed October 22, 2007.

National Center for Health Statistics (2007): *Health United States, 2006* (website): http://www.cdc.gov/nchs/hus.htm. Accessed October 23, 2007.

National Center for Health Statistics (2007b): United States life tables, 2003, *National Vital Statistics Report* 54(14):1, Washington, DC, 2007, Public Health Service.

National Center for Injury Prevention and Control (2007a): *Nonfatal injury reports* (website): http://webappa.cdc.gov/cgi-bin/broker.exe. Accessed October 15, 2007.

National Center for Injury Prevention and Control (2007b): *Fatal injury reports* (website): http://www.cdc.gov/ncipc/wisqars/default.htm. Accessed October 15, 2007.

National Institute of Diabetes and Digestive and Kidney Diseases (2005): *Statistics related to overweight and obesity* (website): http//win.niddk.nih.gov/statistics/index.htm. Accessed February 6, 2005.

National Newborn Screening and Genetics Resource Center (2007): *National screening act sheets and algorithms* (website): http://genes-r-us.uthscsa.edu/. Accessed October 22, 2007.

Olshansky SJ, Passaro DJ, Hershow RC et al: A potential decline in life expectancy in the United States in the 21st century, *N Engl J Med* 352:1138, 2005.

Pourciau CA, Vallette EC: School health. In Nies MA, McEwen M, editors: *Community/public health nursing: promoting the health of populations*, ed 4, St Louis, 2007, Saunders.

Ripa LW: A half-century of community water fluoridation in the United States: review and commentary, *J Public Health Dent* 53(1):17, 1993.

Selekman J: *Pediatric nursing*, Springhouse, Pa, 1993, Springhouse.

Stevenson L, Pappas A: Violence. In Nies MA, McEwen M, editors: *Community/public health nursing: promoting the health of populations*, ed 4, St Louis, 2007, Saunders.

U.S. Department of Agriculture/Food and Consumer Service (2006): *Nutrition program facts: food and nutrition services* (website): http://www.fns.usda.gov/wic/WIC-Fact-Sheet.pdf. Accessed October 9, 2007.

U.S. Department of Health and Human Services: *Healthy people 2010*: conference ed, Washington, DC, 2000, Government Printing Office.

U.S. Department of Health and Human Services (2007): *Overweight and obesity: a vision for the future* (website): http://www.surgeongeneral.gov/topics/obesity/calltoaction/fact_vision.htm. Accessed October 12, 2007.

U.S. Department of Health and Human Services/Office of Disease Prevention and Health Promotion: *Clinician's handbook of preventive services*, ed 2, Washington, DC, 1998, Government Printing Office.

U.S. Department of Health and Human Services/Public Health Services: *Clinician's handbook of preventive services*, ed 2, McLean, Va, 1999, International Medical Publishing.

Vincent JL: Growth and development of the infant. In Potts NL, Mandleco BL: *Pediatric nursing: caring for children and their families*, ed 2, Scarborough, Ontario, Canada, 2007, Delmar.

Chapter 13

Health Promotion and Illness Prevention for Adults

objectives

Upon completion of this chapter, the reader will be able to:

1. Discuss the importance of health-promotion activities in positively influencing the health of adults.

2. Describe the health benefits of regular exercise, and give an example of a recommended exercise program.

3. Discuss problems related to being overweight and obese, and explain basic components of a healthy diet.

4. Describe problems associated with tobacco use, and cite ways to avoid smoking initiation and tips for smoking cessation.

5. Discuss risk factors for heart disease and stroke, and provide ways to minimize them.

6. Discuss risk factors, screening recommendations, and treatment options for the most common types of cancer.

7. Discuss risk factors for diabetes, and describe prevention and management strategies.

key terms

Health promotion	Physical activity and fitness
Illness prevention	Screening
Obesity	Smoking cessation

See Glossary for definitions.

case study

Ben Rogers is a staff nurse at a cardiac rehabilitation center in an urban area. The cardiac center provides comprehensive care to clients with heart disease and services to prevent heart disease. Ben's responsibilities at the center involve assisting in prevention, diagnosis, monitoring, and rehabilitation of cardiovascular disease in adults.

On Monday Ben saw Mr. Ryan, a 50-year-old bank vice president. Although he has never had symptoms indicating a heart condition, Mr. Ryan was referred to the center by his internist because during a recent physical examination, he was determined to be at risk for developing coronary artery disease.

Continued

At the cardiac center each client initially completes a health history and questionnaires that assess known risk factors for heart disease. Among the findings from Mr. Ryan's completed assessments are that he is approximately 30 pounds heavier than the ideal for his height, smokes one to one and a half packs of cigarettes a day (he has cut down from more than two packs a day during the past year), rarely engages in strenuous physical activity, drinks alcohol occasionally, and reports moderate stress in his life. He eats a variety of foods, but admits that he probably eats too many snacks and prefers sweets and bread to fruits and vegetables. He has no history of hypertension or diabetes and his serum cholesterol results over the past 5 years have remained steady, ranging from 200 to 220. He has a positive family history for heart disease. His mother died from a heart attack at age 65. Both grandfathers also died from heart attacks (ages at death unknown). His older brother has had no symptoms of heart disease. His father died in an automobile accident at age 45.

At the cardiac rehab center additional laboratory tests and diagnostic studies were performed to assess risk and determine if Mr. Ryan has evidence of coronary artery disease. Laboratory tests included a lipid profile to assess high-density and low-density lipoprotein values and ratios, an electrocardiogram, and a cardiac stress test. Ben assisted the physicians and technicians with these tests.

Fortunately Mr. Ryan's tests showed no evidence of previous myocardial infarction and no angina. Following the examinations, Ben worked with a team composed of a cardiologist, a dietitian, and an exercise therapist to develop a plan of action for Mr. Ryan to reduce his risk of developing heart disease. Their recommendations were as follows:

1. Stop smoking: Written information on methods to stop smoking was provided and discussed.
2. Dietary changes: Detailed literature on methods to lose weight and reduce dietary fat intake was provided and reviewed.
3. Increase physical activity: A program to improve physical fitness was presented. Detailed instructions to gradually increase daily exercise to at least 30 minutes, 4 to 5 days a week while increasing his heart rate to between 85 and 127 beats per minute were outlined.
4. Reduce stress: Stress management literature was provided. Stress avoidance, relaxation techniques, building supportive relationships, fatigue avoidance, and use of support groups were discussed with Mr. Ryan.
5. Medications: It was determined that Mr. Ryan would not be put on medication to reduce his cholesterol at this time. It was hoped that dietary management would be sufficient to reduce his cholesterol levels. His lipid profile was to be reassessed in 3 months to see if his total cholesterol and low-density versus high-density lipoprotein ratios had improved. Aspirin, 325 mg/day, was prescribed following determination that Mr. Ryan had no allergies or history of bleeding tendencies.

Mr. Ryan agreed to these recommendations, and reasonable goals for each area were set. Finally, he made an appointment to return to the cardiac center in 3 months to assess progress toward his goals.

Health promotion refers to those activities or actions related to encouraging individual lifestyles or personal choices that positively influence health. Physical activity and fitness, nutrition, and substance (e.g., tobacco, alcohol) use and abuse are examples of controllable behaviors or actions that ultimately affect health. In their practice all nurses, particularly those working in community settings, should be prepared for opportunities to assist clients (whether individuals, families, or groups) by providing information, counseling, advocacy, referral, or other interventions that allow the client to make informed choices to promote health.

Primary and secondary prevention refer to those interventions, such as counseling, **screening**, immunization, and education, that directly affect health to prevent acute or chronic disease or disability. This chapter contains assessment and teaching tools and information specific to these concepts. Initially, general health-promotion strategies such as assessment of health risks, promotion of exercise and physical fitness, improving nutrition, and reduction or elimination of harmful substances are described in the discussion of health promotion. Primary and secondary prevention, specifically with regard to several of the leading causes of death and disability (i.e., heart disease and stroke, cancer, and diabetes), are then considered.

CAUSES OF DEATH

Table 13-1 shows the leading causes of death in the United States. As depicted in this table, heart disease, cancer, cerebrovascular disease, and chronic lower respiratory diseases are the top four causes of death. Smoking—particularly cigarette smoking—is a risk factor strongly associated with each of these conditions. Smoking costs approximately $157 billion in annual health-related economic loss (CDC, 2004). In addition, diet and activity patterns were deemed to account for 16.6% of deaths (about 300,000 per year); alcohol contributes to about 3.5% (85,000) of all deaths because it is associated with a significant percentage of accidents, suicides, homicides, and cirrhosis and chronic liver disease (Mokdad, Marks, Stroup, & Gerberding, 2004).

HEALTH PROMOTION AND ILLNESS PREVENTION

Health promotion consists of activities directed toward increasing the level of well-being and actualizing the health potential of individuals, families, communities, and society (Pender, Murdaugh & Parsons, 2006). *Healthy People 2010* (U.S. Department of Health and Human Services [USDHHS], 2000a) identifies health-promotion strategies as those that relate to promoting positive individual lifestyles choices, including physical fitness and good nutrition and limiting or eliminating potentially harmful choices such as tobacco and alcohol use. Likewise, **illness prevention** strategies involve lessening or removing risk factors for specific diseases and early identification of diseases through screening and prompt remediation. Examples of goals in *Healthy*

TABLE **13-1** Estimated Deaths, Death Rates, and Percentage of Total Deaths for the 10 Leading Causes of Death: United States, 2004

CAUSE OF DEATH	RANK	NUMBER	DEATH RATE (PER 100,000)	TOTAL DEATH (%)
All Causes		2,397,615	816.5	100.0
Diseases of the heart	1	652,486	222.2	27.2
Malignant neoplasms	2	553,888	188.6	23.1
Cerebrovascular diseases	3	150,074	51.1	6.3
Chronic lower repiratory diseases	4	121,987	41.5	5.1
Accidents and unintentional injuries	5	112,012	38.1	4.7
Diabetes	6	73,138	24.9	3.1
Alzheimer's disease	7	65,965	22.5	2.8
Influenza and pneumonia	8	59,664	20.3	2.5
Nephritis, nephritic syndrome, and nephrosis	9	42,480	14.5	1.8
Septicemia	10	33,373	11.4	1.4
All other causes	—	414,674	141.2	17.3

From National Center for Health Statistics: Deaths: final data for 2004, *National Vital Statistics Reports* 55(19):1-120, 2007 (electronic version online): http://www.cdc.gov/nchs/data/nvsr/nvsr55/nvsr55_19.pdf.

People 2010 for health promotion and illness prevention are included in the *Healthy People 2010* box.

ASSESSMENT OF HEALTH RISKS AND HEALTH HABITS

To apply the nursing process to health promotion and illness prevention, nurses should begin with assessment. In addition to individual physical, functional, and cognitive assessments that are routinely accomplished, an assessment of behaviors and habits that influence health is also important. An understanding of the client's health beliefs, knowledge, and health habits (both positive and negative) will help the nurse plan appropriate interventions. Appendix B is an example of a tool for general assessment of health risks, lifestyles, and beliefs.

As positive health practices and potential threats to health are identified, nurses can assist individuals, families, and groups by developing plans and programs to promote health and prevent illness. Areas to target should relate to the most common, preventable causes of morbidity and mortality, based on risk factors and identified and potential health threats. This includes such areas as diet, tobacco use, exercise, obesity, substance use, and others. Table 13-2 depicts the relationships among various risk factors and the 10 leading causes of death. The remainder of this chapter describes specific assessments and risk-reduction techniques and provides educational materials and information to equip nurses to assist clients in reducing risks and promoting health. Additional information addressing prevention of problems related to alcohol and substance abuse is provided in Chapter 18, and information addressing prevention of communicable diseases and adult immunizations is provided in Chapter 19.

PHYSICAL ACTIVITY AND FITNESS

Physical activity and fitness are important to good health. The health benefits of regular exercise and physical activity have been thoroughly researched and documented. Indeed, it has been observed that moderate, regular exercise for about half an hour each day, three times a week, can significantly lower death rates for many causes, including cancer and cardiovascular disease (The President's Council on Physical Fitness & Sports, 2007).

Exercise training positively affects health by increasing cardiovascular functional capacity and decreasing myocardial oxygen demand. Exercise helps control blood lipid abnormalities, diabetes, and obesity and can help lower blood pressure. Potential protective benefits from regular physical activity include lowered resting heart rate, more blood pumped with each beat, reduced blood pressure, increased high-density lipoprotein, and improved carbohydrate metabolism. In addition, regular activity helps control weight, increases lean body mass, decreases body fat percentage, produces relief from some symptoms of depression, improves flexibility, increases muscle strength and endurance, and increases bone density. These benefits help reduce or minimize other health threats such as arthritis, diabetes, and osteoporosis (American College of Sports Medicine [ACSM]/American Heart Association [AHA], 2007).

Despite the known benefits, levels of physical activity among Americans remain low. In 2005 23.7% of adults reported no physical leisure-time activity. Women tend to be less active than men, and members of racial and ethnic minorities are more inactive than whites, with those of lower socio-economic levels being less active than those of higher socioeconomic levels (USDHHS/Office of Disease Prevention and Health Promotion [ODPHP], 2007).

The ACSM/AHA (2007) states that persons of all ages should include physical activity as part of a comprehensive health program. A health care provider should be consulted before starting an exercise program, however, if an individual: (1) has been sedentary for a long period of time, (2) is overweight, (3) has a high risk of coronary heart disease, or (4) has a chronic health problem (AHA, 2007a).

An exercise program should be vigorous enough to increase the heart rate to 50% to 80% of the maximum heart rate (220 minus your age). The AHA (2007a) suggests a combination of low-intensity activities and/or moderate intensity activities for 30-60 minutes on most days of the week (4 to 5 times per week). Activities such as walking, hiking, stair climbing, aerobic exercise, jogging, running,

Examples of Objectives for Health Promotion and Illness Prevention for Adults

OBJECTIVE	BASELINE (1998)	TARGET
1.5: Increase the proportion of persons with a usual primary care provider	77%	85%
3.10a: Increase the proportion of physicians (interns) who counsel their at-risk patients about tobacco use cessation	50%	85%
3.13: Increase the proportion of women aged 40 years and older who have received a mammogram within the preceding 2 years	68%	70%
5.4: Increase the proportion of adults with diabetes whose condition has been diagnosed	65%	80%
7.6: Increase the proportion of employees who participate in employer-sponsored health-promotion activities	28%	50%
11.2: Improve the health literacy of persons with inadequate or marginal literacy skills	NA	NA
12.12: Increase the proportion of adults who have had their blood pressure measured within the preceding 2 years and can state whether their blood pressure was normal or high	90%	95%
12.15: Increase the proportion of adults who have had their blood cholesterol checked within the preceding 5 years	68%	80%
15.19: Increase use of safety belts	69%	92%
19.2: Reduce the proportion of adults who are obese	23%	15%
19.8: Increase the proportion of persons aged 2 years and older who consume less than 10% of calories from saturated fat	36%	75%
20.3: Reduce the rate of injury and illness cases involving days away from work from overexertion or repetitive motion	675 injuries per 100,000 workers	338 injuries per 10,000 workers
21.7: Increase the proportion of adults who, in the past 12 months, report having had an examination to detect oral and pharyngeal cancer	14%	35%
22.2: Increase the proportion of adults who engage regularly, preferably daily, in moderate physical activity for at least 30 minutes per day	15%	30%
22.5: Increase the proportion of adults who perform physical activities that enhance and maintain flexibility	30%	40%
26.13: Reduce the proportion of adults who exceed guidelines for low-risk drinking	73%	50%
27.1a: Reduce tobacco use (cigarette smoking) by adults	24%	12%

SIDS, Sudden infant death syndrome.
From U.S. Department of Health and Human Services: *Healthy people 2010,* Conference ed, Washington, DC, 2000, Government Printing Office.

TABLE **13-2** Relationship Between Risk Factors and 10 Leading Causes of Death

CAUSE OF DEATH	PERCENT OF TOTAL DEATHS	SMOKING	HIGH-FAT, LOW-FIBER DIET	SEDENTARY LIFESTYLE	HIGH BLOOD PRESSURE	ELEVATED CHOLESTEROL	OBESITY	DIABETES	ALCOHOL ABUSE
Heart Disease	27.2	X	X	X	X	X	X	X	X
Cancer	23.1	X	X	X			X		X
Stroke	6.3	X	X		X	X	X		
COPD	5.1	X							
Unintentional Injury	4.7	X							X
Diabetes	3.1		X	X			X	X	
Alzheimer's	2.8		X	X					
Pneumonia and influenza	2.5	X							
Kidney disease	1.8	X			X	X	X	X	X
Septicemia	1.4						X	X	

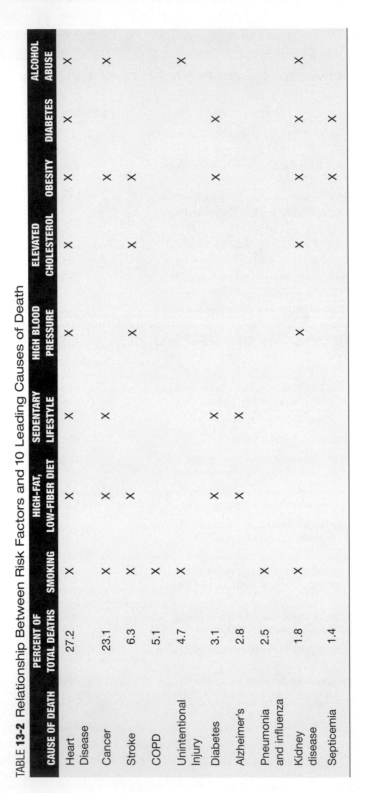

bicycling, rowing, swimming, and sports such as tennis, racquetball, soccer, and basketball are particularly beneficial in improving cardiac fitness. In addition to using aerobic exercises to enhance cardiac fitness, the AHA suggests adding resistance weight training for a minimum of 2 days per week. In addition, the DHHS/ODPHP (1998) suggests that physical activity programs should be as follows:

1. Medically safe (e.g., following physician's advice if one of the risk factors listed previously is a possibility; increasing activities gradually; use of stretching exercise to decrease the risk of musculoskeletal injuries)
2. Enjoyable (e.g., varying activities, exercising with friends or family)
3. Convenient (e.g., flexible, nearby, requiring a minimum of special preparation)
4. Realistic (e.g., gradual increases in intensity, frequency, and duration)
5. Minimally structured (Schedules and goals should be set and maintained when possible, but some flexibility is important because very structured programs may reduce compliance.)

NUTRITION AND WEIGHT CONTROL

Good nutritional practices and maintenance of a desirable weight are essential for good health. However, maintenance of a desirable weight is becoming difficult in the United States, where overweight and obesity are rapidly growing problems. It is estimated that nearly 66% of the U.S. adult population is overweight or obese. The rate of obesity has increased more than 50% in the last two decades, and approximately 25% of U.S. adult females and 20% of adult males are obese (CDC, 2007a). As with children, overweight and obesity in adults is determined by the body mass index (BMI), a number calculated by using weight and height. Table 13-3 presents an example of the BMI designations (normal weight, overweight, obesity) for an adult who is 5′9″ (CDC, 2007b).

Often, the terms overweight and obese are used interchangeably; indeed both indicate a higher weight than is considered to be healthy for a given height, but there are some subtle differences in the use of these terms. An adult who has a BMI between 25 and 29.9 is considered to be overweight.

TABLE **13-3** Example of BMI Designation for Weight Classification

HEIGHT	WEIGHT RANGE	BMI	CONSIDERED
5′ 9″	124 lbs or less	Below 18.5	Underweight
	125 lbs to 168 lbs	18.5 to 24.9	Healthy weight
	169 lbs to 202 lbs	25 to 29.9	Overweight
	203 lbs or more	30 or higher	Obese

From Centers for Disease Control and Prevention (2007): *Defining overweight and obesity* (website): http://www.cdc.gov/nccdphp/dnpa/obesity/defining.htm. Accessed October 19, 2007.

An adult with a BMI of 30 or higher is considered to be obese. These weight ranges have been shown to correlate with an increase in the risk of disease or other health problems. "Obese" is a term that is used to refer to adults or to groups of children. The term is not used to indicate the weight status of a single child.

As a risk factor, **obesity** (BMI of 30 or higher) is associated with hypertension, type 2 diabetes, hypercholesterolemia, coronary artery disease, some types of cancer, gallbladder disease, arthritis, sleep apnea, and stroke. Overweight or obese adults are found in all population groups, but obesity is particularly common among Hispanic, black, Native American, and Pacific Islander women. People residing in the south Atlantic states (West Virginia, North and South Carolina, and Georgia), the east south central region (Kentucky, Tennessee, Alabama, and Mississippi), and the south central region (Arkansas, Louisiana, Oklahoma, and Texas) of the United States have the highest rates of obesity (Centers for Disease Control and Prevention [CDC], 2007a).

Studies have observed that obesity is common among individuals who suffer from "food insecurity," or the lack of readily available nutritious foods. The highest rates of obesity occur in populations with the highest rates of poverty. This correlation may be explained by the reality that these individuals often buy poor quality, high-calorie foods in an attempt to economize. Individuals who are at low socioeconomic levels tend to eat fewer fruits and vegetables and more high-fat, high-calorie foods and foods that are high in sugar. Energy-dense foods taste better than many lower-calorie options, and they tend to cost less, continuing the cycle of consuming poor nutrition and high calories (Drewnowski & Spencer, 2004). When nurses encounter clients who are struggling with obesity, it is important to inquire about the client's income and food availability. If food insecurity is a problem, the nurse should offer the proper referrals and information to assist the client in accessing community resources. Figure 13-1 illustrates the balance between food intake, activity, and weight.

Nurses who work in community settings are frequently in a position to counsel adults on matters related to weight. (See the Community Application box "Fighting Obesity.") To help clients achieve and maintain a healthy weight, nurses can share several recommendations with them. General nutrition guidelines for a healthy diet are as follows:

- Eat a variety of foods.
- Balance the food you eat with physical activity; maintain or improve your weight.
- Choose a diet moderate in sugars.
- Choose a diet moderate in salt and sodium (less than 2400 mg per day).
- Drink only in moderation—no more than one drink daily for women or two drinks daily for

COMMUNITY APPLICATION
Fighting Obesity

In the United States, obesity (which is defined as having a body mass index of 30 or higher) is growing at an alarming rate. Adult obesity increased from 15% in 1976 to 32.9% in 2003.

There is significant concern that as obesity rates continue to grow, the effect will be dramatic increases in related chronic health conditions such as diabetes and cardiovascular disease. Indeed, diabetes increased by 61% between 1991 and 2001. This is widely attributed to the surge in obesity during that same period. To control the obesity epidemic, the CDC makes the following recommendations:

- Health care providers must counsel their obese clients on nutrition and weight reduction.
- Workplaces should offer healthy food choices in their cafeterias and provide opportunities for employees to be physically active on site.
- Schools should offer more physical education that encourages lifelong physical activity.
- Urban policymakers should provide more sidewalks, bike paths, and other alternatives to cars.
- Parents should reduce their children's TV and computer time and encourage outdoor play.

From Centers for Disease Control and Prevention/National Center for Chronic Disease Prevention and Health Promotion (2007): *Overweight and obesity among adults* (website): http://www.cdc.gov/nccdphp/dnpa/obesity/. And from *Diabetes data and trends* (website): http://apps.nccd.cdc.gov/DDTSTRS/default.aspx

men. (One drink is 12 oz of regular beer, 5 oz of wine, or 1.5 oz of 80-proof distilled spirits.)
- Women should consume adequate calcium and folic acid (USDHHS/ODPHP, 1998).

LOWERING FAT AND CHOLESTEROL INTAKE

Because of the association of dietary fat and cholesterol with heart disease, stroke, obesity, and other problems, limitation of these nutrients is one of the main objectives when counseling on nutrition. Dietary guidelines for fat and cholesterol intake are as follows:

- Reduce total dietary fat to 30% or less of total calories.
- Reduce saturated fat intake to less than 10% of calories.

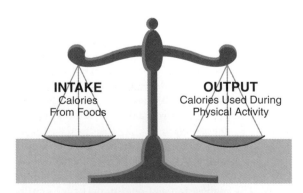

INTAKE
Calories From Foods

OUTPUT
Calories Used During Physical Activity

THE ENERGY BALANCE

Figure 13-1. The Energy Balance.

- Reduce cholesterol intake to less than 300 mg per day (U.S. Department of Health and Human Services [USDHHS], 2000a).

TOBACCO USE

Smoking has been designated the most preventable cause of death in our society. Indeed, tobacco use is responsible for nearly one in five deaths in the United States (American Cancer Society, 2007a). It is estimated that about 438,000 deaths each year in the United States and approximately $167 billion in health care costs are attributable to smoking (CDC, 2007c). Furthermore, almost half of all smokers die from diseases caused by smoking, losing an average of 20 to 25 years of life expectancy. Lung cancer mortality has a particularly strong association with tobacco use because tobacco contributes to 87% of all lung cancers. It is important to realize that lung cancer mortality rates are more than 20 times higher for current male smokers and 12 times higher for current female smokers, compared with persons who have never smoked (ACS, 2007a).

In addition to heart disease, lung cancer, and chronic respiratory diseases (e.g., chronic bronchitis and chronic obstructive pulmonary disease), tobacco use is associated with cancers of the mouth, pharynx, larynx, esophagus, pancreas, uterine cervix, kidney, and bladder, and intrauterine growth retardation, low birth weight, and birth defects (ACS, 2007b).

Per capita cigarette consumption increased annually from 1901 until 1964, when more than 42% of adults were daily smokers. A gradual decline began following the publication of the Surgeon General's Advisory Committee Report on Smoking and Health in the mid-1960s. Consumption varied somewhat over the next decade (1964 to 1974) but has declined steadily since the mid-1970s (USDHHS, 2000b). (See Figure 13-2 for recent trends in cigarette smoking.)

The CDC (2007c) reports that 70% of adults who smoke want to quit, but only about 2.5% per year succeed in quitting smoking permanently. On the positive side, almost half of all living adults who have ever smoked have quit. Programs, tools, medications, and various interventions abound to help with **smoking cessation**. Recognized interventions include self-help groups, videos, and written materials; nicotine chewing gum; nicotine patches; hypnosis; and acupuncture. However, most people who stop (about 90%) do so on their own. The National Cancer Institute has developed a list of tips for smokers to help them quit. These are presented in the Health Teaching box "Tips to Help Smokers Quit."

HEALTH TASK FORCE RECOMMENDATIONS—ILLNESS PREVENTION

The U.S. Preventive Services Task Force (USDHHS/ODPHP, 2007) has published general guidelines or recommendations for periodic individual health examinations based on age. Included in the guidelines is information on the leading causes of death, appropriate screenings, counseling, and immunizations. Special guidelines and frequencies are detailed for those who are identified as being at high risk for a particular health threat or problem. Table 13-4 gives an overview of the specific recommendations for adults younger than 65 years.

PRIMARY AND SECONDARY PREVENTION OF SELECTED CONDITIONS

HEART DISEASE AND STROKE

Heart disease and stroke are the number one and number three leading causes of death in the United States each year. Indeed, each year as many as 1.5 million U.S. residents have a heart attack, and about one third of these die. It is important to note that although heart disease is associated with aging, about 5% of all heart attacks occur in people younger than 40 years, and 32% occur in people younger than 75 (AHA, 2007b). Strokes afflict more than 900,000 U.S. residents each year, and stroke is the leading cause of serious disability in the United States. Risk factors associated with heart disease and stroke are listed in Box 13-1.

Assessment tools for identification of an individual's risk of heart disease can be helpful. Many such tools describe how risks can be lowered or

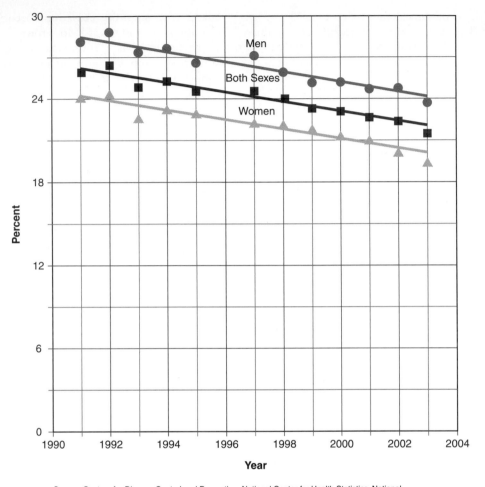

Source: Centers for Disease Control and Prevention, National Center for Health Statistics. National Health Interview Survey. \
Data are age-adjusted to the 2000 standard using age groups: 18-24, 25-34, 35-44, 45-64, 65 and older. Analysis uses the 2000 Standard Population as defined by NCHS (http://www.cdc. gov/nchs/data/statnt/statnt20.pdf).

Figure 13-2. Prevalence of smoking among adults: 1991-2003. (From the National Cancer Institute, 2005 (website): http://progressreport.cancer.gov/doc_detail.asp?pid=1&did=2005&chid=21&coid=201 &mid=#trends).

managed and can be useful in addressing the problem of heart disease. Appendix C shows one example. Nurses and others may use these tools as part of a comprehensive program that includes health teaching and counseling on nutrition, exercise, and smoking cessation, if applicable, to lower risk for all individuals. (See the Health Teaching box "Warning Signs of Heart Attack and Stroke.")

CANCER

Cancer, as has been discussed, is the second leading cause of death in the United States, accounting for about one of every four deaths. More than 1,400,000 new cancer cases are diagnosed each year (excluding basal and squamous cell skin cancers), resulting in more than 550,000 deaths (1500 people each day). There is good news, however, because between 1993

health teaching

Tips to Help Smokers Quit

TIPS FOR PREPARING TO STOP

- Decide positively that you want to stop. Try to avoid negative thoughts about possible difficulties.
- List all the reasons why you want to stop. Every night before going to bed, repeat one of the reasons 10 times.
- Develop strong personalized reasons for stopping. For example, think of all of the time you waste taking cigarette breaks, rushing out to buy a pack, or hunting for a lighter.
- Begin to condition yourself physically. Start a moderate exercise program, drink more fluids, get plenty of rest, and avoid fatigue.
- Know what to expect. Have realistic expectations—stopping isn't easy, but it is not impossible either. More than 3 million people in the United States stop each year. Understand that withdrawal symptoms are temporary and are healthy signs that the body is repairing itself from its long exposure to nicotine. Know that most relapses occur in the first week or two after stopping. At this time, withdrawal symptoms are strongest and your body is still most dependent on nicotine.
- Involve someone else. Make a bet with a friend, ask your spouse or a friend to stop smoking with you, and make a buddy system—tell your family and friends that you are stopping.

TIPS FOR JUST BEFORE STOPPING

- Practice going without tobacco.
- Do not dwell on the fact that you will never use tobacco again. Think of being tobacco-free in terms of 1 day at a time.
- Stop carrying tobacco with you at all times.
- Do not empty your ashtrays or the container that you spit into. This will remind you how much you have used each day, and the sight and smell will be very unpleasant.
- Collect all your cigarette butts into one large glass container as a visual reminder of the mess that smoking represents. Occasionally screw off the lid to smell the foul butt and ash odors.

TIPS FOR THE DAY YOU STOP

- Throw away all of your tobacco, lighters, ashtrays, spittoons, and other tobacco-related paraphernalia.
- Clean your clothes to rid them of the smell of smoke.
- Develop a clean, fresh, smoke-free environment around yourself—at work and at home.
- Schedule an appointment to have your teeth cleaned.
- Make a list of things you would like to buy for yourself or someone else. Estimate your cost of using tobacco and put the money aside to buy yourself a present.
- Keep very busy during the big day. Go to the movies, exercise, take long walks, or go bike riding.

- Buy yourself a treat or do something to celebrate.
- Stay away from other tobacco users.
- Remember that one cigarette or one chew could ruin a successful attempt.
- Remember that alcohol will weaken your willpower. Avoid it.
- Refuse to allow anything to change your mind.

TIPS TO HELP YOU COPE WITH THE PERIODIC URGE TO USE TOBACCO

- First remind yourself that you have stopped and you are a nonuser. Look closely at your urge to use tobacco and ask yourself: "Where was I when I got the urge?" "What was I doing at the time?" "Who was I with?" "What was I thinking?"
- Think about why you stopped. Repeat to yourself your three main reasons for stopping.
- Anticipate triggers and prepare to avoid them. Keep your hands busy, avoid people who smoke or chew, find activities that make smoking difficult, put something other than tobacco in your mouth (e.g., carrots, sunflower seeds, apples, celery, or sugarless gum), and avoid places where smoking is permitted.
- Change your daily routine to break old habits and patterns. After meals, immediately get up from the table, brush your teeth or take a walk; change your morning routine; do not sit in your favorite chair; eat lunch at a different location.
- Use positive thoughts. Remind yourself that you are a nonuser; observe people who do not smoke and remind yourself that they feel normal and healthy without using tobacco and so can you.
- Use relaxation techniques. Breathe in deeply and slowly while you count to five; breathe out slowly, counting to five again.

TIPS FOR COPING WITH RELAPSE

- Stop using tobacco immediately.
- Get rid of any tobacco products that you may have.
- Recognize that you have had a slip or small setback and that a small setback does not make you a smoker or a chewer again.
- Do not be too hard on yourself. One slip does not mean that you are a failure or cannot be a nonuser, but it is important to get yourself back on the nonuser track immediately.
- Realize that many successful former tobacco users stop for good only after more than one attempt.
- Identify triggers. Exactly what was it that prompted you to use tobacco? Be aware of your triggers, and decide how you will cope with them when they come up again.
- Sign a contract with yourself to remain a nonuser.

Adapted from U.S. Department of Health and Human Services/National Institutes of Health/National Cancer Institute: *Clearing the air: how to quit smoking and quit for keeps* (NIH Publication No. 92-1647), Washington, DC, 1991, U.S. Department of Health and Human Services/National Institutes of Health/National Cancer Institute.

TABLE **13-4** Preventive Services Task Force Risk Factors Screening, Referral, and Service for Adults

RISK FACTOR OR GROUP	PREVENTION TARGET CONDITION	PREVENTION SERVICE AND/OR REFERRAL
All adults	Obesity	Obesity screening
	Hypertension	Blood pressure screening
	Coronary heart disease	Cholesterol screening, nutritional counseling, exercise, counseling, smoking cessation counseling, aspirin therapy (if indicated)
	Malnutrition	Nutritional counseling
	Dental disease	Dental check-ups
	Alcohol-related problems	Assess for problem drinking
	Injuries	Counsel about various preventive measures
	Measles, mumps (persons born after 1956 only)	Serology for immune status if no record of vaccination, MMR vaccine if nonimmune
Men 35-65 years and women 45-65 years	Elevated cholesterol	Cholesterol screening, nutritional counseling, exercise counseling, and aspirin therapy (if indicated)
Women ≥40 years of age	Breast cancer	Mammography and clinical breast exam
Persons who are obese	Coronary heart disease and hypertension	Obesity screening, blood pressure screening, cholesterol screening, nutritional counseling, exercise counseling, aspirin therapy (if indicated)
	Diabetes	Fasting glucose, only if symptomatic
Persons undergoing recent divorce or separation, unemployment, or bereavement	Depression	Mental health counseling and possible referral, hospitalization
	Suicide	Question regarding preparatory actions
Persons who received radiation exposure to head and neck during infancy or childhood	Thyroid cancer and hypothyroidism	Palpation of thyroid Thyroid function tests
Persons with a history of dysplastic or congenital nevi; history of immunosuppression; history of severe sunburn in childhood; poor tanning ability; light skin, hair, or eyes; freckles	Skin cancer	Counseling to avoid sun exposure between 10 AM and 3 PM; use protective clothing and sunscreen; consider dermatology referral for those at highest risk
Persons with severe myopia	Glaucoma	Ophthalmology referral for screening

BOX 13-1 Risk Factors Associated with Heart Disease and Stroke

Age: Risk of heart disease and stroke increases steadily with age (about 80% of people who die from heart disease are 65 or older).

Gender: Men have a three to four times greater risk of heart disease than premenopausal women; after menopause, women's rate of heart disease increases sharply, although elderly men have roughly twice the risk as elderly women.

Heredity (including race): Risk increases if a parent or sibling has had a heart attack or stroke or died of heart disease before age 55; blacks have more severe high blood pressure and a higher risk of heart disease. Heart disease is also higher among Mexican Americans, Native Americans, Native Hawaiians, and some Asian Americans.

Smoking: Smoking more than doubles the risk of heart attack and stroke; smokers who have a heart attack are more likely to die and to die suddenly than are nonsmokers.

High blood cholesterol: High blood cholesterol causes narrowing in the arterial walls, thus increasing the possibility of occlusion in the brain or heart.

Hypertension: High blood pressure is a major risk factor in heart attack and is the most important risk factor in stroke.

Physical inactivity: Regular exercise helps prevent heart disease and arteriosclerosis, lessens the development of diabetes and obesity, and helps lower blood pressure in some people.

Large waist circumference: abdominal obesity

Diabetes: Diabetes is linked with increased risk of both heart disease and stroke.

Data from American Heart Association (2006): *Risk assessment for cardiovascular disease* (website): http://www.americanheart.org/presenter.jhtml?identifier=3003499.

---

health teaching

Warning Signs of Heart Attack and Stroke

If you or someone you are with has chest discomfort, especially with one or more of the other signs, or has any of the warning signs of stroke, call for help or get to a hospital immediately.

HEART ATTACK WARNING SIGNS

- Chest Discomfort: Most have discomfort in the center of the chest. The discomfort lasts more than a few minutes or goes away and comes back; it typically feels like uncomfortable pressure, squeezing, fullness, or pain.
- Discomfort in Other Areas of the Upper Body: Discomfort can radiate to one or both arms, the back, neck, jaw, or stomach.
- Shortness of Breath: Shortness of breath often accompanies the chest discomfort, but it can occur before.
- Other signs: Additional indicators are breaking out in a cold sweat, nausea, or lightheadedness.

STROKE WARNING SIGNS

- Sudden numbness or weakness of the face, arm, or leg (especially on one side of the body)
- Sudden confusion, trouble speaking, or understanding
- Sudden trouble seeing in one or both eyes
- Sudden trouble with walking, dizziness, loss of balance, or coordination
- Sudden, severe headache with no known cause

From American Heart Association (2007): *Warning signs* (website): http://www.americanheart.org/presenter.jhtml?identifier=3053. Accessed October 28, 2007.

---

and 2002, cancer deaths decreased by 1.1% per year, and the decline increased to 2.2% between 2002 and 2004 (National Cancer Institute, 2006). Figures 13-3 and 13-4 graphically illustrate trends in cancer death rates for men and women in the United States, and Figure 13-5 depicts recent estimates of newly diagnosed cases and deaths for different types of cancer. These figures demonstrate the dramatic increase in survival rates of individuals diagnosed with cancer and the decreasing incidence of many cancers. The troubling rise of lung cancer among women is also depicted here. As more women adopted the habit of smoking cigarettes, the consequential rise in lung cancer followed. There is one notation of concern, however. The National Cancer Institute predicts that as the U.S. population ages, the number of individuals diagnosed with cancer each year will double in the next 50 years, from 1.3 million to 2.6 million (NCI, 2006).

Prevention and Diagnosis of Selected Cancers

Early detection and treatment of cancer has resulted in improved survival rates for most cancers. For example, cancer of the uterus for women and stomach cancer for men have declined considerably over the decades. In addition, death rates for male lung cancer, female breast cancer, prostate cancer, and colorectal cancers have all decreased significantly in recent years.

Prevention interventions have thus proven to be effective, but more can be done. Many cancers

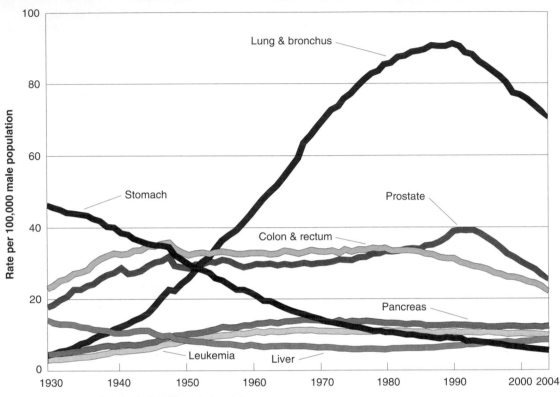

Age-Adjusted Cancer Death Rates,* Males by Site, US, 1930-2004

*Per 100,000, age-adjusted to the 2000 US standard population.

Note: Due to changes in ICD coding, numerator information has changed over time. Rates for cancer of the liver, lung and bronchus, and colon and rectum are affected by these coding changes.

Source: US Mortality Data 1960 to 2004, US Mortality Volumes 1930 to 1959, National Center for Health Statistics, Centers for Disease Control and Prevention, 2006.

American Cancer Society, Surveillance Research, 2008

Figure 13-3. Age-Adjusted Cancer Death Rates–Men by Site, United States, 1930-2003.From the American Cancer Society (website): http://www.cancer.org/downloads/stt/CFF2007AgeAdjDthRatesFem.pdf.

may be prevented through smoking cessation and improved dietary habits (i.e., reducing fat consumption and increasing fruit and vegetable consumption). Physical inactivity and obesity have also been associated with cancer, and positively addressing these issues will be important in further reducing cancer incidence and deaths (NCI, 2007). To assist nurses in teaching and counseling regarding cancer prevention, detection, and treatment, Table 13-5 lists incidence, symptoms, risk factors, and treatment options for some common cancers.

DIABETES

According to the American Diabetes Association (ADA) (ADA, 2006), approximately 20.8 million children and adults in the United States have diabetes (about 7% of the total population). Further, approximately 54 million people are prediabetic, and another one third (6.2 million) are diabetic but undiagnosed. In 2005 alone, 1.5 million people aged 20 and older were diagnosed with diabetes.

Most people with diabetes (90% to 95%) have type 2 diabetes, which usually develops in adults older than 40 years. The remainder (5% to 10%)

Age-Adjusted Cancer Death Rates,* Females by Site, US, 1930-2004

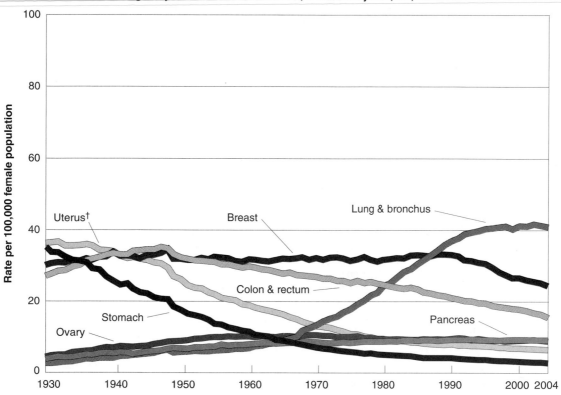

*Per 100,000, age-adjusted to the 2000 US standard population. †Uterus cancer death rates are for uterine cervix and uterine corpus combined.
Note: Due to changes in ICD coding, numerator information has changed over time. Rates for cancer of the lung and bronchus, colon and rectum, and ovary are affected by these coding changes.
Source: US Mortality Data 1960 to 2004, US Mortality Volumes 1930 to 1959, National Center for Health Statistics, Centers for Disease Control and Prevention, 2006.

American Cancer Society, Surveillance Research, 2008

Figure 13-4. Age-Adjusted Cancer Death Rates–Women by Site, United States, 1930-2003. From the American Cancer Society (website): http://www.cancer.org/downloads/stt/CFF2007AgeAdjDthRatesMales.pdf.

of clients have type 1 diabetes, which most often develops in children and young adults. In addition, gestational diabetes develops in 2% to 5% of all pregnancies but disappears when the pregnancy is over. Women who have had gestational diabetes are at increased risk for developing type 2 diabetes later in life (ADA, 2006).

Diabetes is associated with several serious complications such as heart disease and stroke, which account for about 65% of deaths among people with diabetes. Adults with diabetes suffer from heart disease death rates and a risk for stroke two to four times that of individuals who do not have diabetes. Diabetes can also lead to blindness, limb amputation, kidney disease, hypertension, dental disease, and sexual dysfunction. Diabetic retinopathy is the leading cause of new cases of blindness in adults 20 to 74 years of age, and diabetes is the leading cause of kidney failure, accounting for 44% of new cases in 2002. Finally, diabetes accounted for 82,000 amputations in 2002, approximately 60% of all nontraumatic lower limb

Leading Sites of New Cancer Cases and Deaths – 2008 Estimates

Estimated New Cases*		Estimated Deaths	
Male	**Female**	**Male**	**Female**
Prostate	Breast	Lung & bronchus	Lung & bronchus
186,320 (25%)	182,460 (26%)	90,810 (31%)	71,030 (26%)
Lung & bronchus	Lung & bronchus	Prostate	Breast
114,690 (15%)	100,330 (14%)	28,660 (10%)	40,480 (15%)
Colon & rectum	Colon & rectum	Colon & rectum	Colon & rectum
77,250 (10%)	71,560 (10%)	24,260 (8%)	25,700 (9%)
Urinary bladder	Uterine corpus	Pancreas	Pancreas
51,230 (7%)	40,100 (6%)	17,500 (6%)	16,790 (6%)
Non-Hodgkin lymphoma	Non-Hodgkin lymphoma	Liver & intrahepatic bile duct	Ovary
35,450 (5%)	30,670 (4%)	12,570 (4%)	15,520 (6%)
Melanoma of the skin	Thyroid	Leukemia	Non-Hodgkin lymphoma
34,950 (5%)	28,410 (4%)	12,460 (4%)	9,370 (3%)
Kidney & renal pelvis	Melanoma of the skin	Esophagus	Leukemia
33,130 (4%)	27,530 (4%)	11,250 (4%)	9,250 (3%)
Oral cavity & pharynx	Ovary	Urinary bladder	Uterine corpus
25,310 (3%)	21,650 (3%)	9,950 (3%)	7,470 (3%)
Leukemia	Kidney & renal pelvis	Non-Hodgkin lymphoma	Liver & intrahepatic bile duct
25,180 (3%)	21,260 (3%)	9,790 (3%)	5,840 (2%)
Pancreas	Leukemia	Kidney & renal pelvis	Brain & other nervous system
18,770 (3%)	19,090 (3%)	8,100 (3%)	5,650 (2%)
All sites	All sites	All sites	All sites
745,180 (100%)	692,000 (100%)	294,120 (100%)	271,530 (100%)

*Excludes basal and squamous cell skin cancers and in situ carcinoma except urinary bladder.

©2008, American Cancer Society, Inc., Surveillance Research

Figure 13-5. Leading Sites of New Cancer Cases and Deaths–2007 Estimates. From the American Cancer Society (website): http://www.cancer.org/downloads/stt/CFF2007LeadingSites.pdf.

amputations. Therapy to keep the blood sugar levels as close as possible to normal can reduce many of these complications by as much as 70% (ADA, 2006).

Type 2 diabetes is strongly associated with age. Those 65 or older are the most commonly affected; 20.9% of all persons in that age group are diabetic. Diabetes is also highly correlated with race/ethnicity. Being Hispanic, black, or Native American strongly predisposes a person to acquiring type 2 diabetes. Indeed, blacks are 1.8 times as likely to have diabetes as are whites, and 13.3% of blacks are diabetic. Hispanics are almost 1.7 times as likely as whites to have diabetes, and American Indians and Alaska Natives are 2.2 times as likely to have diabetes as are non-Hispanic whites. (See Figure 13-6.) Other significant risk factors for type 2 diabetes include obesity (about 80% of people with type 2

diabetes are overweight) and/or strong family history (ADA, 2006).

The U.S. Preventive Services Task Force (USDHHS/ODPHP, 2007) does not recommend routine diabetes screeing of asymptomatic individuals. All clients, particularly those in high-risk groups, should be taught the following symptoms of diabetes and counseled to contact their primary health care provider should they occur (ADA, 2006):

- Excessive thirst
- Excessive urination
- Blurred vision
- Sensory nerve damage, particularly in the extremities
- Fatigue
- Weight loss
- Slow healing of skin

TABLE **13-5** Incidence, Risk Factors, Symptoms, Early Detection, and Treatment of Selected Cancers

CANCER SITE	INCIDENCE	RISK FACTORS	SYMPTOMS	SCREENING/EARLY DETECTION	TREATMENT
Lung and bronchus	213,380 cases, with 160,390 deaths	Cigarette smoking; occupational or environmental exposure to: secondhand smoke, radon, asbestos, radiation, and other substances	Persistent cough, sputum streaked with blood, chest pain, recurring pneumonia or bronchitis, voice change	Difficult to detect in early stage; chest x-ray, sputum analysis, and low dose CT scan; fiberoptic examination of the bronchial passages when indicated	Usually a combination of surgery, radiation therapy, and chemotherapy
Colon and rectum	153,760 new cases, with 52,180 deaths	Age; personal or family history of cancer; history of polyps of the colon or rectum; inflammatory bowel disease; obesity; frequent alcohol consumption	Rectal bleeding, blood in the stool, change in bowel habits, cramping pain in lower abdomen	Yearly digital rectal examination and stool for occult blood examination; sigmoidoscopy every 5 years; colonoscopy every 10 years	Surgery; surgery and chemotherapy
Breast	180,500 new cases, with an estimated 41,000 deaths (about 0.1% occur in men)	Female; increasing age; personal or family history (mother, sister, daughter); genetic mutation (BRCA1 and BRCA2 genes); long menstrual history (menstrual periods start early and/or end late in life); never had children or late age at first birth (after age 30); high breast tissue density; history of radiation to the chest area; use of postmenopausal hormone therapy; physical inactivity; daily consumption of alcohol; obesity	Changes on mammogram, lump, thickening, swelling, dimpling, skin irritation, distortion, retraction, pain, nipple discharge	Yearly screening mammogram starting at age 40; clinical examination of breasts every 3 years to age 40 and every year thereafter; monthly breast self-examination for all women age 20 and older	Lumpectomy, mastectomy, radiation therapy, chemotherapy, hormone therapy, immunotherapy, or a combination of the above

TABLE **13-5** Incidence, Risk Factors, Symptoms, Early Detection, and Treatment of Selected Cancers

CANCER SITE	INCIDENCE	RISK FACTORS	SYMPTOMS	SCREENING/EARLY DETECTION	TREATMENT
Prostate	218,890 new cases each year, with 27,050 deaths	Age (over 65% are diagnosed in men over age 65); ethnicity (African American men have higher rates than other racial groups); family history; possibly high-fat diet	Weak or interrupted urine flow, inability to urinate, need to urinate frequently, blood in the urine, pain or burning on urination, lower back or pelvic pain	Somewhat controversial. All men 50 and over (45 for men in high risk groups) should be counseled on screening. A digital rectal examination for all men 40 years or older and prostate specific antigen (PSA) test for all men over age 50 should be offered.	Surgery, radiation, and/or hormone treatment
Cervix	11,150 cases annually, with 3670 deaths	Infection with human papillomavirus; early age at first intercourse; multiple sex partners; high parity; cigarette smoking	Abnormal uterine bleeding or spotting, abnormal vaginal discharge	Prevention measures include vaccination against HPV; Papanicolaou test and pelvic examination should be performed annually for women who are sexually active and those age 18 or older	Surgery and or radiation; precancerous (in situ) cases may be treated by cryotherapy or electrocoagulation
Skin Cancer	More than one million cases of basal cell or squamous cell cancer each year; 59,940 cases and 8110 deaths each year from melanoma	Age; excessive exposure to ultraviolet radiation; presence of moles; fair complexion; history of sunburn; use of tanning booths; diseases that suppress the immune system; occupational exposure to coal tar, pitch, ereosote, arsenic compounds, or radium	Change in size or color of a mole or pigmented growth or spot; scaliness, oozing, bleeding, or change in appearance of a bump	Skin self-examination once a month and reporting changes to a physician—ABCD rule for melanoma: A=asymmetry B=border irregularity C=color D=diameter (greater than 6 mm – the size of a pencil eraser)	Surgery, radiation, cryosurgery, and electrodessication; for melanoma, wide margin excision and possible lymph node excision, immune boosting drugs; vaccines and gene therapy are being tested.

Data from American Cancer Society (2007): *Cancer facts & figures–2007*, Atlanta, 2007, American Cancer Society (online): http://www.cancer.org/docroot/STT/content/STT_1x_Cancer_Facts__Figures_2007.asp.

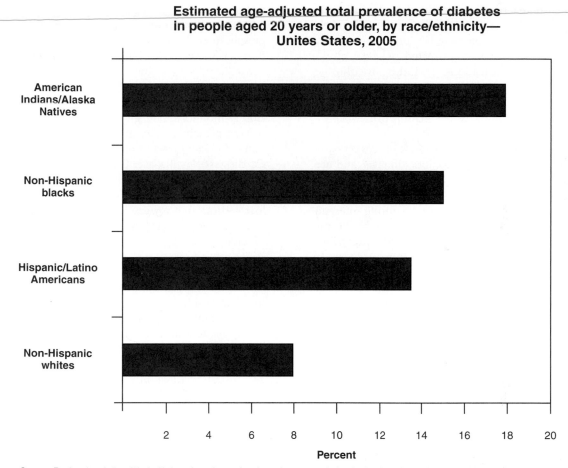

Estimated age-adjusted total prevalence of diabetes in people aged 20 years or older, by race/ethnicity— Unites States, 2005

Source: *For American Indians/Alaska Natives, the estimate of total prevalence was calculated using the estimate of diagnosed diabetes from the 2003 outpatient database of the Indian Health Service and the estimate of undiagnosed diabetes from the 1999-2002 National Health and Nutrition Examination Survey. For the other groups, 1999-2002 NHANES estimates of total prevalence (both diagnosed and undiagnosed) were projected to year 2006.*

* Graph and information obtained from CDC {Center for Disease Control and Prevention} website at http://www.cdc.gov/diabetes/pubs/estimates05.htm#prey4 on December 1,2006.

Figure 13-6. Estimated age-adjusted total prevalence of diabetes in people aged 20 years or older by race/ethnicity–United States, 2005.From American Diabetes Association (2006): *Total prevalence of diabetes and prediabetes* (website): http://www .diabetes.org/diabetes-statistics/prevalence.jsp.

- Gum infection
- Urinary tract infection

Whereas type 1 diabetes is managed with strict adherence to a prescribed diet, intensive monitoring of blood glucose levels, and administration of insulin (often two to four times daily), type 2 diabetes is primarily controlled through diet and other lifestyle changes. Weight loss is strongly encouraged, as is avoidance of alcohol and smoking when indicated. Frequently people with type 2 diabetes must take medication to control blood glucose levels. Usually, oral medications (e.g., oral hypoglycemic/sulfonylureas such as tolbutamide, chlorpropamide, and tolazamide) are sufficient, but many type 2 diabetics eventually need to take insulin to better control serum glucose levels.

Health teaching and counseling for all individuals with diabetes should focus on closely following the recommended diet; monitoring blood glucose levels as directed by their physician; taking medications, including insulin, as prescribed; and carefully observing for complications. Some relatively common complications, prevention methods, and teaching principles include the following:

- Diabetic ketoacidosis (insulin deficiency resulting in hyperglycemia, osmotic diuresis, and acidosis): Ketoacidosis is usually caused by failure to adhere to a program for insulin management or failure to alter insulin intake during intercurrent illnesses. Clients should be taught the importance of compliance with the prescribed medication regimen and how to manage serum glucose levels during illness.
- Hypoglycemia: A low blood glucose level often results from delay or decrease in food intake, vigorous physical activity, or alcohol consumption. Clients should be taught to recognize symptoms of low blood glucose (e.g., apprehension, tremors, sweating, palpitations, fatigue, confusion, headache) and treat with rapidly absorbable carbohydrates (e.g., three to five pieces of hard candy, two to three packets of sugar, or 4 ounces of fruit juice). A family member or friend should be taught to administer oral carbohydrates if the client is unable to treat himself or herself. If this is not possible, the Emergency Medical Service should be notified.
- Periodontal disease: Gingivitis and periodontitis are common in diabetics. Instruction on proper brushing and flossing is essential, and preventive dental care (ideally every 6 months) should be encouraged.
- Eye disease: Diabetes is a major cause of blindness in the United States. Roughly 70% of people with type 1 diabetes develop diabetic retinopathy, and 40% develop macular edema. Clients with diabetes should be taught to report any changes in vision (e.g., blurred vision, "floaters," and flashing lights) immediately. A yearly eye examination is very important because early detection of ophthalmic complications and prompt treatment with laser surgery can reduce visual loss significantly.

- Kidney disease: Diabetic nephropathy is characterized by albuminuria, hypertension, and progressive renal insufficiency. As a result of chronic renal insufficiency, end-stage renal disease may occur. To prevent kidney disease, diabetics must be taught to monitor blood pressure and adhere to treatment of hypertension when indicated; closely monitor blood glucose levels; avoid excessive protein intake; and observe for symptoms of urinary tract infection.
- Cardiovascular disease: Clients should be told that diabetes increases the risk of developing cardiovascular disease. Maintaining a low-fat, low-sodium diet is very important and should be encouraged. Signs and symptoms of cardiovascular disease can be discussed and the client told to report possible symptoms immediately.
- Neuropathy: Clients should be informed about the relationship between poor glycemic control and development of diabetic neuropathy. Complications of neuropathy include orthostatic hypotension, constipation, diabetic diarrhea and fecal incontinence, diabetic bladder dysfunction, and sexual dysfunction. Careful monitoring and maintenance of glucose levels can help reduce neuropathy.
- Foot problems: Persons with diabetes account for approximately 60% of all nontraumatic amputations performed each year. To prevent foot ulcers and potential complications, diabetics should be taught meticulous foot care. Principles include washing and inspecting feet daily, using foot creams or oils, cutting toenails correctly and never cutting corns or calluses, avoiding extremes of temperature, never walking barefoot, wearing appropriate shoes, inspecting the inside of shoes daily, and seeking medical care for all skin lesions (ADA, 2006).

To prevent these and other complications, it is vitally important that all diabetics maintain their diets and treatment regimens, monitor illnesses carefully, and immediately report any complications to their primary care providers. Many organizations and resources are available for clients with diabetes. Health care providers should be aware of these resources and refer clients appropriately.

SUMMARY

Nursing interventions focused on health promotion and illness prevention are largely conducted in community-based settings such as primary health care offices, occupational health settings, clinics, and rehabilitation settings, as illustrated in the opening case study. Like Ben, the nurse from the case study, nurses who practice in these settings should be familiar with current recommendations and guidelines to promote and improve the health of adults.

KEY POINTS

- *Health promotion* refers to activities or actions related to encouraging individual lifestyles or personal choices that positively influence health (e.g., encouraging physical activity and fitness, good nutrition, substance abuse prevention).
- Health benefits of regular exercise and physical activity are well documented. Individuals should work up to moderate-level activities (50% to 80% of maximum heart rate) for a minimum of 30 minutes, four to five times per week, depending on age and presence of existing physical problems. Walking, aerobic dancing, bicycling, jogging, and swimming are examples of recommended activities.
- Good nutritional practices and maintenance of a desirable weight are essential for good health. In the United States, it is estimated that 20% of men and 25% of women are obese. Obesity is associated with hypertension, type 2 diabetes, hypercholesterolemia, coronary artery disease, some types of cancer, and stroke. Nutrition guidelines for a healthy diet include eating a variety of foods; maintaining healthy weight; choosing a diet low in fat, saturated fat, and cholesterol; eating five or more servings daily of vegetables, fruits, and grains; using sugar, salt, and sodium in moderation; and drinking alcoholic beverages in moderation, if at all.
- In the United States, tobacco use is associated with almost 440,000 deaths annually from heart disease, lung cancer, chronic respiratory disease, cancer (mouth, pharynx, larynx, pancreas, and other sites), intrauterine growth retardation, low birth weight, and birth defects. A number of programs, tools, medications, and other interventions are available for clients who want to stop smoking.
- Primary and secondary prevention interventions for heart disease and stroke are essential because these diseases account for the number one and number three causes of death and disability in the United States. Risk factors for heart disease and stroke include smoking, hypertension, hypercholesterolemia, diabetes, obesity, age, sex, and genetic predisposition. Prevention efforts to reduce or eliminate these risk factors include teaching and counseling on nutrition, exercise, and smoking cessation (if applicable).
- Cancer is the second leading cause of death in the United States, resulting in about 550,000 deaths each year. Early detection and treatment of cancer has improved survival rates for most cancers.
- Diabetes affects almost 21 million U.S. residents, about half of whom are not aware they have the disease. Diabetes is one of the leading causes of death and disability and is associated with many health conditions, including blindness, heart disease, stroke, renal failure, nerve damage, amputations, and birth defects. Risk factors for noninsulin-dependent diabetes mellitus include obesity, increasing age, family history, and being a member of certain minority groups (blacks, Hispanics, and Native Americans).

Learning Activities & Application to Practice

In Class

1. With classmates, discuss objectives of *Healthy People 2010* related to health promotion and illness prevention for adults (e.g., improving physical activity and nutrition; quitting use of tobacco; and reducing rates of heart disease, stroke, cancer, and diabetes). Analyze baselines and variations in special populations. What objectives should nurses working in community-based settings address? What health education and anticipatory guidance should be provided?

2. Complete one of the assessment tools located at the back of the book. Share results with classmates. What are areas of strength and weakness? How can tools of this type be used in community settings to help improve the individual's health?

In Clinical

3. Observe for opportunities to share health-promotion and illness-prevention strategies in all settings, particularly as they relate to the leading causes of morbidity and mortality. For example, if you are working with heart disease, stroke, or diabetes patients, provide instruction on minimizing and eliminating risk factors and managing the disease process. How can this be accomplished effectively? How might health teaching be enhanced?

REFERENCES

American Cancer Society (2007a): *Tobacco and cancer* (website): http://www.cancer.org/docroot/PED/ped_10.asp?sitearea=PED. Accessed October 31, 2007.

American Cancer Society (2007b): *Cancer facts & figures–2007*, Atlanta, 2007, American Cancer Society (electronic version online): http://www.cancer.org/docroot/STT/content/STT_1x_Cancer_Facts__Figures_2007.asp. Accessed October 31, 2007.

American College of Sports Medicine/American Heart Association: Physical activity and public health: updated recommendations for adults from the American College of Sports Medicine and the American Heart Association, *Circulation* 116:1081, 2007.

American Diabetes Association (2006): *All about diabetes* (website):http://www.diabetes.org/about-diabetes.jsp. Accessed October 31, 2007.

American Heart Association (2007a): *Exercise and fitness* (website):http://www.americanheart.org/presenter.jhtml?identifier=1200013. Accessed October 31, 2007.

American Heart Association (2007b): *Warning signs* (website): http://www.americanheart.org/presenter.jhtml?identifier=3053. Accessed October 28, 2007.

American Heart Association (2007c): *Heart attack and angina statistics* (website): http://www.americanheart.org/downloadable/heart/1168618073572OLDER07.REV.pdf. Accessed October 22, 2007.

American Heart Association (2006): *Risk assessment for cardiovascular disease* (website): http://www.americanheart.org/presenter.jhtml?identifier=3003499.

Centers for Disease Control and Prevention (2007a): *U.S. obesity trends 1985-2006* (website): http://www.cdc.gov/nccdphp/dnpa/obesity/trend/index.htm. Accessed October 19, 2007.

Centers for Disease Control and Prevention (2007b): *Defining overweight and obesity* (website): http://www.cdc.gov/nccdphp/dnpa/obesity/defining.htm. Accessed October 19, 2007.

Centers for Disease Control and Prevention (2007c): State-specific prevalence of cigarette smoking among adults and quitting among persons aged 18-35 years–U.S. 2006, *MMWR Morb Mortal Wkly Rep* 56(38):993, 2007.

Centers for Disease Control and Prevention (2004): *The surgeon general's report on the health effects of smoking* (website): http://www.cdc.gov/tobacco/data_statistics/sgr/sgr_2004/00_pdfs/executivesummary.pdf. Accessed October 16, 2007.

Centers for Disease Control and Prevention/National Center for Chronic Disease Prevention and Health Promotion (2007): *The importance of physical activity and good nutrition* (website): http://www.cdc.gov/nccdphp/publications/aag/dnpa.htm. Accessed October 16, 2007.

Drewnowski D, Specter SE: Poverty and obesity: the role of energy density and energy costs, *Am J Clin Nutr* 79:6, 2004.

Mokdad AH, Marks JS, Stroup DF, Gerberding JL: Actual causes of death in the United States, 2000, *J Am Med Assoc* 29:1238, 2004 (electronic version online): www.jama.com. Accessed October 16, 2007.

National Cancer Institute (2006): *United States cancer statistics:* 2003, incidence and mortality (website): http://www.cdc.gov/cancer/npcr/npcrpdfs/US_Cancer_Statistics_2003_Incidence_and_Mortality.pdf. Accessed October 22, 2007.

National Cancer Institute (2007): *Cancer prevention overview* (website): http://www.cancer.gov/cancertopics/pdq/prevention/overview/healthprofessional. Accessed October 26, 2007.

National Center for Health Statistics: Deaths: final data for 2004, *National Vital Statistics Reports* 55(19):1, 2007 (electronic version online): http://www.cdc.gov/nchs/data/nvsr/nvsr55/nvsr55_19.pdf.

National Heart, Lung and Blood Institute: *Healthy heart I.Q.* (NIH Publication No. 92-2724), Washington, DC, 1992, National Heart, Lung and Blood Institute.

Office of Disease Prevention and Health Promotion: *Healthstyle: a self-test.* (Publication No. H0012), Washington, DC, 1981, National Health Information Clearinghouse.

Pender NJ, Murdaugh CL, Parsons MA: *Health promotion in nursing practice*, ed 5, Norwalk, Conn, 2006, Prentice Hall.

President's Council on Physical Fitness & Sports (2007): *Pep up your life: a fitness book for mid-life and older persons* (website): http://www.fitness.gov/pepup.htm. Accessed October 16, 2007.

U.S. Department of Health and Human Services (2000a): *Healthy people 2010*: conference ed, Washington, DC, 2000, Government Printing Office.

U.S. Department of Health and Human Services (2000b): *Reducing tobacco use: a report of the surgeon general*, Atlanta, 2000, USDHHS/CDC.

U.S. Department of Health and Human Services/ National Institutes of Health/National Cancer Institute: *Clearing the air: how to quit smoking and quit for keeps* (NIH Publication No. 92-1647), Washington DC, 1991, U.S. Department of Health and Human Services/National Institutes of Health/ National Cancer Institute.

U.S. Department of Health and Human Services/Office of Disease Prevention and Health Promotion (USDHHS/ ODPHP): *Clinician's handbook of preventive services*, ed 2, Washington, DC, 1998, Government Printing Office.

Issues in Women's Health Care

Upon completion of this chapter, the reader will be able to:

1. Discuss issues related to family planning, including contraception options, treatment of infertility, preconception counseling, and prenatal care.

2. Explain the issue of teen pregnancy and suggest ways to decrease problems associated with it.

3. Discuss prevention efforts related to common women's health problems, including breast and gynecologic cancers, osteoporosis, and domestic violence.

key terms

Assisted reproductive technology	Emergency contraception	Teenage pregnancy
Breast cancer	Family planning services	
Contraception	Infertility	
Domestic violence	Osteoporosis	
	Prenatal care	*See Glossary for definitions.*

case study

Lisa Lewis is a registered nurse (RN) practicing in a public-sponsored, comprehensive obstetric and family clinic in an urban area. The clinic is staffed by physicians, gynecologic nurse practitioners (NPs), certified nurse-midwives, RNs, and social workers. In her role Lisa performs various services, including health teaching, obtaining health histories, taking vital signs (including fetal heart rate assessment and measuring fundal height), counseling, performing screenings and skilled tasks (e.g., injections, venipuncture), and assisting the primary care providers in other services (e.g., performance of Papanicolaou [Pap] smears, colposcopy, ultrasonography, and biopsies).

On a recent Friday, Lisa cared for Patty Smith, a 25-year-old mother of two who was being seen for her yearly gynecologic examination and to discuss family planning options. Because Lisa completed Patty's health history, she learned that Patty's last Pap test was 2 years ago while she was pregnant with her second child. That Pap test and all previous tests have been normal. Since the birth of her last child, Patty reports that she and her

Continued

husband have been using condoms and foam to prevent pregnancy, but she would like to explore other forms of contraception. Her vital signs were as follows: blood pressure 110/68, pulse 76, and respirations 16; her weight was appropriate for her height. Patty reports no serious health problems and states that both of her parents are living and in good health.

Lisa briefly explained the contraceptive options available, including the effectiveness and pros and cons of each. Surgical sterilization for Patty or her husband was also discussed, but she reported that she and her husband have not yet decided whether they want any more children, so sterilization was not considered. After learning about benefits and potential side effects of each of her options, Patty decided to return to using "the pill" as she had before her first child.

Lisa assisted the NP with the general physical examination, breast examination, and Pap test. No abnormalities were noted. The NP gave Patty a prescription for oral contraceptives and reviewed how to take them. She reinforced the teaching with a pamphlet.

Before leaving, Lisa informed Patty that she would receive the results of her Pap test in the mail in about 2 weeks. She was reminded to come back in 2 years if she did not have problems.

Nursing practice in community settings encompasses diverse areas of women's health, including family planning, pregnancy, childbearing and infant care, cancer detection, detection and prevention of **domestic violence**, and prevention of osteoporosis. *Healthy People 2010* (U.S. Department of Health and Human Services [USDHHS], 2000) lists several objectives related to women's health, including specific objectives to encourage breastfeeding, discourage smoking, reduce unplanned pregnancies, and improve access to prenatal care. Reducing domestic violence and complications arising from osteoporosis are also among the stated objectives. The *Healthy People 2010* box presents some examples of objectives related to women's health.

This chapter discusses a number of topics related to women's health. Presented here is information on family planning, including available contraception options, women's health care (e.g., screening for reproductive diseases, breast care), prenatal care, and infertility. Finally, prevention and intervention in teenage pregnancy and domestic violence are described.

FAMILY PLANNING

Approximately one half (49%) of pregnancies in the United States are unintended (mistimed or unwanted) (Finer & Henshaw, 2006). This is attributed to lack of knowledge, failure to translate knowledge into behavior, or lack of family planning services and information. **Family planning services** offer health and medical care and counseling that provide women with the information and care they need to make informed choices about whether and when to become parents. Comprehensive family planning includes consideration of factors regarding childbearing, adoption, abstinence from sexual activity outside of a monogamous relationship, use of contraceptives, natural family planning, treatment of infertility, and preconception counseling.

Without effective contraception, 85% to 89% of couples who regularly engage in sexual intercourse will conceive within 1 year (USDHHS, 2000). As stated earlier, an estimated 49% of all pregnancies in the United States are unintended, but there are significant differences based on demographic variables such as race/ethnicity, education, and income (Finer & Hinshaw, 2006). For example, black women (69%) and Hispanic women (54%) experience higher rates of unplanned pregnancy than white women (40%). Education level is also somewhat predictive. Women who have less than a high school education, those who have completed high school, and those with "some college" all report that 50% of their pregnancies are unintended. This contrasts sharply with women who are college graduates; only 24% of their pregnancies are unintended. Similarly, the association between income and whether pregnancies are intentional is notable. Among women whose income is at least 200% above the poverty level (about $42,000 in 2007 for a family of four), only 38% of

healthy people 2010

Examples of Objectives for Family Planning, Maternal/Infant/Child Health, Domestic Violence, and Women's Health

OBJECTIVE	BASELINE (1998)	TARGET
FAMILY PLANNING		
9.1: Increase the proportion of pregnancies that are intended	51%	70%
9.3: Increase the proportion of females at risk of unintended pregnancy (and their partners) who use contraception	93%	100%
9.7: Reduce pregnancies among adolescent females	72 pregnancies per 1000 females 15-17 years	46 pregnancies per 1000 females 15-17 years
9.12: Reduce the proportion of married couples whose ability to conceive or maintain a pregnancy is impaired	13%	10%
MATERNAL/INFANT/CHILD HEALTH		
16.4: Reduce maternal deaths	8.4 per 100,000 live births	3.3 per 100,000 live births
16.5a: Reduce maternal complications during labor and delivery	32.1 per 100 deliveries	20 per 100 deliveries
16.6b: Increase the proportion of pregnant women who receive early and adequate prenatal care	83%	90%
16.11a: Reduce preterm births	11.4%	7.6%
INTIMATE PARTNER VIOLENCE		
15.34: Reduce the rate of physical assault by current or former intimate partners	4.5 physical assaults per 1000 persons	3.6 physical assaults per 1000 persons
WOMEN'S HEALTH		
2.9: Reduce the number of cases of osteoporosis	16% of females	8% of adults
3.3: Reduce breast cancer death rate	27.7 deaths per 100,000	22.2 deaths per 100,000
3.4: Reduce death rate from cervical cancer	3 deaths per 100,000	2 deaths per 100,000
3.11b: Increase the proportion of women 18 years of age and older who have received a Pap test within the preceding 3 years	79%	90%

From U.S. Department of Health and Human Services: *Healthy people 2010*: conference ed, Washington, DC, 2000, Government Printing Office.

pregnancies are unintended, compared with 62% for those below poverty level.

Several recommendations have been made to reduce rates of unintended pregnancy. These include encouraging the postponement of sexual activity (particularly in adolescents) and providing health education to improve the understanding of fertility and promote the appropriate use of available family planning options. Improved access to providers of family planning services is essential.

CONTRACEPTION

At present there are a number of methods available to prevent pregnancy. Abstinence is the most effective means of avoiding unintended pregnancy and is a key method of contraception for many (e.g., teenagers). Other methods of **contraception** include barriers (e.g., condoms, diaphragm, cervical cap), hormonal methods (e.g., oral contraceptives, Depo-Provera, NuvaRing, "the patch"), IUDs, spermicides, sterilization, and natural family planning (USDHHS/Office on Women's Health [OWH], 2005). These methods vary in effectiveness, and each has positive and negative consequences. Table 14-1 compares available contraceptives.

Emergency Contraception

In 1997 the Food and Drug Administration (FDA) recommended approval of the use of high doses of standard birth control pills as postcoital contraception or "morning-after pills." Depending on the stage in the woman's reproductive cycle, **emergency contraception** prevents pregnancy by prevention of ovulation, prevention of fertilization of the egg, or prevention of transportation of the egg to the uterus. In addition, it may render the uterine lining unfavorable to implantation (USDHHS/OWH, 2006).

There are two types of emergency contraception. "Plan B," a two-pill dose of progestin, is marketed for use as "emergency contraception." One pill is taken as soon as possible following intercourse, and the second is taken 12 hours later, although both pills may be taken immediately. The second emergency contraception option is to take a high dose of regular birth control pills, which contain both estrogen and progestin. There is some variation of the dose, based on the type of oral contraceptive used, and some brands may not be used for emergency contraception. The recommended dose is between two and five oral contraceptive pills (depending on the brand) taken up to 72 hours after sex, followed by a repeat of the same dose 12 hours later. (See http://ec.princeton.edu/info/combecp.html for specific information.) If initiated within 72 hours after intercourse, this regimen reduces the risk of pregnancy by 75% for the combination estrogen/progestin pills and 89% for the Plan B (progestin-only) option. Nausea and vomiting are the most common side effects.

PRENATAL CARE

A country's infant mortality rates and maternal mortality rates are often cited as an indicator of the overall health of the country and the efficacy of its health care system. Although U.S. infant and maternal mortality rates have improved during the past several decades, the United States ranks an astonishingly poor twenty-fifth among industrialized countries (USDHHS, 2000).

In 2004 the overall infant mortality rate in the United States was 6.8 per 1000, which although relatively high, demonstrates steady improvement over the past several decades. There is significant disparity, however, based on race and geography. For example, the infant mortality rate for black infants is 13.6 per 1000, compared with 5.7 among non-Hispanic whites and 5.5 for Hispanic women whose country of origin was Mexico. Similarly there are wide variations by state. Indeed, infant mortality rates range from 10.3 per 1000 in Mississippi to 4.7 per 1000 in Vermont (CDC, 2007a).

The higher rate for black infants has long been attributed to lack of access to health care, poverty, teen pregnancy, and several other factors. Black babies have almost twice the risk for low birth weight (LBW) as white babies. In 2004 13.6% of black infants were born with LBW compared with 7% of white infants (USDHHS/NCHS, 2006). Risk factors associated with LBW are younger or older maternal age, high parity, multiples (twins, triplets, etc), poor reproductive history, low socioeconomic status, low level of education, late entry into prenatal care, low pregnancy weight gain, and smoking and other substance abuse.

Prenatal care is effective in preventing, identifying, and addressing pregnancy threats or complications and is particularly important for women at increased medical and/or social risk. Prenatal

TABLE **14-1** Methods of Contraception—Effectiveness, Risks, Benefits, Convenience, and Availability

METHOD	EFFECTIVENESS (TYPICAL USE)	POTENTIAL COMPLICATIONS AND SIDE EFFECTS	POTENTIAL BENEFITS	CONVENIENCE/USE	AVAILABILITY AND COST
Oral contraceptive pills	95%-99.9% (92%-99.9% for 'mini-pills')	*Side effects:* water retention, nausea, headaches, spotting, missing periods, breast tenderness, depression, mood changes *Complications:* blood clots, heart attack, stroke (associated with smoking), hypertension, gallbladder disease, liver tumors; may increase risk of ovarian tumors	May reduce volume and pain of menstruation; periods are regular; may protect women from cancer of the ovary and endometrium and benign breast disease; protects against anemia and ectopic pregnancy	Must be taken daily; effectiveness declines when pills are missed	Prescription required; costs vary, depending on source(retail approximately $30-$35 per month)
Condom	84%-98%	Decreases sensation, loss of spontaneity; a few people are allergic to latex or to spermicide; condoms may break	Helps protect both partners against transmission of STDs and HIV if used properly	Must be put onto the erect penis before the penis comes into contact with the vagina; use a new condom for each act of intercourse	Easy availability; minimal cost
Patch	98%-99% (less effective in women who weigh more than 198 pounds)	Similar to oral contraceptives	Similar to oral contraceptives	A new patch is put in place every week for 3 weeks; no patch is worn during week 4	Prescription is required
IUD	98%-99%	*Side effects:* cramping, bleeding, anemia *Complications:* pelvic inflammatory disease, infertility, perforation of uterus (rare)	IUDs with progestin decrease menstrual cramping in some users	Requires no preparation for intercourse; at least once a month (usually after menstruation), user must check in vagina for strings to ensure IUD is in place	Requires insertion by a trained health professional

Method	Effectiveness	Side Effects/Complications	Advantages	Special Considerations	Availability
Injectables (Depo-Provera)	97%	*Side effects:* amenorrhea, weight gain, headaches, mood changes; should not be used for more than 2 years	May be used when lactating; may have protective effects against endometrial cancer	Effective almost immediately; requires no preparation for intercourse	Requires prescription; one injection every 3 months
Barriers (diaphragms, cervical caps/shield, sponges)	84%-90% for women who have never had a baby; 68%-80% for women who have borne children	*Side effects:* cervical, vaginal irritation; pelvic pressure; vaginal discharge if left in too long; difficulty in removal *Complications:* cervical, vaginal, or bladder infection; toxic shock syndrome (very rare)	Provides some protection against STDs	Requires preparation to insert devices before intercourse (diaphragm and cervical cap, up to 6 hours before intercourse; sponge up to 24 hours before intercourse); should be left in place for 6-8 (but not more than 24) hours after intercourse; should not be used by women who have recently given birth	Diaphragm and cervical cap require a prescription and fitting by a trained health care provider; sponge is available without prescription
Periodic abstinence (natural family planning)	Very variable (53%-86%)	None	Careful monitoring can help determine timing for a planned pregnancy; requires no drugs or devices	Requires frequent monitoring of body functions and periods of abstinence	No prescription; obtain instructions from a trained health care provider; basal thermometers and charts available at drugstores and family planning clinics

Continued

TABLE **14-1** Methods of Contraception—Effectiveness, Risks, Benefits, Convenience, and Availability—cont'd

METHOD	EFFECTIVENESS (TYPICAL USE)	POTENTIAL COMPLICATIONS AND SIDE EFFECTS	POTENTIAL BENEFITS	CONVENIENCE/USE	AVAILABILITY AND COST
Spermicides (foam, gel, cream)	70%-80%	*Side effects:* allergic reaction	Provides some protection against STDs	Must be inserted immediately before intercourse; some find the products messy; no douching for 6-8 hours after intercourse	No prescription necessary; relatively inexpensive
Sterilization	99+%	*Side effects:* pain at surgical site, psychologic reactions *Complications:* infection, regret that the procedure was performed	No interference with sex drive or sexual functioning	Must be certain there is no desire for future pregnancies; surgery must be done by a trained physician; postsurgery instructions must be followed; men must return for sperm checks until all sperm have been cleared from the system	*Vasectomy:* minor surgical procedure for men; usually performed in a physician's office under local anesthesia *Tubal ligation:* minor procedure for women, requires general anesthesia (fairly expensive); most health insurance plans cover sterilization
Abstinence	100%	None	Prevention of STDs and HIV; avoids drugs and devices; safest method of contraception	May be hard to avoid pressure to have intercourse	Prepare responses; talk about decision with partner

Data from: U.S. Department of Health and Human Services/Office on Women's Health: *Birth control methods* (website): www.womenshealth.gov. Accessed November 8, 2007; American Academy of Family Physicians: *Birth control: choosing a method that's right for you* (website): http://familydoctor.org/online/famdocen/home/women/contraceptive/016.html. Accessed November 15, 2007.

care dramatically reduces the likelihood of having a baby with LBW; an expectant mother with no prenatal care is three times more likely to have a baby with LBW than an expectant mother who begins prenatal care during the first trimester. Despite this, about 15% of all pregnant women and 25% of pregnant black women do not receive early (within the first trimester) and adequate prenatal care (USDHHS/National Center for Health Statistics [NCHS], 2006). Goals of prenatal care include assessing the health status of the mother and baby, monitoring fetal development, identification of women at risk for complications and minimizing risks when possible, and providing appropriate education and counseling (Zdanuk, 2007). Most of the women who receive delayed or no prenatal care are poor, lack a high school education, or are very young. Box 14-1 outlines barriers to prenatal care.

In addition to LBW, lack of prenatal care has been associated with prematurity, maternal complications, and infant mortality (USDHHS, 2000). Comprehensive and early prenatal care reduces rates of infant death and LBW. Improving prenatal care beginning in the first trimester of pregnancy is one of the objectives cited in *Healthy People 2010*. This can best be accomplished through removing or lessening barriers.

To reduce the incidence of infants with LBW and other complications, prenatal care should include:
1. Initial and ongoing assessment with risk identification
2. Individualized care based on case management principles
3. Nutritional counseling
4. Education to reduce or eliminate unhealthy habits
5. Stress reduction
6. Social support services
7. Health education

These are discussed briefly in the following sections.

RISK IDENTIFICATION AND CASE MANAGEMENT

Routine health care visits should monitor normal progression of the pregnancy (Figure 14-1). This would include assessment of: (1) fetal growth and development (e.g., measurement of fundal height, listening to fetal heart tones, assessing fetal movement); (2) maternal response to the pregnancy; and (3) possible

BOX 14-1 Barriers to Use of Prenatal Care

I. SOCIODEMOGRAPHIC
- Poverty
- Residence: inner city or rural
- Minority status
- Age: <18 or >39
- High parity
- Non-English speaking
- Unmarried
- Less than high school education

II. SYSTEM-RELATED
- Inadequacies in private insurance policies (waiting periods, coverage limitations, coinsurance and deductibles, requirements for up-front payments)
- Absence of either Medicaid or private insurance coverage of maternity services
- Inadequate or no maternity care providers for Medicaid-enrolled, uninsured, and other low-income women (long wait to get appointment)
- Complicated, time-consuming process to enroll in Medicaid
- Availability of Medicaid poorly advertised
- Inadequate transportation services, long travel time to service sites, or both
- Difficulty obtaining childcare
- Weak links between prenatal services and pregnancy testing
- Inadequate coordination among such services as Women, Infants, and Children (WIC) and prenatal care
- Inconvenient clinic hours, especially for working women
- Long waits to see physician
- Language and cultural incompatibility between providers and clients
- Poor communication between clients and providers, exacerbated by short interactions with providers
- Negative attributes of clinics, including rude personnel, uncomfortable surroundings, and complicated registration procedures
- Limited information on exactly where to get care (phone numbers and addresses)

III. ATTITUDINAL
- Pregnancy unplanned, viewed negatively, or both
- Ambivalence
- Signs of pregnancy not known or recognized
- Prenatal care not valued or understood
- Fear of doctors, hospitals, procedures
- Fear of parental discovery
- Fear of deportation or problems with the Immigration and Naturalization Service
- Fear that certain health habits will be discovered and criticized (smoking, eating disorders, drug or alcohol abuse)
- Selected lifestyles (drug abuse, homelessness)
- Inadequate social supports and personal resources
- Excessive stress
- Denial or apathy
- Concealment

Reproduced with permission of The Alan Guttmacher Institute, from Brown SS: Drawing women into prenatal care, *Fam Plann Perspect* 21(2):73-78, Table 4, 1989.

Figure 14-1. A community-based nurse conducts a prenatal evaluation during a home visit. (Courtesy of Caroline E. Brown.)

complications such as hypertension, gestational diabetes, or multiple fetuses. Identification of risk factors and developing and implementing interventions to eliminate, reduce, or manage the risk factors is essential in producing good pregnancy outcomes. To help nurses who work with women of childbearing age identify women at risk, Box 14-2 lists some factors that contribute to high-risk pregnancy.

Once a possible risk or complication has been identified, a comprehensive plan of care should be outlined to monitor and minimize risks. This plan or program may include detailed case management if the risk factors are significant. For example, if gestational diabetes is diagnosed, the pregnant woman should receive comprehensive education on this condition and receive ongoing monitoring and intervention as indicated. Likewise, if other complications such as pregnancy-induced hypertension, multifetal pregnancy, or preexisting maternal health problems dictate the need, a case management plan should be implemented. For pregnant teenagers, a structured case management program should be encouraged to help minimize the risks associated with teenage pregnancy. These are described later in this chapter.

NUTRITION COUNSELING

Maintenance of good nutrition during pregnancy is vital to the health of both the mother and the developing baby. In general, pregnant women need to increase their caloric intake by about 15%

(about 340 calories/day in the first two trimesters and about 460 calories/day during the final trimester) (Moore, 2007). Basic recommendations include three to four servings of dairy products, five servings of meat or other protein source, six or more servings of breads and cereals, one serving of dark green or orange/yellow vegetables, two or more servings of other vegetables, and at least one serving of fruit high in vitamin C. Of particular concern in pregnant women is ensuring adequate iron and folic acid intake. To obtain sufficient vitamins and minerals, most pregnant women are encouraged to take a multivitamin/multimineral supplement.

Iron supplementation is recommended for virtually all pregnant women. Moore (2007) noted that all pregnant women should receive a supplement of 30 mg of iron daily, starting by the 12th week. Iron is needed to promote fetal and placental growth, increase maternal red blood cell mass, and compensate for basal losses. However, the use of iron supplements may produce unwanted side effects; abdominal discomfort and constipation are the most common. Nurses who care for pregnant women should counsel them on minimizing these side effects. Suggestions may include taking the supplements at bedtime to decrease nausea, increasing fluids and daily exercise, and eating high-fiber foods to reduce constipation.

Research has shown that folic acid is essential to the developing fetus and that supplementation

BOX **14-2** Factors Associated with High-Risk Pregnancy

ECONOMIC

Poverty
Unemployment
Uninsured, underinsured
Poor access to prenatal care

CULTURAL-BEHAVIORAL

Low educational status
Poor health care attitudes
No care or inadequate prenatal care
Cigarette, alcohol, drug use
Age less than 16 or over 35 years
Unmarried
Short interpregnancy interval
Lack of support group
Stress (physical, psychologic)

BIOLOGIC-GENETIC

Previous low-birth-weight infant
African-American race
Low maternal weight at her birth
Low weight for height
Poor weight gain during pregnancy
Short stature
Poor nutrition
Inbreeding (autosomal recessive)
Intergenerational effects
Hereditary diseases

REPRODUCTIVE

Prior cesarean section
Prior infertility
Prolonged gestation
Prolonged labor
Prior infant with cerebral palsy, mental retardation, birth trauma, congenital anomalies
Abnormal lie (breech)
Multiple gestation
Premature rupture of membranes
Infections (systemic, amniotic, extraamniotic, cervical)
Preeclampsia or eclampsia
Uterine bleeding
Parity (0 or more than 5)
Uterine or cervical anomalies
Fetal disease
Abnormal fetal growth
Idiopathic premature labor
Iatrogenic prematurity
High or low levels of maternal serum alpha fetoprotein

MEDICAL

Diabetes
Hypertension
Congenital heart disease
Autoimmune disease
Sickle cell anemia
TORCH infection
Intercurrent surgery or trauma
Sexually transmitted diseases

Adapted from Clemen-Stone S, McGuire SL, Eigsti DG: *Comprehensive community health nursing*, ed 6, St Louis, 2002, Mosby; Data from Nelson WE, Behrman RE, Kliegman RM, Algin AM: *Nelson textbook of pediatrics*, ed 15, Philadelphia, 1996, Saunders.

is effective in reducing fetal abnormalities, particularly neural tube defects (NTDs). Consequently, the benefits of ensuring adequate dietary intake of folic acid should be presented to all women of childbearing age. Even if pregnancy is not being contemplated, women should maintain a daily intake of 0.4 mg of folic acid. This may be obtained through diet or supplementation. Foods high in folic acid include dark green leafy vegetables (e.g., broccoli, spinach), oranges, bananas, whole wheat products, liver, black beans, pinto beans, peanuts, potatoes, and fortified breads and cereals. Pregnant women should be encouraged to eat these foods in addition to taking their daily vitamin/mineral supplement.

Weight gain during pregnancy and the birth weight of the infant are strongly correlated, and low maternal weight gain is a risk factor for having an infant with LBW. An estimated one third of all mothers gain inadequate weight during their pregnancies, a complication particularly common in teenagers and black women (USDHHS, 2000). Because of this, pregnant women should be taught the importance of sufficient weight gain. Weight should be measured with each prenatal visit and monitored closely for indicators of complications (e.g., failure to gain or sudden weight gain suggestive of pregnancy-induced hypertension) (Corbett, 2007).

General recommendations on total weight gain for pregnant women are 25 to 35 pounds for women whose prepregnancy weight is low to normal for height, and 15 to 25 pounds for women whose weight for height is high or who are obese. The rate of weight gain should be 2 to 5 pounds during the first trimester and an additional 0.9 pounds per week thereafter (Moore, 2007).

ELIMINATION OF UNHEALTHY HABITS

The detrimental effects of smoking, alcohol consumption, and use of recreational drugs on the developing fetus have been definitively established. Smoking alone is associated with 20% to 30% of all LBW births in the United States (Askin, 2007; USDHHS, 2000). In addition to LBW, smoking during pregnancy is associated with premature delivery, stillbirth, delayed neurologic and intellectual development, spontaneous abortion, premature rupture of membranes, placenta previa, abruptio placentae, bacterial infection, and infant mortality (CDC, 2004; Fishel, 2007). Therefore maternal smoking should be strongly discouraged throughout pregnancy.

Maternal consumption of alcohol is known to cause defects in the developing fetus, as well as longterm postnatal complications for the child. One of the most serious effects of alcohol use during pregnancy is fetal alcohol syndrome, which is characterized by growth retardation, facial malformations, and central nervous system dysfunction (USDHHS, 2000). Even as little as two drinks per day is associated with developmental delays. As a result, it is recommended that women consume no alcohol during pregnancy.

Recreational or illegal drug use during pregnancy can cause a number of problems for the infant and the mother. The potential effects depend on the substance used and the amount. In general, illicit drug use may cause growth retardation, withdrawal symptoms, and physical anomalies. In addition, maternal use of intravenous drugs is associated with human immunodeficiency virus (HIV) infection, which may in turn be transmitted to the developing fetus. To eliminate these potential problems, all women who are planning on becoming pregnant or who are pregnant should be counseled to avoid illicit drug use before and during pregnancy. Furthermore, testing for HIV is now recommended for all pregnant women (Agency for Healthcare Research and Quality [AHRQ], 2007).

The effect of caffeine on the developing baby has not been determined. Heavy maternal caffeine consumption may be associated with intrauterine growth retardation. Therefore pregnant women should be encouraged to limit their intake of caffeine (Fishel, 2007).

STRESS REDUCTION

Pregnancy and childbirth are stressful for all concerned because the expectant mother and father must face new experiences and pressures that may produce anxiety. Stress is often higher near the end of pregnancy, and many pregnancy-related concerns are shared with the nurse during the third trimester. Common concerns are fear of childbirth, major life changes, negative self-concept, previous loss of a fetus, terminating work, future pregnancies, apprehension about pain in labor and delivery, and effects of birth on the baby, finances, and family. Other stressors more commonly seen in multiparous women include increased fears for the unborn baby with each successive pregnancy, stress from too much company or interfering relatives, concerns about weight reduction following delivery, concern about housework and family routines, fatigue during the postpartum period, increased depression, fear of not having enough time for self and others, disillusionment with parenting and child care, and concern about her own emotional ability to meet the needs of all family members (Matteson, 2001; Zdanuk, 2007).

Nurses who work with pregnant women and their families should be alert to signs and comments indicating increased stress. Adaptive changes related to the pregnancy and impending birth can be promoted. To this end the nurse should provide information on childbirth, refer clients to prepared childbirth classes, and provide literature on recognizing and managing postpartum depression and other potential problems. Encouraging healthful behaviors such as getting adequate rest and good nutrition can help reduce stress. A referral to a psychologist, counselor, or social worker might be necessary to assist with more serious problems (e.g., depression, financial difficulties, or abuse). Nurses should be prepared in advance to provide these referrals by maintaining a list of providers, addresses, and telephone numbers.

SOCIAL SUPPORT SERVICES

Serving as an advocate and referral source for social programs for eligible mothers and children is one of the most important roles of nurses in community-based practice. Many expectant mothers are eligible for at least one social program such as WIC, Medicaid, Aid to Families with Dependent Children, or food stamps. Nurses caring for expectant mothers and infants should be aware of area social programs for pregnant clients and be prepared to refer those who might need social services.

HEALTH EDUCATION

General health education for pregnant women includes providing anticipatory guidance and health teaching about the normal course of pregnancy, labor and delivery, and the postpartum period. Management of common discomforts associated with pregnancy (e.g., nausea and vomiting, constipation, heartburn, urinary frequency, sleep pattern disturbances) should be discussed. The pregnant woman should be encouraged to get adequate rest and regular exercise. Preparation for labor and delivery should include several discussions on signs and symptoms indicating that labor has begun and when to go to the hospital or birthing center for delivery. Finally, signs and symptoms of possible complications (e.g., vaginal bleeding, abdominal cramping, severe headache) should be described, and the mother-to-be should know when to call her physician or clinic and when to seek emergency care.

PRENATAL SCREENING

The U.S. Preventive Services Task Force has developed specific guidelines for periodic health examinations for pregnant women. These recommendations are summarized in Table 14-2. In addition, prenatal screening and counseling for detection of fetal abnormalities is sometimes warranted. These screenings allow for initiation of interventions to ameliorate the consequences of disorders through counseling and specialized obstetric and neonatal care (USDHHS, 2000). Table 14-3 lists some prenatal screening and diagnostic tests.

INFERTILITY

Infertility refers to the inability to conceive after 1 year of regular sexual intercourse without contraception. Approximately 10% to 15% of couples report experiencing problems with conception (CDC/American Society for Reproductive Medicine [ASRM], 2006; Lowdermilk, 2007).

In general, for about 12% to 20% of infertile couples, the cause of infertility is unexplained or idiopathic (CDC/ASRM, 2006; Lowdermilk, 2007). When the cause(s)/contributing factors can be identified, factors related to the female partner account for 40% to 50% of infertility problems, and factors related to the male account for about 20% to 30%; a combination of factors of both partners accounts for another 20% (CDC/ASRM, 2006; Lowdermilk, 2007). In women the most common causes of infertility are problems in ovulation, blocked or scarred fallopian tubes, endometriosis, and endocervical problems (e.g., issues with vaginal or cervical pH, amount and characteristics of vaginal mucous, development of sperm antibodies). Delay of childbirth until after the optimal age for fertility has also been identified as contributing to problems with conception.

In men, abnormal or too few sperm is the most frequent cause of infertility. Factors that contribute to problems with sperm and thus male infertility include underlying disease processes, structural disorders such as undescended testes, trauma, poor nutrition, prolonged exposure to high temperature in the scrotal area (e.g., associated with wearing tight briefs, use of hot tubs), low testosterone levels, and varicocele (Lowdermilk, 2007).

The process of trying to discover the cause of infertility can be expensive, painful, embarrassing, and emotionally draining. To diagnose infertility, both partners must undergo testing, including complete health history and physical examination. A detailed sexual history of both partners is also necessary. Based on information from the histories and physical examination, one or more diagnostic tests may be performed. Table 14-4 lists some tests that may be conducted to diagnose the cause of infertility.

Following identification of the reason for infertility, the couple is counseled on treatment options.

TABLE 14-2 Preventive Services Task Force Risk Factors Screening, Referral, and Service for Pregnant Women

RISK FACTOR OR GROUP	PREVENTION TARGET CONDITION	PREVENTION SERVICE AND/OR REFERRAL
All pregnant women	Asymptomatic bacteriuria, pyelonephritis	Urinalysis and culture
	Anemia	CBC
	Rh incompatibility	Blood typing and antibody testing
	Preeclampsia	Periodic blood pressure measurement
	Domestic Violence	Direct questioning about abuse, using screening instrument; referral for counseling; referral to crisis center, shelter, and social services; notify protective authorities
	Problems related to substance abuse, including alcohol, tobacco, and illicit drugs	Screen for use and counsel regarding personal hazards, effects on fetus, and potential to transmit drugs through breast milk
	Nutritional and immunologic deficiencies	Counsel regarding adequate calcium intake and breast feeding
	Vertical transmission of hepatitis B and HIV	Hepatitis B surface antigen and HIV serology
	Obstetric complications related to STDs	STD/HIV screening and counseling
	Hemoglobinopathy	Hemoglobin electrophoresis and counseling
Periconception period with prior pregnancy affected by NTD	NTD	Referral for amniocentesis with alpha fetoprotein measurement; folic acid supplementation
Pregnant women <35 years of age with no prior pregnancy affected with Down syndrome	Down Syndrome	Serum multiple-marker screening and counseling
Pregnant women >35 years of age or prior pregnancy affected with Down syndrome	Down syndrome	Referral for amniocentesis or chorionic villus sampling or multiple-marker screening and counseling
Pregnant women >35 years of age with obesity or glucosuria on screening urinalysis	Gestational diabetes, fetal macrosomia, birth trauma	Glucose tolerance test
Postpartum period	Thyroid dysfunction	Thyroid screening

From U.S. Department of Health and Human Services/Office of Disease Prevention and Health Promotion: *Clinician's handbook of preventive services*, ed 2, McLean, Va, 1998, International Medical.

TABLE **14-3** Types of Prenatal Genetic Testing

TEST	PURPOSE	ADVANTAGES	DISADVANTAGES	RISKS
Maternal serum alpha fetoprotein (MS-AFP)	Screening test for NTDs, ventral wall defects, trisomy pregnancies	Identifies women at higher risk who otherwise would not receive diagnostic testing	Is not diagnostic; only indicates need for further testing False-positive and false-negative results occur	Venipuncture Minimal risk
Ultrasonography	Assesses gestational age, fetal growth, placental sufficiency Detects multiple gestation and structural anomalies Screening and diagnostic	Detects structural anomalies and effects of intrauterine environment that may not be detected by chromosome analysis	Accuracy depends on skill of ultrasonographer, quality of equipment, and size of defect Does not detect biochemical abnormalities	Noninvasive
Amniocentesis	Chromosome analysis of fetal cells DNA analysis AFP analysis, other biochemical analyses	Diagnostic for chromosome abnormalities Provides DNA for direct and indirect testing for single-gene disorder High accuracy for detection of NTDs by biochemical analysis	Does not detect structural anomalies not caused by chromosome abnormalities, except for neural tube or ventral wall defects Usually not performed until second trimester (14-16 weeks) Results are usually available in 1-3 weeks Relatively expensive	Invasive 0.5% risk of spontaneous abortion Nongrowth of fetal cells requires repeat procedure
Chorionic villus sampling (CVS)	Chromosome analysis of chorionic (fetal) cells DNA analysis	Diagnostic for chromosome abnormalities Provides DNA for direct and indirect testing for single-gene disorders Test is done earlier than amniocentesis (9-12 weeks); therefore results are available earlier	Diagnostic accuracy may be less because of greater risk of maternal cell contamination and false evidence of mosaicism, which may require subsequent amniocentesis Relatively expensive Less available than amniocentesis	Invasive Risk of spontaneous abortion about 2% Controversial evidence of limb-reduction defects

From Hockenberry, M and Wilson D: *Wong's nursing care of infants and children*, ed 8, St. Louis, 2006, Mosby.

TABLE **14-4** Tests for Impaired Fertility

TEST/EXAMINATION	TIMING (MENSTRUAL CYCLE DAYS)	RATIONALE
Hysterosalpingogram	7-10	Late follicular, early proliferative phase; will not disrupt a fertilized ovum; may open uterine tubes before time of ovulation
Postcoital test	1-2 days before ovulation	Ovulatory late proliferative phase; look for normal motile sperm in cervical mucus
Sperm immobilization antigen-antibody reaction	Variable, ovulation	Immunologic test to determine sperm and cervical mucus interaction
Assessment of cervical mucus	Variable, ovulation	Cervical mucus should have low viscosity, high spinnbarkeit
Ultrasound diagnosis of follicular collapse	Ovulation	Collapsed follicle is seen after ovulation
Serum assay of plasma progesterone	20-25	Midluteal midsecretory phase; check adequacy of corpus luteal production of progesterone
Basal body temperature (BBT)	Chart entire cycle	Elevation occurs in response to progesterone; documents ovulation
Endometrial biopsy	21-27	Late luteal, late secretory phase; check endometrial response to progesterone and adequacy of luteal phase
Sperm penetration assay	After 2 days but no more than 1 week of abstinence	Evaluation of spermatozoa's ability to penetrate an egg

From Lowdermilk DL: Infertility. In Lowdermilk DL, Perry SE, editors: *Maternity and women's health care*, ed 9, St Louis, 2007, Mosby.

Treatment of infertility can be very expensive, and outcomes are far from certain. If the problem is related to ovulation, medications such as clomiphene citrate, human menopausal gonadotropin (HMG), or follicle stimulating hormone (FSH) may be given to increase or regulate ovulation. Endometriosis may be treated medically through use of hormones or in more severe cases, surgical repair of the uterus or fallopian tubes (Lowdermilk, 2007).

Similarly, treatment of male infertility may involve the use of drug therapy and lifestyle changes (e.g., improved nutrition, wearing boxer shorts, no hot baths or hot tubs, stopping smoking). Surgery may be required if a varicocele is detected.

If initial therapies are unsuccessful, several other options are available for infertile couples. Again, the possible treatments depend on the identified cause of the problem. For example, if the cervical mucus is not supportive of sperm, artificial insemination with the partner's sperm is an option. Artificial insemination with donor sperm is an option if the male's sperm are insufficient in number or motility.

Assisted reproductive technology (ART) refers to several therapies that have been developed to treat infertility. Success rates for the different procedures vary significantly among centers where the procedures are performed and are based on such factors as age, physical status, and whether the embryos are fresh or frozen or from donor or nondonor eggs. Some of the available options include the following (Lowdermilk, 2007):

- In vitro fertilization (IVF; "test tube" fertilization): the woman's eggs are laparoscopically collected from her ovaries and fertilized in the laboratory, then transferred back to her uterus after normal embryo development has begun.
- Gamete intrafallopian transfer (GIFT): the eggs are harvested from the ovary and placed in a catheter with washed, motile sperm and immediately transferred into the end of the fallopian tube(s). Fertilization occurs in the fallopian tube rather than in the laboratory.
- Zygote intrafallopian transfer: a combination of IVF and GIFT in which the ova are fertilized in the laboratory and then transferred to the fallopian tube for development and transport to the uterus. Success rates are comparable with those of GIFT and IVF.
- Donor ovum transfer: ova from a donor are fertilized in the laboratory by the male partner's sperm and then transferred into the recipient's uterus, which has been hormonally prepared with estrogen and progesterone therapy.
- Donor embryo (embryo adoption): a donated embryo is transferred to the uterus of an infertile woman at the appropriate time (normal or induced) of the menstrual cycle.
- Gestational carrier (surrogate mothers/embryo host): the infertile couple undergoes IVF, but the embryo(s) are transferred to another woman's uterus (the carrier) who will carry the baby to term. The carrier does not provide ova.
- Therapeutic donor insemination: donor sperm are used to inseminate the female partner.

Nurses who work with couples experiencing problems with fertility should be prepared to discuss their options. Information on these options and resources for referral should be made available.

TEENAGE PREGNANCY

Pregnancy and childbearing rates for teenagers remain high in the United States despite well-documented associated adverse health, social, and economic consequences for both the teens and their children. In the United States, **teenage pregnancy** is one of the most serious, complicated, and far reaching of all public health problems. The statistics are astonishing. Consider the following (CDC, 2004; USDHHS/NCHS, 2006; USDHHS, 2000):

- The United States has the highest rate of teenage pregnancy among developed countries.
- Each year, about 900,000 girls between 15 and 19 years of age become pregnant, and 415,000 give birth.
- By age 18, 24% of teenage girls have become pregnant at least once; 18% have given birth.
- More than 80% of teenage pregnancies are unintended.
- Approximately 75% of teenagers report that they use no contraception or use contraception inconsistently.
- More than 27% of non-Hispanic black teens and 35% of Hispanic teens give birth before age 20.

CONSEQUENCES

Teenage pregnancy is associated with serious problems. Teenage mothers are more likely to experience complications of pregnancy, largely because of delayed or no prenatal care, poor nutrition, and other lifestyle factors. They are more likely to experience maternal complications, including pregnancy-induced hypertension, toxemia, anemia, nutritional deficiencies, and urinary tract infections. They are more prone to deliver prematurely, experience rapid or prolonged labor, and have fetal and maternal infections. Infants born to teenage mothers are more likely to have LBW and suffer associated problems (e.g., respiratory problems, neurologic defects) and are more likely to be stillborn (Maurer, 2005).

Probably the most significant factor, however, is the socioeconomic impact of teenage pregnancy. Many pregnant girls and teenage mothers fail to complete high school. This in turn is associated with unemployment and underemployment, resulting in living below the poverty level and reliance on welfare programs.

CONTRIBUTING FACTORS

Higher teenage pregnancy rates are directly tied to reports that teenagers are becoming sexually active at younger ages. In 1970 28.6% of adolescent women

(15 to 19 years) were sexually active. In 2002 about 46% of adolescent females reported they had had sexual intercourse; this was down from a high of 55% in 1995 (CDC, 2004).

Several factors contribute to early engagement in sexual activity. These include peer pressure; pervasive sexually explicit media (e.g., television, movies, music, music videos, information on the Internet); need for love, acceptance, and approval; efforts to gain independence; increased acceptance of unmarried mothers; present rather than future orientation; and lack of maturity (Aretakis, 2004; Maurer, 2005).

COUNSELING TEENAGERS ON ISSUES OF SEXUALITY

The benefits of practicing sexual abstinence should be stressed to all teenagers by health care providers. Providing information on reasons to avoid initiation of sexual intercourse and how to say "no" has been shown to be helpful. Resources that provide materials on sexuality issues for adolescents are available for health care providers and educators who work with teenagers. To assist nurses working with teenagers, the Health Teaching box "Counseling Guidelines to Prevent Adolescent Pregnancy" offers suggestions by the Preventive Services Task Force (USDHHS/Office of Disease Prevention and Health Promotion [ODPHP], 1998).

In addition to these guidelines, nurses who care for sexually active and pregnant teenagers should be aware of their state's laws regarding age of consent for engaging in sexual activity and statutory rape. Although there is no firm consensus on how and when to notify child protective services or other authorities, agencies that work with sexually

---

health teaching

Counseling Guidelines to Prevent Adolescent Pregnancy

1. All adolescents should be asked about their sexual experiences and use of contraceptives. The clinician should maintain a nonjudgmental, empathetic manner and should be willing to answer questions and provide contraceptive advice or refer to another clinician for prescriptions as appropriate. Information should include consequences of pregnancy and STDs and effective methods to prevent them.
2. State laws vary regarding minimum age for minors to consent to treatment and receive contraceptives. Clinicians should familiarize themselves with the laws in their state regarding these issues. Adolescents should be informed about issues of confidentiality regarding pregnancy prevention, STD testing, and treatment, as directed by state regulations and agency policy.
3. Parents should be counseled about the emerging sexuality in teenagers' lives and options for contraception. Clinicians should encourage effective communication between adolescents and their families regarding responsible sexual behavior.
4. Adolescents who are sexually abstinent should be supported in remaining abstinent and should be counseled in methods to resist unwelcome or coercive sexual relationships.
5. Within the parameters set by the state and the agency, adolescents who are sexually active should be assisted in choosing an effective, appropriate method of contraception. Considerations include their personal preferences and motivation, religious beliefs, cultural norms, and relationship

with their partner(s). The most popular contraceptive methods among adolescents are birth control pills and condoms; injectable contraceptives may be appropriate choices for teens. Diaphragms, cervical caps, and periodic abstinence are difficult for teens to use effectively, and IUDs are not recommended for adolescents.
6. All sexually active adolescents should be taught that hormonal contraception (e.g., pills, injections) does not protect against STDs and HIV. The use of condoms in addition to these contraceptives should be encouraged to reduce STDs in sexually active individuals. It should be stressed that condoms are not 100% effective.
7. Adolescents of both genders should be encouraged to talk frankly with their partners about STDs, HIV, and use of contraceptives. Assertiveness with partners about the use of contraception and protective measures against STDs should be supported. It should be stressed that saying "no" is every person's right.
8. Boys should be provided with as much counseling as girls about contraception and STD prevention. Young adolescent males should be taught at an early age about the benefits of abstinence, the importance of responsible sexual behavior, and the importance of condom use if engaging in sexual intercourse.
9. Adolescents using prescribed contraceptives should be followed closely to determine proper use and to monitor for side effects.

HIV, Human immunodeficiency virus; *IUD*, intrauterine device; *STD*, sexually transmitted disease.
Adapted from U.S. Department of Health and Human Services: *Clinician's handbook of preventive services*, ed 2, Washington, DC, 1998, Government Printing Office.

active and pregnant minors should have or should develop policies describing circumstances under which to notify authorities and the process that is involved. For example, in some states girls younger than 15 years cannot legally consent to sex, and adults who engage in sexual intercourse with these teenagers are subject to prosecution. Other states base age of consent on age differences between the girl and her partner (e.g., the older partner cannot be more than 3 years older than the younger one). It may be legally permissible for a 15-year-old girl to have intercourse with a 17-year-old boy, but not with a 24-year-old man. Finally, the nurse should always consider the possibility of sexual child abuse and assess appropriately—particularly when caring for younger girls.

PRENATAL CARE FOR PREGNANT TEENS

For all of the reasons cited, pregnant teenagers need early and comprehensive prenatal care. Case management is preferred. It is particularly important that teenagers be counseled on good nutritional practices, getting plenty of rest, and recognition of signs and symptoms of complications. Pregnant teenagers should be encouraged to stay in school. Because of the extent of this problem, many school districts have developed special programs designed to meet the educational, developmental, maturational, and social needs of the pregnant teenager. On-site health care is frequently a component of school programs. In addition, many programs offer childbirth education, parenting classes, and after-delivery childcare (Figure 14-2).

POSTDELIVERY NEEDS

After delivery, teenagers need ongoing social support and encouragement to complete their education. Financial assistance is also frequently a need, and nurses who practice in community-based settings should know how to refer new mothers to obtain social services such as Aid to Families with Dependent Children, WIC, and food stamps.

Finally, all pregnant teenagers should be counseled regarding sexual activity and contraception choices following delivery. Somewhat surprisingly, repeat pregnancy is frequently a problem. All teenagers who have experienced one pregnancy should be emphatically encouraged to avoid another

Figure 14-2. A teacher and student in a school-based childbirth and parenting class for pregnant teenage girls. (From Matteson PS: *Women's health during the childbearing years: a community-based approach*, St Louis, 2001, Mosby.)

pregnancy and supported in their contraceptive choices.

WOMEN'S HEALTH CARE

In addition to health needs related to childbearing and family planning, several health promotion- and illness-prevention issues should be addressed by health care professionals who care for women of all ages in community settings. The following sections discuss screening recommendations for breast cancer and diseases of the reproductive organs, prevention of osteoporosis, and prevention and identification of and interventions for domestic violence.

SCREENING RECOMMENDATIONS FOR BREAST CANCER

Breast cancer is the most common cancer among women in the United States (excluding skin cancer) and the second leading cause of cancer deaths in women. In the United States a woman's average lifetime risk for developing breast cancer is approximately one in eight (American Cancer Society [ACS], 2007).

Risk factors for breast cancer are age (over 50); personal or family history (e.g., mother, sister); high breast tissue density; high-dose radiation to the chest during medical procedures; first pregnancy after 30 years of age; having had no children; menarche before age 12; menopause after age 50; postmenopausal obesity; alcohol consumption (more than 1 or 2 drinks per day); and a personal history of breast, ovarian, or endometrial cancer (ACS, 2007). Mortality from breast cancer is strongly influenced by its stage at detection; therefore early detection is critical to promoting a good outcome. Mammography and regular breast examination by a clinician are the most commonly used tools to screen women for breast cancer. Breast self examination (BSE) can also be useful, although it is not necessarily recommended at this time.

The American Cancer Society (2007) recommends that all women have a screening mammogram every year beginning at age 40. A clinical breast exam should be performed by a health professional at least every 3 years for women in their 20s and 30s and every year after age 40. High-risk women (e.g., women with a family history of premenopausally diagnosed breast cancer in a first-degree relative) should talk with a clinician about starting mammograms at a younger age and having routine ultrasound examinations or MRIs in addition to mammography. Genetic testing may also be recommended for women with a strong family history. Any palpable breast lump, even if not detected on a mammogram, should be carefully evaluated.

When breast cancer is suspected, a surgical biopsy or needle biopsy is performed. If the lump is confirmed as breast cancer, treatment is typically a combination of surgery (e.g., lumpectomy, simple mastectomy, modified radical mastectomy) and radiation and/or chemotherapy or hormone therapy. All treatment options should be discussed thoroughly with the client, including potential outcomes, side effects, benefits, and negative consequences. Again, the nurse should assist in informed decision making by providing literature on breast cancer and referral to organizations and agencies (e.g., ACS, Reach for Recovery) that provide information on the treatment of breast cancer.

SCREENING RECOMMENDATIONS FOR CANCERS OF THE FEMALE REPRODUCTIVE TRACT

Cancers of the cervix, ovary, and endometrium are relatively common and are treatable if caught early. Screening recommendations for each are described briefly here.

Cancer of the endometrium is the most common gynecologic malignancy and the fourth most common malignancy in women (after breast, colorectal, and lung cancer) (ACS, 2007). Endometrial cancer most often occurs in postmenopausal women between the ages of 50 and 65 years. Risk factors include nulliparity, infertility, late menopause, early menarche, obesity, a family history of breast cancer, higher socioeconomic status, pelvic irradiation, and endometrial hyperplasia (Lowdermilk, 2007b). Hormone replacement therapy also strongly increases the risk of uterine cancer. Abnormal vaginal bleeding and an enlarged uterus are the most common symptoms of endometrial cancer. If postmenopausal bleeding occurs, an endometrial biopsy is usually performed.

Total abdominal hysterectomy and bilateral salpingo-oophorectomy is the treatment of choice for cases of endometrial cancer. Radiation, chemotherapy, hormone therapy, or a combination may be considered (ACS, 2007; Lowdermilk, 2007b).

Although cases have declined in recent years, cancer of the cervix remains a relatively common cancer in women. The major risk factor for cervical cancers is infection with human papillomavirus (HPV). Other risk factors for cervical cancer are early age at first intercourse, having had multiple sexual partners, a history of exposure to diethylstilbestrol, long-term use of oral contraceptives (longer than 5 years), and smoking (ACS, 2007). Cervical carcinoma in situ is most commonly seen in women between 20 and 30 years of age; cases of invasive cervical carcinoma increase with age.

In 2006 the FDA approved the first vaccine to prevent the most common HPV infections that cause cervical cancer; approval for another vaccine is pending. The CDC (2007b) recommends that the vaccine be given to all girls between 11 and 12 years of age, with "catch up" vaccines being given to all girls and women up to age 26 to prevent HPV infection. It is believed that vaccination against HPV will greatly reduce the incidence of cervical cancer in years to come.

Symptoms of cervical cancer include vaginal bleeding or discharge, often associated with sexual intercourse. The widespread use of the Pap test for early detection of cervical cancer has contributed greatly to the decline in deaths from cervical cancer. Recommendations by the ACS (2007) for cervical cancer are as follows:

- Screening approximately 3 years after a woman begins having vaginal intercourse (no later than 21 years of age).
- Screening should be done every year with a regular Pap test or every 2 years using liquid-based tests. At or after age 30, women who have had three normal tests in a row may get screened every 2 to 3 years.
- Women with certain risk factors (e.g., HIV infection) should be screened more frequently.
- Women over 70 years of age may stop screening if they have had three or more consecutive normal Pap tests in the last 10 years.

For cervical changes and abnormal Pap results, one of several diagnostic examinations and treatment options may be chosen. Colposcopy and directed cervical biopsies, cone biopsy (by cold knife, laser, or loop excision), endocervical curettage, and/or loop electrosurgical procedure may be performed. Following treatment, Pap tests every 4 months for the first year and every 6 months thereafter are recommended. If invasive cervical cancer is detected, a total abdominal hysterectomy is usually performed. Additional therapy (e.g., radiation and/or chemotherapy) may be recommended for advanced disease (ACS, 2007; Dambro, 2006).

Cancer of the ovary is quite rare, affecting 1 out of 67 (1.5%) of women; however, it is the most deadly of the cancers of the reproductive organs (ACS, 2007). The high death rate is largely attributable to delay in diagnosis because ovarian cancer rarely produces symptoms until it reaches advanced stages. Early cancers of the ovaries tend to cause somewhat vague symptoms. These symptoms might include: swelling of the stomach (abdomen) or bloating caused by a buildup of fluid, pelvic pressure or stomach (abdominal) pain, trouble

eating or feeling full quickly, having to urinate often or feeling like you have to "go" right away. Women experiencing these symptoms for more than 2 weeks should see their health care provider for evaluation.

Risk factors for ovarian cancer include age (most occur after menopause), family history, nulliparity, older age at the first pregnancy, fewer pregnancies, obesity, and a personal history of breast, endometrial, or colorectal cancer. The pelvic examination is the most common screening examination for ovarian cancer. Treatment is usually a combination of surgery and radiation and/or chemotherapy.

PREVENTION OF OSTEOPOROSIS

Osteoporosis is a very common skeletal disease characterized by decreased bone mass, which leads to increased skeletal fragility and subsequent tendency to fracture. Osteoporosis affects about 10 million U.S. residents, including an estimated 18% of women older than 50 years and 90% of women older than 75 (National Osteoporosis Foundation, 2007). The implications of these high numbers are serious; each year approximately 1.5 million osteoporosis-related fractures occur in the United States. The most common sites of atraumatic fractures are the vertebral column, upper femur, distal radius, and proximal humerus. The most serious fractures are hip fractures, which affect about 250,000 U.S. residents each year. It is estimated that about 17% of women and 6% of men experience a hip fracture by the time they reach 90 years of age (USDHHS, 2000). Further, as the population of the United States ages, the incidence of osteoporosis-related fractures is expected to increase.

Risk factors for osteoporosis include age, female gender, family history, low bone mass, being thin/having a small frame, estrogen deficiency, diet (inadequate calcium and vitamin D and excessive protein and phosphate), decreased activity, sedentary lifestyle, use of alcohol and caffeine, smoking, some medications (corticosteroids, excess thyroid replacement, long-term heparin therapy, chemotherapy, and anticonvulsants), being white or Asian, and radiation therapy (Dambro, 2006; National Osteoporosis Foundation, 2007). At greatest risk for osteoporosis-related fractures are women who are older, white, and slender and who have had a bilateral oophorectomy or early menopause. In addition to increased risk of fractures, osteoporosis is associated with both acute and chronic back pain, kyphosis, and loss of height.

Prevention measures to reduce bone loss include maintaining a diet rich in calcium and vitamin D, regular weightbearing and resistance training exercise, not smoking, and limiting alcohol intake. Women with several risk factors should be encouraged to have bone density testing; pharmacologic therapy may be indicated to prevent and/or treat osteoporosis.

Other preventive measures to reduce osteoporosis include increased calcium intake (1500 mg/day), adequate vitamin D intake (600 to 1000 IU/day), and avoiding excess meat and phosphoric acid-containing beverages (Dambro, 2006). Premenopausal women, particularly those in high-risk groups, should be taught the benefits of calcium supplementation, with the recommended dosage being 1000 mg/day. Encouragement of weightbearing exercise is also very important.

Medications to prevent or reduce bone loss include alendronate (Fosamax), ibandronate (Boniva), risedronate (Actonel), calcitonin, raloxifene (Evista), and zoledronic acid (Reclast). Hormone therapy (estrogen) has also been approved for prevention of osteoporosis in postmenopausal women.

INTIMATE PARTNER VIOLENCE

Studies indicate that between 1.5 and 2 million women in the United States are physically abused by an intimate partner each year (Langford, 2005; Stevenson and Pappas, 2007). It has been noted that abuse is the leading cause of injury in women. In addition, abused women use health services much more frequently than women who have not been abused (Langford, 2005).

Once the pattern of domestic violence begins in a relationship, it tends to recur and become more severe over time. Furthermore, intrafamilial homicide accounts for almost one of six homicides and is often preceded by a history of physical and emotional abuse. Therefore prevention of homicide among spouses and intimates should be linked to the prevention of abuse of women.

Nurses working in community settings are often in a position to identify and intervene in cases of domestic violence. Although there may be considerable variation, there are commonalities in the characteristics of the abuser and the victim. For example, the abuser often has poor impulse control, an unpredictable temper, and an inability to tolerate frustration. He typically is egocentric, is emotionally dependent, has poor social skills, and has a need to dominate. The batterer may also be excessively jealous and may have unrealistic expectations. Frequently he has been a victim of child abuse and is often unemployed or underemployed. Finally, alcohol use may facilitate aggression or may be used as an excuse for aggression (Langford, 2005; Smith-McKenna and Grant, 2003; Stevenson and Pappas, 2007).

In general, victims of domestic violence have low self-esteem. They are typically poorly educated and economically and emotionally dependent on the abuser. They often marry young and have children early; risk increases during pregnancy. They may experience constant fear and gradual isolation from friends and family. Many were victims of child abuse. They often report a hope that "things will get better," but many have a history of suicide attempts.

To help nurses identify suspected cases of domestic violence, Box 14-3 lists physical and behavioral signs and symptoms that might indicate abuse, and the Community Application box "Nursing Interventions for Victims of Domestic Violence" offers strategies for supporting these women and getting them help.

SUMMARY

Lisa, the nurse from the opening case study, worked in a women's health clinic; she was familiar with the many health issues commonly encountered in this group. However, all nurses who work with women of any age in community-based settings, including worksites, schools, practitioner offices, and clinics, should understand the scope of women's health care and be prepared to intervene as appropriate to prevent health problems and promote health.

Health care for women goes beyond issues related to reproduction and encompasses a variety of

BOX 14-3 Injuries, Signs, and Symptoms Suggestive of Domestic Violence

IN AN OFFICE OR CLINIC

- Presenting complaints related to chronic stress or anxiety (e.g., hyperventilation, gastrointestinal disturbances, hypertension, panic attack, headache, chest pain, choking sensation)
- Depression or stress-related conditions (e.g., insomnia, anxiety, fatigue)
- Evidence of fear, embarrassment, or humiliation
- Poor grooming or inappropriate attire
- Any suspicious physical injuries (e.g., bruises, lacerations, scars, burns, swelling, fractures, ear or eye problems secondary to injury, clumps of hair missing)
- Any evidence of physical injury during pregnancy

IN AN EMERGENCY ROOM

- Bleeding injuries, particularly to the head and face
- Perforated eardrum, eye injuries (e.g., black eye, orbital fracture)
- Broken or fractured jaw, arms, ribs, and legs
- Internal injuries; concussion
- Severe bruising, particularly on the back, buttocks, breasts, abdomen, and upper extremities

- Genital/urinary or rectal trauma
- Strangulation marks on the neck
- Burns from cigarettes, liquids, or acids
- Evidence of psychologic trauma (e.g., anxiety, panic attacks, heart palpitations)
- Suicide attempt
- Miscarriage

IN ANY SETTING

- Reports domestic problems; reports being trapped or powerless
- History of hospitalization for traumatic injuries
- Increased anxiety in presence of spouse/partner
- Inappropriate or anxious nonverbal behavior; uncontrolled crying
- Injuries in various stages of healing
- Injuries indicating failure to seek immediate care
- Timid and evasive behavior
- Inconsistent description of the cause of the injury
- Accompanied by male partner who does not wish to leave her alone

Data from: Stevenson L, Pappas A: Violence. In Nies MA, McEwen M: *Community/public health nursing: promoting the health of populations*, ed 4, St Louis, 2007, Saunders; Smith-McKenna L, Grant C: The client who survives violence. In Antai-Otong D, editor: *Psychiatric nursing: biological and behavioral concepts*, Clifton Park, NY, 2003, Delmar; Langford DR: Violence: a social and family problem. In Maurer FA, Smith CM, editors: *Community/public health nursing: health for families and populations*, ed 3, St Louis, 2005, Saunders.

COMMUNITY APPLICATION
Nursing Interventions for Victims of Domestic Violence

1. Interview women with suspicious symptoms or injuries to confirm or refute abuse.

Talk with the woman in a quiet, private area.

Be professional, direct, and honest in questioning.

Be understanding; do not express anger, shock, or disapproval.

2. If abuse is confirmed, assess safety and explore the victim's options to reduce danger.

Affirm to the woman that battering is unacceptable.

Assess the seriousness of the circumstances.

Assist in calling and explaining the situation to friends or family when appropriate.

Assure the victim that disclosed information will be kept confidential to the maximal extent possible.

Counsel the victim about the dynamics of domestic violence, and provide information on potential danger to the woman and her children.

3. If the woman wants to leave the situation and no other options are feasible, provide information on shelters or safe houses.

Obtain information (telephone numbers, criteria, and process for admittance to the shelter) in advance.

Offer to contact the shelter and make arrangements for transportation.

Offer to contact legal authorities to report the abuse and press charges.

4. If the woman chooses to stay in the relationship, encourage and assist her to develop a safety plan for fast escape should violence recur.

Include ways to identify the signs of escalation of violence, and select a sign that will be a cue to leave.

Suggest that she keep a bag packed for herself and her children (include clothing, toiletries, medications, money) and ask a friend or neighbor to store the bag.

Advise her to save money if possible.

Suggest that she take important financial records, such as rent or mortgage receipts and/or the car title.

Provide a list of shelters and the appropriate telephone numbers—know exactly where to go and how to get there.

5. Encourage follow-up care; individual and family therapy should be encouraged when possible.

Data from U.S. Department of Health and Human Services/Office of Disease Prevention and Health Promotion: *Clinician's handbook of preventive services*, ed 2, Washington, DC, 1998, Government Printing Office.

topics. This chapter has covered several areas related to the unique health care needs of women. Primary and secondary prevention strategies and health education for diverse topics of family planning, prenatal care, teenage pregnancy, early detection of cancers, and prevention of osteoporosis were described. The chapter concluded with information on detection and prevention of domestic violence. Nurses in community-based practice should maintain a list of local resources related to women's health and be prepared to refer their clients as needed.

KEY POINTS

- Nursing practice in community settings includes several issues pertaining to women's health. These are family planning, prenatal care, infertility, general health care (e.g., screening for reproductive diseases, breast care, prevention of osteoporosis), detection and prevention of domestic violence, and prevention and intervention in teenage pregnancy.
- Around half of all pregnancies in the United States are unintended; therefore comprehensive family planning is an important component of health care. Family planning includes consideration of factors regarding childbearing, such as abstinence from sexual activity, use of contraceptives, treatment of infertility, and preconception counseling.
- Several methods can be used to prevent pregnancy. Contraception options include barriers (e.g., condoms, diaphragm), hormonal methods (e.g., oral contraceptives, Depo-Provera, Norplant), sterilization, natural family planning, and abstinence. Each method has positive and negative consequences, which should be discussed and considered.
- Prenatal care is important for good pregnancy outcomes. Lack of prenatal care is associated with maternal complications, babies with LBW, prematurity, and infant mortality. Removing or lessening barriers to early and comprehensive prenatal care is important in improving infant mortality rates.
- Infertility affects between 10% and 15% of married couples. Diagnosis of infertility should include testing of both partners to determine the cause of infertility. Following identification of the reason(s) for infertility, the couple is counseled on treatment options, which may include medications, surgery, lifestyle changes, artificial insemination, and more dramatic interventions such as variations of IVF.
- Teenage pregnancy rates in the United States remain higher than those in most industrialized countries and contribute to a number of health and social problems. Teenage pregnancy is associated with complications of pregnancy (both fetal and maternal), failure of the mother to complete high school, unemployment, poverty, and reliance on government assistance.
- Health promotion and illness prevention for women should also include various screenings and health education. Routine screenings for breast cancer include periodic examination by a health care provider and routine mammography for women older than 40. Screening for cancer of the cervix through yearly or biyearly Pap tests is important.
- Osteoporosis affects about 18% of all women older than 50 years and 90% older than 75, and many develop complications such as atraumatic fractures. Strategies to reduce or prevent osteoporosis should be shared with all women as they age.
- Domestic violence is a major cause of injury to women. Nurses working in community settings are often in a position to identify and intervene in cases of domestic violence and should be aware of characteristics of the victim, the batterer, and the family. They should recognize injuries and signs suggestive of domestic violence and be prepared to intervene.

Learning Activities & Application to Practice
In Class

1. Research one of the issues described in this chapter (e.g., infertility, osteoporosis, domestic violence, contraception, cancer screening). What additional information were you able to identify and how should the information be used in providing care to women in community-based settings?

2. Examine the problem of teenage pregnancy in your area. How does it compare with other areas? What efforts have been made to reduce teenage pregnancy and minimize the long-term associated problems?

In Clinical

3. Provide care in a prenatal/postpartum clinic or private practice for several days. Prepare by reviewing relevant material (e.g., nutrition, developmental milestones in pregnancy, breastfeeding) to be ready for opportunities for health promotion and education.
4. Observe contraception counseling. What issues are discussed between the counselor and the client? What factors appear to determine the woman's choice? Are all relevant factors (e.g., effectiveness of method, possible complications and side effects, cost, proper use) presented and discussed?
5. Participate in screening activities for women. Opportunities include teaching BSE, assisting with Pap smears, and observing for signs of domestic violence. Record impressions in a log or diary and share with other members of the clinical group.

REFERENCES

Agency for Healthcare Research and Quality: The guide to clinical preventive services–2007: recommendations of the U.S. Preventive Services Task Force, *AHRQ Pub No 07-05100*, 2007.

American Academy of Family Physicians: *Birth control: choosing a method that's right for you* (website): www.aafp.org. Accessed November 15, 2007.

American Cancer Society: *Cancer facts & Figures–2007*, Atlanta, 2007, American Cancer Society.

Aretakis DA: Teen pregnancy. In Stanhope M, Lancaster J, editors: *Community & public health nursing*, ed 6, St Louis, 2004, Mosby.

Askin DF: Acquired problems of the newborn. In Lowdermilk DL, Perry SE, editors: *Maternity & women's health care*, ed 9, St Louis, 2007, Mosby.

Brown SS: Drawing women into prenatal care, *Fam Plann Perspect* 21(2):73, 1989.

Centers for Disease Control and Prevention/National Center for Health Statistics (2004): *Teenagers in the United States: sexual activity, contraceptive use, and childbearing, 2002* (website): http://www.cdc.gov/nchs/data/series/sr_23/sr23_024.pdf. Accessed November 15, 2007.

Centers for Disease Control and Prevention (2007a): *Overall infant mortality rate in the United States largely unchanged: rates among black women more than twice that of white women* (website): http://www.cdc.gov/print.do?url=http://www.cdc.gov/od/oc/media/pressrel/2007/r070502.htm. Accessed November 8, 2007.

Centers for Disease Control and Prevention (2007b): Quadrivalent human papillomavirus vaccine, *MMWR Morb Mortal Wkly Rep* 56(RR02):1, 2007.

Centers for Disease Control and Prevention (2004): *2004 Surgeon General's report–the health consequences of smoking* (website): http://www.cdc.gov/tobacco/data_statistics/sgr/sgr_2004/index.htm. Accessed November 8, 2007.

Centers for Disease Control and Prevention/American Society for Reproductive Medicine (2006): *Assisted reproductive technology success rates: national summary and fertility clinic reports–2004* (website): http://www.cdc.gov/ART/ART2004/index.htm. Accessed November 7, 2007.

Corbett RW: Nursing care during pregnancy. In Lowdermilk DL, Perry SE, editors: *Maternity & women's health care*, ed 9, St Louis, 2007, Mosby.

Dambro MR: *Griffith's 5-minute clinical consult*, Philadelphia, 2006, Lippincott Williams & Wilkins.

Finer LB, Henshaw SK: Disparities in rates of unintended pregnancy in the United States, 1994 and 2001, *Perspect Sex Reprod Health* 38(2):90, 2006.

Fishel AH: Mental health disorders and substance abuse. In Lowdermilk DL, Perry SE, editors: *Maternity & women's health care*, ed 9, St Louis, 2007, Mosby.

Langford DR: Violence: a social and family problem. In Maurer FA, Smith CM, editors: *Community/public health nursing: health for families and populations*, ed 3, St Louis, 2005, Saunders.

Lowdermilk DL (2007a): Infertility. In Lowdermilk DL, Perry SE, editors: *Maternity & women's health care*, ed 9, St Louis, 2007, Mosby.

Lowdermilk DL (2007b): Structural disorders and neoplasms of the reproductive system. In Lowdermilk DL, Perry SE, editors: *Maternity & women's health care*, ed 9, St Louis, 2007, Mosby.

Maurer FA: Adolescent sexual activity and teenage pregnancy. In Maurer FA, Smith CM, editors: *Community/public health nursing: health for families and populations*, ed 3, St Louis, 2005, Saunders.

Moore MC: Maternal and fetal nutrition. In Lowdermilk DL, Perry SE, editors: *Maternity & women's health care*, ed 9, St Louis, 2007, Mosby.

National Osteoporosis Foundation: *Fast facts about osteoporosis* (website): http://www.nof.org/osteoporosis/diseasefacts.htm. Accessed November 15, 2007.

Smith-McKenna L, Grant C: The client who survives violence. In Antai-Otong D, editor: *Psychiatric nursing: biological and behavioral concepts*, Clifton Park, NY, 2003, Delmar.

Stevenson L, Pappas A: Violence. In Nies MA, McEwen M, editors: *Community/public health nursing: promoting the health of populations*, ed 4, St Louis, 2007, Saunders.

U.S. Department of Health and Human Services/National Center for Health Statistics: *Health, United States, 2006*,

Hyattsville, Md, 2006, National Center for Health Statistics (electronic version online): http://www.cdc.gov/nchs/hus.htm. Accessed November 8, 2007.

U.S. Department of Health and Human Services/Office on Women's Health (2006): *Emergency contraception* (website): http://www.4women.gov/FAQ/econtracep.htm. Accessed November 8, 2007.

U.S. Department of Health and Human Services/Office on Women's Health (2005): *Birth control methods* (website): http://www.4women.gov/FAQ/birthcont.htm. Accessed November 8, 2007.

U.S. Department of Health and Human Services: *Healthy people 2010*: conference ed, Washington, DC, 2000, Government Printing Office.

U.S. Department of Health and Human Services/Office of Disease Prevention and Health Promotion: *Clinician's handbook of preventive services*, ed 2, Washington, DC, 1998, Government Printing Office.

Zdanuk JL: Assessment and health promotion. In Lowdermilk DL, Perry SE, editors: *Maternity & women's health care*, ed 9, St Louis, 2007, Mosby.

Health Promotion and Illness Prevention for Elders

objectives

Upon completion of this chapter, the reader will be able to:

1. Discuss the impact of changing demographics and the "Aging of America" on the health care delivery system and explain why it is important to promote the health of this population.

2. Describe the range of conditions to be assessed in older adults, including assessment of physical health, health history, functional ability, cognitive and mental state, and nutritional status.

3. Explain the importance of promoting functional independence, and give examples of related interventions.

4. Discuss health-promotion and illness-prevention guidelines for older adults, including recommendations on immunizations, safety concerns, and elder abuse.

5. Recognize common health problems in older adults, and give examples of interventions for each.

6. Discuss care assistance arrangements for older adults, including nursing homes, home health agencies, adult day care, and respite care.

key terms

Activities of daily living (ADL)	Functional independence	Polypharmacy
Adult immunization	Hearing deficit	Vision deficit
Alzheimer's disease	Incontinence	
Cognitive impairment	Instrumental activities of	*See Glossary for definitions.*
Elder abuse	daily living (IADL)	

case study

Frank Jefferson is a registered nurse (RN) working in a senior health clinic in a small city. The clinic provides comprehensive, integrated, and systematic care for individuals aged 65 years and older. In addition to three RNs, the clinic employs two physicians, two nurse practitioners, a dietitian, a pharmacist who specializes in geriatrics, laboratory and radiology technicians, and a social worker. Services are individualized, and clients are seen in the clinic, at home, or in the hospital, as warranted.

On Friday, Frank sees Mr. Peterson, a 75-year-old retired postal worker, for his annual physical examination. Mr. Peterson lives with his wife in a small house not far from the clinic. Five years

Continued

earlier, Mr. Peterson had a mild heart attack and was hospitalized for several days. He has been hospitalized on two other occasions: 10 years ago for a cholecystectomy and a year ago for prostate surgery. He takes daily medication for hypertension, a multivitamin, and 325 mg of aspirin. He has occasional bouts of constipation that he states are relieved with over-the-counter laxatives. Mr. Peterson has no physical limitations, drives without difficulty, and wears glasses.

Physical findings show that his weight is unchanged from 1 year ago, blood pressure is 138/86, pulse rate is 76 beats per minute and regular, and respiration rate is 20 breaths per minute. Mr. Peterson is given a complete physical examination, including a complete blood count with a blood lipid profile, an electrocardiogram (ECG), and test for fecal occult blood. Mr. Peterson reports no problems with depression; because his mental and cognitive states are appropriate, no formal assessments are performed. According to clinic records Mr. Peterson had received a pneumococcal immunization 3 years earlier. To further bring him up to date on immunizations, Frank informs him of the CDC's recent recommendation that all persons over the age of 60 receive one dose of herpes zoster vaccine. After discussing possible risks and benefits, Mr. Peterson consents to the shot. He is reminded to return in a couple of months, near the beginning of the influenza season, to receive his yearly vaccination.

Physical examination reveals a relatively healthy older adult. Mr. Peterson's blood pressure appears controlled, the ECG shows no new changes, and the fecal occult blood test is negative. The eye examination, however, shows some degree of cataract formation, and he is referred to an ophthalmologist. In addition, several small lesions are detected on his hands and face, so he is referred to a dermatologist for evaluation.

Health teaching performed by Frank and other members of the clinic staff focuses on diet and physical activity, prevention of falls, signs and symptoms of heart attack, and warning signs of cancer. Before Mr. Peterson leaves, Frank gives him a herpes zoster vaccine injection, informing him that the results of the blood tests will be available early next week, and that he will call with the results.

In 1900, people over 65 years of age constituted 4% of the population. In 2005, 12.4% of the population was over 65, and by 2030 it is projected that that proportion will have increased to 19.7%. The large group of people born between 1946 and 1964 (the Baby Boomers) will begin to reach age 65 in 2011, doubling the population of Americans aged 65 and over. Further, due to improvements in medical care and nutrition during the last 100 years, those 85 years of age and older or the "oldest old" are becoming a larger proportion of the elder population. Indeed, the most rapid population increase over the next decade is expected to be among those over age 85 years (U.S. Census Bureau, 2005a; U.S. Census Bureau, 2006a).

Like in most industrialized countries, in the United States older women are more numerous than older men. Though male births outnumber female births, males have higher mortality rates at almost every age, accounting for more women by age 35. This trend expands with age, and females outnumber males in the population age 65+ by approximately 6.2 million (U.S. Census Bureau, 2005a).

The rapid growth in the number and percentage of elders is very significant. Because of the increase in older Americans, the nation's health care spending is projected to increase by 25% within two decades. Older people, especially the oldest old, are dependent upon the support of family and government sources for financial, physical, and emotional support. Most elders depend on social services such as Social Security and Medicare. These services are largely financed through the contributions of working-age adults. As the number of elders increases, the number of working-age adults responsible for their support decreases in relative terms. Thus it has been noted repeatedly that the United States will be fiscally stressed when the entire Baby Boom generation has reached older age in or about 2030 (U.S. Census Bureau, 2005b).

A major goal for the health of the nation is to increase the years of healthy life for all Americans (USDHHS, 2000). For older adults, achieving *Healthy People 2010* objectives will be confirmed by the presence of active elders who continue to make a valuable contribution to all aspects of community life.

Seeking to improve health and limit disabilities of older Americans are key components of *Healthy People 2010*. The *Healthy People 2010* box presents examples of related objectives.

Due to the complex and unique health needs of the aging population, the anticipated growth in this aggregate, and the resulting impact on the health care delivery system, all nurses should be knowledgeable about health care needs of elders. To offer a better understanding of this population, Box 15-1 presents some facts about older Americans.

Chronic health problems are common among older persons. Arthritis and other orthopedic impairments, hypertension, hearing loss, heart conditions, and visual impairments are the most common chronic conditions among older adults (see Table 15-1). These conditions in turn are often accompanied by functional disabilities. As a result almost 41% of those

healthy people **2010**

Examples of Objectives for Older Adults

OBJECTIVE	BASELINE (1998)	TARGET
2.9: Reduce the overall number of cases of osteoporosis	10%	8%
3.12a: Increase the proportion of adults 65 years of age and older who have received a fecal occult blood test within the preceding 2 years	34%	60%
6.11: Reduce the proportion of people with disabilities who report not having the assistive devices and technology needed	NA	NA
7.12: Increase the proportion of older adults who have participated during the preceding year in at least one organized health-promotion activity	12%	90%
12.6b: Reduce hospitalizations of adults between 75 and 84 years of age with heart failure as the principal diagnosis	26.9 per 1000	13.5 per 1000
14.5b: Reduce invasive pneumococcal infections in adults 65 years of age and older	62 per 100,000	42 per 100,000
14.29a: Increase the proportion of adults aged 65 years and older who are vaccinated annually against influenza	63%	90%
15.28a: Reduce hip fractures among females 65 years of age and older	1121 per 100,000	491 per 100,000
18.14: Increase the number of states, territories, and the District of Columbia with an operational mental health plan that addresses mental health crisis interventions, ongoing screening, and treatment services for elderly persons	24 states	50 states and the District of Columbia
24.2c: Reduce hospitalizations for asthma among adults aged 65 years and older	19.3 per 10,000	10 per 10,000
28.15: Increase the number of people who are referred by their primary care physician for hearing evaluation and treatment	NA	NA

From Department of Health and Human Services: *Healthy people 2010*: conference ed, Washington, DC, 2000, Government Printing Office.

BOX 15-1 Facts About the Elderly

LIFE EXPECTANCY AND POPULATION TRENDS

The life expectancy at birth for Americans is almost 79 years.
Persons 65 years of age can expect to live for 18.5 more years.
About 12.4% of the population is over age 65.
Persons aged 85+ years, America's "oldest old," constitute the most rapidly growing segment of the population.
By 2040, the United States may have more persons aged 65 and older than persons younger than 20 years of age.

LIVING PATTERNS

Most men older than 65 years live with their wives (72%).
Many women older than 65 years are widows (43%).
Less than 5% of the older population is institutionalized at any given time; however, about one in four older adults will spend some time in a nursing home during the last years of their lives.
California, New York, Florida, Pennsylvania, and Texas have the greatest *numbers* of older adults. Florida, Iowa, West Virginia, and Arkansas have the greatest *percentages* of older adults, and populations are rising most dramatically in Nevada, Alaska, Hawaii, and Arizona.
More than 66% of the elderly live in a family setting; about 30% live alone.

RETIREMENT, INCOME, AND POVERTY

About two thirds of American workers retire before age 65 and spend more than 20% of their lives in retirement.
Social Security benefits are the major source of income for the elderly, providing more than half of the monthly income for the majority of recipients.
More than 10% of elderly persons live below the poverty level, and another 6.6% of elders are classified as "near-poor."

HEALTH AND HEALTH CARE

The leading causes of death for persons aged 65 years and older are (in order): heart disease, cancer, cerebrovascular accident, chronic obstructive pulmonary disease, pneumonia/influenza, diabetes, and accidents.
Elderly persons use 32% of all prescription medications.
Adults over 65 years of age average about 6.5 visits to a physician annually.
Medicare is the major source of payment for health care of the elderly and pays approximately 93% of hospital costs for this population.

Data from: Administration on Aging: *A statistical profile of older Americans aged 65+* (website): http://www.aoa.dhhs.gov/press/fact/pdf/ss_stat_profile.pdf. Accessed January 18, 2008.

TABLE **15-1** Prevalence of Selected Chronic Conditions by Age: Prevalence per 1000 People

CONDITION	AGE 65 TO 74 YEARS	AGE 75+ YEARS
Hypertension	456	521
Arthritis/gout (physician diagnosed)	428	505
Heart conditions (including ischemic heart disease and heart rhythm disorders)	246	324
Any cancer	175	228
Diabetes	166	158
Chronic sinusitis	145	142
Asthma	103	96
Stroke	48	105

From Centers for Disease Control and Prevention: *Trends in health and aging* (website): http://209.217.72.34/aging/TableViewer/tableView.aspx. Accessed January 18, 2008.

65 years of age and older report having some kind of disability (U.S. Census Bureau, 2006a).

Improving functional independence through prevention and effective management of chronic illnesses (e.g., heart disease, cancer, stroke, chronic obstructive pulmonary disease, arthritis, osteoporosis) and dealing with conditions associated with aging (e.g., vision and hearing impairments, incontinence, dementia) are goals for all older adults. Promoting regular, moderate physical activity (e.g., walking, gardening, swimming) can help control or limit chronic conditions. Enhanced clinical services directed at prevention of illnesses (e.g., immunization against pneumonia and influenza) and screening for cancer and heart disease can help prevent serious conditions and may provide early diagnosis and referral for prompt treatment when they are detected. In addition, enhanced primary care can assist in the management of chronic problems such as hypertension, arthritis, and diabetes. Improving social networks can promote independence and reduce social isolation, thereby decreasing depression, nutritional deficits, and other related conditions associated with aging.

Nurses practicing in community settings frequently have an opportunity to work with older people and their families and to address these and related issues. This chapter describes assessment of older adults and provides information and materials for health education for this population.

ASSESSMENT OF OLDER ADULTS

The Standards of Gerontological Nursing Practice require regular assessment in a comprehensive, accurate, and systematic manner (American Nurses Association [ANA], 2001). A comprehensive assessment should include gathering information on the individual's physical health, health history, functional ability, cognitive and mental state, and nutritional status. Consistent with use of the nursing process in other areas, interventions should be based on assessment findings and anticipated or potential threats to the health and well-being of the client.

GENERAL ASSESSMENT

A thorough health history is necessary to learn as much about the client as possible, discover issues and problems that might require attention, and assign priority. Most agencies have health history tools and assessment guides available for collecting this information. At the very least, information should include the following (Luggen, 1996):

- Biographical data (name, age, date of birth, sex, race)
- Informant identification (self, relative, friend)
- Chief complaint (reason the client is seeking help)
- History of present illness (onset, location, and severity of symptoms; treatment or control methods; precipitating factors; associated symptoms)
- Past history (allergies, drug reactions, past illnesses, hospitalizations, current prescription and over-the-counter medications)

- Family history (diseases, particularly heart disease, diabetes, tuberculosis [TB], hypertension, arthritis, and cancer, in near relatives [i.e., parents, siblings, children])
- Psychosocial history (marital status; occupation; retirement history; current life situation; nutritional history; alcohol, smoking, or drug use; immunization history; education; leisure and exercise activities)
- Review of systems and history of concerns, symptoms, or illnesses; for example, cardiovascular system (palpitations, murmur, hypertension), gastrointestinal system (nausea, abdominal pain, hemorrhoids), neurologic problems (headache, syncope, seizures), and psychologic problems (depression, memory loss, insomnia)
- Functional capacity (**activities of daily living [ADL]**, such as bathing, toileting, feeding) and **instrumental activities of daily living [IADL]**, such as driving, using the telephone, preparing meals)

COMMON HEALTH PROBLEMS

The process of aging brings about physical changes that often contribute to development of chronic illnesses and conditions. Nurses who frequently care for older adults in community settings should be able to detect unusual or abnormal findings during the assessment process. Table 15-2 presents some of the most common health problems encountered in older people, including etiology, symptoms, risk factors, identification, and clinical management.

NUTRITION

When assessing nutritional status in older people, the nurse must recognize physical changes and other factors that can influence dietary intake. Table 15-3 describes some factors and potential clinical manifestations of poor nutrition. Nurses who routinely work with older clients should assess for signs of nutritional deficiencies and develop interventions to minimize or correct them.

Several warning signs may indicate poor nutritional health. These include the presence of a disease or chronic condition (e.g., depression or diabetes) that changes the way the individual eats or makes it difficult to eat; economic hardship; reduced social contact; multiple medicines; involuntary weight loss or gain; needing assistance with IADL; and very old age (80+).

TABLE **15-2** Common Health Problems in Later Maturity

DISEASE/CONDITION	DEFINITION	RISK FACTORS	SIGNS/SYMPTOMS	MANAGEMENT/TREATMENT
CARDIOVASCULAR SYSTEM				
Coronary artery disease (CAD); angina	Progressive obstruction of blood flow through one or more coronary arteries caused by a build-up of plaque (cholesterol and lipids) on interior artery walls	Age (increases with age), gender, race, and genetic inheritance; elevated serum lipids, hypertension, smoking, obesity, diabetes, stress, sedentary lifestyle	Substernal chest pain that may radiate to the left arm, neck, jaw, or shoulder; tachycardia or bradycardia; apprehension; dyspnea; diaphoresis; nausea and vomiting; syncope; fatigue	Dependent on degree of damage and physical findings Medications; coronary artery angioplasty, stent placement; coronary artery bypass graft
Congestive heart failure (CHF)	Condition of altered cardiac function in which cardiac output is insufficient to meet demands of tissue metabolism	Age, hypertension, arteriosclerosis, CAD, other heart and lung conditions (arrhythmia, pneumonia, mitral stenosis, endocarditis)	Rales (crackles), difficulty breathing, tachypnea, confusion, insomnia, agitation, depression, nausea, anorexia, dyspnea, orthopnea, weight gain, bilateral ankle edema	Medications Other interventions: reduction in sodium intake, bed rest
Arrhythmias	Cardiac conduction irregularities characterized by chaotic electrical activity	Age, hypertension, CAD, valvular heart disease, CHF, diabetes, pulmonary embolus, hyperthyroidism	Irregular pulse, tachycardia, palpitations, light-headedness, fatigue, dyspnea, syncope, angina	Avoidance of risk (ethanol, caffeine, nicotine), management of underlying disease, prevention of complications (embolus) Medications; surgery (pacemaker implantation, implantable defibrillator)
Peripheral vascular disease (atherosclerotic occlusive disease)	Obstruction or narrowing of the arteries, causing interruption of blood flow to extremities (most commonly to feet and legs)	Complications of atherosclerosis, smoking, hyperlipidemia, diabetes, hypertension, and physical stress	Intermittent claudication, diminished or absent pulses, affected limb is cold and pale	Smoking cessation, foot and limb care, exercise program, weight control, cholesterol management, management of diabetes Surgery (bypass surgery, angioplasty, stent placement, amputation in extreme cases)

RESPIRATORY SYSTEM

Chronic obstructive pulmonary disease (COPD)	Consists of chronic bronchitis (increased mucus production and recurrent cough), emphysema (destruction of interalveolar septa)	Cigarette smoking, passive smoking, aging, air pollution, occupational exposure, severe viral pneumonia early in life	Chronic bronchitis: cough, sputum production, frequent infections, dyspnea, cyanosis, wheezing, diminished breath sounds Emphysema: minimal cough, scant sputum, dyspnea, weight loss, occasional infections, barrel chest, use of accessory muscles for respiration, pursed-lip breathing, diminished breath sounds	Smoking cessation, aggressive treatment of infections, treat reversible bronchospasm, pulmonary rehabilitation Medications; supplemental oxygen when necessary
Asthma	Reversible airway disease characterized by bronchial constriction, mucosal edema, and increased mucus production	Allergic factors (pollens, molds, dust mites, animal dander), smoke and other pollutants, viral infections, exercise, family history	Abnormal pulmonary function tests, wheezing, cough, prolonged expiration, hyperresonance, decreased breath sounds, nocturnal dyspnea, cyanosis, use of accessory respiratory muscles	Medications; monitoring of peak expiratory flow (PEFR); identify and eliminate irritants
Pneumonia	Acute inflammation of the lungs caused by bacterial, viral, fungal, chemical, or mechanical agents; most commonly caused by viral or bacterial infection in adults	Age, viral infection, alcoholism, immunosuppression, smoking, COPD, diabetes, malnutrition, mechanical ventilation, altered consciousness	Cough; fever; chest pain; chills; dark, thick, or bloody sputum; anorexia; anxiety; chest dull to percussion; crackles (rales); cyanosis; diminished breath sounds; dyspnea; pleuritic pain; rhonchi; tachypnea; tachycardia; weakness	Medication, antibiotic therapy; bed rest; in severe cases, oxygen therapy, mechanical ventilation, chest physiotherapy when necessary

Continued

TABLE **15-2** Common Health Problems in Later Maturity—cont'd

DISEASE/CONDITION	DEFINITION	RISK FACTORS	SIGNS/SYMPTOMS	MANAGEMENT/TREATMENT
MUSCULOSKELETAL SYSTEM				
Osteoporosis	Progressive bone loss predisposing to atraumatic fractures, particularly of vertebra, upper femur, distal radius, humerus, and ribs	Gender (more common in women), age, family history, race/ethnicity, inadequate calcium and vitamin D intake, sedentary lifestyle, alcohol use, caffeine, smoking, steroid use, chemotherapy, radiation therapy	Acute or chronic back pain, kyphosis, scoliosis, atraumatic fractures, loss of height, absence of peripheral bone deformities	Weight reduction if appropriate; increase calcium intake; avoid excess phosphate or protein intake; encourage ambulation and weight-bearing exercise; medications
Osteoarthritis	Degeneration of articular cartilage and hypertrophy of bone	Age, obesity, prolonged occupational or sports stress, injury	Slowly developing joint pain, pain following use of joint, stiffness (particularly in the morning), joint enlargement, decreased range of motion, tenderness	Weight reduction, fitness program, heat, physical therapy, protection of joints Medications; surgery (e.g., joint replacement, debridement) may be indicated with advanced disease
GENITOURINARY TRACT				
Prostate conditions	Benign prostatic hyperplasia (BPH) is the benign growth of the prostate, which may result in bladder outlet obstruction	Gender (male), age, family history	Obstructive symptoms: decrease in force of urine stream, hesitancy, postvoid dribbling, incomplete bladder emptying, overflow incontinence, urinary retention, inability to voluntarily stop stream, frequency, nocturia, urgency, urge incontinence	Medications Surgery: transurethral resection of prostate (TURP), open prostatectomy, other procedures

GASTROINTESTINAL TRACT

Periodontal disease (gingivitis)	Degeneration of tissues supporting the teeth	Malnutrition, aging, inadequate plaque removal, diabetes, poor dental hygiene, faulty dental restoration, irritation by faulty bridges or dentures	Mouth odor, gum swelling, redness and bleeding, loose teeth, tooth loss	Removal of irritating factors (plaque, faulty dentures), promoting good oral hygiene, regular dental check-ups, smoking cessation Medication sometimes indicated in severe cases
Diverticulosis, Diverticulitis (diverticular disease)	*Diverticulum of colon:* herniation of colon mucosa through the muscular layer; more common in sigmoid and distal colons *Diverticulitis:* an abscess or inflammation of diverticula	Low-fiber diet, defects in colon wall strength, age (>40 yr), low-residue diet, family history	*Diverticulosis:* 10%-25% of individuals with diverticula have symptoms, pain, diarrhea, constipation, but no signs of inflammation *Diverticulitis:* pain (acute, localized in left lower quadrant), fever, anorexia, nausea, vomiting. constipation or diarrhea, rebound tenderness, abdomen distended and tympanic	Liquids and bland diet during acute diverticulitis; all clients with diverticula should increase dietary fiber intake Medications during acute phase Surgery: colon resection in severe cases
Constipation	Decrease in frequency from usual bowel elimination pattern or difficulty in defecating	More common with age, sedentary lifestyle, electrolyte abnormalities, concomitant illness, inadequate fluid intake, inadequate fiber or bulk, side effects of drugs, chronic abuse of laxatives; psychologic, emotional, and environmental factors	Less frequency of bowel movements than the client perceives as normal (typically 3-5 times/wk), change in baseline defecating pattern, smaller stools than normal, impaction of stool, difficulty expelling feces from the rectum, painful evacuation, sensation of incomplete emptying of bowel, abdominal fullness	Encourage measures to improve bowel habits, routine time for toileting, avoid straining, respond to urge to defecate, daily physical exercise, increase fluid intake, increase dietary fiber Medications: bulk-forming agents (Metamucil, Citrucel), laxatives, stool softeners, suppositories, cathartics, enemas

Continued

TABLE **15-2** Common Health Problems in Later Maturity—cont'd

DISEASE/CONDITION	DEFINITION	RISK FACTORS	SIGNS/SYMPTOMS	MANAGEMENT/TREATMENT
ENDOCRINE SYSTEM				
Diabetes	Type 2 diabetes accounts for 70%-80% of all cases; hyperglycemia and glucose intolerance from defects in insulin secretion and peripheral insulin action	Family history, obesity, age, race/ethnicity; almost 50% of elderly may have glucose intolerance	Polyuria, polydipsia, and polyphagia (however, classical symptom triad may be absent in Type 2 diabetes); weight loss; constipation; numbness and tingling in peripheral extremities; diminished peripheral pulses; headache; weakness; fatigue; frequent infections; abnormal plasma glucose levels	Diet management; weight loss when appropriate; regular exercise; home monitoring of blood or urine glucose; instruction in self-monitoring for and management of complications Medications (oral hypoglycemic agents or insulin when necessary)
NEUROLOGIC SYSTEM				
Alzheimer's disease	Degenerative organic mental disorder characterized by progressive brain deterioration and dementia; cause unknown	Family history, age, head trauma, low education level, Down syndrome; hypothesized causes include: excessive amount of an amyloid protein (beta-amyloid peptide) tissue; a virus; exposure to metals (particularly aluminum and mercury); an autoimmune disorder; plaque formation	Progressive cognitive impairment. *Early symptoms:* memory loss, distractible, forgets names or events, gets lost in familiar surroundings, aware of mental decline. *Progressive symptoms:* increased memory loss, wanders, confabulates; experiences bowel and bladder incontinence; decreased ability to understand and express language. *Late symptoms:* hallucinations and delusions; inability to perform ADL, little response to stimuli, loss of body functions	Medications: cholinesterase inhibitors or memantine for cognitive symptoms; antidepressants, antipsychotics or anxiolytics for behavioral symptoms; Provide comfort measures; avoid change (i.e. maintain stable surroundings)

Parkinson disease	Neurodegenerative disorder of extrapyramidal system	Age; slightly more common in males; cause unknown, although possibly the result of exposure to a toxin or infectious agent or loss of dopamine neurons	Rhythmic tremors of fingers, feet, lips, and head, with progressive rigidity of facial and trunk muscles; characteristic sign is shuffling gait while client is leaning forward at the trunk	Maintain activity to highest degree possible, use cane for walking, avoid tension and frustration, minimize emotional upsets; physical and occupational therapy may be indicated; medications
Cerebrovascular accidents (CVAs)	Sudden onset of a focal neurologic deficit resulting from infarction or hemorrhage within the brain	Age, arteriosclerosis, hypertension, smoking, diabetes, race/ethnicity, family history	Symptoms depend on the site of CVA and include: hemianesthesia, aphasia, visual field defects, headache, seizure, amnesia, confusion, diplopia, vertigo, ataxia, facial paresis, dysphagia, dysarthria, impaired consciousness, behavioral changes	Maintain oxygenation; monitor cardiac rhythm; control hypertension; promote physical therapy, occupational therapy, and speech therapy when indicated; medications (e.g., antithrombotics); surgery (e.g., carotid endarterectomy)
SENSORY DISORDERS				
Cataract	Clouding or opacity of lens; may be congenital, related to metabolic or systematic conditions, or traumatically induced	Aging; exposure to ultraviolet B rays	Blurred vision, problems with visual acuity in bright light or at night, falls, or accidents; lens opacity on eye examination; pupil may appear cloudy or white	Surgery, commonly with lens implantation

Continued

TABLE **15-2** Common Health Problems in Later Maturity—cont'd

DISEASE/CONDITION	DEFINITION	RISK FACTORS	SIGNS/SYMPTOMS	MANAGEMENT/TREATMENT
Glaucoma	Damage to optic nerve and loss of visual field and visual acuity associated with high intraocular pressure	Race/ethnicity (more common among Native Alaskan/Inuits and African Americans), family history; some medications	*Acute:* severe eye pain, blurred vision, halos around lights, nausea and vomiting, elevated intraocular pressure *Chronic:* none until advanced, then gradual loss of peripheral vision, headaches, misty vision	Medications to lower pressure Surgery if glaucoma not managed through medication
Hearing loss	Hearing loss may be complete or partial; may be classified as conductive or sensorineural	Eustachian tube obstruction, exposure to loud noise levels for extended periods; ototoxic medications; heredity; aging; cerumen impaction; perforation of tympanic membrane	Difficulty hearing (may be gradual or sudden); other symptoms include tinnitus, dizziness, pain	Dependent on cause. As appropriate: remove cerumen with suction and irrigation; for serous otitis: decongestants; surgery may be required for some conditions (e.g., tympanic membrane perforation); use of assistive devices

Data from Dambro MR: *Griffith's 5-minute clinical consult*, Philadelphia, 2006, Lippincott Williams & Wilkins; Eliopoulos C: *Gerontological nursing*, ed 6, Philadelphia, 2004, Lippincott Williams & Wilkins; Luggen AS: *Core curriculum for gerontological nursing*, St Louis, 1996, Mosby; Murray RB, Zentner JP, Pinnel N: Assessment and health promotion for the person in later maturity. In Murray RB, Zentner JP, editors: *Nursing Assessment and health promotion: strategies through the life span*, ed 5, Norwalk, Conn, 1993, Appleton & Lange.

TABLE **15-3** Factors that May Affect Nutrition in Later Maturity

FACTOR AND PROCESS	EFFECT	CLINICAL MANIFESTATION
INGESTION		
Loss of teeth; poor dentures; atrophy of jaws	Improper mastication; deletion of important foods from diet	Irritable bowel syndrome; constipation; malnutrition
Dietary habits	Overeating; eccentric diets	Obesity; malnutrition
Psychologic losses and changes; changes in social environment; lack of socialization	Poor appetite	Anorexia; weight loss
Reduced income; difficulty with food preparation and ingestion	Excessive ingestion of carbohydrates	Obesity; malnutrition
Decreased fluid intake	Dry feces	Impacted stools
DIGESTION AND ABSORPTION		
Decreased secretion of hydrochloric acid and digestive enzymes	Interference with digestion	Dietary deficiencies
Hepatic and biliary insufficiency	Poor absorption of fats	Fat-soluble vitamin deficiency; flatulence
Atrophy of intestinal mucosa and musculature	Poor absorption; slower movement of food through intestine	Vitamin and mineral deficiencies; constipation
Decreased secretion of intestinal mucus	Decreased lubrication of intestine	Constipation
METABOLISM		
Impaired glucose metabolism and use	Diabetic-like response to glucose excesses	Hyperglycemia; hypoglycemia
Decrease in renal function	Inability to excrete excess alkali	Alkalosis
Impaired response to salt restriction	Salt depletion	Low-salt syndrome
Decline in basal metabolic rate	Lower caloric requirements, but same amount of food eaten	Obesity
Changes in iron and calcium (phosphorus, magnesium) metabolism	Iron deficiency; increased requirements for calcium	Anemia; demineralization of bone; osteoporosis
Changes in vitamin metabolism	Deficiency in vitamins K and C especially	Peripheral neuropathy, sensorimotor changes; easy bruising and bleeding tendencies

From Murray RB, Zentner JP, Pinnell NN, Boland MH: Assessment and health promotion for the person in later adulthood. In Murray RB, Zentner JP, editors: *Nursing assessment and health promotion: strategies through the life span*, ed 7, Upper Saddle River, NJ, 2001, Prentice Hall.

Missing or loose teeth and poor-fitting dentures may also contribute to poor nutrition in elders. Although the percentage of adults with complete tooth loss is decreasing, tooth loss remains a prominent concern of older adults. Indeed, approximately 20% of adults aged 65 and older suffer complete tooth loss. Older adults with lower educational levels suffer the highest percentage of complete tooth loss, with women, Black seniors, and those with low income levels having the highest prevalence of tooth loss (National Oral Health Surveillance System, 2007). Nurses who work with the elderly should routinely ask about their client's oral health and make referrals as needed to a dentist or dental laboratory.

Obesity, a body mass index equal to or above 30, is becoming more prominent among adults, including adults over 65. Obesity has increased dramatically among older adults, with 33.4% of men aged 65 to 74 and 38.8% of women in this age group being obese. Among those aged 75 and over, 20% of men and 20% of women were obese (US Census Bureau, 2005a). Sociodemographic factors such as lower educational level and race have been found to be associated with obesity (Black women are considerably more likely to be obese than white women).

Exercise, in addition to decreasing the risk for cardiovascular disease, cancer, and diabetes, is helpful in decreasing body fat and maintaining a healthy weight. Exercise increases muscle and bone mass, which increases muscle strength and activity tolerance. Increased bone and muscle mass can help prevent falls among older adults and the injuries that accompany falls. Despite the benefits of exercise, few older adults get the recommended 30 minutes or more of moderate physical exercise five or more days a week. Physical activity tends to decrease with age. Those 65 and older are about five times more likely to never be physically active than those aged 18 to 24. Walking is the most common type of activity among seniors, with older women being more likely to be physically active than older men (U.S. Census Bureau, 2005a).

Nurses in the community should encourage older adults to eat five or more servings of fruits and vegetables daily and decrease the amount of fat and carbohydrates consumed. Referrals to community resources that provide healthful foods (food pantries, Meals on Wheels, food stamps) can assist older Americans on limited incomes to enjoy better nutrition. Single seniors may find eating out more convenient and enjoyable than eating at home alone and may begin to eat out frequently, leading to increased food consumption and weight gain. Referrals to senior citizens' lunch programs may help these persons eat more healthfully.

In addition to referral to providers or community resources that address specific access problems, interventions for nutritional deficits might include obtaining a referral for Meals on Wheels if the client is not able to cook or obtaining dental care or dentures for clients with poor or missing teeth. Nutrition education is vitally important, and the nurse might suggest the use of specially enriched dietary supplements (e.g., Ensure) and offer tips on how to manage constipation.

Promoting Functional Independence

Functional independence refers to the extent to which the individual (in this case the older adult) is able to complete normal ADLs and IADLs without assistance from others. Activities of daily living generally include bathing, dressing, eating, getting in and out of bed and chairs, walking, going outside, and toileting. The ability to perform necessary functions of life such as taking transportation, preparing meals, shopping, and using the telephone are examples of IADLs. Managing money and accomplishing routine housework are additional examples.

In older adults functional impairment can be caused by cognitive, physical, social, and/or psychologic disorders. The prevalence and incidence of disability increases with age. With each 10 years after the age of 65, the odds of losing mobility double (U.S. Census Bureau, 2005b). Disabilities affect 29% of older persons. It is estimated that about 10% of those over 70 years of age have difficulty performing at least one ADL (e.g., bathing, eating, dressing), and approximately 20% of elders have difficulty going outside of the home (U.S. Census Bureau, 2005b). In addition, about 10% have difficulty performing at least one IADL (e.g., making meals, shopping, cleaning). The percentage of persons needing help with ADLs increases significantly with age, rising from 15% for ages 65 to 69 years to 50% for those over age 85 years. Similarly the percentage of persons needing help with IADL increases with age to approximately 55% by age 85 years (U.S. Census Bureau, 2006b).

Several objectives of *Healthy People 2010* address screening and referral of elderly clients for threats to functional independence (see the *Healthy People 2010* table earlier in the chapter). Areas specifically targeted include the following:

- Hearing deficits
- Vision deficits
- Cognitive impairment
- Depression
- Urinary incontinence

It is essential that all nurses working with older populations recognize threats and limitations to functional independence, as well as associated health problems. Tools, health information, and teaching tips to prevent or manage problems with functional independence are described next.

HEARING DEFICITS

Some 33% of individuals aged 65 years and over and more than half of those over 85 have some degree of **hearing deficit** (USDHHS, 2000). Because of embarrassment or frustration, hearing loss in the elderly can contribute to social isolation, depression, and exacerbation of coexisting psychologic problems. The most common types of hearing loss and associated factors are the following:

- Presbycusis (most common in older adults): results from changes in the inner ear manifested by slow decline that begins with lost ability to hear high-pitched tones
- Tinnitus: auditory ringing or roaring; may be caused by cerumen, infection, aspirin, certain antibiotics, or a nerve disorder
- Conductive hearing loss: results from fluid in the middle ear, abnormal bone growth, or middle ear infection
- Sensorineural hearing loss: results from damage to parts of the inner ear or auditory nerve; may be from birth defects, head injuries, tumors, illnesses, certain prescription drugs, hypertension, or stroke (National Institute on Aging [NIA], 2005).

All older adults should be questioned about hearing loss. If hearing loss is suspected or confirmed, a pure-tone test using an audiometer may be recommended. Clients with evidence of hearing loss should be referred to a specialist because medical or surgical treatment may improve or restore hearing function. Hearing aids, when appropriate, are prescribed by specialists, but nurses in community settings may be in a position to assist the client explore resources to help obtain a hearing aid and later provide instruction for its proper use and maintenance.

VISION DEFICITS

Vision loss in adults is common, and the prevalence increases with age. It is estimated that 20.3 million people in the United States have some vision impairment. Approximately 1 in 28 Americans over the age of 40 is affected by low vision or blindness (Gohdes, Balamurugan, Larsen, and Maylahn, 2005). Cataracts, glaucoma, macular degeneration, and diabetic retinopathy often cause visual problems in the elderly. Loss of vision in turn may result in trauma from falls, automobile crashes, and other injuries and may significantly affect quality of life (U.S. Census Bureau, 2005a). Because most **vision deficits** can be successfully managed through medical or surgical treatment or use of corrective lenses, early detection and prompt treatment are very important.

A comprehensive eye examination, including screening for visual acuity and glaucoma, should be performed yearly for individuals aged 65 and over. A Snellen wall chart or a tumbling "E" chart at 20 feet is used for basic screening. The client should wear corrective lenses, if prescribed, during screening.

To determine the impact of visual impairment, the nurse should ask about limitations to ADL and IADL associated with poor vision. For example, the nurse might ask, "Does your vision make it difficult for you to feed yourself, read medication labels, groom yourself, handle money, or find your way around places outside of your home?" Discovering whether the client is using visual assistance devices (glasses, contact lenses, magnifying lenses, large print books) can help determine the degree of adaptation. After a complete assessment the nurse should refer clients to an eye care specialist for further evaluation if they report significant changes in visual acuity or visual acuity of 20/40 or less with corrective lenses. In addition to identifying clients with visual difficulties and referring them for follow-up treatment, the nurse may be able to help the client obtain needed treatment, visual aids (magnifying lenses, portable lights, large print books), or corrective lenses.

COGNITIVE IMPAIRMENT

Some degree of **cognitive impairment** is common among older individuals and often increases with age. An estimated 5% to 20% of individuals older than 65 and almost 50% of those over 85 experience some degree of mental impairment (U.S. Census Bureau, 2005). Alzheimer's disease, vascular infarctions, and pharmaceuticals are frequently implicated as inducing cognitive changes.

Screening for cognitive function should include orientation, short-term memory, receptive and expressive language ability, attention, and visual-spatial ability. Use of a short screening instrument such as the Mini Mental State Examination (Figure 15-1) may be helpful in eliciting important information quickly. If cognitive impairment is noted, consultation with family members and referral to a specialist may be indicated.

In regard to care of individuals with cognitive impairments, **Alzheimer's disease** is of particular concern for nurses who routinely work with the elderly. It is estimated that Alzheimer's disease accounts for more than half of the cases of dementia in older adults. Other potential causes of dementia are stroke, Parkinson's disease and other progressive diseases, medication reactions, endocrine abnormalities, metabolic disturbances, infections, and

Mini Mental State Examination Sample Items

Orientation to Time

"What is the date?"

Registration

"Listen carefully,

I am going to say three words.

You say them back after I stop.

Ready? Here they are...

HOUSE (pause), CAR (pause), LAKE (pause).

Now repeat those words back to me."

[Repeat up to 5 times, but score only the first trial.]

Naming

"What is this?"

[Point to a pencil or pen.]

Reading

"Please read this and do what it says."

[Show examinee the words on the stimulus form.]

CLOSE YOUR EYES

Figure 15-1. Mini Mental State Examination sample items. (Reproduced by special permission of the Publisher, Psychological Assessment Resources, Inc., 16204 North Florida Avenue, Lutz, Florida 33549, from the Mini Mental State Examination, by Marshal Folstein and Susan Folstein, Copyright © 1975, 1998 by Mini Mental LLC, Inc. Published 2001 by Psychological Assessment Resources, Inc. Further reproduction is prohibited without permission of PAR, Inc. The Mini Mental State Examination can be purchased from PAR, Inc. by calling 800-331-8378 or 813-968-3003.)

nutritional deficiencies (Family Caregiver Alliance, 2005).

Alzheimer's disease is a degenerative mental disorder characterized by progressive brain deterioration, resulting in impaired memory and thought and behavioral changes. The Community Application box "Intervention Guidelines for Alzheimer's Disease" presents a review of the risk factors, manifestations, and clinical management. Box 15-2 lists current statistics and should help nurses who work with older people better understand the scope and significance of the problem.

DEPRESSION

Depression in older adults causes distress and suffering and leads to mental and physical impairments and social isolation. Although depression is common in older adults, it is often missed, untreated, or undertreated because as a person ages the signs of depression are likely to be overlooked or ignored. Confusion or attention problems caused by depression can mimic Alzheimer's disease or other brain disorders. In addition, mood changes and other signs of depression can be caused by medications (NIA, 2007a).

While depression is prevalent among older adults in general, depression rates are highest among older adults who have a physical health problem. Indeed, between 8% and 20% of older adults in the community and up to 37% of older adults in health care institutions experience symptoms of depression (USDHHS/NIMH, 1999). To assess for depression, older adults should be evaluated for the following (NIA, 2007a):

- An "empty" feeling, ongoing sadness, and anxiety
- Tiredness, lack of energy
- Loss of interest or pleasure in everyday activities, including sex
- Sleep problems, including trouble getting to sleep, very early morning waking, and sleeping too much
- Eating more or less than usual
- Crying too often or too much
- Aches and pains that don't go away when treated
- A hard time focusing, remembering, or making decisions

COMMUNITY APPLICATION
Intervention Guidelines for Alzheimer's Disease

Direct goals toward helping the client experience the highest possible physical, emotional, intellectual, and social functions for as long as possible.

CLIENT AND CAREGIVER EDUCATION SHOULD FOCUS ON:

Manifestations of the disease
Stages and progression of the disease (what to expect)
Pharmacologic management (provide information on clinical drug trials)
Behavioral management
Provision of a consistent routine
Avoiding chemical or physical restraints
Communication strategies
Simple commands and directions
Monitoring for acute illnesses and effects of medications

CAREGIVER AND CLIENT COUNSELING AND REFERRAL SHOULD INCLUDE:

Locating community resources
Legal/financial issues

Durable power of attorney
Conservatorship or guardianship
Establishment of trusts
Advance directives and living will
Financial assistance
Medicare
Medicaid
Long-term care insurance
Social Security Disability Insurance
Supplemental Security Income
Long-term care options (home care, respite care, nursing homes, Alzheimer's disease units)
Family and social support
Management of stress and lifestyle changes

Data from American Association of Retired Persons: *Coping & caring: living with Alzheimer's disease*, Washington, DC, 1993, American Association of Retired Persons; Lukacs K.: Neurological/Alzheimer's disease. In Luggen AS, editor: *Core curriculum for gerontological nursing*, St Louis, 1996, Mosby.

BOX 15-2 Alzheimer's Disease: Statistics

- More than 5 million Americans have Alzheimer's disease, and almost 8 million Americans will have it by the year 2030 unless a cure or prevention is found.
- Alzheimer's disease is a leading cause of death among adults.
- One in 8 persons over age 65 (13%) and nearly half of those over 85 have Alzheimer's disease.
- A person with Alzheimer's disease lives an average of 8 years after the onset of symptoms.
- Most people with Alzheimer's disease live at home, with care provided by family and friends.
- Half of all nursing home patients have Alzheimer's disease or a related disorder; this care costs an average of $75,000 per person per year.
- The direct and indirect costs of Alzheimer's and other dementias amount to more than $148 billion annually.
- States with the largest numbers of deaths due to Alzheimer's disease in 2003 were (in order): California, Florida, Texas, Pennsylvania, and Ohio.

Modified from Alzheimer's Disease Association: *Alzheimer's Facts and Figures, 2007* (website): http://www.alz.org/national/documents/report_alzfactsfigures2007.pdf. Accessed January 15, 2008.

- Feeling guilty, helpless, worthless, or hopeless
- Being irritable
- Thoughts of death or suicide; a suicide attempt

Counseling and antidepressants can help alleviate many of the problems associated with depression. Medications should be managed with care, however, because side effects, drug-drug interactions, comorbidities, and barriers to compliance may exist.

Along with depression, older adults are at risk for suicide. In the United States, suicide rates increase dramatically with age. Indeed, older white men have a suicide rate almost five times that of the general population, and individuals 65 years and older account for 16% of all suicides. Furthermore the suicide rate for individuals 85 years and older is the highest in the country (NIMH, 2007).

Prevention and treatment of depression in older adults are essential to their overall health and sense of well-being. For example, grief counseling for widows and widowers and promoting participation in self-help groups can ameliorate problems and improve social adjustment. In addition, counseling and pharmacologic treatment can be effective adjuncts.

INCONTINENCE

Incontinence (the involuntary loss of urine) is a significant cause of disability and dependency in older adults and contributes to social isolation, embarrassment, feelings of loss of control, and low self-esteem. An estimated 45% of older American women and a significant number of older men experience urinary incontinence, but despite its prevalence, urinary incontinence is widely underdiagnosed and underreported (Specht, 2005). Reasons cited are inadequate education about the condition on the part of health care providers and shame or embarrassment on the part of affected individuals.

The most common types of urinary incontinence are:

- Stress incontinence (most common): involuntary loss of urine associated with movements that put pressure on the bladder (e.g., exercise, coughing, sneezing, laughing, and lifting heavy objects)
- Urge incontinence: involuntary urine leakage before reaching a toilet; most often found in those with enlarged prostate, diabetes, infection, stroke, dementia, Parkinson's disease, multiple sclerosis, or those taking certain pharmaceuticals
- Overflow incontinence: involuntary urine leakage from an overdistended bladder; usually from urethral obstruction in older men or uterine prolapse in older women
- Functional incontinence: urine leakage that occurs in older adults who have a hard time getting to the toilet because of restricted mobility
- Transient incontinence: sudden onset and temporary incontinence generally caused by treatable factors such as delirium or confusion, infection, metabolic conditions (e.g., hyperglycemia, hypercalcemia), and fecal impaction (Specht, 2005).

Treatment of incontinence can improve ADL and IADL for most clients, and community health professionals should be aware of the problem, including its effects, causes, and treatment options. To identify individuals at risk or who suffer with this common problem, health care providers should routinely ask older clients about bladder control, using questions such as, "Do you have trouble with your bladder?" or "Do you have trouble holding your urine (water)?" If urinary incontinence is identified through questioning, detection of an odor, visualization of wetness, or client complaint, and if it represents a problem for the client or caregiver, further evaluation is needed.

A thorough health history should include questions regarding elimination patterns. Diagnosis is based on physical examination, measurement of urinary residual volume, and urinalysis. Blood testing may be done to assess renal function and rule out diabetes. Treatment options are related to etiology and include a variety of behavior techniques, pharmacologic therapy, surgery, or a combination of these health care interventions.

HEALTH PROMOTION AND ILLNESS PREVENTION

Although health-promotion- and illness-prevention interventions for older adults can be very beneficial in reducing death and disability and improving quality of life, the health care system has not systematically encouraged or provided preventive health services for this population. Many older adults seek out medical care only in response to illness and are unlikely to see health care providers when they have no symptoms. They rely on health care professionals to recommend preventive tests and screenings. Because older clients may be unaware of activities that would improve their health and well-being, it is incumbent on providers in community settings to seek opportunities to provide health teaching, perform screenings, and encourage other preventive services.

Healthy People 2010 encourages providers to improve access to primary care; to work to remove barriers to preventive care; and to provide clients with prescribed screening, counseling, and immunization services. Health care providers who routinely work with older clients in community settings should be prepared to perform assessments, laboratory tests, counseling, and immunizations as appropriate. A list of specialties and specialists for referral should be compiled in advance of client visits, and mechanisms for timely, systematic, and streamlined care through interagency and interdisciplinary collaboration and communication should be strongly encouraged.

IMMUNIZATION RECOMMENDATIONS

Although primary prevention through immunization against a variety of illnesses is strongly encouraged (if not mandated) for children, immunization recommendations for older adults are sometimes overlooked. As a result, deaths from vaccine-preventable diseases sometimes occur among older people. For example, the vast majority of influenza deaths occur in individuals 65 years or older, particularly older

adults with underlying health problems such as pulmonary or cardiovascular disorders.

Improving the immunization status of Americans older than 65 is addressed by several of the objectives of *Healthy People 2010* (see the *Healthy People 2010* box in this chapter). The Immunization Practices Advisory Committee recommends that all older adults complete a primary series of diphtheria and tetanus toxoids (Centers for Disease Control and Prevention [CDC], 2007a). In addition, a single dose of pneumococcal polysaccharide vaccine, a single dose of herpes zoster vaccine, and annual vaccination against influenza should be strongly encouraged for all adults over age 65, particularly those with preexisting chronic health conditions. Table 15-4 summarizes **adult immunization** recommendations.

SAFETY CONCERNS FOR OLDER ADULTS

Several objectives from *Healthy People 2010* concerning older adults relate to safety. The document specifically addresses injuries from falls and poisoning caused by drug interactions and inadvertent overdosing. In addition, encouraging health care providers to identify, treat, and refer victims of elder abuse is discussed as a component of the objectives to decrease violent and abusive behaviors.

FALLS

Falls are the leading cause of death from injury for people aged 65 and older, and in 2004 almost 15,000 elderly persons died as a result of falls. Fall-related injuries contributed to about 1.8 million visits to emergency departments and more than 433,000 hospital admissions for this age group. Further, more than one third of all elderly people have reported a fall during the previous 12 months (CDC, 2006). Falls and fall-related injuries are of special concern in older adults because of two factors: (1) the severity of injuries and (2) longer recovery periods and resultant threats to long-term health and functioning. In addition to the immediate pain and disability caused by the injury, falls are associated with loss of confidence in ability to function independently, restriction of physical and social activities, increased dependence, and increased need for long-term care.

TABLE **15-4** Immunizations Recommended for Adults

IMMUNIZATION	RECOMMENDATION
Tetanus/diphtheria	All adults should be screened and given boosters every 10 years
Influenza	Annually for all adults 50+; other adults in high-risk groups (e.g., those with chronic illnesses, health care providers)
Pneumococcal vaccine	Adults 65+; one dose; those who received pneumococcal vaccine before age 65 should be revaccinated if it has been more than 5 years since the first vaccine
Herpes zoster	Adults aged 60+, even if they report a prior episode of herpes zoster
Hepatitis B	Adults in high-risk groups (e.g., persons with occupational risk, hemodialysis patients, household contacts of those infected with hepatitis B virus [HBV], men who have sex with men)
Varicella	Any person without a reliable history of varicella disease or vaccination or who is seronegative for varicella
Measles/mumps/rubella	Anyone born after 1956 without written documentation of immunization on or after the first birthday should be given at least one dose; health care personnel born after 1956 who are at risk of exposure to clients with measles should have documentation of two doses of vaccine on or after their first birthday
Hepatitis A	Adults in high-risk groups (e.g., persons traveling to or working in countries with high or immediate endemicity of infection; men who have sex with men; persons with chronic liver disease)

From Centers for Disease Control and Prevention: *Recommended adult immunization schedule, United States, October 2007-September, 2008* (website): http://www.cdc.gov/mmwr/pdf/wk/mm5641-Immunization.pdf. Accessed January 14, 2008.

Most falls occur in the home, although 30% to 40% occur in public places. Whereas most falls do not result in serious injury, between 5% and 15% of those who fall sustain fractures or other significant injuries. Fracture of the hip, femur, humerus, wrist, and ribs are the most common severe injuries from falls (Eliopoulos, 2004). Meiner (2006) reported that falls are the leading cause of hip fracture and that women sustain about 80% of all hip fractures.

A number of risk factors for falling have been identified. Nurses working with older adults in any setting should be aware of risk factors for falls and should direct interventions accordingly. Intrinsic factors that contribute to falls include:

- Age-related changes in vision, posture, and gait
- Emotional/mental state (agitated, depressed, rushed, distracted, confused, anxious)
- Weakness
- Fear of incontinence
- Denial of illness
- Pain
- Podiatric conditions (ingrown toenails, corns, bunions)
- Adjusting to a new environment (recent move, recent admission or transfer)
- Diagnosis of conditions that affect stability, mobility, and cognitive functions
- Alcohol
- Medications (sedatives/hypnotics, tricyclic antidepressants, antihypertensive agents, analgesics, and diuretics) (Ebersole and Hess, 2001; Meiner, 2006)

Extrinsic or environmental factors that may contribute to falls in elders include inappropriate lighting (dark, dim, glare, shadows); uneven, wet walking surfaces; inadequate handrails and poor step design on stairways; and furniture that is too low, too soft, or tips easily. In the bathroom a slippery tub or shower and lack of rails for the tub or toilet often cause falls. Other factors include clothing that is too long or loose or shoes that are too large or have soles that are smooth and slippery (Meiner, 2006; Stone and Chenitz, 1991). The Health Teaching box "Guidelines for Prevention of Falls in the Home" offers strategies for making the physical environment safer for elders.

health teaching

Guidelines for Prevention of Falls in the Home

LIGHTS AND LIGHTING

1. Eyes tire quickly in improper lighting. Illuminate reading material or the object worked on. Illuminate steps, entranceways, and rooms before entering. Use 70- or 100-watt bulbs, not 60-watt bulbs.
2. Avoid glaring light caused by highly polished floors or large expanses of uncovered glass. Use sunglasses to avoid the glare of highway driving, but use light tints or photoray lenses.
3. Allow more time to adjust to changes in light levels. When going from a dark to a light room or vice versa, allow a minute or two for the eyes to accommodate to the change in light before proceeding.
4. Dirty glasses or outgrown prescription lenses inhibit vision. Keep glasses clean. Have regular eye examinations to identify changes and to get new glasses when needed. If possible, do not use bifocals when walking because it is difficult to see the ground clearly.
5. Ability to see up, down, and sideways decreases with age. Observe the lay of the land; learn to look ahead at the ground to spot and avoid hazards such as cracks in sidewalks. Use canes, walking sticks, and walkers as prescribed.
6. At night, keep a nightlight on in your bedroom and bathroom. When getting out of bed at night, put the light on and wait a minute or two for the eyes to adjust before getting up. Have a telephone near the bed to eliminate the need to get up to answer the phone. Before going out in the evening or late afternoon, turn on a light.

ACTIVITY

1. Get up from a chair slowly.
2. When getting out of bed, sit up, then wait a minute or two. Move to the side of the bed and wait another minute. Rise after sitting for a few minutes.
3. If dizzy, sit down immediately. Sit on a step or a chair, or ease to the sidewalk if outdoors.

4. Avoid tipping the head backward (extending the neck). Activities to avoid that extend the neck are washing windows, hanging clothes, and getting things from high shelves.
5. Use shelves at eye level. Avoid rapid turning of the head.
6. If weather is rainy and windy, avoid going out.
7. Use alcohol and tranquilizers with caution.
8. Exercise programs keep bodies limber. Consult a physician and then enroll in a senior exercise program.
9. Shoes and slippers should be flat and rubber-soled. Avoid clothing such as long robes and loose-fitting garments that may catch on furniture or door knobs.

AROUND THE HOUSE

1. Avoid scatter rugs and small bathroom mats that can slide. Repair loose, torn, wrinkled, or worn carpet.
2. Avoid slick, high polish on floors.
3. Put things in easy reach and avoid reaching to high shelves.
4. Use nonskid treads on stairs and nonskid mats in tub.
5. Install a grab rail in the bath, and shower and also by the toilet as needed.
6. Install handrails on both sides of the stairs. Paint stair edge in bright contrasting color.
7. Remove door thresholds.
8. Remove low-lying objects, such as coffee tables and extension cords.
9. Wipe up spills immediately.
10. Watch for pets underfoot and scattered pet food.
11. Check for even, nonglare lighting in every room, with easily accessible light switches.
12. Avoid floor coverings with complex patterns.
13. Avoid clutter in living areas.
14. Select furniture that provides stability and support, such as chairs with arms.
15. Check walking aids routinely, such as rubber tips on canes and screws on walkers.

From Chenitz WC, Kussman HL, Stone JT: Preventing falls. In Chenitz WC, Stone JT, Salisbury SA, editors: *Clinical gerontological nursing: a guide to advanced practice*, Philadelphia, 1991, Saunders.

COMPLIANCE WITH MEDICATION

Another threat to the safety of older people is the use and misuse of medications. Elders consume more than one-third of all prescription medications, and as a result they are at risk for adverse drug reactions. Reactions commonly arise from such factors as normal aging changes that affect absorption, metabolism, and excretion of drugs in the body; conditions that affect the body's response to drugs (e.g., bed rest, dehydration, stress); and the use of multiple drug regimens to treat concurrent health problems (Murray, 2005).

An estimated 25% to 50% of elderly persons are not compliant with their medication regimens (Murray, 2005). Nurses who work with older clients should be aware of factors that contribute to medication noncompliance and try to anticipate and recognize both actual and potential problems and be prepared to intervene. Box 15-3 provides a list of factors that can contribute to medication misuse.

Polypharmacy refers to the prescribing of multiple drugs for a client; it is a fairly common practice that affects many older people. Both prescription and nonprescription medications contribute to problems

BOX **15-3** Factors that Interfere with Medication Regimen Compliance in Elders

- Physiologic changes associated with aging that affect absorption, metabolism, and excretion of drugs
- Lack of knowledge or information about the reason for taking the medication and the prescribed regimen; stopping the medication when symptoms subside
- Inaccessibility to pharmacy services
- Problems with self-administration, such as failure to take the medication as prescribed, inability to open drug containers, forgetfulness, vision problems
- Multiple prescriptions or related medications for the same condition from different providers

- Lack of financial resources to purchase necessary medications (medications are not covered by Medicare)
- Complexity of drug regimens and volume of drugs needed
- Desire to avoid unpleasant side effects
- Fear of drug dependency
- Failure to discard discontinued or outdated medications
- Sharing of prescription medications with spouse or others
- Failure to report self-medication with over-the-counter drugs
- Interactions between different medications

Data from Eliopoulos C: *Gerontological nursing*, ed 6, Philadelphia, 2004, Lippincott Williams & Wilkins; Graves M: Drug use and abuse. In Hogstel MO, editor: *Nursing care of the older adult*, ed 2, New York, 1988, Wiley; Murray TA: Elderly persons in the community. In Maurer FA, Smith CM, editors: *Community/public health nursing: health for families and populations*, ed 3, St Louis, 2005, Saunders.

encountered in polypharmacy. To avoid problems associated with use of multiple medications, the nurse should:

- Help the client make and maintain a list of all prescription and over-the-counter medications, including purpose, dosage, frequencies, dates of use, and side effects.
- Simplify the medication regimen as much as possible.
- Ensure that the client brings all medications when seeing a practitioner.
- Evaluate potential medication interactions whenever a new medication is prescribed.
- Inform the client about possible side effects and symptoms of toxicity and explain what to do in the event of an occurrence.
- Use a medication box that can be filled weekly, and distribute the medications based on the day (Sunday through Saturday) and time of day (morning, noon, evening, before bed).

ELDER ABUSE

Elder abuse refers to neglect, physical injury, or exploitation that results in harm to an older adult. As a result of widespread underreporting, the incidence of elder abuse is difficult to determine, but estimates are that each year 3% to 6% of older Americans are victims of abuse and neglect (Clark, 2008; Stevenson and Pappas, 2007). Elder abuse can take several forms. The most common types of elder abuse are listed in Table 15-5.

Probably only a fraction of cases of elder abuse are reported. Reasons for failure to report abuse include:

- Reluctance of older people to admit that their child or loved one might abuse them

- Love for abuser
- Dependence on the abuser
- Fear of further injury
- Inability to report the abuse

Even health care providers may neglect to report elder abuse, often because of failure to recognize the problem, ignorance of their legal responsibility to report suspected cases, or failure to adequately assess at-risk situations.

In most cases the abuser is a caregiver, either a close family member or provider in a nursing home. Among family members the spouse is most often the abuser (58% of cases), followed by children (23% to 30% of cases) (Murray, 2005). Risk factors common to victims of elder abuse include the following:

- The victim's dependency on the caregiver (physical, emotional, or financial)
- Confusion
- Incontinence
- Frailty
- Illness
- Mental disabilities
Characteristics of the abuser include:
- A previous history of violence
- Being overwhelmed by the burden of providing care
- Feelings of frustration and resentment

Whenever working with older people in community or long-term settings, nurses should be aware of indicators of possible elder abuse and direct interventions accordingly. Indicators may include the following (Landenburger & Campbell, 2004; Murray, 2005):

- Unexplained or repeated injury
- Discrepancies between injury and explanation

TABLE **15-5** Types of Elder Abuse

TYPE OF ABUSE	EXAMPLE
Physical	Beating, slapping, rape and sexual molestation, murder
Confinement	Use of physical or chemical (sedatives) restraints, confinement to bed
Psychologic or emotional	Verbal assault, isolation, exclusion, threats of abuse or abandonment, insults, humiliation, intimidation
Financial or material	Taking resources and possessions without consent; forcing or coercing elders to sign over properties and possessions
Neglect	Withholding food, adequate clothing, shelter, health care, or medications; deprivation of dentures or eyeglasses; failure to assist with ADL; abandonment; neglect may be passive or active
Abandonment	Desertion of elder by an individual who is the primary caregiver or person who has assumed responsibility for providing care

Data from Ballard D: Legal and ethical issues. In Meiner SE, Lueckenotte AG, editors: *Gerontologic nursing*, ed 3, St Louis, 2006, Mosby; Stevenson L, Pappas A: Violence. In Nies M, McEwen M, editors: *Community/public health nursing: promoting the health of populations*, ed 4, St Louis, 2007, Saunders.

- Inappropriate use of medication (overuse or underuse)
- Fear of the caregiver
- Untreated wounds (decubitus ulcers)
- Evidence of poor care (an unclean or malnourished client)
- Withdrawal and passivity
- Failure to seek appropriate medical care
- Contractures resulting from immobility or restraints
- Unwillingness or inability of caregiver to meet the client's needs
- An unsafe home situation

In all states, nurses and other health care professionals have a legal responsibility to report suspected cases of elder abuse. Typically the nurse should report possible cases to the adult protective services department of the area social services agency.

Usually interventions are directed toward recognizing and reducing risks. Prevention activities for elder abuse are presented in the Community Application box "Elder Abuse Prevention." Referral to appropriate community agencies can assist in alleviating some of the stresses on caregivers and thereby reduce the possibility of neglect and abuse. Respite care providers and adult day care centers can give the caregiver an opportunity to have time away from constant duty while alternative supervision for the client is provided. Meals on Wheels can deliver nutritious meals for individuals, and senior citizens centers and

COMMUNITY APPLICATION
Elder Abuse Prevention

Each year hundreds of thousands of older persons are abused, neglected, and exploited by family members and others. Many victims are people who are older, frail, vulnerable, and depend on others to meet their most basic needs. In response the Administration on Aging recommended several prevention activities to address the problem of elder abuse. These include the following:

- Enhancing professional training through providing workshops for adult protective services personnel and other professional groups, by encouraging statewide conferences for all service providers with an interest in elder abuse, and developing training manuals, videos, and other materials for professional education
- Coordinating health service systems and service providers through creation of elder abuse hotlines for reporting, formation of statewide coalitions and task forces, and creation of local multidisciplinary teams and coalitions
- Providing technical assistance through development of policy manuals and protocols that outline the proper or preferred procedures for elder abuse protection, detection, and management
- Enhancing efforts to develop public education campaigns, including public service announcements, posters, flyers, and videos
- Supporting adult protective service agencies
- Providing crisis intervention and social and health services that older persons need

From Administration on Aging: *Elder abuse prevention* (website): http://www.aoa.gov/press/fact/alpha/fact_elder_abuse_pf.asp. Accessed January 14, 2008.

state or local offices on aging can provide information and resources for older clients and their caregivers.

CARE ASSISTANCE FOR OLDER ADULTS

Only about 5% of older Americans reside in institutional settings (e.g., nursing homes) (Westley and Fletcher, 2004). The remainder live in their own homes, typically with their spouse or alone. If individuals have health problems or need assistance with ADL or IADL, they may reside with someone who can assist them, usually a child, sibling, or other relative.

Whether a person lives at home or with someone else, assistance from an external organization or agency can be beneficial in certain circumstances. This care assistance might be temporary (e.g., home health care following hip replacement surgery) or more permanent (e.g., adult day care for a frail individual who lives with an adult child who is employed). Table 15-6 describes several types of community-based providers and agencies that assist in caring for older adults. Long-term care in a nursing home may ultimately be needed. See the Community Application box "Choosing a Nursing Home."

Referrals for assistance or services can be one of the most important interventions nurses who work with older clients can initiate. Each nurse should assemble a list of local providers and services for quick referral for these individuals and their caregivers. For example, the nurse should have readily available the phone numbers for Meals on Wheels, a nearby respite care provider or adult day care center, and organizations that provide financial assistance to older people.

TABLE **15-6** Long- and Short-Term Care Providers and Facilities for Older Adults

SETTING/PROVIDER	CAREGIVERS	SERVICES
Home	Informal caregivers (spouses, children, neighbors)	Variable, depending on needs of the elder; assist with ADL, health care, meals
Home health agencies	Professionals and paraprofessionals (nurses, therapists, aides)	Intermittent skilled nursing; various therapies; assistance with ADL, shopping, transportation, chores
Nursing homes (skilled nursing facilities and intermediate care facilities)	Professionals and paraprofessionals (nurses, therapists, aides)	Skilled nursing, monitoring, various therapies, assistance with ADL, supervision as needed
Community-based services	Professional and volunteer staff	Preventive health care, on-site and delivered meals, legal and tax services, transportation, recreation
Adult day care	Professionals, paraprofessionals, and volunteers	Temporary care for elders who live at home with family or friends but need supervision and assistance during care provider's workday
Respite care	Professionals, paraprofessionals, and volunteers	Temporary care (few hours, day, week) for disabled or frail older person for the purpose of relieving the family or principal care provider
Housing services (retirement communities, assisted living, board-and-care, halfway houses, congregate living)	Professionals, paraprofessionals	Services variable, based on individual need and functional ability; include room, meals, assistance with ADL, medication management, some protective oversight

COMMUNITY APPLICATION
Choosing a Nursing Home

Approximately 1.5 million Americans, or about 5% of those 65 years of age or older, reside in nursing homes. Choosing a nursing home is very difficult, and the Health Care Financing Administration (HCFA) presented the following 8-step process for this task:

Step 1: Talk to People You Trust—Seek advice from family, friends, and health professionals (e.g., doctors, social workers, hospital discharge planners).

Step 2: Look at Options—Various living arrangements offer different levels of care. Options include subsidized senior housing, assisted living arrangements, board-and-care homes, continuing care homes, and retirement communities.

Step 3: Gather Information—Gather as much information about homes in the area as possible. Talk with health care professionals, ask friends, and look in the phone book. Also, speak with someone from the Long-term Care Ombudsman programs in the area and check Medicare's website.

Step 4: Evaluate Selection Factors—Factors to consider include location, availability, staffing, acceptance of Medicare and Medicaid reimbursement, services and fees, religious and cultural preferences, and special needs.

Step 5: Paying for Care—Paying for care is a major concern, and several payment methods are possible. Medicare pays for some costs under certain circumstances; Medicaid pays most costs for people with limited income and assets. About half of nursing home residents pay costs from savings. Other possible sources are managed care plans, Medicare supplemental insurance, and long-term care insurance.

Step 6: Visit Nursing Homes—Visit potential nursing homes, talk with staff and residents, and request a copy of the most recent inspection.

Step 7: Follow-up Visits—Make several visits at different times of the day and on different days of the week. Critically examine the quality of life of the residents and the quality of care, nutrition, and safety.

Step 8: After Admission—Ensure that you are treated with dignity and respect. Important issues include use of restraints, money management, privacy, respect of property, and guardianship and advance directives.

From U.S. Department of Health and Human Services/Health Care Financing Administration: *Your guide to choosing a nursing home* (Publication No. HCFA-02174-B), Baltimore, Md, 2000, HCFA.

SUMMARY

The population of Americans over age 65 keeps growing at an astonishing rate. As a result the United States needs many more health care professionals, nurses in particular, who are educationally prepared to work with older adults. In the case study, Frank provided nursing care in a senior health clinic and worked with clinic staff to address the many potential and actual health problems commonly found among elders. In addition, the client in this example was very typical of older adults seeking care in community settings.

Because most health care for elders is provided in community settings, nurses should be trained and equipped to manage older adult care appropriately, focusing special attention on health promotion, illness prevention, and recognition of the unique needs of this population.

KEY POINTS

- Because almost 20% of Americans will be older than 65 years by 2030, improving older adult health and limiting disabilities are essential components of health care practice.

- Assessment of older adults should be comprehensive and include evaluation of physical health, health history, functional ability, cognitive and mental state, and nutritional status.

- *Functional independence* refers to the extent to which an individual is able to perform ADL and IADL without assistance from others.

- To promote functional independence, the nurse should identify and manage potential threats and limitations and associated health problems. Areas of assessment and intervention include hearing deficits, vision deficits, cognitive impairment, depression, and urinary incontinence.

- Health-promotion and illness-prevention interventions should include immunization, addressing safety concerns (falls and medication compliance), and assessment and intervention in elder abuse.

- Common health problems in older adults include cardiovascular conditions, respiratory diseases (chronic obstructive pulmonary disease, asthma), musculoskeletal problems (osteoporosis, arthritis), genitourinary conditions (prostate enlargement, incontinence), gastrointestinal problems, endocrine disorders (diabetes), neurologic conditions (Alzheimer's disease, cerebrovascular accidents), sensory disorders (cataracts, hearing impairment), and mental health problems (depression).

- Care assistance arrangements for older adults include nursing homes, home health agencies, adult day care providers, and respite care providers.

Learning Activities & Application to Practice
In Class
1. Discuss *Healthy People 2010* objectives that address older adults. What progress has been made in achieving the objectives? Outline strategies and interventions that nurses can implement to contribute to achieving the objectives.

In Clinical
2. Visit providers of assistive care for elders (a local adult day care center, nursing home, or retirement center). What services are provided, and who is the provider? What activities are available? How are services funded? Share findings with the group.
3. In a log or diary, record the chronic conditions identified in clinical practice. What percentage of elders encountered have more than one chronic condition? What are common combinations (e.g., chronic obstructive pulmonary disease and asthma, diabetes, peripheral vascular disease, CAD)? Share observations with members of the group.
4. Assess the home of an older client for threats to safety, particularly falls. Develop a plan or strategy to reduce identified threats.

REFERENCES

Administration on Aging (2006): *A statistical profile of older Americans age 65+* (website): http://www.aoa.dhhs.gov/press/fact/pdf/ss_stat_profile.pdf. Accessed January 10, 2008.

American Nurses Association: *Scope and standards of gerontological nursing practice*, ed 2, Washington, DC, 2001, American Nurses Association.

Ballard D: Legal and ethical issues. In Meiner SE, Lueckenotte AG, editors: *Gerontologic nursing*, ed 3, St Louis, 2006, Mosby.

Centers for Disease Control and Prevention (2007a): *Ambulatory medical care utilization for 2005* (website): http://www.cdc.gov/nchs/data/ad/ad388.pdf. Accessed January 14, 2008.

Centers for Disease Control and Prevention (2007b): *Recommended adult immunization schedule, United States, October 2007-September 2008* (website): http://www.cdc.gov/mmwr/pdf/wk/mm5641-Immunization.pdf. Accessed January 14, 2008.

Centers for Disease Control and Prevention (2006): *Falls among older adults: an overview* (website): http://www.cdc.gov/ncipc/factsheets/adultfalls.htm. Accessed January 14, 2008.

Chenitz WC, Kussman HL, Stone JT: Preventing falls. In Chenitz WC, Stone JT, Salisbury SA, editors: *Clinical gerontological nursing: a guide to advanced practice*, Philadelphia, 1991, Saunders.

Clark MJ: *Nursing in the community*, ed 3, Upper Saddle River, NJ, 2008, Prentice Hall.

Dambro MR: *Griffith's 5-minute clinical consult*, Philadelphia, 2006, Lippincott Williams & Wilkins.

Eliopoulos C: *Gerontological nursing*, ed 6, Philadelphia, 2004, Lippincott Williams & Wilkins.

Family Caregiver Alliance (2005): *Dementia* (website): http://www.caregiver.org/caregiver/jsp/content_node.jsp?nodeid=569&expandnodeid=480. Accessed January 14, 2008.

Gohdes DM, Balamurugan A, Larsen B, Maylahn C: Age-related eye diseases: an emerging challenge for public health professionals, *Prev Chronic Dis* 2(3):A17, 2005 (electronic journal online): www.cdc.gov/PCD/.

Graves M: Drug use and abuse. In Hogstel MO, editor: *Nursing care of the older adult*, ed 2, New York, 1988, Wiley.

Hashizume S: Home health care. In Chenitz WC, Stone JT, Salisbury SA, editors: *Clinical gerontological nursing: a guide to advanced practice*, Philadelphia, 1991, Saunders.

Landenburger K, Campbell J: Violence and human abuse. In Stanhope M, Lancaster J, editors: *Community & public health nursing*, ed 6, St Louis, 2004, Mosby.

Langford DR: Violence: a social and family problem. In Maurer FA, Smith CM, editors: *Community/public health nursing: health for families and populations*, ed 3, St Louis, 2005, Saunders.

Luggen AS: Aging process. In Luggen AS, editor: *Core curriculum for gerontological nursing*, St Louis, 1996, Mosby.

Meiner SE: Safety. In Meiner SE, Lueckenotte AG, editors: *Gerontologic nursing*, ed 3, St Louis, 2006, Mosby.

Murray R, Zentner J, Pinnell N: Assessment and health promotion for the person in later adulthood. In Murray RB, Zentner JP, editors: *Nursing assessment and health promotion: strategies through the life span*, ed 7, Upper Saddle River, NJ, 2001, Prentice Hall.

Murray TA: Elderly persons in the community. In Maurer FA, Smith CM, editors: *Community/public health nursing: health for families and populations*, ed 3, St Louis, 2005, Saunders.

National Institute on Aging (2005): *Age page: hearing loss* (website): http://www.niapublications.org/agepages/hearing.asp. Accessed January 14, 2008.

National Institute on Aging (2007a): *Age page: depression* (website): http://www.niapublications.org/agepages/depression.asp. Accessed January 14, 2008.

National Institute on Aging (2007b): *Elder abuse* (website): http://www.aoa.gov/press/fact/alpha/fact_elder_abuse.asp. Accessed January 14, 2008.

National Institute of Mental Health (2007): *Older adults: depression and suicide facts* (website): http://www.nimh.nih.gov/

health/publications/older-adults-depression-and-suicide-facts.shtml. Accessed January 14, 2008.

National Oral Health Surveillance System, The Centers for Disease Control and Prevention (2007) (website): http://apps.nccd.cdc.gov/nohss/DisplayV.asp?DataSet=2&nkey=7931. Accessed December 23, 2007.

Specht JKP: 9 myths of incontinence in older adults, *Am J Nurs* 105(6):58, 2005.

Stevenson L, Pappas A: Violence. In Nies M, McEwen M, editors: *Community/public health nursing: promoting the health of populations*, ed 4, St Louis, 2007, Saunders.

Stone JT, Chenitz WC: The problem of falls. In Chenitz WC, Stone JT, Salisbury SA, editors: *Clinical gerontological nursing: a guide to advanced practice*, Philadelphia, 1991, Saunders.

U.S. Census Bureau (2006a): *2006 American community survey data profile highlights* (website): http://factfinder.census.gov/servlet/ACSSAFFFacts?_submenuId=factsheet_1&_sse=on. Accessed November 5, 2007.

U.S. Census Bureau (2006b): *Population aged 65 and older United States* (website): http://factfinder.census.gov/servlet/STTable?_bm=y&-geo_id=01000US&-qr_name=ACS_2006_EST_G00_S0103&-ds_name=ACS_2006_EST_G00_. Accessed November 11, 2007.

U.S. Census Bureau (2005a): *Interim population projections by age and sex: 2004-2030* (website): http://www.census.gov/population/www/projections/projectionsagesex.html. Accessed November 5, 2007.

U.S. Census Bureau (2005b): *Age 65+ in the United States: 2005* (website): http://www.census.gov/prod/2006pubs/p23-209.pdf. Accessed November 5, 2007.

U.S. Department of Health and Human Services: *Healthy people 2010*, conference ed, Washington, DC, 2000, Government Printing Office.

U.S. Department of Health and Human Services, National Institute of Mental Health: *Mental health: report of the surgeon general*, Rockville, Md, 1999, USDHHS, SAMHSA, CMHS, NIH, NIMH.

Westley CJ, Fletcher KR: Health of older adults. In Stanhope M, Lancaster J, editors: *Community health nursing: promoting health of aggregates, families and individuals*, ed 6, St Louis, 2004, Mosby.

Health Promotion and Illness Prevention for Families

1. Discuss the concept of family, and explain the different types of families.

2. Describe characteristics common to all families, and identify the purpose of the family.

3. Describe the stages of the family life cycle, and give examples of tasks to be accomplished at each stage.

4. Perform a family assessment, and develop a plan of care for a family, including construction of a genogram, ecomap, and/or family health tree.

5. Discuss nursing interventions to promote health and prevent disease for families at various developmental stages.

key terms

Blended family	Family health tree	Stages of family
Ecomap	Family roles	development
Extended family	Genogram	
Family	Nuclear dyad	
Family assessment	Nuclear family	
Family crises	Single-parent family	*See Glossary for definitions.*

case study

Jessica Richardson is a registered nurse (RN) employed by a visiting nurse association (VNA) affiliated with a public health department in a large city. She specializes in caring for high-risk infants and their families. Most of the babies Jessica sees are low-birth-weight babies, or they had complications following birth. In addition, several of the infants in her caseload have birth anomalies or genetic disorders.

On a recent Monday, Jessica admitted a new family into service. Jeffrey Smith was born 7 weeks prematurely and weighed just under 3 pounds at birth. His mother Sarah is an unmarried 16-year-old high school junior who lives with her mother, grandmother, and two siblings. Jeffrey spent almost 2 weeks in the neonatal intensive care unit (NICU) because

Continued

of breathing problems before moving to the regular nursery. He was discharged at 6 weeks of age at 4.5 pounds. Because of his history of breathing difficulties and two episodes of apnea, Jeffrey needs to wear an apnea monitor 24 hours a day.

Jessica scheduled the initial home visit to occur within a few hours of the baby's discharge. She wanted to spend time with as many of the immediate family members as possible to do a thorough assessment of the family and the home environment. Jessica learned that Sarah and Jeffrey live with Sarah's mother Maggie (34 years of age), Maggie's mother Lucille (60 years of age), and Sarah's younger brother Pete (15 years of age) and sister Abby (13 years of age). Sarah's parents have been divorced for 10 years, and the family moved to Lucille's home at that time so she could help care for the three grandchildren, then ages 3, 5, and 6 years.

Maggie is the primary breadwinner for the family. She is employed as a supervisor at a local paper mill, and her income is adequate to meet the basic needs of the family. After the divorce Mr. Smith relocated to another state. He is a construction worker, but is only periodically employed and rarely sends child support money. Lucille does not work outside the home because she is partially disabled as the result of a back injury. Pete and Sarah contribute to the family finances by working in fast food establishments, although Sarah has not worked since going into premature labor. Jeffrey's father is a high school student named Jimmy. Jimmy is no longer involved with Sarah and has shown minimal interest in the child; he provides no financial support.

For the initial meeting, Jessica interviewed Sarah and her mother and grandmother. Jessica was told that Lucille would be the primary caretaker of Jeffrey during the day while Sarah is completing her last 2 years of high school and Maggie works. Sarah will provide most of his care during the evenings and on weekends.

The family lives in a three-bedroom, one-bath frame house. The sleeping arrangements have changed since the baby came home. Lucille has one bedroom alone and Maggie and Abby share another. Sarah and the baby have the third room, and Pete sleeps on the couch. Jessica observed that the kitchen was clean and that there were ample supplies (e.g., diapers and bottles) for the infant. There is a baby bed in Sarah's room, and Sarah acknowledged that Jeffrey will ride in a car seat at all times.

From her interview Jessica learned that health care for the family is paid through insurance provided by Maggie's employer. Lucille receives Medicaid and Medicare because of her disability. They receive no other social services.

Sarah recovered from Jeffrey's birth without incident and stated that she has no current health problems. Maggie reported that she is in good health, although she smokes about two packs of cigarettes a day. She is also about 20 pounds overweight. In addition to her chronic back problem, Lucille is diabetic, and Jessica observed that she is about 50 pounds overweight. Maggie and Lucille explained that the other teenagers are all in good health, with no significant health problems. Jessica gained additional information about the extended family's health history.

Maggie reported that the family attends church weekly. Sarah is behind in school, but should be able to catch up and graduate. She hopes to go to beauty college after graduation and become a hair stylist. Pete is an adequate student, but Maggie expressed concern over some of his friends, who she knows smoke and drink and may be involved in drugs and gang activity. Abby is an excellent student and hopes to go to college to become a lawyer.

Jessica performed a complete physical assessment on Jeffrey. He had gained 1 ounce from the previous day and was breathing normally. The apnea monitor was attached and working properly. Her interventions for the first visit were directed toward teaching Sarah, Maggie, and Lucille how to care for Jeffrey. She focused on recognizing breathing problems and apnea and other health problems common to low-birth-weight and premature infants. She explained how to maintain the apnea monitor and what to do when the alarm sounds, and she gave detailed instructions on emergency procedures and how to manage them, including when to call for assistance. She also provided the three women with instructional materials that supplemented what she taught.

The women asked questions and were able to repeat the instructions, indicating comprehension. Jessica made an appointment to return the following day for follow-up and additional teaching.

The **family** is the most basic social unit. Some form of family can be found in all human societies. The family is the primary social group for each individual and contributes to his or her growth and experiences. The family impacts how the individual adapts and responds to changes and threats and directly influences health. The family has a major role in shaping the person.

Although the individual is usually the primary recipient of health care, many nurses, particularly those working in community settings, recognize the importance of providing interventions directed at the family level. For example, a nurse who works in a primary care pediatric clinic cares for several children from one family simultaneously, understanding that both acute and chronic illnesses can affect the entire family. Likewise a home health nurse caring for an elderly diabetic man works with his spouse and extended family as she teaches the important points of managing diabetes. Finally, a hospice nurse cares for the entire family of a dying client, knowing that each member is affected by the illness and death of their loved one.

This chapter describes issues related to families and family health. It focuses on helping nurses who work in community settings understand the different types and stages of families and how to recognize both healthy and unhealthy family characteristics. Last, the process of assessment and intervention for families is covered.

THE CONCEPT OF FAMILY

When many people think of a family, they think of a husband/breadwinner and wife/homemaker with one or more children living in the home. Sometimes they include extended family members, in particular, grandparents, children living away (either single or married), and grandchildren. Others may consider aunts and uncles, cousins, godparents, and even very close friends to be part of their immediate family.

But what constitutes a family is not easily explained because family means different things to different people. It has been pointed out that culture, not biology, determines family organization; therefore the meaning of family is different for people from different cultures (Murray et al., 2001). In addition, the concept of family is dynamic and

evolving. In contemporary American society, conceptualizations of family have moved from a vision of the nuclear family and extended family to include a variety of households, such as unmarried adults living together with or without children, single-parent households, divorced couples who combine households with children from previous marriages, and homosexual couples with or without children (Box 16-1).

DEFINITIONS OF FAMILY

Many definitions for family can be found in the literature. According to Vaughn-Cole and colleagues (1998), traditional definitions of family are based on

BOX 16-1 Types of Families

Nuclear family: mother, father, and child(ren) living together but apart from both sets of the father's and mother's parents

Nuclear dyad: husband and wife or other couple living alone without children

Single-parent family: mother or father living with either biologic or adopted children; they may be tied emotionally, but not legally, to a partner

Extended family: nuclear family plus other relatives of one or both spouses; relatives may or may not live with the nuclear family and may include great-grandparents and great-great-grandparents

Stepfamily (blended family): one divorced or widowed adult with all or some of his or her children and a new spouse with all or some of his or her children; may include the children born to this union so that parents, stepparents, children, and stepchildren or stepsiblings live together

Three generational family: any combination of the first, second, and third generation members living within a household

Grandparent-headed family: a three generational family in which the grandparent is often responsible for care of the grandchildren

Single adult: never married, separated, divorced, or widowed individual living alone or with other single adults in a nonsexual relationship

Cohabiting couple: unmarried couple living together

Compound family: one man or woman with several spouses

Same-sex family: gay or lesbian partners living together; may have children

From Cooley M: A family perspective in community/public health nursing. In Maurer FA, Smith CM, editors: *Community/public health nursing practice: health for families and populations*, ed 3, St Louis, 2005, Saunders; Murray RB, Zentner PP, Brockhaus JPD, Brockhaus R, Sullivan E: The family: basic unit for the developing person. In Murray RB, Zentner JP, editors: *Health promotion strategies through the life span*, ed 7, Upper Saddle River, NJ, 2001, Prentice Hall.

persistent myths. One of these myths is that the typical family is a nuclear family consisting of parents and children. Another myth relates to the ideal of the extended family of several generations working toward a common family goal. The authors pointed out that these are now the exception rather than the rule.

Definitions for family are varied and numerous. The U.S. Census Bureau (2006) provides a definition reflective of social change, stating: "A family group is any two or more people (not necessarily including a householder) residing together and related by birth, marriage, or adoption. A household may be composed of one such group, more than one, or none at all. The count of family groups includes family households, related subfamilies, and unrelated subfamilies." Other basic definitions for family include the following:

> "A cluster of people whose relationship is stipulated by law in terms of marriage and descent, and whose precise membership varies according to the circumstances" (Farber, 1973, p. 2).

> "A primary group of people living in a household in consistent proximity and intimate relationship" (Helvie, 1981, p. 64).

> "An aggregate made up of a body of units, the individuals that represent the whole or the family" (Siegrist, 2007, p. 361).

More complete or complex definitions can also be found. For example, Allender and Spradley (2005a) stated that a "family consists of two or more individuals who share a residence or live near one another; possess some common emotional bond; engage in interrelated social positions, roles and tasks; and share a sense of affection and belonging" (p. 496).

A similar definition is proposed by Murray and others (2001) who explained that a family is "a small social system and primary reference group made up of two or more persons living together who are related by blood, marriage, or adoption or who are living together by agreement over a period of time" (p. 158).

Finally, Craft and Willadsen (1992) wrote that the family is a "social context of two or more people characterized by mutual attachment, caring, long-term commitment, responsibility to provide individual growth, supportive relationships, health of members and of the unit, and maintenance of the organization and system during constant individual, family, and societal change" (p. 519).

Stuart (1991) summarized the following conceptualizations of family:

- The family is a system or unit.
- Family members may or may not be related and may or may not live together.
- The unit may or may not contain children.
- Commitment and attachment exist among unit members and include future obligation.
- The unit caregiving functions consist of protection, nourishment, and socialization of unit members.

TYPES OF FAMILIES

Defining family is difficult because families can assume many different forms. Traditional families include the nuclear family, the nuclear dyad (husband and wife with no children or with grown children), and single adult families where one adult lives alone. Other variations include multigenerational families, in which several generations or age groups live together in the same household; kin networks, in which several nuclear families live in the same household or near one another and share goods and services; blended families, in which single parents marry and raise children from one or both previous relationships; and single-parent families, in which one adult cares for a child or children as a result of a temporary relationship or a legal separation, divorce, or death of a spouse (Allender and Spradley, 2005a). Some types of both traditional and nontraditional families are described here and are summarized in Box 16-1.

Nuclear Family

The conjugal **nuclear family** is composed of a married husband and wife and children. The children may be either biologic offspring or adopted. Several factors, such as the high rate of divorce, increased sexual freedom, decreased social stigma attached to illegitimacy, and alternative sexual lifestyles have contributed to the changing form of the nuclear family. As a result, the nuclear family is becoming less common. Indeed, only about 22% of American families consist of a married couple with children living at home (U.S. Census Bureau, 2007).

Nuclear Dyad

A **nuclear dyad** (a married couple without children in the home) occurs by choice, because of infertility, or because children are grown and away from home

(Clark, 2008). The nuclear dyad is the most common household arrangement, with somewhat less than half of all families (40%) being nuclear dyads.

Single-Parent Family

A **single-parent family** consists of an adult woman or man and children. Single-parent families result from divorce, out-of-wedlock pregnancies, absence or death of a spouse, or adoption by a single person. Most (81%) single-parent families are headed by women (U.S. Census Bureau, 2007).

The number of single-parent families has risen sharply in the past few decades. Between 1970 and 2005, births to single women increased from 11% to 27% of all births, and the proportion of single-mother households more than doubled from 10% to 23% of households with children (U.S. Census Bureau, 2007).

Extended Family

An **extended family** consists of the family kin network and includes grandparents, aunts, uncles, and cousins. Like the nuclear family, the extended family has been greatly affected by social changes. In the past, members of an extended family often lived in close proximity, but because of increased mobility, families are more likely to live away from their extended kin network.

Stepfamily or Blended Family

A stepfamily or **blended family** is composed of two adults, at least one of whom has remarried following divorce or death of a spouse. Blended families can include children from either adult's previous marriage(s) and offspring from the new marriage.

Like single-parent families, blended families have increased rapidly in the United States over the last several decades. This is because it is estimated that 40% to 50% of marriages end in divorce, and two thirds of divorces involve children. Most divorced adults eventually remarry, contributing to the formation of thousands of stepfamilies each year (Clark, 2008).

Cohabitating Family

A cohabitating family consists of a man and woman living together without being married. Increasingly, unmarried couples have children, with four out of ten cohabiting couples having children in their household. Cohabitation is becoming increasingly

prevalent in the United States, and the number of unmarried couples increased from 3.2 million households in 1990 to 5.4 million households in 2000 (U.S. Census Bureau, 2007).

Gay or Lesbian Family

A gay or lesbian family is a form of cohabitation in which a couple of the same sex lives together and shares a sexual relationship. Approximately 10% of unmarried-partner households consist of partners of the same sex, with about half being male partners and half female partners (Clark, 2008).

Grandparent-Headed Family

In many instances in the United States grandparents are raising their grandchildren. Grandparent-headed families typically occur because of working parents, divorce, AIDS, drug or alcohol abuse, or child abuse or abandonment (Clark, 2008). Immigration also effects the living arrangements of children, with grandparents providing housing for immigrant relatives. Approximately 7% of all U.S. households are headed by grandparents (U.S. Census Bureau, 2007). The Community Application box "Grandparents Raising Grandchildren" presents some of the adaptive dynamics of a grandparent-headed family.

Although all families are unique, they all possess certain common qualities or characteristics. This is true regardless of whether they are nuclear families, nuclear dyads, foster families, gay/lesbian families, or other family types (Allender and Spradley, 2005a). For example, each family can be thought of as a small social system in which each individual is a subsystem. The family system as a whole and each individual subsystem interact with other subsystems and the larger suprasystem in multiple ways.

Each family has a basic structure and function; these are dynamic and change with time and circumstances. Families are interdependent, meaning that family members rely on other members for assistance and to meet a variety of needs such as affection, love, loyalty, and financial commitment. In addition, families set and maintain boundaries (generation boundaries and family community boundaries), which result from shared experiences and expectations. Finally, all families create and maintain their own set of values, rules, and goals (Allender and Spradley, 2005a; Murray et al., 2001).

COMMUNITY APPLICATION
Grandparents Raising Grandchildren

Many older Americans approaching or in retirement suddenly find themselves raising their grandchildren. According to the U.S. Census Bureau, in the year 2000 3.9 million children were living in homes maintained by their grandparents—a 76% increase since 1970. At some point more than 10% of grandparents raise a grandchild for at least 6 months, and typically grandparents are caregivers for much longer periods. The reasons for the increase in the number of grandparents caring for their grandchildren include death of parents, incarceration of parents, unemployment of parents, substance abuse by parents, teen pregnancy, family violence, and human immunodeficiency virus (HIV)/AIDS.

This phenomenon has important health consequences. Grandparents in the caregiving role are more prone to psychologic and emotional strain and feelings of helplessness and isolation. Many grandparent caregivers face financial dificulties, and grandparent caregivers are 60% more likely to live in poverty than are grandparents not raising grandchildren. Grandparent caregivers often neglect their own physical and emotional health because they give priority to the needs of their grandchildren.

In addition, the grandchildren in their care often have unmet physical, emotional, and developmental needs that may require special assistance. There may be legal issues because grandparents often must obtain legal authority to get their grandchildren medical care; enroll them in school; and enable them to receive immunizations, public assistance, and supportive services. Finally, grandparents may need respite services, affordable housing, and access to medical care.

From Administration on Aging (2007): *Grandparents raising grandchildren* (website): http://www.aoa.gov/prof/notes/notes_grandparents.asp. Accessed October 21, 2007.

PURPOSES OF FAMILIES

Families exist to serve several purposes. For example, according to Murray and colleagues (2001), families provide physical safety and meet the economic needs of family members. The family helps members develop physically, emotionally, intellectually, and spiritually and creates a healthy environment for the family's well-being. The family should also help members develop a personal identity and a value system. This value system is generally built on spiritual and philosophic beliefs and the cultural and social system with which the family identifies.

Families also teach members social skills and how to communicate effectively. They teach gender roles and appropriate behaviors. Families provide security, support, encouragement, and motivation. Finally, families help members cope with crises and societal demands (Allender and Spradley, 2005a; Murray et al., 2001).

ROLES IN THE FAMILY

Roles are socially expected behavior patterns that are determined by a person's position or status. In families, roles are the assigned or assumed parts that members play during day-to-day living; they are bestowed and defined by the family. In a given family, the specific roles to be played vary, depending on the family's structure, needs, and patterns of functioning (Allender and Spradley, 2005a).

Within a family, each person occupies several roles by virtue of his or her position. For example, the adult woman in the house typically occupies the role of wife and mother. She may also be the cook, laundress, and housekeeper, as well as being a bread winner. The adult male in the house may be the primary bread winner. He may also be the disciplinarian and teacher.

Family roles may be well defined (formal) or less well defined (informal). Formal roles are expected sets of behaviors associated with family positions (i.e., husband, wife, mother, father, brother, sister, son, daughter). Informal roles are those behaviors not associated with a particular position, but which influence how and by whom emotional needs are met. Children and adults take on multiple roles, both formal and informal (Clark, 2008).

Role conflict occurs when the demands of fulfilling several roles contradict or compete with each other. Role conflict can also occur when one individual's definition of a role does not correspond with someone else's definition of the same role (Clark, 2008). For example, a husband may see his wife as the cook/housekeeper and child care provider and the wife might expect her husband to help out around the house and take care of the children. Alternatively a child might be responsible for caring for a younger sibling and need supervision himself.

DEVELOPMENTAL STAGES OF FAMILIES

Just as an individual grows through a series of developmental stages (i.e., infancy, toddlerhood, childhood), a normal family also evolves through a series of several stages. Indeed, the typical family goes through the following stages: beginning family (marriage); early childbearing family; preschool children, school-age children, teenage children, launching family, middle-age family, and aging family (Siegrist, 2007).

Alterations in family development may occur that inhibit movement through these stages. Divorce and remarriage, for example, dramatically redefine the **stages of family development**. Likewise, having a late baby when other children are adolescents changes the family development cycle. Other alterations to the family life cycle occur with single parenting, infertility, and early, unexpected death. Table 16-1 provides a summary of tasks to be accomplished in each stage of the family's life cycle. In addition, each stage of family development is described briefly.

ESTABLISHMENT STAGE (BEGINNING FAMILY)

In the establishment stage, a couple goes through courtship and engagement. A commitment to a partner is made, usually through marriage. The new couple must develop and define their relationship and become free of parental domination. They establish their own home and life patterns and focus on the new lifestyle with the partner. At some point, the beginning family discusses parenting issues.

EARLY CHILDBEARING STAGE

In the early childbearing stage, the couple must resolve feelings and issues about pregnancy and parenthood. At some point, the woman becomes

TABLE **16-1** Stages and Tasks of Middle-Class North American Family Life Cycle

STAGE	TASK
Launching: the single young adult leaves home	Coming to terms with the family of origin Development of intimate relationships with peers Establishment of self; career and finances
Marriage: the joining of families	Formation of identity as a couple Including spouse in realignment of relationships with extended families
Families with young children	Integration of children into family unit Adjusting tasks: childbearing, financial, and household Accommodation of new parenting and grandparenting roles
Families with adolescents	Development of increasing autonomy for adolescents Reexamining midlife marital and career issues Initial shift toward concern for the older generation
Families as launching centers	Establishment of independent identities for parents and grown children Renegotiation of marital relationship Readjusting relationships to include in-laws and grandchildren Dealing with disabilities and death of older generation
Aging Families	Maintaining couple and individual functioning while adapting to the aging process Supporting role of middle generation Supporting yet allowing autonomy of older generation Preparation for own death and dealing with the loss of spouse and/or siblings and other peers

From Siegrist BC: Family health. In Nies M, McEwen M, editors: *Community/public health nursing: promoting the health of populations*, ed 4, St Louis, 2007, Saunders; Wright LM, Leahey M: *Nurses and families: a guide to family assessment and intervention*, ed 2, Philadelphia, 1994, FA Davis.

pregnant or the couple decides to adopt. This stage requires significant adjustment to changes in lifestyle, and the couple must work through a number of related developmental tasks. When the infant arrives, they must adjust to caring for it. In addition, they need to renegotiate marital and extended family relationships.

FAMILIES WITH PRESCHOOL-AGE CHILDREN

In families with preschool-age children, the couple learns to adjust to family life, concentrating on adapting to the needs and interests of small children. They must learn to cope with energy depletion and lack of privacy as parents. Financial issues may be prevalent if the wife leaves the workforce or the family must pay for child care.

FAMILIES WITH SCHOOL-AGE CHILDREN

Families with school-age children need to adjust to growing children's activities. They should promote development of joint decision making by children and parents and encourage and support the children's education achievements.

FAMILIES WITH ADOLESCENTS

During the adolescent stage of family development, the family should strive to maintain open communication among family members. This is a good time to strengthen the family unit to support and encourage ethical and moral values. During this stage it is important to balance freedom with responsibility as teenagers mature.

LAUNCHING FAMILIES

As children become adults and leave home, the family must cope with different types of changes. They should be ready to release the young adults with appropriate rituals and assistance, while continuing to maintain a supportive home base. During this stage the husband and wife reestablish their relationship as a couple.

MIDDLE-AGE FAMILIES

In the middle-age years, the family (possibly now a dyad) prepares for retirement. During this stage a significant focus is on maintaining kin ties with both older and younger generations. In many cases, the middle-age family is called on to provide significant assistance to their own aging parents and to their children who have been launched and begun their own families.

AGING FAMILIES

As the family ages, it is important to adjust to retirement. Other significant changes include loss of spouse, siblings, close friends, and possibly the loss of aging children. Often the family must decide to close the family home or adapt it for elderly members (McCarthy and Mandle, 2000).

FAMILY HEALTH

Family health refers to the health status of a given family. Family health is concerned with how well the family functions together as a unit and considers the health of each family member and how each member relates to other members. Family health also involves how well the family relates to and copes with the community outside the family. Because of the interactions between and among the family members and the interactions with the larger community, it is important for nurses who work in community settings to be aware of, and prepared to intervene in, issues that relate to family health.

HEALTHY PEOPLE 2010 AND FAMILY HEALTH

Although *Healthy People 2010* (U.S. Department of Health and Human Services [USDHHS], 2000) does not address families per se, a number of objectives related to families and family health can be found. In addition, other objectives can or should be addressed at the family level. The *Healthy People 2010* box lists several objectives related to family health.

CHARACTERISTICS OF HEALTHY FAMILIES

In healthy families, the family is the stable source for sustenance, nurturance, growth, and development of each member. There is mutual support as members share in problem solving and decision making. There is also recognition that the family is dynamic and that each member will become part of another family system at some point in time.

Healthy families maintain flexible boundaries that support and encourage exchange between the family and the larger society. There is a defined power structure, which results from clear role definitions and appropriate rules. In healthy families,

healthy people **2010**

Objectives Related to Family Health

OBJECTIVE	BASELINE (1998)	TARGET
1.1: Increase the proportion of persons with health insurance	86%	100%
1.6: Reduce the proportion of families that experience difficulties or delays in obtaining health care or do not receive needed care for one or more family members	12%	7%
6.5: Increase the proportion of adults with disabilities reporting sufficient emotional support	70%	79%
7.7: Increase the proportion of health care organizations that provide client and family education	NA	NA
8.23: Reduce the proportion of occupied housing units that are substandard	6.2%	3%
9.4: Increase the proportion of pregnancies that are intended	51%	70%
9.12: Reduce the proportion of married couples whose ability to conceive or maintain a pregnancy is impaired	13%	10%
11.1: Increase the proportion of households with access to the Internet at home	26%	80%
15.34: Reduce the rate of physical assault by current or former intimate partners	4.5 assaults per 1000	3.6 assaults per 1000
22.11: Increase the proportion of children and adolescents who view television 2 or fewer hours per day	60%	75%
27.9: Reduce the proportion of children who are regularly exposed to tobacco smoke at home	27%	10%

From U.S. Department of Health and Human Services: *Healthy people 2010*: conference ed, Washington, DC, 2000, USDHHS.

power is shared among members, within parental roles, and appropriate with age. Also there is an open communication system in which there is honest, clear, and direct communication. Finally, the healthy family is adaptable, flexible, and resilient; this allows for coping with changing demands (Cooley, 2005).

The following specific characteristics or traits can be observed in healthy families:

- Members interact with each other repeatedly in many contexts (Figure 16-1).
- Members are encouraged to grow and develop as individuals and members of the family.
- Members are enhanced and fulfilled by maintaining contacts with a wide range of community groups and organizations.
- Members make efforts to master their lives by becoming members of groups, finding information and options, and making decisions.
- Members support and maintain a healthy environment and lifestyle.
- Members engage in flexible role relationships, share power, respond to change, support growth and autonomy of others, and engage in decision making that affects them.
- Members support mastery of developmental tasks leading to interdependence, progressive differentiation, and transformation to meet the requisites for survival of the system.
- Members provide nurturance and resources for growth and sustenance (Allender and Spradley, 2005b; Murray et al., 2001; Siegrist, 2007).

Figure 16-1. Family celebrations and traditions strengthen the role of the family. (From Potter PA, Perry AG: *Fundamentals of nursing*, ed 5, St Louis, 2001, Mosby.)

CHARACTERISTICS OF UNHEALTHY FAMILIES

Just as there are characteristics common to healthy families, patterns that are not adaptive and might be termed *unhealthy* can be identified among families as well. Some of these characteristics include the following:

- Maladaptation: signs of strained or destructive family relationships
- Lack of understanding, communication, and helpfulness between members
- Each family member alternately acts as if the other did not exist or harasses others through arguments
- Lack of family decision making and lines of authority
- Parent's possessiveness of the children or the mate
- Children's derogatory remarks to the parents or vice versa
- Extreme closeness between husband and his mother or family, or between the wife and her mother or family
- Members not maintaining individuality, being too close or enmeshed, or too distant with each other
- Parents being domineering about performance of household tasks
- Few outside friends for parents or children
- Scapegoating or blaming each other for difficulties
- High level of anxiety or insecurity present in the home
- Lack of creativity and stability
- Pattern of immature or regressive behavior in parents or children
- Boundaries between generations not maintained (children carrying out parental roles because of parental inability or abandonment) (Murray et al., 2001)

When observing or assessing families, the nurse should watch for signs or indications that might show the family has unhealthy traits or characteristics. Table 16-2 lists some risk factors for unhealthy families, based on life cycle stage.

FAMILY CRISIS

Family crises are experienced in all families. Two basic types of family crises are the maturational crisis and the situational crisis. A maturational crisis is a normal transition point in which old patterns of communication and old roles must be exchanged for new patterns and roles. Every family experiences maturational crisis points, whether or not a crisis is actually experienced. Examples of transitional periods in which maturational crises may occur are adolescence, marriage, and parenthood (Clark, 2008).

A situational crisis can occur when the family experiences an event that is sudden, unexpected, and unpredictable. Such events threaten biologic, psychologic, or social integrity and lead to disorganization, tension, and severe anxiety. Examples of situational crises include illness, accidents, death, and natural disasters (Clark, 2008).

TABLE **16-2** Family Stage-Specific Risk Factors and Related Health Problems

STAGE	RISK FACTORS	HEALTH PROBLEMS
Beginning childbearing family	Lack of knowledge about family planning Adolescent marriage Lack of knowledge concerning sexual and marital roles and adjustments Low-birth-weight infant Lack of prenatal care Inadequate nutrition Poor eating habits Smoking, alcohol, drug abuse Unmarried status First pregnancy before age 16 or after 35 History of hypertension and infections during pregnancy Rubella, syphilis, gonorrhea, and acquired AIDS Genetic factors Low socioeconomic and educational levels Lack of safety in the home	Premature baby Birth defects Birth injuries Accidents SIDS Respiratory distress syndrome Sterility Pelvic inflammatory disease Fetal alcohol syndrome Mental retardation Child abuse Injuries Birth defects Underweight or overweight
Family with school-age children	Working parents with inappropriate use of resources for child care Poverty Abuse or neglect of children Generational pattern of using social agencies as a way of life Multiple, closely spaced children Low family self-esteem Children used as scapegoats for parental frustration Repeated infections, accidents, or hospitalizations Parents immature, dependent, and unable to handle responsibility Unrecognized or unattended health problems Strong beliefs about physical punishment Toxic substances unguarded in the home Poor nutrition	Behavior disturbances Speech and vision problems Communicable diseases Dental caries School problems Learning disabilities Cancer Injuries Chronic diseases Homicide Violence
Family with adolescents	Racial and ethnic family origin Lifestyle and behavior patterns leading to chronic disease Lack of problem-solving skills Family values of aggressiveness and competition Family values rigid and inflexible Daredevil risk-taking attitude Denial behavior Conflicts between parents and children Pressure to live up to family expectations	Violent deaths and injuries Alcohol and drug abuse Unwanted pregnancies Sexually transmitted diseases Suicide Depression

STAGE	RISK FACTORS	HEALTH PROBLEMS
Family with middle-age adults	Hypertension Smoking High cholesterol level Physical inactivity Genetic predisposition Use of oral contraceptives Sex, race, and other heredity factors Geographical area, age, occupational deficiencies Habits (e.g., diet with low fiber, pickling, charcoal use, and broiling) Alcohol abuse Social class Residence	Cardiovascular disease, principally coronary artery disease and cerebrovascular accident (stroke) Diabetes Overweight Cancer Accidents Homicide Suicide Abnormal fetus Mental illness Periodontal disease and loss of teeth Depression
Family with older adults	Age Drug interactions Metabolic disorders Pituitary malfunctions Cushing syndrome Hypercalcemia Chronic illness Retirement Loss of spouse Reduced income Poor nutrition Lack of exercise Past environments and lifestyle Lack of preparation for death	Mental confusion Reduced vision Hearing impairment Hypertension Acute illness Infectious disease Influenza Pneumonia Injuries such as burns and falls Depression Chronic disease Elder abuse Death without dignity

From Rentfro AR: Health promotion and the family. In Edelman CL, Mandle CL, editors: *Health promotion throughout the lifespan*, ed 6, St Louis, 2006, Mosby.

A crisis state is associated with high stress and tension levels. The result of a crisis can be either resolution (resulting in a healthier, more positive state of being) or loss of well-being and a higher potential for recurrent crisis. Temporary relief can be gained from the use of defense mechanisms, environmental action, or both. During periods of crisis, families are more susceptible to change and are usually more open to help (Clark, 2008).

Bergman (1993) identified the following key family characteristics that influence how people recover from and function during and after crises:

- Family cohesion: emotional bonding of family members and the degree of individual autonomy of each person in the family
- Family adaptation: the degree of flexibility evidenced by the ability to change roles, relationships, and power structures in response to stress

- Family social integration: the degree of social network with neighbors, friends, other family members, and religious or social organizations
- Degree of stress experienced by the family: includes combinations of stressors that may influence the family

If these characteristics are strong, in most cases the family can respond appropriately or positively to the crisis and adapt effectively. If the family characteristics are weak, the crisis may be more difficult to manage or resolve.

NURSING CARE OF FAMILIES

The concept of family nursing is not new. It has been taught in schools of nursing since Nightingale's time. Indeed, the National League for Nursing (NLN) has emphasized the importance of caring for the family in standard curricula guides for schools of nursing since 1917. Furthermore, many modern nurse theorists (Newman, King, Orem, Roy) extensively discuss the family and its importance to individuals and society (Siegrist, 2007).

FAMILY NURSING

Nurses working in community settings should be aware that the individual can best be understood within the social context of the family. Nurses can approach family health care in two ways. The first is viewing the family as the context of care; the second is viewing the family as client. When families are treated as the context within which individuals are assessed, the emphasis is primarily on the individual, keeping in mind that he or she is part of a larger system, the family (family as context). Conversely, when the nurse treats the family as a set of interacting parts and emphasizes assessment of the dynamics among these parts rather than the individual parts themselves (family members), the family as a whole rather than the individual members becomes the client (family as client) (Hitchcock, 2003).

In family nursing, care may focus on the individual family member within the context of the family, on the family unit, or in some cases both. The nurse establishes a relationship with each family member within the unit and understands the influence of the unit on the individual and larger group or community (Siegrist, 2007). Birthing, parent-child relationships, adult day care, chronic illness, and home care are best addressed using nursing practice models emphasizing the family.

Friedman (2003) presented some reasons that nurses should work with families. This list included the following ideas:

- Within the family unit, any dysfunction that affects one or more family members will probably affect other family members and the family as a whole.
- The wellness of the family is highly dependent on the role of the family in every aspect of health care, from prevention to rehabilitation.
- The level of wellness of the whole family can be raised through care that reduces lifestyle and environmental risks by emphasizing health promotion, self-care, health education, and family counseling.

- Commonalities in risk factors and diseases shared by family members can lead to case finding within the family.
- A clear understanding of the functioning of the individual can be gained only when the individual is assessed within the larger context of the family.
- The family as a vital support system to the individual member needs to be incorporated into treatment plans.

FAMILY NURSING INTERVENTIONS

The nurse can provide several interventions to promote family health. For example, the nurse can act as a collaborator, helping the family to assess, improve, enhance, and evaluate their current health practices. The nurse can also assist the family in identifying high-risk behaviors and helping them make decisions about lifestyle choices. The nurse can provide information about health issues and give reinforcement for positive health practices. Finally, the nurse can act as a liaison for referral or collaboration between the family and community resources (Rentfro, 2006). The Community Application box "Possible Nursing Roles in Health Promotion and Disease Prevention Through Stages of Family Development" lists other nursing roles and interventions for the family, based on the various family developmental stages.

FAMILY ASSESSMENT

A comprehensive **family assessment** should be the basis for promoting the health of a family. Several factors influence the assessment of the family: (1) the nurse's perception of what constitutes a family, (2) knowledge of theories, norms and standards, and (3) ability to put the family at ease. When performing a comprehensive assessment of the family, Allender and Spradley (2005b) suggest that the nurse do the following:

1. Focus on the family as a total unit
2. Ask goal-directed questions
3. Allow adequate time for data collection
4. Combine quantitative and qualitative data
5. Exercise professional judgment

In addition, Friedman (2003) lists 12 data-collection categories for family health assessment. These are shown in Box 16-2.

COMMUNITY APPLICATION
Possible Nursing Roles in Health Promotion and Disease Prevention Through Stages of Family Development

STAGE	POSSIBLE NURSING ROLE
Couple	Counselor on sexual and role adjustment
	Teacher of and counselor on family planning
	Teacher of parenting skills
	Coordinator for genetic counseling
	Facilitator in interpersonal relationships
Childbearing family	Monitor of prenatal care and referrer for problems of pregnancy
	Counselor on prenatal nutrition
	Counselor on prenatal maternal habits
	Supporter of amniocentesis
	Counselor on breastfeeding
	Coordinator with pediatric services
	Supervisor of immunizations
	Referrer to social services
	Assistant in adjustment to parental role
Family with preschool and school-age children	Monitor of early childhood development; referrer when indicated
	Teacher of first-aid and emergency measures
	Coordinator with pediatric services
	Counselor on nutrition and exercise
	Teacher of dental hygiene
	Counselor on environmental safety in the home
	Facilitator in interpersonal relationships
Family with adolescents	Teacher of risk factors on health
	Teacher in problem-solving issues regarding alcohol, smoking, diet, and exercise
	Facilitator of interpersonal skills with adolescents and parents
	Direct supporter of, counselor on, or referrer to mental health resources
	Counselor on family planning
	Referrer for sexually transmittable disease
Family with young or middle-age adults	Participant in community organizations involved in disease control
	Teacher in problem-solving issues regarding lifestyle and habits
	Participant in community organizations for environmental control
	Case finder in the home and community
	Screener for hypertension, Pap smear, breast examination, cancer signs, mental health, and dental care
	Counselor on menopausal transition

Continued

COMMUNITY APPLICATION
Possible Nursing Roles in Health Promotion and Disease Prevention Through Stages of Family Development—cont'd

Family with older adults	Facilitator in interpersonal relationships among family members
	Referrer for work and social activity, nutritional programs, homemakers' services, and nursing home
	Monitor of exercise, nutrition, preventive services, and medications
	Supervisor of immunization
	Counselor on safety in the home
	Counselor on bereavement

From Rentfro AR: Health promotion and the family. In Edelman CL, Mandle CL, editors: *Health promotion throughout the lifespan*, ed 6, St Louis, 2006, Mosby.

 16-2 Data Collection Categories for a Comprehensive Family Assessment

1. Family demographics: family composition, socioeconomic status, education, ages, occupation, ethnicity, and religious affiliation of its members
2. Physical environment data: geography, climate, housing, space, social structures, food availability, and dietary patterns
3. Psychologic and spiritual environment: relationships, mutual respect, and support; promotion of members' self-esteem, spiritual development, and goals
4. Family structure and roles: family organization, socialization processes, division of labor, authority, and power patterns
5. Family function: Ability to carry out appropriate developmental tasks and provide for members' needs
6. Family values and beliefs: how to raise children, how to make and spend money, and emphasis on education, religion, work, health, and community involvement
7. Family communication patterns: frequency and quality of communication within a family and between the family and its environment
8. Family decision-making patterns: how decisions are made and implemented
9. Family problem-solving patterns: how the family handles its problems
10. Family coping patterns: how a family handles conflict and life changes; nature and quality of support systems and perception and responses to stressors
11. Family health behavior: family health history, current physical health status of members, use of health resources, and health beliefs
12. Family social and cultural patterns: family discipline and limit-setting practices; promotion of members' initiative, creativity, and leadership; family goals; and development of meaningful relationships within and outside the family

FAMILY HEALTH ASSESSMENT TOOLS

Completion of a family health assessment instrument may help the nurse identify the health status of individual members of the family and aspects of family composition, function, and process. A family health assessment may elicit information about the environment or community context of the family and enables the community health nurse to plan interventions appropriately (Siegrist, 2007).

The family assessment should be as comprehensive as possible. Many tools are available to assist the nurse in assessing the family. One family assessment tool is provided in Appendix E. An assessment tool of this type helps the nurse gather data on family characteristics, structure, and processes, and the environment (i.e., residence, neighborhood, and community). Not all information is appropriate for every family, however, and the assessment instrument should be modified and adapted as necessary to fit the individual family (Siegrist, 2007). Other tools for family assessment include the genogram, the family health tree, and the ecomap, described in the following sections.

GENOGRAM

A **genogram** is a tool that helps the nurse outline the family's structure. It is a way to diagram the family to view family patterns. The genogram may be developed during an early family interview and includes births, deaths, divorces, and remarriages. It might also identify other characteristics (race, social class), occupations, and places of family residence (Allender and Spradley, 2005b). Figure 16-2 shows commonly used genogram symbols and Figure 16-3 depicts a genogram that Jessica, the nurse from the opening case study, constructed from her assessment of the Smith family.

FAMILY HEALTH TREE

A **family health tree** is another tool that nurses in community-based practice may use. By expanding on the genogram, the family health tree provides a way to record pertinent data about a family's medical and health histories. Causes of death of deceased family members, when known, are important. Genetically linked diseases, including heart disease, cancer, diabetes, hypertension, sickle cell anemia, allergies, asthma, and mental retardation, are particularly important to assess. Environmental and occupational diseases, psychosocial problems (i.e., mental illness), obesity, and infectious disease should be noted.

From the health problems depicted in the family health tree, familial risk factors can be drawn. The family health tree can also be used to plan or enhance positive familial influences on risk factors such as diet, exercise, coping with stress, or pressure to have a physical examination (Siegrist, 2007). Figure 16-4 is the family health tree Jessica developed for the Smith family.

ECOMAP

An **ecomap** is a tool that can be used to explain a family's linkages to their suprasystems or the larger environment. The ecomap visually illustrates the dynamic family-environment interactions and shows the connections between the family and the world. The ecomap depicts the important nurturing connections and conflicts or areas of stress between family members. Figure 16-5 presents Jessica's ecomap of the Smith family. An ecomap can also demonstrate the flow or lack of resources; therefore it may help point to areas for conflict resolution or to where additional resources are needed (Siegrist, 2007).

An ecomap should be completed during an early family interview, noting persons, institutions, and agencies significant to the family. In constructing an ecomap a central circle is drawn to represent the family, and smaller circles in the periphery represent people and systems (school, work, friends, church, health care) whose relationships with the family are significant (Allender and Spradley, 2005b).

APPLICATION OF THE NURSING PROCESS TO CARING FOR FAMILIES

When caring for families in community settings, typically one member of the family is identified as the client who is the primary recipient of nursing care. This client may have an identified health problem, a chronic illness that needs continued monitoring, or a significant potential problem. Often, however, a family has more than one member with actual or potential health problems. Because family members are interconnected, the health of each is a concern to the nurse, and all family members may benefit from interventions (Cooley and Smith, 2005).

ASSESSMENT

Using the tools or instruments described earlier as a guide, the nurse should assess and reassess the family in their own environment and within the neighborhood. Data about the family should be collected from as many members of the family as possible. The nurse should assess verbal and nonverbal cues and environmental and behavioral information. When possible the nurse should observe family dynamics, including communication patterns among family members, roles taken, and division of labor. Assessment should also include what is available to the family in terms of social support, schools, recreation, and religious activities.

Jessica, the nurse in the opening case study, performed a thorough assessment on the Smith family. She completed a family assessment instrument (much like the one in Appendix E) by interviewing each of the adult family members and by observing the

**Genogram
Symbols**

Figure 16-2. Genogram symbols.

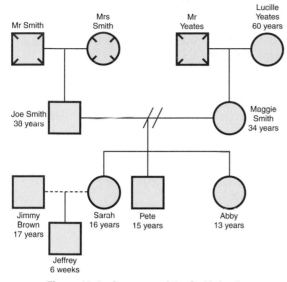

Figure 16-3. Genogram of the Smith family.

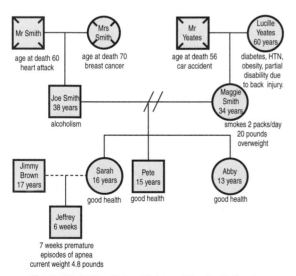

Figure 16-4. Family health tree of the Smith family.

family's environment. In addition, she drew a genogram, ecomap, and family health tree (Figures 16-3 to 16-5), illustrating her impression of relationships among family members and relationships between the family members and the larger society.

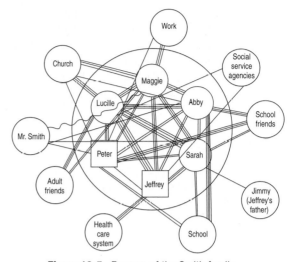

Figure 16-5. Ecomap of the Smith family.

ANALYSIS AND DIAGNOSIS

Family assessments may provide massive amounts of data and are often complex and confusing. The information must be integrated and analyzed before decisions about the plan of care can be made. When analyzing data, the nurse might determine what style the family uses in day-to-day functioning (i.e., are they receptive, distant, resistant, disorganized, rigid, ordered, dependent?). The nurse would also identify family strengths and weaknesses and identify and prioritize health needs or areas of concern. For example, is the family dealing with normal growth and development issues? Is the family coping with illness or loss? Is the family dealing with external stressors? Does the family have adequate resources and support? (Cooley and Smith, 2005)

Following review and analysis, nursing diagnoses can be made for each individual family member and/or for the family as a whole. In addition to actual and potential health problems and developmental issues, nursing diagnoses may stem from problems in communication or roles and value conflict.

In the chapter opening case study, Jessica identified several areas that needed intervention. First there was evidence of knowledge deficit on the part of Sarah, Lucille, and Maggie with regard to caring for a new infant with a chronic health problem. This is a priority issue.

Jessica also determined that several family processes were altered because the family had to adapt to the introduction of a new family member whose presence would affect the others. There was also a potential for parental role conflict in Sarah because she wanted to help care for the infant but needed to spend a great deal of time in school.

Maggie and Lucille both demonstrated health-seeking behaviors as they questioned Jessica about personal health issues—Maggie wanted to stop smoking and Lucille requested information on diet and exercise. Finally, Maggie shared with Jessica concerns over Pete's friend network and worried that he might become involved with drugs or gangs.

INTERVENTION

As explained, interventions are based on assessment and analysis. They are offered by the nurse to address actual and potential health problems of individuals within the family and the family as a whole.

In the case study, Jessica's primary interest is on helping the family adapt to the new infant and to meet his special needs. As mentioned, she taught the women how to care for the child, how to identify and manage potential problems, and emergency procedures. She also gave them information on social service programs they might be eligible for, including Women, Infants, and Children (WIC) and a community-sponsored day care program.

To address possible role conflicts with Sarah, Jessica talked at length with her about how she would help her grandmother care for the baby. Sarah recognized the importance of completing her education and knew that it was essential for her and Jeffrey's future. In confidence Jessica also talked with Sarah about sexuality and contraception, explaining that it is common for teen mothers to become pregnant again. She left literature for Sarah on all of the issues they discussed.

For Maggie and Lucille's questions, Jessica stated that she would gather some literature from the health department on healthy lifestyles. She would also provide a referral for Maggie to attend a smoking cessation program. Finally, she suggested that Maggie make an appointment with Pete's school counselor to gather more information about drug and alcohol problems in the school and to see how Pete was doing in school. She also strongly encouraged Maggie to work to open communication patterns with Pete.

EVALUATION

Evaluation is the ongoing process of observing family progress toward meeting goals identified by the nurse and family. Evaluation is not merely a terminal phase, but should be ongoing within nursing care.

In the case study Jessica continually evaluated responses to her health teaching. She encouraged questions and had the women verbally repeat her instructions. She also evaluated responses to her counseling and planned on following up to see if the family members complied with suggestions. For example, on a subsequent visit, she would ask Maggie if she had started her smoking cessation program and if she had met with Pete's counselor.

SUMMARY

Families are vital to promoting and preserving health. It is acknowledged that individuals can best be understood within the context of their family, and the family can be essential in helping address individual health needs. Furthermore, the family itself may be healthy or unhealthy and may possess a number of risk factors that affect each member and the family as a whole. These health threats and risk factors are often best addressed at the family level. As a home health nurse working with high-risk infants, Jessica, the nurse from the opening case study, understood the impact of serious health problems and threats on the family and recognized the necessity of caring for the entire family in many cases.

This chapter has covered issues important to family health care. Through understanding the concept of family, recognizing the different types of families, and knowing the stages in a family's developmental life cycle, the nurse can more effectively assess, plan, implement, and evaluate family health. Nurses who work in community settings are frequently in a position to care for clients within the context of their family and to care for the family as a unit. They should be prepared to intervene appropriately.

KEY POINTS

- Many definitions of family are found in the literature. In general, families are social units or systems consisting of two or more persons in a committed relationship. The family provides protection, nourishment, and socialization for family members.
- Several different types of families can be identified: the nuclear family, nuclear dyad, single-parent family, extended family, blended family, grandparent-headed family, single adult, cohabitating couple, and homosexual family.
- Certain characteristics or traits are common to all families. For example, all families are social systems, families change, families are interdependent, families meet a variety of needs, and families create and maintain their own set of values, rules, and goals.
- Families exist to serve several purposes, including providing physical safety and meeting the economic needs of family members. They also help members develop physically, emotionally, intellectually, and spiritually and teach social skills and how to communicate.
- Each family member has both formal and informal roles within the family unit. Role conflict may occur when roles contradict or compete with each other or when one person's role definition does not correspond with another's definition.
- Most families grow through a series of developmental stages: beginning family stage, early childbearing family stage, preschool children stage, school-age children stage, teenage children stage, launching family stage, middle-age family stage, and aging family stage.
- Family health refers to the health status of a given family at a point in time; it is concerned with how well the family functions together as a unit and how the family copes with the outside community.
- Healthy families share common characteristics, including interaction with other family members, encouraging members to grow and develop, enhancing and fulfilling family members, maintaining a healthy environment, having flexible role relationships and shared power, and providing nurturance.

- Unhealthy families share common characteristics, including lack of understanding, poor communication between members, lack of defined lines of authority, possessiveness of the children or mate, members not maintaining individuality, parents being domineering, few outside friends, high levels of anxiety or insecurity in the home, and immature or regressive behavior in parents or children.
- Family crises are experienced in all families and include *maturational crises* (related to normal developmental stages or transitions) and *situational crises* (related to sudden, unexpected and unpredictable events).
- Family nursing interventions should promote family health and include providing information, acting as a referral source, collaborating, and counseling.
- A family assessment should be thorough, covering such issues as demographics, the physical environment, the psychologic environment, family roles, family function, family values, communication patterns, coping patterns, and family health behavior. Tools that nurses can use include a family assessment instrument, a genogram, a family health tree, and an ecomap.
- In family nursing, the nurse should apply each step of the nursing process to caring for an individual within the context of his/her family or caring for the family as a unit.

Learning Activities & Application to Practice
In Class
1. Compose a definition of family. In groups of five or six, discuss criteria for a family.
2. Complete a genogram, family health tree, and/or ecomap for your own family. Identify potential areas for intervention at the individual and family level. Share with the rest of the class on a voluntary basis.

In Clinical
3. Identify a family from your clinical experience who is at risk for dysfunction. If the family is agreeable, complete a family health assessment and make nursing diagnoses and recommendations. Share findings with the clinical group.

REFERENCES

Allender J, Spradley B (2005a): Theoretical bases for promoting family health. In Allender JA, Spradley BW, editors: *Community health nursing: promoting and protecting the public's health*, ed 6, Philadelphia, 2005, Lippincott.

Allender J, Spradley B (2001b): Assessment of families. In Allender JA, Spradley BW, editors: *Community health nursing: promoting and protecting the public's health*, ed 6, Philadelphia, 2005, Lippincott.

Bergman A: High-risk indicators for family involvement in social work in health care: a review of the literature, *Soc Work* 38:282, 1993.

Clark MJ: *Community health nursing: advocacy for population health*, ed 5, Upper Saddle River, NJ, 2008, Prentice Hall/Pearson.

Cooley M: A family perspective in community/public health nursing. In Maurer FA, Smith CM, editors: *Community/public health nursing practice: health for families and populations*, ed 3, St Louis, 2005, Saunders.

Cooley M, Smith CM: Nursing process and families. In Maurer FA, Smith CM, editors: *Community/public health nursing practice: health for families and populations*, ed 3, St Louis, 2005, Saunders.

Craft MJ, Willadsen JA: Interventions related to family, *Nurs Clin North Am* 27:517, 1992.

Farber B: *Family and kinship in modern society*, Glenview, Ill, 1973, Scott Foresman.

Friedman M, Bowden VR, Jones E: Family nursing: research, theory and practice, ed 5, Upper Saddle River, NJ, 2003, Prentice Hall.

Helvie CO: *Community health nursing: theory and process*, New York, 1981, Harper & Row.

Hitchcock JE: Frameworks for assessing families. In Hitchcock JE, Schubert PE, Thomas SA, editors: *Community health nursing: caring in action*, ed 2, Clifton Park, NY, 2003, Delmar.

Murray RB et al: The family: basic unit for the developing person. In Murray RB, Zentner JP, editors: *Health promotion strategies through the life span*, ed 7, Upper Saddle River, NJ, 2001, Prentice Hall.

Rentfro AR: Health promotion and the family. In Edelman CL, Mandle CL, editors: *Health promotion throughout the lifespan*, ed 6, St Louis, 2006, Mosby.

Siegrist BC: Family health. In Nies M, McEwen M, editors: *Community/public health nursing: promoting the health of populations*, ed 4, St Louis, 2007, Saunders.

Stuart M: An analysis of the concept of family. In Whall A, Fawcett J, editors: *Family theory development in nursing: state of the science and art*, Philadelphia, 1991, FA Davis.

U.S. Census Bureau (2006): *Current population survey (CPS)–definitions and explanations* (website): http://www.census.gov/population/www/cps/cpsdef.html. Accessed October 4, 2007.

U.S. Census Bureau (2007): *Statistical abstract of the U.S.: 2007* (website): http://www.census.gov/compendia/statab/population/. Accessed October 21, 2007.

U.S. Department of Health and Human Services: *Healthy people 2010*: conference ed, Washington, DC, 2000, USDHHS.

U.S. Department of Health and Human Services (2004): *Indicators of child, family and community connections* (website): http://aspe.dhhs.gov/hsp/connections-charts04/index.htm. Accessed October 21, 2007.

Vaughn-Cole B, Johnson MA, Malone JA: *Family nursing practice*, Philadelphia, 1998, Saunders.

Wright LM, Leahey M: *Nurses and families: a guide to family assessment and intervention*, ed 2, Philadelphia, 1994, FA Davis.

Five

Nursing Care of Clients with Special Needs in Community Settings

Vulnerable Groups

1. List several risk factors that can lead to vulnerability, and describe the interaction of multiple risk factors.

2. Discuss the concept of poverty, and explain how poverty affects health.

3. Explain health threats common to homeless men, women, adolescents, and children, and describe nursing interventions to address actual and potential health problems in this vulnerable group.

4. Explain health threats common to migrant workers and their families, and describe nursing interventions to address actual and potential health problems in this vulnerable group.

5. Explain health threats common to disabled persons, and describe nursing interventions to address actual and potential health problems in this vulnerable group.

key terms

Disability	Impairment	Poverty threshold
Disasters	Marginalization	Vulnerability
Disempowerment	Migrant health centers	Vulnerable groups
Disenfranchisement	(MHCs)	
Handicap	Migrant workers	*See Glossary for definitions.*
Homeless	Poverty	

case study

Sandra Dunn, RN, is a school nurse in a large high school. One of her responsibilities is to monitor the condition of each of the students with disabling conditions. One of the special needs children enrolled in the school is Molly Franklin, an 18-year-old female who has Down syndrome and type I diabetes. Molly and her family receive services to assist with her care. Though Molly is 18, she has the cognitive ability of a 6-year-old child and will be unable to live independently. Currently Molly lives with her parents and depends upon them for financial support and help with some activities of daily living.

Continued

Molly understands that she must be on a limited diet because of her diabetes, and she is compliant, eating only the lunch and snacks packed daily by her mother. Molly is proficient in performing blood glucose measurements, but she does not fully comprehend the implications of the results and cannot take corrective action unless monitored.

Recently Mrs. Dunn sought out Sandra to discuss Molly's future. She stated that she and her husband realized that Molly will never be able to live on her own, and their other grown children did not feel that they would be able to provide the care she needs.

Because she has worked with Molly for several years, Sandra is aware that the Dunns do not have the financial resources to hire someone to care for her. During their discussion Sandra gave Mrs. Dunn contact information for representatives from several agencies and organizations in the area that provide services for disabled persons. She also referred Mrs. Dunn to the school district's social worker for follow-up, recognizing that the Dunns would need long-term and potentially comprehensive assistance to help Molly.

Everyone is at risk for health problems or health threats related to some personal characteristic, a lifestyle habit, where they live, what they do, their education level, their family income, or a host of other factors. Men are at risk for heart disease, women are at risk for breast cancer, elders are at risk for problems related to aging, smokers are at risk for lung cancer, coal miners are at risk for black lung disease, and the list goes on. But some groups are at greater risk than others because of multiple risk factors; these are termed **vulnerable groups**.

Health issues related to some vulnerable groups (i.e., children, members of racial/ethnic minorities, elders, those with mental illnesses) are described in other chapters. This chapter is concerned with describing health problems and health threats pertaining to certain particularly vulnerable groups. These are persons in extreme **poverty**, the homeless, migrant workers, and disabled persons.

VULNERABLE GROUPS

As has been described previously, the interaction of many factors, both internal and external, can increase a person's risk of developing a health problem. These factors can include such things as genetic makeup, lifestyle patterns, and the physical and social environments in which one lives and works. **Vulnerability** applies to a person or group more likely to develop a health-related problem or problems and to have more serious outcomes stemming from their exposure to multiple risks (Bushy, 2005).

Vulnerable groups are those people "who have an increased relative risk or susceptibility to adverse health outcomes" (Flaskerud and Winslow, 1998, p. 69). A vulnerable group is a subgroup of the population that is more likely to develop health problems as a result of exposure to risk(s) or to have worse outcomes from those health problems than the population as a whole (Sebastian, 2004).

Vulnerable groups share common risks or combinations of common risks and their own personal risk factors (i.e., personal habits, social environment, physical environment), which make it more likely that they will develop a particular health problem or problems. It is the cumulative and interactive aspects of multiple risk factors that leave persons vulnerable (Bushy, 2005).

Healthy People 2010 (U.S. Department of Health and Human Services [USDHHS], 2000) recognizes that significant health disparities exist among different segments of the population. The objectives highlight the fact that differences occur based on combinations of factors such as age, gender, race/ethnicity, education, income, disability, location, and sexual orientation, among others. Very often, vulnerable individuals and families belong to more than one of these at-risk groups. For example, a pregnant adolescent may be poor and Hispanic, or a rural elderly woman may be blind. The *Healthy People 2010* box gives examples of some of the objectives related to vulnerable groups.

Vulnerability is multidimensional and is exacerbated by the combined effects of limited resources, including physical and environmental

healthy people 2010

Objectives Related to Vulnerable Groups

OBJECTIVE	BASELINE (1998)	TARGET
POVERTY AND HOMELESSNESS		
1.6: Reduce the proportion of families below poverty level that experience difficulties or delay in obtaining health care or do not receive needed care for one or more family members	17%	7%
8.23: Reduce the proportion of occupied housing units that are substandard	6.2%	3%
18.3: Reduce the proportion of homeless adults who have serious mental illness	25%	19%
19.12: Reduce iron deficiency among young children (lower income <130% of poverty threshold)	12%	5%
21.12: Increase the proportion of children and adolescents under age 19 years at or below 200% of the federal poverty level who received any preventive dental service during the past year	20%	57%
RURAL AND MIGRANT HEALTH		
8.5: Increase the proportion of persons serviced by community water systems who receive a supply of drinking water that meets the regulations of the Safe Drinking Water Act	73%	95%
8.13: Reduce pesticide exposures that result in visits to a health care facility	27,156	13,500
20-1e: Reduce deaths from work-related injuries (agriculture, forestry, and fishing)	24.1 per 100,000	16.9 per 100,000
21.14: Increase the proportion of community-based health centers, including migrant and homeless health centers that have an oral health component	34%	75%
DISABILITIES		
2.5: Increase the employment rate among adults with arthritis in the working-age population	67%	78%
6.5: Increase the proportion of adults with disabilities reporting sufficient emotional support	70%	79%
7.1: Increase high school completion of persons with disabilities	79%	90%
16.14a: Reduce the occurrence of developmental disabilities (mental retardation)	131 per 10,000	124 per 10,000

From U.S. Department of Health and Human Services: *Healthy people 2010*: conference ed, Washington, DC, 2000, USDHHS.

resources (e.g., working and/or living in a hazardous environment); personal resources (e.g., poverty, limited social support); and biologic, psychologic, and social resources (e.g., presence of illness, genetic predisposition, family support). Contributing factors include disempowerment, disenfranchisement, and marginalization.

Vulnerability is a power issue because it involves a lack of control over critical resources needed to function effectively. **Disempowerment** is the loss of power or control over individual circumstances. Vulnerable groups often develop an external locus of control, and they may believe that events are outside their control. An external locus of control makes it more difficult for people to initiate action or seek care for health problems. Health promotion and illness-prevention activities are not important or are ineffective (Sebastian, 2004).

Similarly, persons who are marginalized live on the margins, or edges, of society rather than in the mainstream. Persons who are experiencing **marginalization** have limited control and power and often are overlooked by those in control.

Disenfranchisement refers to a feeling of separation from mainstream society in which the individual does not have an emotional connection with any group in particular or the larger social fabric in general. Vulnerable groups may be invisible to society and forgotten in health and social planning. Disenfranchisement, marginalization, and disempowerment suggest that vulnerable groups do not have the social supports necessary to effectively manage an emotionally and physically healthy lifestyle. Indeed, many vulnerable individuals have limited support networks because they do not have well-established linkages with formal organizations in their communities; nor do they have other sources of support (family, friends, neighbors).

Social and economic factors predispose people to vulnerability. Poverty and social isolation are particularly associated with risk and vulnerability, and being poor affects the health and well-being of individuals of all ages. Vulnerability results from individual and family efforts to do what is necessary to manage. Social isolation is related to vulnerability (Bushy, 2001; Sebastian, 2004).

Being at the extremes of age (very young or very old) can increase vulnerability. In addition, disease processes (e.g., human immunodeficiency virus [HIV] infection, cancer) and physiologic problems that result from injuries or congenital abnormalities or mental or physical disability can lead to vulnerability. Box 17-1 gives examples of vulnerable groups of special concern to nurses in community settings.

Vulnerable families are at risk because of an intensity or clustering of multiple stressors associated with life events. High-risk families include those who have a chronically ill or disabled family member or who have a family member who has a serious mental illness or abuses alcohol or drugs. In addition, special or unexpected events can promote vulnerability in some families. This includes diagnosis of a fatal disease, sudden death, unemployment,

---

BOX 17-1 Particularly Vulnerable Groups

Disabled persons
Homeless persons
Migrant workers
Persons in extreme poverty
Persons who are HIV positive
Persons with serious health problems
Pregnant adolescents
Refugees and recent immigrants
Severely mentally ill individuals
Substance abusers
Very young or very old individuals
Victims of disasters
Victims of violence

---

and **disasters**. Finally, trauma-related events such as accidents, domestic violence, and sexual abuse can predispose a family to subsequent health problems (Bushy, 2001).

PERSONS IN SEVERE POVERTY

A significantly large vulnerable group in the United States consists of those persons who are severely impoverished. Severe poverty affects health and well-being in a number of ways. People who are poor are more likely to live in hazardous environments that are overcrowded and have inadequate sanitation. Poverty is more likely to affect women, children, and the elderly, with more than 80% of those in poverty being among these groups (Sebastian, 2004). Those who are poor frequently work at high-risk jobs, eat poorly, and have multiple stressors. Furthermore, poverty often reduces access to health care.

This section examines the health implications of poverty and focuses on two particularly vulnerable groups—the homeless and migrant workers. It provides information that helps nurses in community-based practice develop and implement effective interventions as they encounter persons from these vulnerable groups.

DEFINITION OF POVERTY

To be poor is to have few or no material possessions and to have inadequate access to family and community resources. Low socioeconomic status in American society is characterized by social and economic deprivation that combines poor income, no accumulated assets, no access to power, poor education, and a low-status occupation. People are indigent when they are impoverished and deprived of basic comforts.

Sebastian (2004) noted that poverty may be acute, such as cases occurring suddenly after a crisis (job loss or illness), or poverty may be chronic and persist over many years. Poverty may also be described as absolute, such as when food, shelter, and clothing are lacking, or relative, such as when individuals or families must subsist on less than adequate resources.

In most cases in the United States, poverty is established by measuring and comparing family income with a predetermined index. Each year the Census Bureau provides a set of income thresholds that vary by family size and composition to determine who is poor. If a family's total income is less than the federally defined poverty threshold, then that family is considered poor. For example, in 2006 the **poverty threshold** for a family of four with two children was $20,614; the poverty threshold for a family of three with two children (single-parent family) was $16,079 (U.S. Census Bureau, 2006). The poverty threshold is updated each year and affects eligibility to such programs as Medicaid, Head Start, subsidized housing, and food stamps.

Characteristics of the Poor

According to the Census Bureau (2006), about 12.3% of the general population, or 36.5 million persons, lived in poverty in 2006; this represented a slight decrease from 2005. Those who are extremely poor (less than half the official poverty threshold) are slightly less than half of the total, or 14.6 million Americans.

In terms of numbers, most impoverished Americans are white; however, a disproportionate number of racial and ethnic minority members are poor. For example, 20.6% of Hispanics and 24.3% of Blacks are poor, compared with 8.2% of non-Hispanic whites. Children represent 40% of the poor population, with 17.4% of Americans under the age of 18 living in poverty. The majority of children under 6 who are poor live with single mothers, with 28.3% of families with female heads living below the poverty level (U.S. Census Bureau, 2006).

Both urban and rural localities have significant poor populations. Statistics show that 15.2% of people in rural areas are poor, and 16.1% of people in urban areas are poor. Poverty rates differ by region of the country. In 2006 poverty was greatest in the south (13.8%). In the Midwest, the Northeast, and the West, poverty levels were 11.2%, 11.5%, and 11.6%, respectively. Finally, the states with the greatest percentage of people in poverty include New Mexico (17.1%), Louisiana (17.4%), Washington, DC (18.8%), Mississippi (19.8%), Alabama (16%), and Kentucky (17.4%) (Institute for Research on Poverty [IRP], 2007).

Many of the poor are employed; however, only a small fraction have full-time jobs year round. Others have part-time employment, often in low-paying retail service industries or as migrant farmworkers or day laborers.

Poverty and Health

Poverty directly affects health and well-being. Persons living in poverty and near-poverty have higher rates of chronic illness, higher infant morbidity and mortality, shorter life expectancy, more complex health problems, and more significant complications and physical limitations resulting from chronic diseases. These poor health outcomes are often secondary to barriers that impede access to health care, such as inability to pay for health care, lack of insurance, geographic location, language, maldistribution of providers, transportation difficulties, and negative attitudes of health care providers.

HOMELESSNESS

Poverty can lead to homelessness. Homelessness is a rather complex concept and not easily defined. Although it is easily agreed upon that persons living in bus stations, under bridges, or in shelters run by relief organizations (e.g., Salvation Army) are **homeless**, there is some disagreement in other cases. For example, are a woman and her children living temporarily in a shelter for abused women considered homeless? Is a teen runaway living in a friend's basement homeless? What about an autistic adult who is in a halfway house awaiting a permanent residence?

In general, a person is considered homeless if they lack a fixed, regular address and adequate sleeping arrangements. This includes people who have a primary nighttime residence that is: (1) a supervised publicly or privately operated shelter, (2) an institution that provides a temporary residence (e.g., halfway house), or (3) a public or private place not designated for sleeping (e.g., park benches). This definition addresses the circumstances of those persons who are literally homeless (living under bridges or in shelters), but does not include those who are living with relatives or in substandard housing (Bolla, 2004; Maurer, 2005).

The following types or stages of homelessness have been identified (Belcher, Scholler-Jaquish, and Drummond, 1991):

1. *Episodic homelessness* refers to individuals who live below or slightly above the poverty line and are socially stigmatized and vulnerable. Connection to a home is tenuous and may be episodic as persons move in and out of poverty.
2. *Temporary homelessness* refers to people who have recently become homeless. They still identify with the mainstream of their communities and view living on the streets or relying on shelters as an unacceptable lifestyle; most are attempting to regain a lost home, job, and social standing.
3. *Chronic homelessness* refers to people who have been homeless for a significant time and don't identify with most members of society. They accept their lives on the streets as normal and are more easily and clearly identifiable as homeless.

Homeless people are found in both rural and urban areas. Many sleep at night in shelters, streets, parks, alleys, shopping centers, libraries, and other places. They often seek shelter in public buildings, single-room occupancy hotels, all-night movie theaters, abandoned buildings, and vehicles, therefore it is difficult to accurately estimate their numbers.

Since the 1980s the number of homeless people has surpassed that of the Great Depression. Joining the traditional homeless, predominately composed of single males, are the new homeless. Today the homeless include families with children, single women, adults who are unemployed and underemployed, immigrants, substance abusers, abandoned children, adolescent runaways, elders, persons who are mentally ill, and Vietnam-era veterans (Droes and Hatton, 2007).

Factors that contribute to homelessness include unemployment, underemployment, poverty, a decrease in the number of affordable housing units, emergency demands on income, alcohol and drug addiction, and deinstitutionalization of chronically mentally ill persons. Other factors include a shift from goods production to services, which has changed the labor market and increased joblessness, lack of affordable health care, and domestic violence (Bolla, 2004; Droes and Hatton, 2007; Maurer, 2005).

Characteristics of Homelessness

Throughout most of the twentieth century, the homeless were predominately men. Most were white, and the vast majority had mental health problems, particularly alcoholism. At the beginning of the twenty-first century, the face of homelessness has changed. Although single men still make up the majority of the homeless, families with children now account for 33% of the homeless population (The National Coalition for the Homeless [NCH], 2007). Box 17-2 shows characteristics that describe the homeless population.

Characteristics of the homeless and causes of homelessness vary, based on location. For example, racial and ethic minorities account for approximately 60% of the urban homeless population; the rural homeless are mostly white. The large number of minorities among urban homeless are associated with poverty, unemployment, lack of low-income housing, and racial discrimination. Chronic home-

---

BOX **17-2** Characteristics of the Homeless

41% are single men
41% are families with children (75% are headed by single women)
13% are single women
25% are children
5% are unaccompanied minors (largely teenage runaways)
50% are Black
35% are white
13% are Hispanic
2% are Native American
1% are Asian
32% are substance abusers
10% are veterans
22% are severely mentally ill
20% are employed

Source of data: Droes NS, Hatton DC: Homeless populations. In Nies M, McEwen M, editors: *Community/public health nursing: promoting the health of populations*, ed 4, St Louis, 2007, Saunders; Maurer FA: Vulnerable populations. In Maurer FA, Smith CM, editors: *Community/public health nursing: health for families and populations*, ed 3, St Louis, 2005, Saunders.

lessness for the white urban population is more likely to be related to substance abuse and mental illness (Maurer, 2005).

Homeless men make up the largest and most visible group of the homeless population. Most homeless men are mentally ill and/or substance abusers. Interestingly at least 10% of urban homeless are military veterans (Maurer, 2005).

Homeless women are not as visible as are homeless men, yet they account for 17% of the homeless population (NCH, 2007). There are many types of homeless women, including single women with a history of drug and alcohol abuse and "bag ladies" who are mostly white, over the age of 40, and mentally ill. These groups tend to seek refuge in public buildings or areas. The largest group of homeless women, however, consists of mothers with dependent children in their care. This group tends to be young, and many have mental illnesses and/or substance abuse problems. Domestic abuse has been cited as the primary cause for homelessness for mothers and children. Battered women are often forced to choose between abuse and homelessness. In a 2003 study 25% of women who were interviewed stated that they had been physically abused in the last year (NCH, 2007). Further, women with children are more likely to be found in shelters or welfare hotels than on the streets.

As many as half a million teenagers leave home each year. Most are runaways, but others are "throwaways." Homeless teenagers have significant psychologic issues and a high rate of drug abuse. Homeless youths tend to come from dysfunctional and single-parent homes, and many report that their parents are substance abusers. There is often a history of family violence and physical and sexual abuse. Homeless youths typically live in neighborhoods among drug users and prostitutes, and they often resort to such activities as prostitution and selling drugs to survive. Because of this lifestyle, they frequently have serious and complex health problems (Maurer, 2005).

Homeless children make up almost 39% of the total homeless population, with 42% of these children under the age of 5 (NCH, 2007). Most are preschoolers who live in overcrowded apartments or shelters. Many homeless children suffer from depression, anxiety, and learning disabilities (Maurer, 2005).

Health Problems of the Homeless

It is interesting to note that health problems are both a cause and effect of homelessness. Indeed, some health problems contribute to homelessness. Often these health problems lead to lack of employment and severance of support systems, resulting in a downward spiral toward homelessness. Examples of such problems are schizophrenia, dementia and personality disorders, substance abuse, and acquired immunodeficiency syndrome (AIDS) (Butts, 2001).

Other illnesses or health problems are the result of living on the streets or in shelters. These include skin problems, respiratory disorders, communicable diseases, malnutrition, physical assault, periodontal disease, and sexually transmitted diseases (STDs). Skin problems are often related to continual walking in inadequate or improper fitting shoes, lack of hygienic measures, and exposure to infections and parasites. Respiratory problems and communicable diseases are related to continued exposure to weather and crowded conditions in shelters. Malnutrition and poor dental health result from lack of regular, nutritious meals and lack of dental care. Physical assault is commonplace because sleeping in shelters and on the street leaves persons open to victimization (Butts, 2001).

Chronic health problems are exacerbated by homelessness. Successful management of such diseases as AIDS, diabetes, hypertension, renal disease, and liver disease is very difficult if not impossible, and complications are common. Mental illnesses, in particular schizophrenia and depression, are seriously complicated by homelessness (Droes and Hatton, 2007). Approximately 16% of the single adult homeless population suffers from severe and persistent mental illness, and about 30% of the homeless population suffers from some form of addiction (NCH, 2007).

Health problems among the homeless vary by gender and age. For example, homeless men experience acute physical health problems, respiratory infections, trauma, and skin disorders at higher rates than do men in the general population. Chronic disorders, such as hypertension, musculoskeletal conditions, gastrointestinal problems, peripheral vascular disease, chronic obstructive pulmonary disease (COPD), neurologic disorders (e.g., seizures), poor dental care, HIV/AIDS, and tuberculosis, also occur at higher rates than in the general population. Many health conditions are exacerbated by alcoholism, which occurs more frequently among homeless than nonhomeless men. Mental illness and drug abuse are also much more common (Droes and Hatton, 2007).

Homeless women have more physical health problems such as asthma, anemia, and ulcers compared with their nonhomeless counterparts. The incidence of STDs is about twice that of women in the general population. Pregnancy rates are higher, and the outcomes of pregnancy are worse. Homeless women have more mental-health-related problems, including anxiety, panic disorders, depression, substance abuse, eating disorders, self-mutilation, and suicidal behaviors. About 20% of homeless women are alcoholics, and 10% to 20% suffer from other drug problems (Droes and Hatton, 2007).

Among homeless adolescents, frequent health problems include pregnancy, STDs (including HIV/AIDS), alcohol and drug abuse, depression, and suicide (Droes and Hatton, 2007). Homeless children are more likely to be low birth weight and experience immunization delays, upper respiratory tract and ear infections, asthma, skin disorders, and anemia. Homeless children are also more likely to lack personal and social skills, language skills, and gross- and fine motor skills compared with poor but housed preschoolers (Droes and Hatton, 2007).

Health Care for the Homeless

Health care for the homeless should address both the specific and general needs of this group. Primary prevention measures may include working to improve living conditions in shelters, reducing exposure to communicable diseases, and enhancing efforts to improve hygiene to eliminate parasitic skin conditions such as lice and scabies. Providing a good supply of socks and shoes (particularly athletic shoes) is important, as are coats and other warm clothing in the winter. Flu shots should be offered in the fall, and if feasible, immunization against pneumonia and hepatitis B should be provided. Other primary prevention activities include provision of nutritious meals and dental care in shelters.

Secondary prevention efforts for the homeless can involve screening and referral for both acute and chronic health conditions, including tuberculosis, HIV, hypertension, and diabetes. Tertiary prevention

generally centers on management of chronic mental health problems (e.g., schizophrenia, depression, substance abuse) and physical problems (e.g., cirrhosis, diabetes, renal disorders, HIV/AIDS).

MIGRANT WORKERS

Few Americans consider the labor needed to produce the bounty of fruit and vegetables they enjoy daily. Without the labor provided by migrant farm workers, the daily diet of average Americans would be lacking in fresh produce. **Migrant workers** are individuals whose principal employment is in agriculture on a seasonal basis and who establish a temporary residence for such employment while traveling from location to location. In contrast, seasonal farmworkers live in one geographic location and work in the fields of that particular area.

Migrant farmworkers comprise a vulnerable population with regard to health risks because they have a low income and migratory status. Additional variables, including cultural, linguistic, economic, and mobility factors, contribute to the nature and magnitude of health problems common among farmworkers (Chafey, Hill, and Burg, 2007). This population is vulnerable to isolation and neglect. Fear of deportation, poverty, and limited education intensify feelings of distrust of various segments of society; in many areas, nurses provide the only source for health care for migrant workers.

Demographics of Migrant Workers

The Office of Migrant Health estimates that in the United States 4.2 million persons are in migrant and seasonal farmwork (Napolitano and Jones, 2004). The average age of a migrant farmworker in the United States is 31 years, and 81% of farmworkers are men. Another important characteristic of this population is that 84% speak Spanish, with 12% unable to speak English. The median level of education among farmworkers is the sixth grade (National Center for Farmworker Health [NCFH], 2007).

Most migrant farmworkers spend June to September doing seasonal harvesting, traveling from farm to farm to work. After harvest time, they are typically unemployed, unless nonagricultural work can be found. Income for migrant workers is well below the poverty level, and most earn about $7500 per year. Though the income for migrant workers has increased over the last decade, when adjusted for inflation, migrant worker incomes have actually *decreased* by 5% (NCFH, 2007).

Migrant farmworkers usually have their permanent residence in one of the border states (California, Texas, Arizona, Florida, New Mexico) or in Puerto Rico or Mexico. They move from place to place along predetermined routes called *migrant streams*. The eastern stream originates in Texas, Puerto Rico, and Florida and extends up the east coast to states east of the Mississippi River, reaching as far north as New York. This stream is ethnically diverse and includes Mexicans, Blacks, whites, Haitians, and Jamaicans. The midwestern stream begins in Texas and reaches across the southwestern and midwestern states, moving into Canada and covering areas both east and west of the Mississippi. The western stream is the largest and originates in California and Arizona. This stream moves up the West Coast to all the western states. The midwestern and western streams are largely composed of Mexicans, but groups of Native Americans and Southeast Asians are in certain areas (Allendar, 2005a).

Characteristics of Migrant Workers

Most migrant farmworkers are multigenerational, and their families have been farmworkers for several generations. Farmwork provides the income that the family lives on for the entire year. Pay is hourly, at or below minimum wage, and only for the duration of the season (Spencer and Morgan, 2001).

Migrant farmworkers live in temporary housing for days or weeks. Housing is often substandard and crowded and typically consists of shacks and mobile homes. Sanitation and drinking water are variable and often not available in the fields. Although employers recognize the need for adequate housing, housing is expensive and is used for short periods of time. Substandard housing for migrant farmworker families is often adjacent to pesticide-treated fields and may cost workers up to 30% of their income (NCFH, 2007).

Health Problems of Migrant Workers

Migrant workers face a wide a variety of risk factors, including occupational risks associated with hazardous work and poor working conditions and socioeconomic risks from poverty and homelessness. Crowded living conditions, travel, and malnutrition are other risk factors. Migrant workers are at risk for communicable diseases such as tuberculosis, hepatitis A, and hepatitis B (Sebastian, 2004). Although they are at high risk for health problems, farmworkers lack sick leave benefits and are reluctant to miss work (NCFH, 2007). Box 17-3 gives additional information about the health problems of migrant workers.

Work-Related Issues for Migrant Workers

Agriculture shares the highest rates of worker fatality for any U.S. industry, and it accounted for 13% of all job-related fatalities from 1994 to 1999. In 2001, the rate of fatal injury for those employed in agriculture was 22.8 per 100,000 workers, compared with a rate of 5 per 100,000 for all types of U.S. workers. Agricultural machinery is the most common cause of fatalities and nonfatal injuries of U.S. farmworkers; tractor-related accidents are the most frequent events associated with loss of life (NCFH, 2007).

Work-related health conditions arise from the physical demands of working 12- to 14-hour days. Injuries are not uncommon and result from working on ladders when harvesting fruit trees or using other equipment. Pesticide exposure is a particular concern. Associated health effects of exposure to pesticides include memory loss, difficulty with concentration, mood changes, abdominal pain, nausea,

---

BOX 17-3 Health Problems of Migrant Farmworkers

Migrant life expectancy is 49 years.
Migrant infant mortality is 125% higher than the national average.
The death rate from flu and pneumonia is 20% higher than the national average.
The rate of parasitic infection is 11 to 59 times higher than the general population.

The death rate from tuberculosis and other communicable diseases is 25 times higher than the general population.
Poor nutrition often results in infant deaths, anemia, dental problems, vision problems, and poor mental and physical development of children.

Data from Allender JA: Migrant families and seasonal workers. In Allender JA, Spradley BW, editors: *Community health nursing: concepts and practice*, ed 6, Philadelphia, 2005, Lippincott.

vomiting, diarrhea, headache, malaise, skin rashes, and eye irritation. Chronic exposure may lead to cancer, blindness, infertility, liver damage, polyneuropathy, and neurobehavioral problems (Napolitano and Jones., 2004).

Other major health care problems include women's health issues, high infant mortality, malnutrition, diabetes, hypertension, respiratory illness, anemia, parasites, and delayed immunization. Mental and social problems include high rates of substance abuse and family violence. Specific occupational health problems include risk of motor vehicle accidents (caused by high annual mileage), pesticide exposure, poor sanitation, farm accidents, skin diseases, and exposure to temperature extremes (Spencer and Morgan, 2001).

Dental problems are epidemic in migrant populations, and many studies cite oral disease as the most frequent health problem among migrant workers. Despite this, dental care is a very low priority. Indeed, migrant families may seek to have teeth extracted when they become painful; little consideration is given to dental repair or restoration. Many migrant families do not even own a toothbrush, and most have limited knowledge of dental care (Allendar, 2005a).

Health Care for Migrant Workers

Migrant farmworkers experience limited access to health care. Financial, cultural, transportation, mobility, language, and occupational factors are frequently cited as the major barriers that limit access to health care. Access to dental, mental health, and pharmacy services are even more problematic.

The Migrant Health Act (1962) authorized federal aid for clinics serving migrant and agricultural workers and families (Allendar, 2005a). The Migrant Health Act funds migrant health care in more than 360 sites across the country, but only about 20% of eligible migrant workers are reached (Napolitano and Jones, 2004). The population served by **Migrant Health Centers (MHCs)** is limited to migratory and seasonal agricultural workers and their families. Services in an MHC are usually on a fee-for-service basis, and a sliding-fee schedule is used for those without insurance. In most areas MHCs offer environmental health services (e.g., rodent control, field sanitation, sewage treatment), infectious and parasitic disease screening and control, and accident prevention programs (including prevention of excessive pesticide exposure).

Nursing care for migrant workers is typically broad-based and general. Care is variable, and services can include prenatal care, infant and childcare, home care for both acute and chronic illnesses, hospice care, school health, and mental health care. Goals identified for working with migrant populations include the following:

- Reducing abuse of alcohol and other drugs
- Improving nutrition
- Improving mental health and preventing mental illness
- Reducing environmental health hazards
- Improving occupational safety and health
- Preventing unintentional injuries
- Reducing violence and abusive behavior
- Prevention and control of HIV infection and AIDS
- Immunizing against infectious diseases
- Improving maternal and infant health
- Improving oral health
- Reducing adolescent pregnancy
- Improving reproductive health
- Prevention, detection, and control of chronic diseases
- Improving access to health services (Allendar, 2005a)

In caring for these very vulnerable populations, the nurse can work to evaluate and improve services. Nurses can help improve health care by using unique methods of health care delivery such as mobile health vans, migrant ministries, and vouchers to address gaps in health care. It is important that nurses network with other providers and use information tracking systems to ensure continuity of care. Finally, it can be helpful to use lay personnel from the ethnic groups served to enhance services and promote community outreach (Allendar, 2005b).

PERSONS WITH DISABILITIES

Disability is a concept that is not well understood. Indeed, due to the many different causes of disability, it is often not recognized or acknowledged by nurses and other health care providers. Some disabled persons, such as blind persons, those with spinal cord injuries, and the severely mentally retarded, are easily identifiable. Others, such as persons with AIDS, serious asthma, schizophrenia, a severe heart condition, or a hearing difficulty, might not be recognized as being disabled.

Migrant farmworkers and the homeless, the vulnerable groups described previously, are very small groups in specific locations, and most health care providers rarely if ever encounter them. Disabled persons, on the other hand, are extremely common. Based on the most common definitions of disability, as many as 20% of the population could be considered disabled. However, the commonality of being disabled may lead to vulnerability. This section describes ways in which nurses in community settings can be aware of the many factors that may cause or contribute to disability and ways that they may direct the planning and providing of care for this vulnerable group.

DEFINITIONS RELATED TO DISABILITY

A *disability* involves any restriction on or lack of ability to perform an activity in a normal manner or within the normal range. Disability may result from a physical or psychologic limitation. Other related but different terms are *impairment* and *handicap*. It is important, however, to distinguish among these concepts. An anatomic, mental, or psychologic loss or other abnormality is an **impairment** and can lead to disability. A **handicap** is a disadvantage resulting from an impairment or disability

(Treloar and Artinian, 2007). Table 17-1 presents an overview of terminology for impairment, disability, and handicap.

Limitations in functional activities (e.g., seeing, hearing, talking, walking, climbing, lifting items), activities of daily living (ADLs) (e.g., bathing, dressing, eating, toileting), and instrumental activities of daily living (IADLs) (e.g., shopping, banking, light housecleaning, preparing meals) determine disability. In short, disability is a measure of limitations in activity.

Disability indicates that an individual has some functional limitation from an alteration in anatomy (internal or external physical condition) or physiology. The 1990 Americans with Disabilities Act (ADA), PL 101-336, defines disability as a physical or mental impairment that substantially limits one or more of the major life activities of an individual who has a record of such an impairment or is regarded as having such an impairment. Physical impairment is any physiologic disorder or condition, cosmetic disfigurement, or anatomic loss affecting one or more of the body systems. Impairments include orthopedic abnormalities, visual and hearing difficulties, cerebral palsy, epilepsy, muscular dystrophy, multiple sclerosis, and HIV. Mental impairment is any serious or sustained mental or psychologic disorder such as mental retardation, emotional or mental illness, or a specific learning disability (DeCoux and McDowell, 2001).

TABLE **17-1** Terminology for Impairment, Disability, and Handicap

CHARACTERISTIC	IMPAIRMENT	DISABILITY	HANDICAP
Definition	Physical deviation from normal structure, function, physical organization, or development	Restricted ability to perform an activity in a normal or expected manner; what activity the person cannot perform	Disadvantage imposed by impairment or disability related to environment
Measurability	Objective and measurable	May be objective and measurable	Not objective or measurable; is an experience related to the responses of others
Illustrations	Spina bifida, spinal cord injury, amputation, detached retina	Cannot walk unassisted; uses crutches and/or a manual or power wheelchair; blindness	Reflects physical and psychologic characteristics of the person, culture, and specific circumstances
Level of analysis	Microlevel (e.g., body organ)	Individual level (e.g., person)	Macrolevel (e.g., societal)

From Treloar LL, Artinian B: Populations affected by disabilities. In Nies M, McEwen M, editors: *Community/public health nursing: promoting the health of populations*, ed 4, St Louis, 2007, Saunders.

CHARACTERISTICS OF DISABLED PERSONS

A national study conducted in 2002 provided data on the characteristics of disabled persons. Approximately 19% of the noninstitutionalized population (more than 50 million people) had a disabling condition that interfered with life activities; more than half of these had a severe disability. Approximately 51.2 million people aged 6 and older needed personal assistance with activities of daily living, and 2.7 million people aged 15 and over used a wheelchair. Approximately 7.9 million people suffered from some degree of visual disability, and an estimated 7.98 million people suffered from some degree of hearing disability. Disability is age-related, rising from approximately 6.5% of the population aged 5 to 20 years to 13% of the population aged 21 to 64 years to over 40% of the population aged 65 and over (Steinmetz, 2004). Chronic, disabling conditions cause major limitations in activity for more than 1 out of 10 Americans (CDC, 2005). The majority of people with disabilities are female (28.2 million), but 23 million males are also affected by disability. Asians and Pacific Islanders have the lowest rate of disability, with Blacks having the highest rates.

CONDITIONS RELATED TO DISABILITY

As mentioned, there is a huge variety in the health problems and conditions associated with disability. These include AIDS-, alcohol-, or drug-related problems; arthritis or rheumatism; back or spine problems; blindness or other visual impairment; broken bones; cancer; cerebral palsy; deafness or serious trouble hearing; diabetes; epilepsy; head or spinal cord injury; heart trouble; high blood pressure; chronic renal disease; learning disability; lung or respiratory trouble (asthma, chronic bronchitis, COPD); mental retardation; missing limbs, hands, or fingers; paralysis; senility, dementia, or Alzheimer's disease; speech disorder; stiffness or deformity of the foot, leg, arm, or hand; stomach trouble; and stroke (McClellan, 2004; Treloar and Artinian, 2007).

The U.S. Census Bureau separates the causes of disability into three domains: physical, communication, and mental. In 2002 approximately 2.7 million people had a communication disability, 18.9 million had a physical disability, and 4.4 million had a mental disability. A further 17.2 million people had disabilities in two domains, with 4.4 million having disabilities in all three domains (Steinmetz, 2004).

Arthritis is the greatest cause of disability in the United States, followed by disorders of the back or spine and heart disease. Arthritis accounted for 7.2 million cases of disability among persons aged 15 years and older during 1991 and 1992. Heart disease, the leading cause of death, accounted for 4.6 million cases of disability during that same time. (CDC, 2005).

People with orthopedic disabilities represent 38% of the total number of Americans with disabilities. The two leading causes of disabilities include orthopedic impairment and arthritis, which inhibit a person's ability to work and function independently. Asthma, diabetes, mental disorders, and learning disabilities are also frequent causes of limitation (Raimondi, Corasaniti, and Hardinger, 2005; Treloar and Artinian, 2007).

Some conditions are more likely to be severely disabling than others. Arthritis is statistically the leading disabling condition, but mental retardation, cerebral palsy, and paralysis of the extremities, although they affect many fewer people, are nonetheless much more disabling to the individuals affected. Studies show that regardless of their disabling condition, most disabled people marry and live with a spouse. However, those with disabilities who are unmarried are more likely to live with nonrelatives than are nondisabled persons.

MAJOR LEGISLATION RELATED TO DISABILITIES

As mentioned, the ADA defined disability according to the limitations in a person's ability to carry out major life activities. Physical disabilities, sensory disabilities (e.g., being deaf or blind), intellectual disabilities, serious emotional disturbances, learning disabilities, significant chemical and environmental sensitivities, and health problems such as AIDS and asthma are examples of disabilities that may substantially limit at least one major life capacity (i.e., ability to breathe, walk, see, hear, speak, work, care for self, and learn) (Treloar and Artinian, 2007).

The ADA took effect in 1992 and provided a mandate against discrimination toward people with disabilities in everyday activities. The ADA guarantees equal opportunities for people with disabilities related to employment, transportation, public accommodations, public services, and tele-communications (Treloar and Artinian, 2007).

The 1975 Education for All Handicapped Children Act (PL94-142), later renamed the Individuals with Disabilities Education Act (IDEA), was enacted following other legislation and court cases ruling that children with disabilities should receive access to public education. As time passed, IDEA helped eligible children receive free, appropriate public education in the least restricted environment for their individual needs (Treloar and Artinian, 2007). This act has resulted in mainstreaming children with disabilities (many of which are extremely severe) into regular public schools. In addition, the act mandates that the schools provide whatever health and custodial services the children need to function and to learn.

Nursing Care for People with Disabilities

Nurses who work with people with disabilities and their families provide nursing care in a variety of community-based sites. People affected by disabilities have many health care needs common to non-disabled people but other health care needs that are unique because of the disability. For example, a middle-aged blind woman needs health education and preventive services to screen for breast and cervical cancer, diabetes, and heart disease like any other middle-aged woman. Because of her disability, however, the nurse must tailor the delivery of the health care information for the client's use. Many teaching materials are available in alternative formats such as Braille and audio. As with all clients, the nurse must respond to the needs and resources of the individual.

Guiding principles for providing nursing care for persons with disabilities were proposed by Treloar and Artinian (2007). They reported the following:

- Nurses should recognize and understand that the client is an expert in his or her own health status.
- Nurses should listen and learn from the client and gather data from the perspective of the client and family.
- Nurses should work to establish relationships that are responsive to the methods of the person and family for dealing with the disability.
- Nurses should care for the client and family, not the disability.

- Finally, nurses should be well informed about the numerous community resources for disabled persons and should become strong advocates.

SUMMARY

This chapter has presented a great deal of information on vulnerability and vulnerable groups. Some of the groups described (i.e., those with disabilities) are large and have both general and specific health problems. Others, such as migrant workers and the homeless, are relatively small and have more easily defined and identified health risks and health problems. Nurses who work in community settings should be aware of the risks and needs of these groups and recognize how multiple risks factors can interact to increase health problems and make them more difficult to manage.

KEY POINTS

- Vulnerable groups are those people who have an increased risk or susceptibility to adverse health outcomes; risk factors tend to be cumulative and interactive.
- Vulnerability is exacerbated by the combined effects of limited resources. Contributing factors include disempowerment, disenfranchisement, and marginalization.
- Poverty is established by comparing family income with the federally defined poverty threshold. In 2006 the poverty threshold for a family of four with two children was $20,614; the poverty threshold for a family of three with two children (single-parent family) was $16,079 (U.S. Census Bureau, 2006).
- About 12.3% of Americans have incomes below the poverty threshold. The majority of the poor are white, but members of racial and ethnic minority groups are overrepresented among the poor. Families headed by single mothers are likely to live in poverty.
- Persons in poverty have poorer health than those not impoverished. Health problems include higher rates of chronic illness, higher infant morbidity and mortality, shorter life expectancy, more complex health problems, and more significant complications from chronic diseases.
- Persons are considered homeless if they sleep in a supervised shelter, an institution that provides

a temporary residence, or in a public or private place not designated for sleeping.

- Factors that contribute to homelessness include unemployment, underemployment, poverty, a decrease in the number of affordable housing units, emergency demands on income, alcohol and drug addiction, domestic violence, and deinstitutionalization of chronically mentally ill persons.
- The largest group of homeless is composed of single men; however, the number of homeless single women and families with children is growing.
- Health problems are a cause and an effect of homelessness. Health problems that can contribute to a person becoming homeless include schizophrenia and other severe mental disorders, substance abuse, and AIDS. Health problems that result from living on the streets or in shelters include skin problems, respiratory disorders, communicable diseases, malnutrition, physical assault, periodontal disease, and STDs.
- Migrant farmworkers are individuals whose principal employment is in agriculture on a seasonal basis and who establish a temporary residence for employment while traveling from location to location.
- Migrant farmworkers are at risk for a number of health problems related to hazardous work and poor working and living conditions and socioeconomic risks of poverty.
- Health care for migrant farmworkers is often provided in MHCs, which are supported by the Migrant Health Act (1962).
- Almost one in five Americans has some type of disability that limits their ability to perform an activity in a normal manner. Limitations in functional activities, ADL, and IADL determine disability.
- Disability is age-related, rising from approximately 6.5% of the population aged 5 to 20 years to 13% of the population aged 21 to 64 years to over 40% of the population aged 65 and over (U.S. Census Bureau, 2006). The most common causes of disability are heart disease and orthopedic problems, including arthritis. Other common causes of disability are asthma, hearing or visual impairment, cerebral palsy, and head or spinal cord injury.
- The ADA (1990) prohibits discrimination toward people with disabilities in everyday activities

and affects such areas as employment, transportation, public accommodations, public services, and telecommunications.

Learning Activities & Application to Practice
In Class
1. In groups of four to six, work with classmates to become familiar with organizations that serve the populations discussed.
2. Discuss the various experiences that class members have had with persons from each of the populations discussed. Are the experiences positive or negative? What biases are noted in discussion? Are there assumptions made about vulnerable groups that might be erroneous?

In Clinical
3. If feasible, spend at least one clinical day working in a setting that provides health care for one of the vulnerable groups described (the homeless, migrant workers). What health problems were observed that are related to risk factors?

REFERENCES

Allender JA (2005a): Migrant families and seasonal workers. In Allender JA, Spradley BW, editors: *Community health nursing: concepts and practice*, ed 6, Philadelphia, 2005, Lippincott.

Allender JA (2005b): Urban health care, poverty and homelessness. In Allender JA, Spradley BW, editors: *Community health nursing: concepts and practice*, ed 6, Philadelphia, 2005, Lippincott.

Belcher JR, Scholler-Jaquish A, Drummond M: Three stages of homelessness: a conceptual model for social workers in health care, *Health Soc Work* 16(2):87, 1991.

Bolla CD: Poverty and homelessness. In Stanhope M, Lancaster J, editors: *Community & public health nursing*, ed 6, St Louis, 2004, Mosby.

Bushy A: Rural health. In Smith CM, Maurer FA, editors: *Community/public health nursing: health for families and populations*, ed 3, St Louis, 2005, Saunders.

Bushy A: Vulnerability: an overview. In Lundy KS, Janes S, editors: *Community health nursing: caring for the public's health*, Boston, 2001, Jones and Bartlett.

Butts JB: Urban and homeless populations. In Lundy KS, Janes, S, editors: *Community health nursing: caring for the public's health*, Boston, 2001, Jones and Bartlett.

Centers for Disease Control and Prevention (2005): *Chronic disease overview* (website): http://0-www.cdc.gov.mill1.sjlibrary.org/nccdphp/overview.htm. Accessed September 25, 2007.

Chafey K, Hill WG, Burg GR: Rural and migrant health. In Nies M, McEwen M, editors: *Community/public health nursing: promoting the health of populations*, ed 4, St Louis, 2007, Saunders.

DeCoux VM, McDowell LG: Disabilities and health. In Lundy KS, Janes S, editors: *Community health nursing: caring for the public's health*, Boston, 2001, Jones and Bartlett.

Droes NS, Hatton DC: Homeless populations. In Nies M, McEwen M, editors: *Community/public health nursing: promoting the health of populations*, ed 4, St Louis, 2007, Saunders.

Flaskerud JH, Winslow BJ: Conceptualizing vulnerable populations health-related research, *Nurs Res* 47(2):69, 1998.

Institute for Research on Poverty (2007): *Frequently asked questions about poverty* (website): http://www.irp.wisc.edu/. Accessed September 13, 2007.

Lundy KS, Butts JB: The role of the community health nurse in disasters. In Lundy KS, Janes S, editors: *Community health nursing: caring for the public's health*, Boston, 2001, Jones and Bartlett.

Maurer FA: Vulnerable populations. In Maurer FA, Smith CM, editors: *Community/public health nursing: health for families and populations*, ed 3, St Louis, 2007, Saunders.

McClellan MA: The physically compromised. In Stanhope M, Lancaster J, editors: *Community & public health nursing*, ed 6, St Louis, 2004, Mosby.

Napolitano M, Jones KD: Migrant health issues. In Stanhope M, Lancaster J, editors: *Community & public health nursing*, ed 6, St Louis, 2004, Mosby.

National Center for Farmworker Health (2007): *Overview of America's farmworkers* (website): http://www.ncfh.org/aaf_01.php. Accessed September 24, 2007.

National Coalition for the Homeless (2007): *Who is homeless?* http://www.nationalhomeless.org/publications/facts/Whois.pdf. Accessed September 24, 2007.

Raimondi DS, Corasaniti RP, Hardinger ME: Rehabilitation clients in the community. In Maurer FA, Smith CM, editors: *Community/public health nursing: health for families and populations*, ed 3, St Louis, 2005, Saunders.

Sebastian JG: Vulnerability and vulnerable populations: an overview. In Stanhope M, Lancaster J, editors: *Community & public health nursing*, ed 6, St Louis, 2004, Mosby.

Spencer GA, Morgan LL: Rural populations. In Lundy KS, Janes S, editors: *Community health nursing: caring for the public's health*, Boston, 2001, Jones and Bartlett.

Steinmetz E: Americans with disabilities: 2002, *Curr Popul Rep* Series P70-107, U.S. Census Bureau, 2004.

Treloar LL, Artinian B: Populations affected by disabilities. In Nies M, McEwen M, editors: *Community/public health nursing: promoting the health of populations*, ed 4, St Louis, 2007, Saunders.

U.S. Census Bureau: *Poverty in the United States: 2000*, Washington, DC, 2006, Government Printing Office.

U.S. Department of Health and Human Services: *Healthy people 2010*: conference ed, Washington, DC, 2000, USDHHS.

Mental Health Issues

Upon completion of this chapter, the reader will be able to:

1. Explain the concept of mental health, and discuss the importance of mental health promotion.

2. Describe some of the most common types of mental illnesses encountered in community settings, including depression, anxiety disorders, eating disorders, and attention deficit hyperactivity disorder.

3. Discuss the different types of substance abuse, and explain risk factors and treatment.

4. Discuss the problem of suicide and recognize risk factors.

5. Describe different types of treatment for mental disorders, including use of psychotherapeutic medications, psychotherapy, and behavior therapy.

12-step programs	Depression	Psychotherapeutic
Agoraphobia	Mental health	medications
Anorexia nervosa	Mental illness	Psychotherapy
Anxiety disorders	Obsessive-compulsive	Substance abuse
Attention deficit	disorder (OCD)	Suicide
hyperactivity disorder	Panic disorder	
(ADHD)	Phobia	*See Glossary for definitions.*
Behavioral therapy	Posttraumatic stress	
Bulimia nervosa	disorder (PTSD)	

Kay Morton is a registered nurse (RN) working in a public-sponsored primary care clinic for indigent and homeless people in a large southwestern city. The clinic is housed in a center that provides comprehensive care for the poor. The center provides two meals a day, counseling, and assistance with job training and employment, housing, child care, and a number of other services. In addition to administrative and support personnel, the center employs five social workers, two psychologists, two RNs, and a physician's assistant. Residents

Continued

from an area medical school provide psychiatric and medical care, and other local physicians periodically volunteer their services. In addition to primary medical care, other related services offered at the center include drug and alcohol counseling and 12-step programs, psychologic counseling, and psychiatric care.

Recently Kay saw Jeannie Smith for follow-up psychiatric care. Jeannie is 22 years old and a participant in the center's intensive case management program. Jeannie has three children (ages 6, 5, and 2 years) and has been receiving public assistance for more than 6 years. During that time her children have been in foster care on several occasions. She admits to using crack cocaine, marijuana, and several other street drugs in addition to alcohol. She was diagnosed with bipolar disorder 2 years ago and is currently on medication. Since beginning the program, Jeannie has been clean, has passed a high school equivalency examination, is enrolled in a local community college, and works part time as a cashier. She and her children live in a subsidized apartment, and the center assists her with child care.

At the center Jeannie was first seen by her caseworker for her weekly visit; after that Jeannie went to the clinic. Following routine clinic procedures, Kay admitted Jeannie and asked her about compliance with her medication regimen, about any observed side effects and use of illicit drugs, and whether she had any other problems, questions, or concerns.

Jeannie replied that she had been taking her medications as prescribed and had noticed no side effects. Also she had not been using any substances prohibited in the program. She reported that her children have been well, her job is satisfactory, and school is fairly difficult, but she is managing. Kay took Jeannie's vital signs and weighed her. The weight and vital signs were all consistent with previous readings. Following agency protocols and a physician's order, Kay collected a urine specimen from Jeannie to be sent for drug screening.

After Kay completed her assessment, the psych-iatric resident talked with Jeannie for about 20 minutes. To ensure that Jeannie's lithium levels were within therapeutic range, the physician asked Kay to obtain a blood sample. Kay drew a small sample from Jeannie's right arm, using careful sterile technique and giving attention to universal precautions. She reviewed the purpose of the test with Jeannie and explained that the results would be back in a day or two. Jeannie verbalized understanding and left to keep her appointment with her psychologist.

Mental health has been defined as "a state of successful performance of mental function, resulting in productive activities, fulfilling relationships with other people, and the ability to adapt to change and to cope with adversity" (U.S. Department of Health and Human Services/Substance Abuse and Mental Health Services [USDHHS/SAMHS], 2000, p. 18-3). Mental health refers not only to the absence of mental disorders, but also to the ability of an individual to negotiate daily challenges and social interactions of life without experiencing cognitive, emotional, or behavioral dysfunction. Mental health and mental disorders can be affected by numerous factors such as biologic and genetic vulnerabilities, acute or chronic physical dysfunction, environmental conditions, and stressors. Consider the following statistics:

- Mental disorders affect approximately 20% of the U.S. population.

- Each year almost 10% of the adult population will experience serious psychologic distress.
- About 20% of children and adolescents (9 to 17 years of age) have a diagnosable mental disorder (e.g., depression, autism, attention deficit hyperactivity disorder [ADHD]) during a given year.
- Schizophrenia affects about 1% of the adult population at any one time.
- Major depression is a leading cause of disability (measured by the number of years lived with a disabling condition) among persons age 5 and older.
- Depression and associated affective/mood disorders affect about 5% of the population of the United States at any one time; approximately 14.7% of the population has experienced at least one episode of major depression.
- Suicide, a potential outcome of mental illness and mental disorders, is the eleventh leading

cause of death in the United States (2004), and the third leading cause of death among 15- to 24-year-olds.

- Only about 25% of people with a mental disorder obtain help for their illness in the health care system.
- Persons hospitalized with major depression account for more bed days than any impairment except cardiovascular disorders.
- Individuals with job-related stress and depression miss an average of 16 work days annually. (USDHHS/SAMHSA,2006;USDHHS/SAMHSA, 2007)

The use and abuse of illicit drugs and alcohol are strongly related to mental disorders. They are both a cause and effect of mental illness. Use of drugs and alcohol is directly associated with violence, suicide, birth defects (including mental retardation), accidental injury, and long-term health problems (e.g., liver disease, heart disease, some forms of cancer, and acquired immunodeficiency syndrome [AIDS]). The impact of drug and alcohol abuse in the United States is evident in the following statements (USDHHS/ SAMSHA, 2007):

- More than 8% of Americans aged 12 and older report that they are current users of illicit drugs.
- More than half of Americans aged 12 and older report that they are current drinkers of alcohol.
- Ten million persons aged 12 and older (about 4.2% of the adolescent/adult population) reported driving under the influence of illicit drugs during the past year; 12.4% of persons aged 12 and older admitted to driving under the influence of alcohol at least once during the previous year.

- More than 23 million people (9.6% of the population) need treatment for an illicit drug or alcohol use problem.
- Substance abuse is the cause of 120,000 deaths each year (100,000 attributed to alcohol and 20,000 attributed to drug use and associated AIDS).
- Alcohol and drug problems cost U.S. citizens some $276 billion per year, or more than $1000 for each citizen.
- Alcohol is implicated in nearly half of all deaths caused by motor vehicle crashes.
- Alcohol use during pregnancy is the leading preventable cause of birth defects.

Table 18-1 gives an overview of the prevalence rates for the major groups of mental disorders. Early identification, appropriate treatment, and rehabilitation can significantly reduce the duration and level of disability associated with mental disorders and decrease the possibility of relapse. Interventions to promote mental health and decrease mental disorders include focusing on decreasing stressors and/ or increasing the capacity of the individual to cope with stress. Other interventions include the use of pharmacologic agents and psychosocial interventions, such as strengthening interpersonal, psychologic, and physical resources through counseling, support groups, and training.

Two focus areas of *Healthy People 2010* (USDHHS, 2000) address the related issues of mental health and problems associated with substance abuse. Mental Health and Mental Disorders (Focus Area #18) and Substance Abuse (Focus Area #26) contain a number of objectives concerning mental health and related issues. The *Healthy People 2010* box lists selected objectives from these focus areas.

TABLE **18-1** One-Year Prevalence Rates for Mental Disorders

Any substance disorder	3.8%
Anxiety disorders (e.g., phobias, general anxiety disorder, obsessive compulsive disorder, posttraumatic stress disorder)	18.2%
Mood disorders (e.g., manic depressive episode, dysthymia, schizophrenia, anorexia)	9.5%
Impulse-control disorders (e.g. ADD/ADHD, oppositional-defiant disorder, conduct disorder)	8.9%
Any disorder	26.2%

From U.S. Department of Health and Human Services/Substance Abuse and Mental Health Services Administration (2006): *Mental Health– United States, 2004* (website): http://download.ncadi.samhsa.gov/ken/pdf/SMA06-4195/CMHS_MHUS_2004.pdf. Accessed Sept 17, 2007.

healthy people 2010

Objectives Related to Mental Health

OBJECTIVE	BASELINE (1998)	TARGET
18.1: Reduce the suicide rate	10.8 suicides per 100,000	6 suicides per 100,000
18.5: Reduce the relapse rates for persons with eating disorders, including anorexia nervosa and bulimia nervosa	NA	NA
18.9a: Increase the proportion of adults aged 18 to 54 years with serious mental disorders who receive treatment	47%	55%
26.1a: Reduce deaths caused by alcohol-related motor vehicle crashes	6.1 per 100,000	4 per 100,000
26.2: Reduce cirrhosis deaths	9.4 per 100,000	3 per 100,000
26.3: Reduce drug-induced deaths	5.1 per 100,000	1 per 100,000
26.6: Reduce the proportion of adolescents who report that they rode during the previous 30 days with a driver who had been drinking alcohol	37%	30%
26.9c: Increase proportion of high school seniors never using alcoholic beverages	19%	29%
26.11b: Reduce the proportion of college students engaging in binge drinking during the past 2 weeks	39%	20%

From U.S. Department of Health and Human Services: *Healthy people 2010*: conference ed, Washington, DC, 2000, USDHHS.

Over the last 50 years psychiatry and mental health services have changed dramatically. Until the mid-1900s, treatment of the mentally ill was largely carried out in long-term psychiatric hospitals. The development of psychotropic drugs in the 1950s led to dramatic breakthroughs in the treatment of mental illness and enabled thousands of clients to be treated on an outpatient basis (Shoemaker and Caverly, 2006). The process of deinstitutionalization began in the early 1960s in response to legislation intended to move mental health care into the community. The Mental Retardation Facilities and Community Mental Health Centers Construction Act of 1964 (PL 88-164) was written to improve inpatient, outpatient, emergency, and day treatment and consultation and education services for persons with mental disorders. As a result of these developments, between 1955 and 1980 the census of state and county mental hospitals declined from 559,000 to 138,000 (Sharfstein, Stoline, and Koran, 2002).

In 1955 75% of patient care for mental illnesses took place in state hospitals. Today 75% of client care for mental disorders occurs in community-based settings (Sharfstein et al., 2002). Ambulatory, or outpatient, care for mental disorders can be provided in many settings and by a variety of professionals, paraprofessionals, and volunteers. Persons with mental problems may seek assistance from physicians and other professional clinicians (e.g., psychologists, counselors) in private practice, hospital outpatient departments, mental health centers or clinics, alcohol and drug units or outpatient clinics, emergency departments, family or social service agencies, crisis centers, volunteer services such as self-help programs (e.g., Alcoholics Anonymous [AA], Narcotics Anonymous [NA]), and clergy or religious counselors.

The number of health professional visits a client needs varies greatly, depending on the mental health problem, diagnosis, or disorder. Therapeutic mental health services include individual, family, and group psychotherapy; individual psychoanalysis; cognitive therapy; behavioral therapies (e.g., modeling, operant conditioning, aversion therapy); hypnosis; expressive therapies (e.g., art therapy); milieu therapy; medications; electroconvulsive therapy; and psychosurgery (Carson and Trubowitz, 2006; Sharfstein et al., 2002).

This chapter discusses some of the most common mental disorders encountered by nurses in community-based practice. The correlating and contributing health problems and risks posed by the use of alcohol and illicit drugs are also described. Nursing roles and interventions are included throughout.

MENTAL HEALTH AND MENTAL ILLNESS

As discussed, mental health is more than absence of mental illness. There are varying degrees of mental health, and no one characteristic is indicative of good mental health, nor can lack of one characteristic indicate a mental illness. In general, mental health is determined by how a person feels about himself or herself, how they feel about others, and how they meet the demands of everyday life (National Mental Health Association, 1996). Mental health refers to the ability to adapt to distress by mobilizing internal and external resources to minimize tension. Mentally healthy individuals are independent, have high self-esteem, and are able to form meaningful interpersonal relationships (Antai-Otong, 2008; Stuart and Laraia, 2005).

In contrast, **mental illness** refers to maladaptive responses to distress and an inability to mobilize resources. The mentally ill person is often dependent, has low self-esteem, and has difficulty forming interpersonal relationships (Antai-Otong, 2008). In the Diagnostic and Statistical Manual of Mental Disorders IV (DSM-IV), (American Psychiatric Association [APA], 2000) the APA has classified mental illnesses and outlined diagnostic criteria for some 300 mental disorders. Some of the most common disorders are discussed here. These include depression, anxiety disorders, ADD, eating disorders, and substance abuse. In addition, suicide, a consequence of mental illness, is also addressed. Assessment and treatment of mental disorders concludes the chapter.

DEPRESSION

Depression affects almost 21 million Americans (9.5% of the adult population) each year (NIMH, 2003). Estimates are that 25% of all women and 12% of all men will suffer at least one episode of depression during their lifetime. Approximately 3% to 5% of teenagers experience clinical depression each year. Most people (almost two thirds) with a depressive illness do not seek treatment, although most, even those with the most severe disorders, can be helped (National Institute of Mental Health [NIMH], 2002). Estimates of the cost of depression in the United States are about $34 billion each year. In addition to direct costs, factors to be considered include the value of lost work days and impact on productivity (National Alliance on Mental Illness, 2007).

The most prevalent types of depression are major depression, dysthymia, and bipolar disorder. Major depression is diagnosed when an individual experiences symptoms that interfere with the ability to work, sleep, eat, and enjoy once pleasurable activities for a period of at least 2 weeks (APA, 2000). These symptoms may include depressed mood, diminished interest in most activities, significant weight loss or weight gain, and diminished ability to think or concentrate.

Dysthymia is chronic, mild depression that lasts a minimum of 2 years. In dysthymic disorder, the individual experiences depressive symptoms that are not disabling but keep him or her from functioning or from feeling good. As with major depression, persons with dysthymia may have poor appetite or may overeat; they often have insomnia or hypersomnia, and experience low energy or fatigue. In dysthymia, the symptoms cause significant distress or impairment in social, occupational, or other areas of functioning, and some people with dysthymia also experience major depressive episodes (APA, 2000).

Bipolar disorder (manic-depressive illness) produces cycles of depression and mania. During a manic episode, the individual will experience a period of abnormally and persistently elevated expansive or irritable mood that lasts for a week or longer. During this period, the individual often experiences inflated self-esteem or grandiosity. He or she may have a decreased need for sleep and may be more talkative than usual. The person may also experience racing thoughts, have difficulty concentrating, and be easily distractible. Lastly, during a manic episode, the individual may pursue pleasurable activities (e.g., drug abuse, spending sprees, irresponsible sexual activity) that have a high potential for negative consequences. Bipolar disorder is diagnosed if the mood disturbance is severe enough to impair occupational functioning or necessitates hospitalization to prevent harm to self or others (APA, 2000).

RISK FACTORS AND SYMPTOMS

Nurses working in community-based settings should be aware of risk factors for developing depression and symptoms that might indicate a depressive episode. They can then work to reduce risk factors and teach others to be aware of these symptoms. Health education should also include information on when and how to obtain treatment. Symptoms of depression and mania are included in Box 18-1. The following are risk factors for depression as outlined by the USDHHS/Office of Disease Prevention and Health Promotion (ODPHP) (1998):

- Prior episode(s) of depression
- Family history of depressive disorder
- Prior suicide attempt(s)
- Female gender
- Postpartum period
- Medical comorbidity
- Lack of social support
- Stressful life events
- Personal history of sexual abuse
- Current substance abuse

The accompanying Health Teaching box presents risk factors specifically for depression in women.

The highest rates of depressive disorders are found among those 25 to 44 years of age, with rates apparently increasing among those born after 1945. This trend may be the result of psychosocial factors (e.g., single parenting, changing roles, stress). Married people and those in ongoing intimate relationships have a lower rate of clinical depression than do those living alone. Overall, however, unhappily married people have the highest rates, whereas happily married men have the lowest. About 32% of clinically depressed individuals have some form of substance abuse or dependence.

BOX 18-1 Symptoms of Depression and Mania

DEPRESSION

Persistent sad, anxious, or "empty" feelings
Feelings of hopelessness and/or pessimism
Feelings of guilt, worthlessness, and/or helplessness
Irritability, restlessness
Loss of interest in activities or hobbies once pleasurable, including sex
Fatigue and decreased energy
Difficulty concentrating, remembering details, and making decisions
Insomnia, early-morning wakefulness, or excessive sleeping
Overeating or appetite loss
Thoughts of death or suicide, suicide attempts
Persistent aches or pains, headaches, cramps or digestive problems that do not ease even with treatment

MANIA

Abnormally elevated mood
Irritability
Decreased need for sleep
Grandiose notions
Increased talking
Racing thoughts
Increased activity, including sexual activity
Markedly increased energy
Poor judgment that leads to risk-taking behavior
Inappropriate social behavior

From National Institute of Mental Health (2007): *Depression* (NIH Publication No. 07-3561), Rockville, Md, 2007, National Institute of Mental Health and National Institute of Mental Health (2008). *Symptoms of depression and mania* (website): http://www.nimh.nih.gov/health/publications/depression-what-every-woman-should-know/symptoms-of-depression-and-mania.shtml. Accessed April 15, 2008.

DEPRESSION IN CHILDREN AND ADOLESCENTS

According to the National Mental Health Association (2006), between 2% and 4% of prepubertal children and as many as 12% of adolescents may have depression. A family history of depression is a major risk factor for childhood depression. Other associated factors that may increase the risk of depression in children and adolescents include a history of verbal, physical, or sexual abuse; frequent separation from or loss of a loved one; poverty; mental retardation; ADD/ADHD; hyperactivity; and chronic illness. Complications of depression in children and adolescents include poor school performance, poor peer relations, alcohol and drug abuse, promiscuity, teenage pregnancy, other psychiatric illnesses, and suicide. It should be noted that suicide is the third leading cause of death among persons 10 to 24 years

---

health teaching

Risk Factors for Depression in Women

DEVELOPMENTAL ROLES

Adolescence: Female high school students have higher rates of depression, anxiety disorders, eating disorders, and adjustment disorders than male students. Contributing factors may include changes in roles and expectations and physical, intellectual, and hormonal changes.

Adulthood: Multidimensional stresses (e.g., responsibilities at home and work, single parenthood, caring for children and aging parents); lack of an intimate, confiding relationship; and marital disputes increase depression.

REPRODUCTIVE EVENTS

Menstruation and premenstrual syndrome: Depressed feelings, irritability, and other behavioral and emotional changes may occur; these symptoms usually begin after ovulation and worsen until menstruation begins. Premenstrual syndrome is probably attributable to the variations in estrogen and other hormones.

Pregnancy: Pregnancy (if desired) seldom contributes to depression. Having an abortion does not appear to lead to a higher incidence of depression. Women with infertility problems may be subject to extreme anxiety or sadness.

Postpartum depression: Many women experience sadness ranging from transient "blues" to major depression to severe, incapacitating psychotic depression. Many women who experience depressive illness after childbirth have had prior depressive episodes (although they may have not been diagnosed).

Maternal depression: Maternal depression may negatively affect a child's behavioral, psychologic, and social development.

Menopause: In general, menopause is not associated with an increased risk of depression.

ABUSE

Women molested as children are more likely to have clinical depression at some time in their lives than are those with no history of abuse. There may be a higher incidence of depression among women who were raped as adults and women who experience physical abuse and/or sexual harassment; this may be the result of fostering low self-esteem, helplessness, self-blame, and social isolation.

POVERTY

Low economic status contributes to isolation, uncertainty, frequent negative events, and poor access to resources. Although sadness and low morale are more common among those with low income, it is not known if depression is more prevalent in low income persons.

CULTURAL CONSIDERATIONS

Depression may be diagnosed less frequently in African American women than white women but slightly more frequently in Hispanic women than white women.

DEPRESSION IN LATER ADULTHOOD

Depression in elderly women may be most often related to widowhood. About one-third of widows meet criteria for major depression in the first month following the death of their spouses; this may persist longer than a year in some women.

Data from National Institute of Mental Health (2005): *Depression: What every woman should know. The many dimensions of depression in women* (website): http://www.nimh.nih.gov/health/publications/depression-what-every-woman-should-know/the-many-dimensions-of-depression-in-women.shtml. Accessed April 16, 2008

(accounting for 4600 deaths), and that the rate of suicide among young males is five times that of young females (CDC, 2007). Health care providers should recognize the symptoms of depression and refer for treatment as appropriate. Box 18-2 summarizes characteristics of depression that may be seen in all age groups.

TREATMENT

Treatment for depression includes pharmacologic therapy, psychotherapy, electroconvulsive therapy, behavior therapy, or a combination of these (NIMH, 2002). Treatment for all mental disorders is addressed in greater detail later in this chapter.

ANXIETY DISORDERS

Anxiety disorders are a group of mental illnesses characterized by feelings of severe anxiety, resulting symptoms, and efforts (sometimes extreme) to avoid those symptoms. Anxiety disorders are the most common of all the mental disorders, affecting as many as 18% of the general population at any given time (USDHHS/SAMSHA, 2006). Anxiety disorders may be attributed to genetic makeup and life experiences of the individual. Some of the more commonly encountered anxiety disorders are generalized anxiety disorder (GAD), panic disorder (sometimes accompanied by agoraphobia), phobias, obsessive-compulsive disorder (OCD), and

18-2 Characteristics of Depression Across the Life Span BOX

CHILDHOOD
Infants and Preschoolers

Insidious onset
Apathy, fatigue, withdrawal
Poor appetite, weight loss
Few spontaneously describe feeling sad

Prepubertal Children

May report sadness, suicidal thoughts
Irritability, self-criticism, weepiness
Decreased initiative and responsiveness to stimulation, apathy
Fatigue, sleep disturbance, enuresis, encopresis, weight loss, anorexia, somatic complaints
Poor school performance
Social withdrawal, increased aggressiveness

ADOLESCENCE

Feelings of sadness less frequent
Unhappy, restlessness, boredom, irritability
Affects are intense and labile
Low self-esteem, hopelessness, worthlessness
Associated anxiety
Feelings of loneliness and being unloved
Pessimism about the future
Loss of interest in friends and activities, apathy
Low frustration tolerance
Poor school performance
Argumentativeness
Increased conflict with peers
Acting-out behavior (e.g., running away, stealing, physical violence)
Sexual activity (promiscuity)
Substance abuse
Complaints of headaches, abdominal pain
Hypersomnia

EARLY AND MIDDLE ADULTHOOD

Depressed mood
Anhedonia
Feelings of worthlessness, hopelessness, guilt
Reduced energy, fatigue
Sleep disturbance, especially early morning awakening and multiple nighttime awakenings
Decreased sexual interest and activity
Psychomotor retardation
Anxiety
Decreased appetite and weight loss or increased appetite and weight gain

LATER ADULTHOOD

Frequently do not complain of depressed mood; may present with tearful affect
Feelings of helplessness
Pessimism about the future
Rumination about problems
Critical and envious of others
Loss of self-esteem
Guilt feelings
Depressions tend to last longer and are more severe than in middle adulthood
Perceived cognitive deficits
Somatic complaints
Constipation
Social withdrawal
Loss of motivation
Change of appetite

CORE SYMPTOMS ACROSS AGE GROUPS

Suicidal ideation
Diminished concentration
Sleep disturbance

From Lewin L: The client with a depressive disorder. In Antai-Otong D, editor: *Psychiatric nursing: biological and behavioral concepts*, Clifton Park, NY, 2003, Delmar.

posttraumatic stress disorder (PTSD). These are discussed briefly here.

GENERALIZED ANXIETY DISORDER

A diagnosis of GAD describes chronic, unrealistic, and exaggerated worry and tension about one or more life circumstances lasting 6 months or longer without anything seeming to provoke it (NIMH, 2006). Approximately half of all cases of GAD begin in childhood or adolescence; it is more common in women than in men.

Symptoms of GAD include trembling, twitching, muscle tension, headaches, irritability, sweating or hot flashes, dyspnea, nausea, and feeling a lump in the throat. It typically fluctuates with periods of increasing symptoms that are usually associated with life stressors or impending difficulties.

PANIC DISORDER

Some 2% to 4% of the population will suffer from panic disorder during their lifetime; women experience approximately double the rate of men (NIMH, 2006). **Panic disorder** can occur at any age, but it most often begins in young adulthood (average age 17 to 30 years). Panic disorder typically develops in three stages, with clients potentially stopping at any stage or progressing through all three. Individuals often have their first attack or cluster of attacks after a variety of life stresses. The initial attack may occur suddenly and unexpectedly while the client is performing everyday tasks. A typical panic attack can include tachycardia, dyspnea, dizziness, chest pain, nausea, numbness or tingling of the hands and feet, trembling or shaking, sweating, choking, or a feeling one is going to die, go crazy, or do something uncontrolled. This can be extremely frightening. A diagnosis of panic disorder is made when attacks occur with some degree of frequency or regularity.

During the second stage, the anxiety attacks become increasingly frequent and severe, and the individual develops anticipatory anxiety (fear of having a panic attack). During this phase, events and circumstances associated with the attack may be selectively avoided, leading to phobic behaviors (e.g., if a woman has an attack while driving, she may become anxious the next time she needs to drive and begin to avoid driving and eventually refuse to drive altogether). In this phase the client's life may become progressively constricted.

As the avoidance behavior intensifies, a third stage may develop. The client begins to withdraw further to avoid being in places or situations from which escape may be difficult or embarrassing or in which help may be unavailable in the event of a panic attack (e.g., church, elevators, movie theaters). The fear of being in these situations or places can lead to **agoraphobia** (literally, fear of the marketplace or open places). Agoraphobics frequently progress to the point where they cannot leave their homes without experiencing anxiety. Agoraphobia is the most common phobia leading to the use of health services, particularly when accompanied by panic attacks. About one third of all people who experience panic attacks eventually develop agoraphobia.

Panic disorder is often accompanied by other conditions. If not treated, approximately 50% to 65% of clients with panic disorder will develop a major depression at some time in their lives (USDHHS/PHS, 1999). Alcoholism is also common. Cognitive-behavioral therapy and medication can help 70% to 90% of people with panic disorder.

PHOBIAS

A **phobia** is an irrational fear of something (an object or situation), and as many as 8% of Americans are affected by phobias at any given time. Adults with phobias realize their fears are irrational, but facing the feared object or situation might bring on severe anxiety or a panic attack. Phobias may begin in childhood but usually first appear in adolescence or adulthood.

Social phobia, or social anxiety disorder, is a persistent and intense fear of and compelling desire to avoid something that would expose the individual to a situation that might be humiliating and embarrassing. Its tendency is familial and may be accompanied by depression or alcoholism. Social phobia often begins in childhood or early adolescence. Individuals suffering from social phobia think that others are very competent in public but that they are not. Small mistakes are exaggerated. The most common social phobia is a fear of public speaking. Other examples include being unable to urinate in a public bathroom and not being able to answer questions in social situations. Most people with social phobias can be treated with cognitive-behavior therapy and medication.

Simple phobias (excluding panic attack or social phobia) involve a persistent fear of and compelling desire to avoid certain objects or situations. Common objects of phobias are spiders, snakes, dogs, cats, and situations such as flying, heights, and closed-in spaces. The person often recognizes that the fear is excessive or unreasonable but nonetheless avoids the situation or endures it with intense anxiety. Systematic desensitization and normal exposure are the most effective treatments for simple phobias.

OBSESSIVE-COMPULSIVE DISORDER

Obsessive-compulsive disorder (OCD) is characterized by anxious thoughts and rituals that the individual has difficulty controlling. The person with OCD is overcome with the urge to engage in some ritual to avoid a persistent frightening thought, idea, image, or event—the obsession. Compulsions are the rituals or behaviors that are repeatedly performed to prevent, neutralize, or dispel the dreaded obsession. When the individual tries to resist the compulsion, anxiety increases. Common compulsions include hand washing, counting, checking, or touching.

Obsessive-compulsive disease is diagnosed only when the compulsive activities consume at least an hour a day and interfere with daily life. Most individuals recognize that what they are doing is senseless but are unable to control the compulsion. About 2% of Americans are afflicted with OCD, which often appears in the teenage years or early adulthood. Depression or other anxiety disorders often accompany OCD. Clomipramine (Anafranil) and fluoxetine (Prozac) have been effective in treating OCD (NIMH, 2006). Behavioral therapy may also help.

POSTTRAUMATIC STRESS DISORDER

Posttraumatic stress disorder (PTSD) is a debilitating condition that follows a terrifying event. Individuals with PTSD have recurring, persistent, frightening thoughts and memories of their ordeal. Traumatic incidents that trigger PTSD may have threatened that individual's life or the life of someone else. Incidents include "shell shock" or "battle fatigue" common to war veterans, violent attack (e.g., kidnapping, rape, mugging), serious accidents, natural disasters (e.g., earthquake, tornado), or witnessing mass destruction or injury, such as an airplane crash. Sometimes the individual is unable to recall an important aspect of the traumatic event. Interestingly, about 19% of Vietnam veterans experienced PTSD at some point after the war (NIMH, 2007).

People with PTSD repeatedly relive the trauma in the form of nightmares and/or disturbing recollections, flashbacks, or hallucinations. As a result, they often have sleep disturbances, depression, and feelings of detachment or emotional numbness, and/or are easily startled. They may avoid places or situations that bring back memories (e.g., a woman raped in an elevator may refuse to ride in elevators), and anniversaries of the event are often very difficult. It occurs at all ages and may be accompanied by depression, substance abuse, and/or anxiety. It usually begins within 3 months of the trauma, and the course of the disorder varies. Some individuals recover within 6 months; the condition becomes chronic in others. Infrequently the illness does not manifest until years after the traumatic event.

Posttraumatic stress disorder is treated with antidepressants, antianxiety medications, and psychotherapy. Support from family and friends can be very beneficial.

EATING DISORDERS

Eating disorders are becoming increasingly prevalent in the United States. Indeed, the most common eating disorders, anorexia nervosa and bulimia nervosa, affect about 3 million U.S. residents. Currently it is estimated that anorexia affects 0.5% to 3.7% of girls and women during their lifetime. In addition, as many as 1.1% to 4.2% of adolescent and college-aged women have some symptoms of bulimia (NIMH, 2001).

Eating disorders almost exclusively affect females; males account for only 5% to 10% of bulimia and anorexia cases. Most clients diagnosed with eating disorders are white. This, however, may be because of socioeconomic factors rather than race because females in middle and upper socioeconomic groups are most frequently affected. Anorexia and bulimia are often triggered by developmental milestones (e.g., puberty, first sexual contact) or crisis (e.g., death of a loved one, ridicule over weight, starting college).

BULIMIA NERVOSA

"The essential features of bulimia are binge eating and inappropriate compensatory methods to prevent weight gain" (APA, 2000, p. 545). A *binge* is defined as eating an abnormal amount of food at a discrete time (usually less than 2 hours) (APA, 2000). For example, a bulimic might eat an entire pie, half a cake, or a half gallon of ice cream at one sitting. Snacking throughout the day is not considered bingeing.

To lose or maintain weight, the bulimic practices purging, which usually involves self-induced vomiting caused by gagging, using an emetic, or simply mentally willing the action. Laxatives, diuretics, fasting, and excessive exercise may also be employed to control weight.

Bulimia nervosa typically begins in adolescence or during the early 20s and usually in conjunction with a diet. Members of certain professions that emphasize weight and/or appearance (e.g., dancers, flight attendants, athletes, actors, models) are at high risk (Ibrahim, 2006).

A number of health problems may result from bulimia. Electrolyte imbalance can result in fatigue, seizures, muscle cramps, arrhythmias, and decreased bone density. Vomiting can damage the esophagus, stomach, teeth, and gums.

ANOREXIA NERVOSA

The person suffering from **anorexia nervosa** becomes obsessed with a fear of fat and with losing weight. Anorexia nervosa often develops with a fairly gradual decrease in caloric intake. However, the decrease in caloric intake continues until the anorexic is consuming almost nothing. Anorexia usually begins in early adolescence (12 to 14 years is the most common age group) and may be limited to a single episode of dramatic weight loss within a few months, followed by recovery, or the illness may last for many years. Anorexia, as well as other eating disorders, may persist into adulthood. Subsequently, women in their twenties and thirties and beyond are increasingly seeking treatment.

As stated earlier, anorexia nervosa almost exclusively affects white adolescent girls. Other characteristics of girls who develop anorexia are that they are well-behaved and eager to please; are perfectionists; may have a poor self-image; are dependent on others' opinions, introverted, and insecure; are overly compliant and deferential to others' wishes; and are emotionally reserved (Ibrahim, 2006).

In response to the severely decreased caloric intake, the body tries to compensate by slowing down body processes. Menstruation ceases; blood pressure, pulse, and respiration rates slow; and thyroid activity diminishes. Electrolyte imbalance can become very severe. Other symptoms include mild anemia, joint swelling, and reduced muscle mass. Health care practitioners should be aware that anorexia nervosa may be life threatening.

TREATMENT

Treatment for eating disorders includes nutrition counseling, psychotherapy, and behavior modification and may take a year or more. Hospitalization may be required for clients with serious complications. Self-help groups and support groups can be very beneficial for both the client and the family. Many bulimics appear to respond to antidepressants. Anorexia nervosa, however, does not appear as responsive to medication.

Nurses who frequently work with adolescent girls and young women in community settings such as schools and clinics should be aware of the risk factors, signs, and symptoms of anorexia and bulimia and be prepared to intervene.

ATTENTION DEFICIT HYPERACTIVITY DISORDER

One of the most common conditions encountered by nurses who work with children in community settings is ADD or **attention deficit hyperactivity disorder (ADHD)**. (Here the disorder is referred to as ADHD.) In the United States ADHD affects 3% to 5% of all children (about 2 million) (NIMH, 2007). Behaviors that might indicate ADHD usually appear before age 7 years and are often accompanied by related problems, such as learning disability, anxiety, and depression. The three major characteristics of ADHD are inattention, hyperactivity, and impulsivity. A diagnosis is made when a child exhibits at least six of the following symptoms for at least 6 months and when the behavior is maladaptive or inconsistent with their developmental level:

- Fails to give close attention to details or makes careless mistakes in schoolwork
- Has difficulty sustaining attention in tasks or activities
- Does not seem to listen when spoken to directly
- Does not follow through on instructions and fails to finish schoolwork, chores, or duties in the workplace
- Has difficulty organizing tasks and activities
- Avoids, dislikes, or is reluctant to engage in tasks that require sustained mental effort
- Loses things necessary for tasks or activities
- Is easily distracted by extraneous stimuli
- Forgetful in daily activities (APA, 2000)

"Hyperactivity" symptoms may or may not be present. These include: fidgets with hands or feet, squirms in seat, runs about or climbs excessively in inappropriate situation, talks excessively, blurts out answers, interrupts or intrudes, and has difficulty awaiting turn (APA, 2000).

The cause of ADHD is not known, but it is important to note that research does not support that it is caused by minor head injuries, birth complications, food allergies, too much sugar, poor home life, poor schools, or too much television. Maternal substance use and abuse (e.g., alcohol, cigarettes, cocaine) may affect the brain of the developing baby and produce symptoms of ADHD later in life. This, however, accounts for only a small percentage of those affected (NIMH, 2007).

Attention disorders appear to run in families because children diagnosed with ADHD usually have at least one close relative who also has ADHD, and at least one third of all fathers who had ADHD as children have children with symptoms. In addition, in the majority of sets of identical twins in which one has the disorder, the other does also (NIMH, 2007). Although parents may notice symptoms and signs, it is often teachers who recognize the behaviors consistent with attention deficit disorders and suggest referral for assessment and treatment.

Experts caution that diagnosis of attention disorders should be made following a comprehensive physical, psychologic, social, and behavioral evaluation and not be based solely on anecdotal reports from parents. The evaluation should rule out other possible reasons for the behavior (e.g., emotional problems, poor vision or hearing, physical problems) and should include input from teachers, parents, and others who know the child well. Intelligence and achievement testing may also be performed to rule out or identify a learning disability.

Symptoms of ADHD are typically managed through a combination of behavior therapy, emotional counseling, and practical support. Use of medication is becoming increasingly commonplace in the management of ADHD. It is very important, however, that children with attention disorders and their families understand that medication does not cure the disorder; it just temporarily controls symptoms.

Stimulants are the medications that have been shown to be successful in treating attention disorders in both children and adults. The most commonly used medications are methylphenidate (Ritalin, Concerta) and amphetamines (Dexedrine, Dextrostat, or Adderall). Most children with ADHD show improvement when taking one of these drugs (NIMH, 2007).

Effective doses vary among children, and drug regimens for treatment of ADHD vary among physicians. Some physicians recommend keeping children on medication only during school and have the child stop taking the medication on weekends and during summer vacation. Others prescribe medication every day, assuming that this regimen is more beneficial in helping establish positive behavior patterns and work habits.

Medications used to treat ADHD have some potential adverse effects. Appetite suppression is fairly common and may contribute to growth retardation. Periodic assessment of height and weight is therefore important. Sleeping difficulties are also possible. There is concern that long-term use of pemoline (Cylert) may affect the liver. Therefore liver function must be assessed periodically in clients taking this medication (NIMH, 2007).

SUBSTANCE ABUSE

Substance abuse refers to patterns of use of alcohol and/or other drugs that result in health consequences or impairment in social, psychologic, and occupational functioning. A diagnosis of substance abuse may be made if an individual brings about hazardous situations from substance abuse (e.g., driving an automobile while impaired) or if the individual experiences substance-related legal problems. Substance dependence occurs when the individual develops a tolerance for the substance and needs increased amounts to achieve the desired effect. In substance dependence, there may be problems associated with withdrawal of the substance, a need to take the substance more often and in larger amounts, and an unsuccessful desire to cut down or control substance use. The person who is substance dependent may spend an inordinate amount of time in activities to obtain the substance or to recover from it and may neglect or abandon social, occupational, or recreational activities because of the substance (APA, 2000).

The toll taken by alcohol and other drugs on society is staggering. The economic costs of alcohol alone are massive. Alcohol and drug use is involved in several of the leading causes of morbidity and mortality in the United States, including accidental injury, suicide, homicide, liver disease, certain types of cancer, and AIDS (USDHHS, 2000). A number of legal and illegal substances used by many Americans, including alcohol, cigarettes, marijuana, heroin, and many others, are harmful.

ALCOHOL ABUSE

Alcoholism is the largest drug problem in the United States today. Indeed, about 10% of the adult population has a chronic, heavy intake of alcohol and shows symptoms of alcoholism. Box 18-3 lists some facts about alcohol abuse.

BOX 18-3 Fast Facts About Alcohol Use and Abuse

Approximately 75,000 deaths in the U.S. each year are attributed to excessive alcohol use; thus alcohol is the third leading lifestyle-related cause of death for the nation.

Slightly more than half (50.9%) of Americans age 12 and over are current drinkers of alcohol.

By eighth grade, almost 70% of adolescents state that they have tried alcohol at least once; the average age of first use is 14 years.

Abuse varies markedly, based on cultural and ethnic groups; males reporting recent binge drinking by race/ethnicity are as follows: Native American/Alaska Native, 31.0%; white, 24.1%; Hispanic, 23.9%; Black, 19.1%; and Asian, 11.8%.

Alcohol consumption is highest between 18 and 34 years of age, when about 62% of individuals report having used alcohol during the last month.

Binge drinking and heavy alcohol use peak between 21 and 25 years of age.

More than 40% of all fatal traffic accidents involve alcohol.

Drinking also contributes to a large percentage of injuries and deaths involving falls, fires or burns, homicides, suicides, and drownings.

Long-term alcohol abuse is associated with neurologic problems (dementia, stroke, neuropathy), cardiovascular problems, psychiatric problems, social problems, and certain cancers (mouth, throat, esophagus, liver, breast).

Data from Centers for Disease Control and Prevention (2008): *General information on alcohol use and health* (website): http://www.cdc.gov/alcohol/quickstats/general_info.htm. Accessed April 15, 2008, and U.S. Department of Health and Human Services/Substance Abuse and Mental Health Services Administration (2007): *Results from the 2006 national survey on drug use and health: national findings* (website): http://www.oas.samhsa.gov/nsduh/2k6nsduh/2k6results.pdf. Accessed September 17, 2007.

ILLICIT DRUG USE

Illicit drugs used in the United States include opioids (e.g., heroin, morphine), cocaine (e.g., crack), amphetamines, hallucinogens (e.g., lysergic acid diethylamide [LSD], phencyclidine [PCP]), marijuana, and inhalants (e.g., airplane model glue, spray paint, nail polish remover, gasoline). Box 18-4 lists a few relevant statistics on the use and abuse of illicit drugs.

RISK FACTORS FOR SUBSTANCE ABUSE

Several risk factors have been identified that can contribute to the likelihood that an individual might abuse alcohol and/or other drugs. Box 18-5 lists these by developmental stage. Nurses who work in community settings such as clinics, physicians' offices, schools, and work sites should be knowledgeable about risk factors that contribute to substance

BOX 18-4 Fast Facts About the Use and Abuse of Illicit Drugs

Drug abuse costs U.S. residents more than $110 billion annually; in contrast to alcohol abuse, much of the costs of illicit drug use are from costs related to crime, property destruction, and public attempts to control their use.

The use of illicit drugs has declined over the last several decades. In the late 1970s, almost 40% of high school seniors reported using drugs, compared with 18.3% in 2006.

Drug use among adolescents dropped slightly between 2002 and 2005; marijuana is the major illicit drug used by this group.

Males are more than three times as likely as females to be heavy drinkers and more than twice as likely to use marijuana weekly; males and females are equally likely to use cocaine.

In 2005, in the U.S. 8.1% of those age 12 years and over reported using an illicit drug during the previous month.

Almost 22% of people in state prisons and 67% of people in federal prisons in 2005 were incarcerated for drug offenses.

Among state prisoners, 33% admitted they were under the influence of drugs at the time of their offense and 57% reported use of illicit drugs during the month prior to their offense.

Deaths from illicit drugs are often from a combination of two or more illicit drugs or drugs combined with alcohol; heroin or cocaine is involved in two thirds of drug deaths; almost 40% of illicit drug deaths are among adults aged 30 to 39 years (perhaps indicating chronic problems due to drug abuse); Blacks are more than twice as likely to die from the effects of illicit drugs as are whites.

About one third of new AIDS cases occur among injecting drug users or people having sexual contact with them.

Data from: Bureau of Justice Statistics (2005): *Probation and parole in the United States, 2004* (website): http://www.ojp.usdoj.gov/bjs/dcf/correct.htm. Accessed April 15, 2008; U.S. Department of Health and Human Services: *Healthy people 2010*: conference ed, Washington, DC, 2000, USDHHS; and U.S. Department of Health and Human Services/Substance Abuse and Mental Health Services Administration (2007): *Results from the 2006 national survey on drug use and health: national findings* (website): http://www.oas.samhsa.gov/nsduh/2k6nsduh/2k6results.pdf. Accessed September 17, 2007.

18-5 Risk Factors for Alcohol and Other Drug Abuse by Stage of Life

CHILDHOOD

Fetal exposure to alcohol and other drugs (AOD)
Parents who are substance abusers
Physical, sexual, or psychologic abuse
Economic disadvantage
Delinquency
Mental health problems such as depression and suicidal
    ideation
Disability

ADOLESCENCE

Parental use of AOD
Low self-esteem
Depression
Psychologic distress
Poor relationship with parents
Low sense of social responsibility
Lack of religious commitment
Low academic performance and motivation
Peer use of AOD
Participation in deviant, aggressive behavior

YOUNG ADULTHOOD

Exposure to drug users in social and work environments
Marital and work instability

Unemployment
Divorce
Psychologic or psychiatric difficulties

MIDDLE ADULTHOOD

Bereavement, especially as a result of loss of spouse or
    significant other
Adverse work conditions or unemployment
Changes in health status or appearance
Socioeconomic stressors
Environmental changes or relocation
Divorce, separation, or remarriage
Difficulties with children or changes in child-rearing
    responsibilities

OLDER ADULTHOOD

Retirement or role status change
Loss of loved ones
Changes in health status and mobility
Increased sensitivity to effects of alcohol and other drugs
Housing relocations
Affective changes (e.g., anxiety and depression)
History of previous misuse or abuse of AOD
Solitude or social contexts that foster use of AOD
Negative self-concept

From U.S. Office of Substance Abuse Prevention: *Nurse training course: alcohol and other drug abuse prevention*, Rockville, Md, 1992, National Training System, U.S. Public Health Service.

abuse and know when to intervene to reduce them whenever possible.

SIGNS AND SYMPTOMS OF SUBSTANCE ABUSE

Nurses should also be aware of the signs and symptoms that might indicate use and/or abuse of alcohol and other drugs. To help nurses recognize these symptoms of substance use and withdrawal and identify appropriate treatment, Table 18-2 describes each.

TREATMENT FOR SUBSTANCE ABUSE

An estimated 18 million people who use alcohol and other drugs are in need of treatment, and less than one fourth will get it. Unlike health care for other conditions, most of the funding for drug and alcohol treatment facilities comes from federal block grants and state and local government funds. Private insurance and Medicaid and other public insurance programs contribute less than a third of the total funding for treatment.

Substance abuse treatment is effective for many people, and most need some kind of treatment to recover from substance abuse. The key to effective treatment is to match the client's needs with the intervention strategy most appropriate for the individual. The vast majority of clients in alcohol and/or drug treatment programs are outpatients. Alcohol and drug treatment services are provided by family practitioners, internists, psychiatrists, and other medical specialists and in emergency rooms. Self-help groups are an important part of recovery for many. Common models of treatment consist of education and participation in twelve-step programs.

Education

To break the abuser's denial, intense and ongoing education about the disease of alcoholism or other drug addiction may be helpful, including the following:

- Initiation of the Twelve Steps of AA
- Required reading of literature from AA or NA (as appropriate)
- Attendance at AA or NA meetings
- Skill building to maintain abstinence

TABLE **18-2** Signs of Intoxication, Indications of Withdrawal, and Treatment Modalities for Selected Psychoactive Substances

SUBSTANCE	SIGNS OF INTOXICATION	INDICATIONS OF WITHDRAWAL	TREATMENT MODALITIES
Alcohol	Decreased alertness, impaired judgment, slurred speech, nausea, double vision, vertigo, staggering, unpredictable emotional changes, stupor, unconsciousness, increased reaction time	Anxiety, insomnia, tremors, delirium, convulsions	Detoxification, psychotherapy, group therapy, family therapy, self-help groups (AA, Al-Anon), pharmacologic therapy, residential programs, referral for vocational rehabilitation and social services as needed
Sedatives, hypnotics, anxiolytics	Slurred speech, slow and shallow respiration, cold and clammy skin, nystagmus, weak and rapid pulse, drowsiness, blurred vision, unconsciousness, disorientation, depression, poor judgment, motor impairment	Anxiety, insomnia, tremors, delirium, convulsions (may occur up to 2 weeks after stopping use of anxiolytics)	Detoxification, psychotherapy, and group therapy (for underlying psychiatric disorders)
Opioids	Sedation, hypertension, respiratory depression, impaired intellectual function, constipation, pupillary constriction, watery eyes, increased pulse and blood pressure	Restlessness, irritability, tremors, loss of appetite, panic, chills, sweating, cramps, watery eyes, runny nose, nausea, vomiting, muscle spasms, impaired coordination, depressed reflexes, dilated pupils, yawning	Pharmacologic therapy (methadone, opioid antagonists), therapeutic communities (Synanon, Odyssey House, Phoenix House), group therapy, assistance with social skills, vocational training and job placement, family therapy, self-help groups (NA, Chemical Dependency Anonymous), psychotherapy
Cocaine	Irritability, anxiety, slow and weak pulse, slow and shallow breathing, sweating; dilated pupils, increased blood pressure, insomnia, seizures, disinhibition, impulsivity, compulsive actions, hypersexuality, hypervigilance, hyperactivity	*Early crash:* agitation, depression, anorexia, high level of craving, suicidal ideation *Middle crash:* fatigue, depression, no craving, insomnia *Late crash:* exhaustion, hypersomnolence, hyperphagia, no craving *Early withdrawal:* normal sleep and mood, low craving, low anxiety *Middle and late withdrawal:* anhedonia, anxiety energy, high level of craving exacerbated by conditioned cues	Hospitalization, self-help groups, contingency contracting (client agreement to urinary monitoring and acceptance of aversive contingencies for positive results), pharmacologic therapy (tricyclic antidepressants)

Substance	Signs/Effects of Use	Withdrawal Symptoms	Treatment
		Extinction: normal hedonic response and mood, episodic craving triggered by conditioned cues	
Amphetamines	Sweating, dilated pupils, increased blood pressure, agitation, fever, irritability, headache, chills, insomnia, agitation, tremors, seizures, wakefulness, hyperactivity, confusion, paranoia	Fatigue, hunger, long period of sleep, disorientation, severe depression	No established treatment guidelines; may be similar to treatment for cocaine abuse
Hallucinogens	Dilated pupils, mood swings, elevated blood pressure, paranoia, bizarre behavior, nausea and vomiting, tremors, panic, flushing, fever, sweating, agitation, aggression, nystagmus (with PCP)	Slight irritability, restlessness, insomnia, reduced energy level, depression	Detoxification, psychotherapy (for underlying psychiatric disorders), group therapy, residential programs
Cannabis (marijuana, hashish)	Reddened eyes, laughter, confusion, panic, drowsiness, increased pulse, respiration, and blood pressure	Insomnia, hyperactivity, decreased appetite	Same as for hallucinogens; self-help groups
Inhalants	Giddiness, drowsiness, increased vital signs, headache, nausea, fainting, stupor, fatigue, slurred speech, disorientation, delirium	None reported	Psychosocial interventions, psychotherapy (for underlying psychiatric disorder), sociodrama, vocational rehabilitation, family therapy, social support services
Nicotine	Headache, loss of appetite, nausea, increased pulse, blood pressure, and muscle tone	Nervousness, increased appetite, sleep disturbances, anxiety, irritability	Aversive conditioning, desensitization, substitution, hypnotherapy, group therapy, relaxation training, supportive therapy, abrupt abstinence

Adapted from Clark MJ: Substance abuse. In Clark MJ, editor: *Community health nursing: advocacy for population health*, ed 4, Upper Saddle River, NJ, 2008, Prentice Hall.

Twelve-Step Programs

Participation in **twelve-step programs** (e.g., NA and AA) gives social support and structure that assists in the recovery process. Nurses who are in a position to identify those in need of these services should be knowledgeable about the programs and ready to supply information and referral. To this end, Box 18-6 presents the Twelve Steps of AA. Further information can be obtained by contacting local programs or national offices.

SUICIDE

Suicide is the most serious potential outcome of mental disorders and the eleventh leading cause of death in the United States. Each year more than 30,000 U.S. residents take their own lives. Depression, schizophrenia, panic disorder, and alcohol and other drug abuse have been implicated in both attempted and completed suicides (USDHHS, 2000). Box 18-7 lists some statistics regarding suicide of which the nurse in community-based practice should be aware.

Risk factors for suicide include a strong family history of psychiatric disorders (e.g., depression or suicidal behavior), previous suicide attempts, serious medical illness, family violence, alcohol and other drug abuse, and accessibility to firearms. To combat the high rates of suicide among adolescents and young adults, the National Center for Injury Prevention and Control outlined general recommendations, which are listed in the Community Application box "Examples of Suicide Prevention Programs."

IDENTIFICATION OF MENTAL DISORDERS

Whether the nurse is working in a physician's office, a clinic, home health, a school, occupational health, or another setting, recognition of signs and symptoms that might indicate a mental disorder is an important component of practice. For example, a student might come to the school nurse's office concerned about a friend who induces vomiting in the bathroom after lunch each day; an occupational health nurse might observe signs consistent with alcohol abuse in an employee; or a client might visit a clinic for a routine visit, but mention that for the last several weeks she has been unable to sleep, has lost several pounds, and is no longer interested in her normal activities. In each of these situations, the nurse should continue to assess for other signs and symptoms that might indicate a mental disorder and be prepared to intervene should concerns be supported.

Often the assessment process includes direct questioning or observation. At other times a standardized assessment tool or questionnaire might be employed. Figures 18-1 through 18-3 contain examples of instruments that are available to elicit information about symptoms of anxiety or depression or conditions such as alcohol abuse. However, whenever using these or other screening tools, the nurse

---

BOX 18-6 The Twelve Steps of Alcoholics Anonymous

1. Admitted we were powerless over alcohol—that our lives had become unmanageable
2. Came to believe that a Power greater than ourselves could restore us to sanity
3. Made a decision to turn our will and our lives over to the care of God as we understood Him
4. Made a searching and fearless moral inventory of ourselves
5. Admitted to God, to ourselves, and to another human being the exact nature of our wrongs
6. Were entirely ready to have God remove all these defects of character
7. Humbly asked Him to remove our shortcomings
8. Made a list of all persons we had harmed and became willing to make amends to them all
9. Made direct amends to such people wherever possible, except when to do so would injure them or others
10. Continued to take personal inventory and, when we were wrong, promptly admitted it
11. Sought through prayer and meditation to improve our conscious contact with God as we understood Him, praying only for knowledge of His will for us and the power to carry that out
12. Having had a spiritual awakening as the result of these steps, we tried to carry this message to alcoholics and to practice these principles in all our affairs.

The Twelve Steps are reprinted with permission of Alcoholics Anonymous World Services, Inc. Permission to reprint this material does not mean that AA has reviewed or approved the contents of this publication, nor that AA agrees with the views expressed herein. AA is a program of recovery from alcoholism—use of the Twelve Steps in connection with programs and activities that are patterned after AA but address other problems does not imply otherwise.

BOX **18-7** Suicide Facts

SUICIDE DEATHS (UNITED STATES, 2004)

Suicide was the 11th leading cause of death in the United States. The total number of suicide deaths was 32,439 (average of 89 suicides per day).

About 1.4% of all deaths were from suicide (in contrast, 26.5% of deaths are from heart disease, 23% are from cancer, and 7% are from cerebrovascular disease—the three leading causes).

There were almost twice as many deaths due to suicide than deaths due to HIV/AIDS (17,453).

Suicide by firearms was the most common method for both men and women, accounting for more than half of all suicides.

More men than women die by suicide; the gender ratio is nearly 4:1.

The highest suicide rates are for males older than 75 years (rate 37/100,000).

Suicide is the third leading cause of death among young people 15 to 24 years of age (following unintentional injuries and homicide in this age group).

ATTEMPTED SUICIDES

There are an estimated 8 to 25 attempted suicides to one completion; the ratio is higher in women and youth and lower in men and the elderly.

More women than men report a history of attempted suicide (gender ratio 2:1).

The strongest risk factors for attempted suicide in adults are depression, alcohol abuse, cocaine use, and separation or divorce.

The strongest risk factors for attempted suicide in youth are depression, alcohol or other drug use disorder, and aggressive or disruptive behaviors.

Adapted from National Institute of Mental Health (2007): *Suicide in the U.S.: statistics and prevention* (website): http://www.nimh.nih.gov/health/publications/suicide-in-the-us-statistics-and-prevention.shtml. Accessed Sept 26, 2007; CDC (2007): *Suicide: facts at a glance* (website): http://www.cdc.gov/ncipc/dvp/suicide/SuicideDataSheet.pdf. Accessed Sept 26, 2007.

COMMUNITY APPLICATION
Examples of Suicide Prevention Programs and General Recommendations for Prevention of Suicide Among Adolescents and Young Adults

SUICIDE PREVENTION PROGRAMS

School gatekeeper training: School staff are taught to identify and refer students at risk for suicide.

Community gatekeeper training: Community members (e.g., clergy, police, recreation staff) and clinical health care providers who see adolescent clients are trained to identify and refer persons who are at risk for suicide.

General suicide education: Students are taught about suicide, including warning signs and how to seek help for themselves or others.

Screening programs: Questionnaires or other screening instruments are used to identify high-risk adolescents and young adults and provide further assessment and treatment.

Peer support programs: Peer relationships and competency in social skills among high-risk adolescents and young adults are encouraged.

Crisis centers and hotlines: Trained volunteers and paid staff provide telephone counseling and other services for suicidal persons.

Restriction of access to lethal means: Activities and programs that restrict access to handguns, drugs, and other common means of suicide are encouraged.

Intervention after a suicide: Focus on friends and relatives of persons who have committed suicide to help prevent or contain suicide clusters and help adolescents and young adults cope effectively with feelings of loss that follow the sudden death or suicide of a peer.

SUICIDE PREVENTION RECOMMENDATIONS

Ensure that suicide prevention programs are linked as closely as possible with professional mental health resources in the community.

Avoid reliance on one prevention strategy: Use of more than one of the types of programs detailed above is recommended.

Expand suicide prevention efforts for young adults.

Incorporate evaluation efforts into suicide prevention programs.

From Centers for Disease Control and Prevention: Programs for the prevention of suicide among adolescents and young adults, *MMWR Morb Mortal Wkly Rep* 43(RR-6):3-8, 1994.

should be prepared in advance to intervene, based on assessment data. Very frequently this will involve referral to other health professionals for further assessment, testing, counseling, and treatment. In addition, the personal and sensitive nature of mental health problems necessitates that the nurse strictly follow professional standards and organizational policies or guidelines related to privacy.

For example, following district and state guidelines to comply with confidentiality requirements, a school nurse who suspects that a student has an eating disorder might talk with the student's

During the Past Week	Rarely or None of the Time (Less than 1 Day)	Some or a Little of the Time (1-2 Days)	Occasionally or a Moderate Amount of the Time (3-4 Days)	Most or All of the Time (5-7 Days)
1. I was bothered by things that don't usually bother me.	0	1	2	3
2. I did not feel like eating; my appetite was poor.	0	1	2	3
3. I felt that I could not shake off the blues even with the help of my family or friends.	0	1	2	3
4. I felt that I was just as good as other people.	3	2	1	0
5. I had trouble keeping my mind on what I was doing.	0	1	2	3
6. I felt depressed.	0	1	2	3
7. I felt everything I did was an effort.	0	1	2	3
8. I felt hopeful about the future.	3	2	1	0
9. I thought my life had been a failure.	0	1	2	3
10. I felt fearful.	0	1	2	3
11. My sleep was restless.	0	1	2	3
12. I was happy.	3	2	1	0
13. I talked less than usual.	0	1	2	3
14. I felt lonely.	0	1	2	3
15. People were unfriendly.	0	1	2	3
16. I enjoyed life.	3	2	1	0
17. I had crying spells.	0	1	2	3
18. I felt sad.	0	1	2	3
19. I felt that people disliked me.	0	1	2	3
20. I could not get "going."	0	1	2	3

Figure 18-1. Center for Epidemiologic Studies depression scale. Interpretation: A total score of 22 or higher is indicative of depression when the scale is used in primary care. (From Radloff LS: The CES-D scale: a self-report depression scale for research in the general population, *Applied Psychologic Measurement* 1:385-401, 1977. Copyright 1977 by West Publishing Company/Applied Psychological Measurement, Inc. Reproduced by permission.)

Rank	Life Event	Mean Value	Rank	Life Event	Mean Value
1	Death of spouse	100	23	Son or daughter leaving home	29
2	Divorce	73	24	Trouble with in-laws	29
3	Marital separation	65	25	Outstanding personal achievement	28
4	Jail term	63			
5	Death of close family member	63	26	Wife begins or stops work	26
6	Personal injury or illness	53	27	Begin or end school	26
7	Marriage	50	28	Change in living conditions	25
8	Fired at work	47	29	Change in personal habits	24
9	Marital reconciliation	45	30	Trouble with boss	23
10	Retirement	45	31	Change in work hours or conditions	20
11	Change in health of family member	44			
12	Pregnancy	40	32	Change in residence	20
13	Sex difficulties	39	33	Change in schools	20
14	Gain of new family member	39	34	Change in recreation	19
15	Business readjustment	39	35	Change in church activities	19
16	Change in financial state	38	36	Change in social activities	18
17	Death of close friend	37	37	Mortgage or loan less than $10,000	17
18	Change to different line of work	36			
19	Change in number of arguments with spouse	35	38	Change in sleeping habits	16
			39	Change in number of family get-togethers	15
20	Mortgage over $10,000	31			
21	Foreclosure on mortgage or loan	30	40	Change in eating habits	15
22	Change in responsibilities at work	29	41	Vacation	13
			42	Christmas	12
			43	Minor violations of the law	11

Life Crisis Categories and LCU Scores*

No life crisis	0-149
Mild life crisis	150-199
Moderate life crisis	200-299
Major life crisis	300 or more

*The LCU score includes those life event items experienced during a 1-year period.

Figure 18-2. Social readjustment rating scale. (Reprinted by permission of the publisher from Holmes TH, Rahe RH: The social readjustment rating scale, *J Psychosom Res* 11:213-217, 1967. Copyright 1967 by Elsevier Science Inc.)

"Have you ever felt you ought to **C**ut down on drinking?"
"Have people **A**nnoyed you by criticizing your drinking?"
"Have you ever felt bad or **G**uilty about your drinking?"
"Have you ever had a drink first thing in the morning to steady your nerves or get rid of a hangover (**E**ye-opener)?"
One "yes" response should raise suspicions of alcohol abuse. More than one "yes" response should be considered a strong indication that alcohol abuse exists.

Figure 18-3. The CAGE questionnaire. (From Ewing JA: Detecting alcoholism: the CAGE questionnaire, *J Am Med Assoc* 252(14):1905-1907, 1984. Copyright 1984 by American Medical Association.)

parents and teachers, the school counselor and principal, or appropriate others so that the best course of action can be followed in getting that student the needed help. If a client in a clinic or doctor's office describes signs and symptoms consistent with depression, the nurse should chart the reported information and consult with the client's physician about the comments that were voiced. When an employee is suspected of alcohol abuse, the occupational nurse should follow company policy on how, when, and under what circumstances the employee and his or her supervisor should be informed of the concerns. The employee should be given information on available treatment options and support groups.

TREATMENT OF MENTAL DISORDERS

The goals of treatment for mental illness are to reduce symptoms, improve personal and social functioning, develop and strengthen coping skills, and promote behaviors to improve the individual's life. Basic approaches to the treatment of mental disorders include pharmacotherapy, psychotherapy, and/or behavior therapy.

PSYCHOTHERAPEUTIC MEDICATIONS

Psychotherapeutic medications do not cure mental illness; they act by controlling symptoms. As with medications for physical health problems, the appropriateness of psychotherapeutic medications and their prescribed regimen depends on the diagnosis, side effects, and client response. Table 18-3 lists some commonly used psychotherapeutic medications. Indications and adverse effects and nursing implications for the different types of medications are briefly discussed.

Antipsychotic Medications

Antipsychotic medications are used to reduce symptoms of schizophrenia. Most antipsychotic medications are neuroleptics. Neuroleptics are quite effective but may produce some side effects. The most common are drowsiness, tachycardia, orthostatic hypotension, weight gain, photosensitivity, and menstrual irregularities. Often side effects diminish after a few weeks.

More serious adverse effects of neuroleptics include "extrapyramidal reactions" (movement disorders resulting from the effect of the drug on the extrapyramidal motor system) (Laraia, 2005). Acute dystonia (characterized by spasms or cramping of the muscles of the tongue, face, neck, or back), parkinsonism (including bradykinesia, masklike face, drooling, tremor, rigidity, shuffling gait), and akathisia (restlessness characterized by constant pacing and squirming) are extrapyramidal reactions sometimes seen early in treatment with antipsychotic drugs (Pearson, 2006; Sherr, 2004; Levi et al., 2003). These adverse effects tend to decrease with time or can be managed with other medications (e.g., antiparkinsonian agents).

The most serious extrapyramidal adverse effect of antipsychotic agents, however, is tardive dyskinesia. Tardive dyskinesia produces involuntary movement of the tongue and face and develops in up to 5% of younger clients during long-term therapy. It may, however, develop in as many as 30% of older clients on long-term therapy (Levi et al., 2003). Eating difficulty and weight loss may result. Tardive dyskinesia is permanent, although some symptoms decline in severity after the dosage is reduced or the drug is withdrawn (Pearson, 2006; Sherr, 2004).

Clozapine (Clozaril), risperidone (Risperdal), olanzapine (Zyprexa), quetiapine (Seroquel), and ziprasidone (Geodon) are termed atypical neuroleptics. These are relatively new medications that have been shown to be more effective than traditional antipsychotic medications for some people with schizophrenia. These medications have less risk of extrapyramidal side effects, including tardive dyskinesia, than other antipsychotics. Other complications or adverse effects are possible, however. Clozapine, the most commonly used atypical neuroleptic, is known to cause agranulocytosis in 1% to 2% of clients. Because this condition is potentially fatal, persons on Clozapine must have weekly white blood cell counts performed to assess for signs of agranulocytosis. Treatment is stopped if the white blood cell count is below 3000 or the granulocyte count is under 1500 (Levi et al., 2003). In addition, olanzapine and clozapine have been identified as potentiating development or exacerbation of type 2 diabetes in some individuals (Cohen, 2004).

TABLE **18-3** Psychotherapeutic Medications

GENERIC NAME	TRADE NAME
Antipsychotic Medications	
Chlorpromazine	Thorazine
Chlorprothixene	Taractan
Clozapine	Clozaril
Fluphenazine	Permitil, Prolixin
Haloperidol	Haldol
Loxapine	Loxitane
Mesoridazine	Serentil
Molindone	Lidone, Moban
Olanzapine	Zyprexa
Perphenazine	Trilafon
Pimozide (for Tourette Syndrome)	Orap
Quetiapine	Seroquel
Risperidone	Risperdal
Thioridazine	Mellaril
Thiothixene	Navane
Trifluoperazine	Stelazine
Triflupromazine	Vesprin
Ziprasidone	Geodon
Antimanic Medications	
Carbamazepine	Tegretol
Divalproex sodium (valproic acid)	Depakote
Gabapentin	Neurontin
Lamotrigine	Lamictal
Lithium carbonate	Eskalith, Lithane, Lithobid
Lithium citrate	Cibalith-S
Topiramate	Topamax
Antidepressant Medications	
Amitriptyline	Elavil
Amoxapine	Asendin
Bupropion	Wellbutrin
Citalopram (SSRI)	Celexa
Clomipramine	Anafranil
Desipramine	Norpramin, Pertofrane
Doxepin	Adapin, Sinequan
Escitalopram (SSRI)	Lexapro

Continued

TABLE **18-3** Psychotherapeutic Medications—cont'd

GENERIC NAME	TRADE NAME
Fluvoxamine (SSRI)	Luvox
Fluoxetine (SSRI)	Prozac
Imipramine	Tofranil
Isocarboxazid (MAOI)	Marplan
Maprotiline	Ludiomil
Mirtazapine	Remeron
Nefazodone	Serzone
Nortriptyline	Aventyl, Pamelor
Paroxetine (SSRI)	Paxil
Phenelzine (MAOI)	Nardil
Protriptyline	Vivactil
Sertraline (SSRI)	Zoloft
Tranylcypromine (MAOI)	Parnate
Trazodone	Desyrel
Trimipramine	Surmontil
Venlafaxine	Effexor
Antianxiety Medications (All of these medications except buspirone are benzodiazepines)	
Alprazolam	Xanax
Buspirone	BuSpar
Chlordiazepoxide	Librax, Libritabs, Librium
Clonazepam	Klonopin
Clorazepate	Azene, Tranxene
Diazepam	Valium
Halazepam	Paxipam
Lorazepam	Ativan
Oxazepam	Serax
Prazepam	Centrax
Stimulants	
Amphetamine with dextroamphetamine	Adderall
Dextroamphetamine	Dexedrine, Dextrostat
Dexmethylphenidate	Focalin
Methylphenidate	Ritalin
Methylphenidate (long-acting)	Concerta
Methylphenidate (extended release)	Metadate ER

Modified from National Institute of Mental Health (2007): *Medications with addendum, 2007* (NIH Publication No. 07-3929, electronic version online): accessed April 15, 2008 from http://www.nimh .nih.gov/health/publications/medications/medications.pdf.

Antimanic Medications

Lithium is the most frequently used medication for treatment of bipolar disorders. Response to treatment with lithium varies somewhat between individual clients. In addition, the range between an effective dose and a toxic dose is small, so serum lithium levels must be monitored closely. It is recommended that levels be checked routinely at the beginning of treatment and every few months thereafter to determine the optimal maintenance dosage (NIMH, 2005; Pearson, 2006).

Side effects are often worse during the initial stage of lithium therapy and include drowsiness, weakness, nausea, vomiting, fatigue, hand tremors, increased thirst, and weight gain. Long-term lithium use may affect thyroid function; therefore thyroid function tests should also be performed periodically.

Anticonvulsants

Anticonvulsants such as valproate (Depakote), carbamazepine (Tegretol) and gabapentin (Neurontin) are also used to treat mania. The most common side effects of anticonvulsants include drowsiness, dizziness, confusion, visual disturbances, memory impairment, and nausea. Periodic blood tests are needed to monitor white blood cell counts and screen for anemia (NIMH 2001b).

Antidepressants

Antidepressants are used most often for serious depression, but they can also be helpful for mild depression and anxiety. The choice of medications is usually based on the individual client's symptoms. Most medications take 1 to 3 weeks before improvement is seen. If little or no change occurs in symptoms after 5 to 6 weeks, a different medication should be tried. Treatment is usually continued for a minimum of several months and may last up to a year and sometimes more.

Tricyclic antidepressants are commonly used for treatment of major depression. Side effects vary somewhat between medications and between individuals. Potential side effects include drowsiness, blurred vision, dry mouth, constipation, weight gain, orthostatic hypotension, dysuria, fatigue, and weakness. Often side effects diminish or disappear during the course of treatment. Tricyclics may interfere with other medications and substances, including thyroid hormone, antihypertensives, oral contraceptives, sleeping medications, antipsychotic

medications, diuretics, antihistamines, aspirin, vitamin C, alcohol, and tobacco.

An overdose of tricyclic antidepressant medications may produce tachycardia, dilated pupils, and flushed face. In extreme cases, overdose may cause agitation, which may progress to confusion, loss of consciousness, seizures, arrhythmias, cardiorespiratory collapse, and death (NIMH, 2007).

Monoamine oxidase inhibitors (MAOIs) are more often used for atypical depression in which symptoms like anxiety, panic attacks, and phobias are present. The MAOIs may cause a serious reaction with certain foods (e.g., aged cheeses, foods containing monosodium glutamate), beverages (e.g., red wines), and medications (e.g., antihistamines, decongestants, local anesthetics, amphetamines, insulin, some narcotics, and antiparkinsonian medications). Reactions may produce hypertension, headache, nausea, vomiting, tachycardia, confusion, psychotic symptoms, seizures, stroke, and coma (NIMH, 2007). Persons taking MAOIs should be given a list of restricted foods, beverages, and medications and be encouraged to strictly comply with the restrictions.

Selective serotonin reuptake inhibitors (SSRIs) are the newest class of antidepressants available in the United States and have a more rapid onset of action than do other antidepressants. Improvement is usually seen in 2 to 4 weeks after initiation of therapy (Pearson, 2006). Gastrointestinal problems, headache, insomnia, anxiety, and agitation are the most common side effects of SSRIs. Ejaculatory delay in men and skin rashes, which may be severe, have also been noted. In addition, SSRIs may decrease appetite (Pearson, 2006; Levi, et al, 2003).

Serious complications have resulted when SSRIs are used in conjunction with other medications. In particular, fluoxetine (Prozac) should not be combined with MAOIs and should only be used with caution with tricyclic antidepressants (Pearson, 2006). The Food and Drug Administration (FDA) issued a "Black Box" warning for SSRIs, suggesting that these drugs may increase suicidal thoughts and behaviors in children and adolescents (U.S. FDA, 2004).

Antianxiety Medications

Benzodiazepines are medications used to treat most anxiety disorders. They have been shown to be safe and effective and have low addictive potential. The most commonly used benzodiazepines are alprazolam (Xanax), diazepam (Valium), clonazepam (Klonopin), and lorazepam (Ativan). Antianxiety medications usually act rapidly. Dosage varies greatly, depending on the symptoms and the individual's body chemistry. Common side effects include drowsiness, loss of coordination, fatigue, and mental slowing or confusion. Combining benzodiazepines and alcohol can produce serious interactions and potentially life-threatening complications, and clients should be warned accordingly.

Stimulants

Stimulants are primarily used to treat symptoms of ADHD and narcolepsy. The most common side effects are decreased appetite and difficulty in falling asleep. Some children report gastrointestinal problems, headache, and depression. Growth retardation has been documented in some children, so careful ongoing assessment of growth patterns is recommended while children are taking stimulants.

PSYCHOTHERAPY

Psychotherapy refers to the process of discovery that helps alleviate troubling emotional symptoms and assists individuals in returning to a healthy life. Psychotherapy is often used in conjunction with medication to treat many mental disorders. Various types of psychotherapy include the following:

- *Individual or interpersonal therapy* focuses on the client's current life and relationships within the family, social, and work environments.
- *Family therapy* involves discussions and problem-solving sessions with every member of a family—sometimes with the entire group, sometimes with individuals.
- *Couples therapy* is used to develop the relationship and minimize problems through understanding how individual conflicts are expressed in the couple's interactions.
- *Group therapy* involves a small group of people with similar problems who, with the guidance of a therapist, discuss individual issues and help each other with problems.
- *Play therapy* is a technique used for establishing communication and resolving problems with young children.

- *Cognitive therapy* works to identify and correct distorted thought patterns that can lead to troublesome feelings and behaviors; often combined with behavioral therapy (NIMH, 1994).

Short-term psychotherapy is often used when situational stresses (e.g., death in the family, divorce, physical illness) produce problems. In these cases therapy may only last a few weeks or months, with the goal of helping the individual resolve the problem as quickly as possible. Long-term therapy may last for several months to several years and emphasize underlying problems.

BEHAVIORAL THERAPY

Behavioral therapy uses learning principles to change thought patterns and behaviors systematically. Behavior therapy is used to encourage the individual to learn specific skills to obtain rewards and satisfaction. Stress management, biofeedback, and relaxation training are examples of behavior therapy .

SUMMARY

As discussed throughout this chapter, mental disorders are very common and are most often identified and treated in community settings. Therefore all nurses who work in the community should be knowledgeable about risk factors and signs and symptoms that might indicate a mental disorder and be prepared to intervene. In the opening case study, Kay, who works in a clinic for indigent persons, understood the types of mental health problems commonly observed in community settings. As a result she was prepared to effectively address the needs of her clients.

This chapter has described some of the more common mental disorders, including assessment of risk factors and symptoms, overview of diagnostic criteria, and basic treatment regimens. Brochures and teaching materials are available free of charge from many organizations, and a supply of appropriate materials can be made available for all who come in contact with the health care provider. For example, a school nurse can display brochures on eating disorders, depression in teenagers, and prevention of alcohol and drug abuse in adolescents in or near the school clinic. Likewise, a variety of educational materials describing mental disorders and threats to mental health should be easily accessible in worksite settings and primary care clinics. These measures can help demystify mental illness and assist those who need treatment to seek care. In addition to these resources, the nurse in community-based practice is strongly encouraged to develop a list of area individuals, groups, agencies, and organizations that provide services for persons with mental disorders and their families.

KEY POINTS

- Mental health refers to the absence of mental disorders and the ability of an individual to negotiate the daily challenges and social interactions of life without experiencing cognitive, emotional, or behavioral dysfunction.
- Approximately 75% of client care for mental disorders occurs in community-based settings. Providers include physicians, psychologists, counselors, clergy, and laypersons. Settings for care include outpatient departments, mental health centers and clinics, alcohol and drug units, emergency departments, family or social service agencies, crisis centers, and volunteer services (self-help programs).
- Depression affects almost 19 million people in the United States each year. Nurses in community-based practice should be aware of risk factors and symptoms of depression and routinely assess those in high-risk groups. Treatment for depression includes pharmacologic therapy, electroconvulsive therapy, behavior therapy, and/or psychotherapy.
- Anxiety disorders are the most common mental disorder, affecting up to 18% of the general population. The most common anxiety disorders are GAD (chronic, unrealistic, and exaggerated worry), panic disorder (sometimes accompanied by agoraphobia), phobias, OCD, and PTSD. Anxiety disorders are treated with antidepressants, antianxiety medications, behavior therapy, and psychotherapy.
- Eating disorders are becoming increasingly prevalent in the United States. Bulimia is characterized by binge eating and purging (self-induced vomiting, use of laxatives, diuretics, fasting, and excessive exercise). Individuals with anorexia nervosa are obsessed with a fear of fat and with

losing weight. Anorexia and bulimia usually develop during adolescence. Nurses who work with adolescents and young adults should be aware of the signs and symptoms of eating disorders and screen those considered to be at risk. Treatment includes counseling, psychotherapy, and behavior modification.
- Attention deficit hyperactivity disorder affects 3% to 5% of all children and is characterized by inattention, hyperactivity, and impulsivity. A diagnosis of ADD or ADHD should be made following a comprehensive physical, psychologic, social, and behavioral evaluation to rule out other possible reasons for the behavior. It is usually managed through a combination of behavior therapy, emotional counseling, practical support, and medication.
- A number of legal and illegal substances used by Americans are potentially harmful. Alcoholism is the greatest drug problem in the United States today. Illicit drugs used include opioids (e.g., heroin, morphine), cocaine, amphetamines, hallucinogens, marijuana, and inhalants. Nurses in community-based settings should be aware of risk factors of substance abuse, signs of intoxication and withdrawal, and treatment of the most common psychoactive substances and refer accordingly.
- Suicide is the most serious potential outcome of mental disorders and is the eleventh leading cause of death in the United States. Risk factors for suicide include a family history of psychiatric disorders, previous suicide attempts, serious medical illness, family violence, alcohol and other drug abuse, and accessibility to firearms.
- Treatment of mental disorders includes use of psychotherapeutic medications (e.g., antipsychotics, antimanics, anticonvulsant medications, antidepressants, antianxiety medications, stimulants), psychotherapy, and behavior therapy.

Learning Activities & Application to Practice
In Class

1. In groups of four to six, discuss one of the commonly encountered mental health problems described in this chapter (e.g., depression, anxiety disorders, eating disorders, substance abuse). Share if you have encountered the problem in

practice, and if so describe how the problem was identified and treated. In the group, devise primary, secondary, and tertiary prevention strategies to address the mental health problem and share ideas with the class.

2. Discuss the *Healthy People 2010* objectives related to "Alcohol and Other Drugs" and "Mental Health and Mental Disorders." Examine differences related to age, race/ethnic group, and gender (e.g., suicide is most common among white males; alcohol-related motor vehicle deaths for American Indians are 400% higher than for the population as a whole). Identify factors that contribute to differences and outline strategies to address these factors.

In Clinical

3. Identify, investigate, and visit area organizations and providers that care for persons with mental disorders or work to improve mental health. During the visit learn what services are available, how services are accessed, what interventions are provided, and what the responsibilities of nurses are. Share findings with the clinical group.

4. Identify the most common mental disorder encountered in the community-based setting in which you are assigned (e.g., if you are in elementary school—ADD; if in a high school—eating disorders or substance abuse; if working with women or elders—depression). Compile or develop materials that could be used for health education in that setting. Develop a forum to share the materials with other health professionals at the setting or with members of the group or community (e.g., a seminar for parents of children diagnosed with ADD/ADHD).

REFERENCES

American Psychiatric Association: *Diagnostic and statistical manual of mental disorders*, ed 4, text rev, Washington, DC, 2000, American Psychiatric Association.

Antai-Otong D: Foundations of psychiatric nursing practice. In Antai-Otong D, editor: *Psychiatric nursing: biological and behavioral concepts* ed 2, Clifton Park, NY, 2008, Delmar.

Carson VB, Trubowitz J: Relevant theories and therapies for nursing practice. In Varcarolis EM, Carson VB, Shoemaker NC, editors: *Foundations of psychiatric mental health nursing: a clinical approach*, ed 5, St Louis, 2006, Saunders.

Centers for Disease Control and Prevention (2007a): Suicide trends among youths and young adults aged 10-24 years– United States, 1990-2004, *MMWR Morb Mortal Wkly Rep* 56(35):905, 2007.

Centers for Disease Control and Prevention (2007b): *Suicide: facts at a glance* (website): http://www.cdc.gov/ncipc/dvp/Suicide/SuicideDataSheet.pdf. Accessed September 17, 2007.

Centers for Disease Control and Prevention: Programs for the prevention of suicide among adolescents and young adults, *MMWR Morb Mortal Wkly Rep* 43(RR-6):3, 1994.

Clark MJ: Substance abuse. In Clark MJ, editor: *Community health nursing: advocacy for population health*, ed 4, Upper Saddle River, NJ, 2008, Prentice Hall.

Cohen D: Atypical antipsychotics and new onset diabetes mellitus: an overview of the literature. *Pharmacopsychiatry* 37(1):1, 2004.

Ewing JA: Detecting alcoholism: the CAGE questionnaire, *J Am Med Assoc* 252(14):1905, 1984.

Holmes TH, Rahe RH: The social readjustment rating scale, *J Psychosom Res* 11:213, 1967.

Ibrahim K: Eating disorders. In Varcarolis EM, Carson VB, Shoemaker NC, editors: *Foundations of psychiatric mental health nursing: a clinical approach*, ed 5, St Louis, 2006, Saunders.

Laraia MT: Biological context of psychiatric nursing care. In Stuart GW, Laraia MT, editors: *Principles and practice of psychiatric nursing*, ed 8, St Louis, 2005, Mosby.

Levi V, Antai-Otong D, Pennebaker DF, Riley J: Psychopharmacologic therapy. In Antai-Otong D, editor: *Psychiatric nursing: biological and behavioral concepts*, Clifton Park, NY, 2003, Delmar.

Lewin L: The client with a depressive disorder. In Antai-Otong D, editor: *Psychiatric nursing: biological and behavioral concepts*, Clifton Park, NY, 2003, Delmar.

National Alliance on Mental Illness (2007): *The impact and cost of mental illness: depression* (website): http://www.nami.org/Template.cfm?Section=Policymakers_Toolkit&Template=/ContentManagement/ContentDisplay.cfm&ContentID=19043. Accessed September 20, 2007.

National Institute of Mental Health: *Helpful facts about depressive illnesses* (NIH Publication No. 94-3875), Rockville, Md, 1994, National Institute of Mental Health.

National Institute of Mental Health (2007): *Attention deficit hyperactivity disorder* (website): http://www.nimh.nih.gov/health/publications/adhd/complete-publication.shtml. AccessedSeptember 20, 2007.

National Institute of Mental Health: *Depression* (NIH Publication No. 07-3561), Rockville, Md, 2007, National Institute of Mental Health (website): http://www.nimh.nih.gov/health/publications/depression/nimhdepression.pdf. Accessed April 15, 2008.

National Institute of Mental Health (2007): *The numbers count: mental disorders in America* (website): http://www.nimh.nih.gov/health/publications/the-numbers-count-mental-disorders-in-america.shtml#SpitzerBinge. Accessed September 20, 2007.

National Institute of Mental Health (2006): *Anxiety disorders* (NIH Publication No. 06-3879, electronic version online): http://www.nimh.nih.gov/health/topics/anxiety-disorders/index.shtml. Accessed September 27, 2007.

National Institute of Mental Health (2003): *Depression: a treatable illness* (website): http://www.nimh.nih.gov/health/

publications/depression-a-treatable-illness.shtml. Accessed September 20, 2007.

National Institute of Mental Health (2001a): *Eating disorders* (NIH Publication No. 01-4901), Rockville, Md, 2001, National Institute of Mental Health.

National Institute of Mental Health (2001b): *Bipolar disorders* (NIH Publication No. 01-3679), Rockville, Md, 2001, National Institute of Mental Health.

National Mental Health Association: *Mental health and you*, Alexandria, Va, 2006, National Mental Health Association.

Pearson G: Psychopharmacology. In Mohr WK, editor: *Psychiatric-mental health nursing*, ed 6, Philadelphia, 2006, Lippincott.

Radloff LS: The CES-D scale: a self-report depression scale for research in the general population, *Applied Psychological Measurement* 1:385, 1977.

Robert Wood Johnson Foundation: *Substance abuse: the nation's number one health problem*, Waltham, Mass, 1993, Institute for Health Policy, Brandeis University.

Sharfstein SS, Stoline AM, Koran L: Mental health services. In Kovner AR, Jonas S, editors: *Jonas & Kovner's health care delivery in the United States*, ed 7, New York, 2002, Springer.

Sherr J: Psychopharmacology and other biologic therapies. In Fortinash KM, Holoday-Worret PA, editors: *Psychiatric and mental health nursing*, ed 3, St Louis, 2004, Mosby.

Shoemaker NC, Caverly S: Mental health nursing in community settings. In Varcarolis EM, Carson VB, Shoemaker NC, editors: *Foundations of psychiatric mental health nursing: a clinical approach*, ed 5, St Louis, 2006, Saunders.

Stuart GW, Laraia MT: *Principles and practice of psychiatric nursing*, ed 8, St Louis, 2005, Mosby.

U.S. Department of Health and Human Services: *Healthy people 2010*: conference ed, Washington, DC, 2000, USDHHS.

U.S. Department of Health and Human Services/Office of Disease Prevention and Health Promotion: *Clinician's handbook of preventive services*, ed 2, Washington, DC, 1998, Government Printing Office.

U.S. Department of Health and Human Services/Public Health Service: *Mental health: a report of the surgeon general*, Rockville, Md, 1999, USDHHS.

U.S. Department of Health and Human Services/Substance Abuse and Mental Health Services Administration: *Findings from the 1999 national household survey on drug abuse*, Washington, DC, 1999, USDHHS.

U.S. Department of Health and Human Services/Substance Abuse and Mental Health Services Administration (2006): *Mental health–United States, 2004* (website): http://download.ncadi.samhsa.gov/ken/pdf/SMA06-4195/CMHS_MHUS_2004.pdf. Accessed Sept 17, 2007.

U.S. Department of Health and Human Services/Substance Abuse and Mental Health Services Administration (2007): *Results from the 2006 national survey on drug use and health: national findings* (website): http://www.oas.samhsa.gov/nsduh/2k6nsduh/2k6results.pdf. Accessed September 17, 2007.

U.S. Food and Drug Administration (2004): *Public health advisory: suicidality in children and adolescents being treated with antidepressant medications* (website): http://www.fda.gov/CDER/DRUG/antidepressants/SSRIPHA200410.htm. Accessed September 25, 2007.

Communicable Disease: Prevention and Intervention

1. Discuss the changes in incidence and prevalence of communicable disease patterns in the United States over the past century, and describe the impact of immunization on those patterns.

2. Discuss the *epidemiologic triangle*.

3. Describe the various ways that communicable disease may be transmitted.

4. Explain the process of reporting communicable diseases.

5. Describe the process of immunization, and explain the pediatric immunization schedule, including contraindications, precautions, and reporting of adverse events.

6. Discuss the incidence and prevalence of sexually transmitted diseases, and present prevention strategies.

7. Identify potential emerging infectious diseases and discuss their prevention.

8. Discuss health issues related to international travel, focusing on prevention of communicable diseases.

9. Discuss the categories of diseases and agents that could be used in bioterrorism.

key terms

Active immunity	Immunity	Vaccine Adverse Event
Bioterrorism	Immunization schedule	Reporting System (VAERS)
Category A agents	Passive immunity	Vaccine-preventable
Direct transmission	Reportable diseases	diseases
Emerging infectious	Sexually transmitted	
diseases	diseases (STD)s	*See Glossary for definitions.*

case study

Mark Mitchell works as a nurse for the public health department in a midsized city. Mark's primary responsibility is investigation and follow-up of suspected cases of reportable diseases. One recent Monday, Mark received a call from a local pediatrician, who reported a
Continued

possible case of measles in a 3-year-old boy named Grant. To gather information about the case, Mark reviewed the child's presenting symptoms with the physician. The symptoms were a fever of over 101°F for 2 days, mild cough, runny nose, conjunctivitis, and a red rash, which his mother reported began on his face and had progressed to his trunk. Upon prompting from Mark, the pediatrician looked inside the child's mouth and discovered small red spots with bluish-white centers on the buccal mucosa (Koplik's spots). In addition, the pediatrician stated that according to her records, Grant's immunization status was incomplete because he had received only his initial diphtheria/pertussis/tetanus (DPT), Haemophilus influenzae b (HIB), and polio vaccinations at her office. The mother denied that the child had received shots at any other clinic. The pediatrician concluded that although Grant was quite ill, he did not need to be hospitalized but would be treated with cough medication, antipyretics, and decongestants as an outpatient.

Mark was aware that during the past 6 weeks, 10 cases of measles had been confirmed in the county and about 20 others were suspected. Because of the presence of the disease in the area, Mark determined that with Grant's symptoms and his incomplete immunization status, it was probable that Grant was ill with measles. Mark instructed the pediatrician to obtain a sample of blood to send to the state laboratory for confirmation of the diagnosis. According to department protocols, Mark obtained the boy's name and address and made a visit to the boy's home later that day.

Grant was the youngest of three (Joseph, 6, and Brittany, 9). While in the home, Mark questioned Grant's parents regarding the immunization status of their other two children and reviewed their immunization records. Both children's records were complete and included two injections of measles/mumps/rubella (MMR) vaccine, as required by the state for all children in school, and both of Grant's parents had been immunized as children.

Next, Mark gathered as much information as the parents could provide pertaining to other children that Grant had been around during the previous 2 weeks. He discovered that Grant had spent a few hours at a babysitter's house on 2 separate days and in the church's nursery for about 3 hours the previous Sunday. Mark called the nursery director at their church. She stated there had been about 10 children in Grant's class on Sunday, and she knew of none that were sick. She agreed to call all of the parents and explain that their children had possibly been exposed to measles. Further, she would instruct them to call their pediatricians to check their children's immunization status.

The babysitter was then called. She reported that one of the children she provided care for on a sporadic basis had been very ill with a fever about 10 days previously, but she did not know what was wrong with the child. Mark obtained that child's name and her parent's telephone number and address and continued the process of communicable disease surveillance.

Caring for individuals with communicable diseases was one of the earliest functions of nurses. Later, prevention of the spread of communicable diseases through advocating cleanliness and the use of immunizations and medications became an integral part of nursing practice. Indeed, the first intervention learned by virtually every nursing student relates to the spread of communicable diseases: "Wash your hands!" The importance of frequent and thorough handwashing is repeatedly stressed and cannot be overstated for preventing the spread of communicable diseases.

Though the mechanism of the spread of disease was poorly understood until the early 1800s, it is now known that a complex interplay of three factors are involved in both the spread and the containment of infectious diseases. The *epidemiologic triangle* (Figure 19-1) illustrates this relationship between the agent, host, and environment.

The *agent* in this illustration is the cause of the disease. Common agents of infectious diseases are bacteria and viruses. When looking for the cause of noninfectious diseases such as heart disease, the agent would be factors such as hypercholesterolemia, hypertension, and overweight. The *host* is the organism, human or animal, that harbors the agent. A community or group of people can also be a host. In the case of heart disease, the host is the person who has

Figure 19-1. The Epidemiologic Triangle.

the causative factors related to heart disease. The *environment* refers to the external conditions of the host that allow the disease to be transmitted. A warm, poorly-ventilated room is a good environment for the transmission of the common cold. In the case of a noninfectious disease, the environment includes those things such as an individual's behavior, culture, and physiologic factors. Ecologic factors of the greater environment, such as air pollution, are also included here. (Merrill & Timmreck, 2006).

The premise of the epidemiologic triangle is that if any of the factors are changed or removed, the disease cannot be transmitted, or in the case of noninfectious diseases, the disease process will not progress. The infectious agent can be killed or rendered harmless by chemical disinfection or antibiotics, or the client's cholesterol level can be lowered so that heart disease does not progress. The host can be treated with rest, good nutrition, and medication to make it impossible for the infectious agent to grow and replicate. In the case of a community host, the community can enact policies to protect the health of its members. Common surfaces can be cleaned, and personnel can wash their hands and cover their mouths when they cough or sneeze to prevent the agent from being transmitted to other clients, where the process of infection can start anew.

Around 1900, communicable diseases accounted for 4 of the top 10 causes of death for Americans. At that time pneumonia and influenza were designated collectively as the leading cause of death,

followed closely by tuberculosis (TB). Diarrhea and enteritis were collectively the third major cause of death, and diphtheria was tenth. A similar list for 2004 contains only one notation of communicable disease. Pneumonia and influenza were collectively the seventh leading cause of death that year, accounting for about 2.7% of all deaths (National Center for Health Statistics [NCHS], 2007). Acquired immunodeficiency syndrome and human immunodeficiency virus (AIDS and HIV) infection are also among the leading causes of death in certain age or ethnic groups. With these exceptions, communicable disease as a cause of mortality has largely been eradicated in the twenty-first century. In terms of morbidity, however, there has not been much improvement. Many Americans are sickened each year by a variety of communicable diseases ranging from mild (colds or stomach flu) to serious and life threatening (influenza or TB). In addition, the possibility of emerging infectious diseases is a continuing threat.

This chapter presents an overview of contemporary health problems and issues that relate to communicable disease prevention, transmission, and management. *Healthy People 2010* (U.S. Department of Health and Human Services [USDHHS], 2000) lists three priority areas that specifically target the prevention and management of communicable diseases. These are HIV Infection (Area 13), Immunization and Infectious Diseases (Area 14), and **Sexually Transmitted Diseases (STDs)** (Area 25). Examples of goals from these priority areas are shown in the *Healthy People 2010* box.

COMMUNICABLE DISEASE TRANSMISSION

Communicable diseases may be transmitted either directly, through physical contact with infected individuals, or indirectly, through a source other than another human. **Direct transmission** can be through physical contact including biting, kissing, and touching (e.g., for influenza, colds, strep throat) or sexual contact (e.g., for HIV, STDs, hepatitis B [HBV]). Indirect transmission can be vehicleborne through fomites (objects that absorb and transmit infectious material, e.g., toys, telephones, money) or substances (e.g., food, water, blood). Communicable disease may

healthy people **2010**

Objectives Related to Epidemiology

OBJECTIVE	BASELINE (1998)	TARGET
13.1: Reduce AIDS among adolescents and adults	19.5 per 100,000	1 per 100,000
13.2: Reduce the number of new AIDS cases among adolescent and adult men who have sex with men	17,847	13,385
13.6: Increase the proportion of sexually active persons who use condoms	23%	50%
14.1d: Reduce or eliminate indigenous cases of HBV in people aged 2 to 18	945	9
14.1g: Reduce or eliminate indigenous cases of pertussis in children under age 7	3417	2000
14.9: Reduce new cases of hepatitis C	2.4 per 100,000	1 per 100,000
14.22d: Achieve and maintain effective vaccination coverage levels for two doses of MMR vaccine	92%	90%
14.29a: Increase the proportion of adults who are vaccinated annually against influenza	63%	90%
25.1b: Reduce the proportion of females aged 15 to 24 attending STD clinics with *Chlamydia trachomatis* infections	12.2%	3%
25.2: Reduce new cases of gonorrhea	123 per 100,000	19 per 100,000
25.6: Reduce the proportion of females who have ever required treatment for PID	8%	5%

From U.S. Department of Health and Human Services: *Healthy people 2010*: conference ed, Washington, DC, 2000, Public Health Service.

also be transmitted indirectly through vectors such as animals (e.g., rabies, anthrax, toxoplasmosis) or arthropods (e.g., malaria, Lyme disease, Rocky Mountain spotted fever). Airborne transmission through dust and droplet and droplet nuclei may be either direct (sprayed body fluids from sneezing or coughing for colds, influenza) or indirect (contaminated dusts or droplet nuclei for legionellosis, TB) (Table 19-1). Figure 19-2 illustrates various methods for communicable disease transmission.

Efforts to prevent the spread of communicable diseases must incorporate primary prevention strategies designed to stop transmission. Encouraging frequent handwashing, use of tissues to cover the mouth and nose when coughing or sneezing, mosquito control, rabies inoculation for all pets, and promoting sexual abstinence or appropriate use of condoms are examples of primary prevention interventions that attempt to stop the spread of communicable diseases.

TABLE **19-1** Types of Transmission

DIRECT TRANSMISSION	INDIRECT TRANSMISSION
PHYSICAL CONTACT	**VEHICLEBORNE**
Biting	Fomites (toys)
Touching	Substances (food, blood)
Spitting	
SEXUAL CONTACT	**VECTORBORNE**
Fecal-oral	Mechanical
Anal intercourse	Biologic
Oral-genital	
AIRBORNE	**AIRBORNE**
Dust and droplets	Dust and droplets
Droplet nuclei	Droplet nuclei

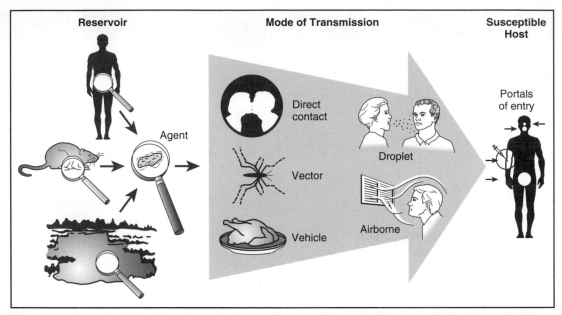

Figure 19-2. Chain of infection. (From Centers for Disease Control and Prevention: *Principles of epidemiology,* ed 2, Atlanta, 1992, Centers for Disease Control and Prevention.)

REPORTABLE COMMUNICABLE DISEASES

Each state has an established reporting system to monitor communicable diseases. Typically state laws or regulations empower the state board or department of health to establish and modify reporting requirements. The individual states are then required to report selected data to the Centers for Disease Control and Prevention (CDC). The CDC monitors communicable diseases and provides aggregate reports and interpretation of trends. In response to findings, it issues recommendations through weekly updates and periodic publications.

According to the CDC (1992), state regulations usually specify:

- The disease and conditions that must be reported
- Who is responsible for reporting
- What information is required on each case of disease reported
- How, to whom, and how quickly the information is to be reported
- Control measures to be taken for specified diseases

REPORTABLE DISEASES

Reportable diseases and those that require notification of authorities vary slightly from state to state. A list of diseases and conditions that are required to be reported nationally is available from the CDC website. A list of the reportable diseases for each state is typically available from the state's health department website. Every nurse, particularly those who work in community-based settings and Emergency Departments (EDs), should be familiar with the diseases that must be reported.

WHO IS RESPONSIBLE FOR REPORTING

Although there may be differences based on state regulations, most states require reporting of known or suspected cases of reportable diseases by physicians, dentists, nurses, and other health professionals (medical examiners, laboratory directors, chiropractors, veterinarians) and administrators of hospitals, clinics, nursing homes, schools, and nurseries (CDC, 1992). Typically organizations (e.g., clinics, doctors' offices, hospitals) designate one individual who is responsible for this activity and who has been trained in the process. State and local public health officials depend on health care professionals in their areas to promptly report cases of communicable diseases to monitor trends and detect unusual occurrences of disease.

WHAT INFORMATION IS REQUIRED

Data to be collected vary, based on the disease. Usually case reports include the name, age, sex, race or ethnicity, date of birth, address, and telephone number of the patient. Case reports then describe the disease, including its date of onset, the attending physician or person reporting the disease, and the method of diagnosis. Some diseases (e.g., chicken pox or influenza during an outbreak) may only be reported by number of cases.

HOW, WHEN, AND TO WHOM TO REPORT

Individual state regulations dictate the process for reporting. Some diseases, such as those that are rare, potentially very infectious, or involved in unusual outbreaks, are to be reported immediately by telephone. These typically include plague, rabies, measles, and poliomyelitis. Others are usually reported on a weekly basis either by telephone or by written report. Examples of illnesses reported weekly include AIDS and other STDs, TB, Lyme disease, and mumps. Most frequently the health professional identifying a reportable disease reports the finding to the local health department. The local health department in turn reports to the state health department, which then reports to the CDC.

STEPS TAKEN TO CONTROL SPREAD

States may have specific instructions to follow when certain diseases are identified. These instructions can include sending out surveillance teams to investigate and confirm reported cases; instruction on collecting of specimens; and specified control techniques such as environmental sanitation, immunization, quarantine, and education on prevention of transmission (CDC, 1992). Nurses working in public health departments, hospital infection control departments, ambulatory settings, schools, and industry should be aware of the most frequently encountered communicable diseases in their settings and learn the appropriate measures to take when a reportable disease is suspected or confirmed.

IDENTIFYING COMMUNICABLE DISEASES

Identifying various communicable diseases can be difficult for new nurses and experienced practitioners alike. *The Red Book,* a publication of the American Academy of Pediatrics (AAP, 2006), is the recognized reference source on communicable diseases. Another excellent source on the identification of communicable diseases is the National Center for Infectious Diseases (NCID) (http://www.cdc.gov/ncidod/). Both of these resources provide information on signs and symptoms, communicability, incubation period, and complications of communicable diseases.

Control of communicable diseases necessitates careful monitoring of trends and disease patterns. Table 19-2 lists several reportable diseases and the number of cases for selected years, dating from 1950. This table graphically illustrates the effectiveness of immunization efforts in the reduction of **vaccine-preventable diseases** and trends in some communicable diseases that are interesting (fluctuation of gonorrhea, relative stability of hepatitis A), troubling (recent rise in pertussis cases), and encouraging (0 cases of diphtheria in 2005).

VACCINE-PREVENTABLE DISEASES

Vaccination against communicable diseases has very dramatically affected morbidity and mortality from infectious diseases, as Table 19-2 shows. The worldwide eradication of small pox in 1980 is an example of the success possible through the use of global efforts to control disease through immunization. Efforts to eradicate other diseases, such as measles and polio, have been less successful to date, primarily because of failure to appropriately immunize all those who are susceptible. Table 19-3 further illustrates the impact of routine vaccinations.

The routine pediatric **immunization schedule** has become very complex in recent years. Recommendations have been modified a number of times since the early 1980s, with the addition of new vaccines, changes in the ages for administration, requirements for informed consent, and reporting of serious side effects. Nurses who primarily work

TABLE **19-2** Selected Reportable Diseases by Year

	NUMBER OF CASES						
DISEASE	**1950**	**1960**	**1970**	**1980**	**1990**	**1999**	**2005**
AIDS	N/A	N/A	N/A	N/A	41,595	45,104	41,120
Diphtheria	5796	918	435	3	4	1	—-
Gonorrhea	286,746	258,933	600,072	1,004,029	690,169	360,076	339,593
Hepatitis A	2820	41,666	56,797	29,078	31,441	17,047	4488
Hepatitis B	Nonspecific	Nonspecific	8310	19,015	21,102	7694	5119
Measles	319,124	441,703	47,351	13,506	27,786	100	66
Mumps	N/A	N/A	104,953	8576	5292	387	314
Pertussis	120,718	14,809	4249	1730	4570	7288	25,616
Poliomyelitis	33,300	3190	33	9	6	—	1
Rubella	N/A	N/A	56,552	3904	1125	267	11
Syphilis	217,558	122,538	91,382	68,832	134,255	35,628	33,278
Tuberculosis	121,742	55,494	37,137	27,749	25,701	17,531	14,097
Varicella	N/A	N/A	N/A	190,894	173,099	46,016	32,242

From Centers for Disease Control and Prevention: Summary of notifiable diseases, United States, 2005, *MMWR Morb Mortal Wkly Rep* 54(53):1-96, 2007.

TABLE **19-3** Impact of Vaccines in the 20th Century

DISEASE	20TH CENTURY ANNUAL MORBIDITY	2005 TOTAL	% DECREASE
Smallpox	48,164	0	100
Diphtheria	175,885	0	100
Pertussis	147,271	25,616	83
Tetanus	1314	27	98
Polio (paralytic)	16,316	1*	>99.9
Measles	503,282	66	>99.9
Mumps	152,209	314	>99
Rubella	47,745	11	99.8
Congenital Rubella	823	1	99.8
Haemophilus influenzae (over 5 years)	20,000 (est)	226 (serotype B or unknown serotype)	

*Imported vaccine-associated polio.
From Centers for Disease Control and Prevention: *Epidemiology & prevention of vaccine-preventable diseases*, Atlanta, 2007, Centers for Disease Control and Prevention.

with children in schools, clinics, and doctors' offices and who administer immunizations must be aware of a number of components of immunization delivery. In addition to a basic understanding of the principles behind immunization, nurses should know the pediatric immunization schedule and standards, contraindications and precautions, requirements for parent education and consent, and the process for reporting adverse vaccine events. Each is discussed here.

IMMUNITY

Immunity refers to protection from infectious disease. There are two basic mechanisms for acquiring immunity: active and passive.

- **Passive immunity** is protection produced by an animal or human and transferred to another human. Passive immunity often provides effective protection, but this protection usually wanes in a few weeks or months.
- **Active immunity** is protection that is produced by the person's own immune system. This type of immunity is generally long-lasting (CDC, 2007a).

Examples of passive immunity include transplacental transfer of immunity from a mother to her infant and injection of constituents of blood products from human donors (e.g., homologous pooled human antibody, immune globulin).

Active immunity occurs following the stimulation of the body's immune system to produce antibodies and cellular immunity, often after a person has had a disease. Active immunity can also be achieved through administration of a vaccine that produces an immunologic memory similar to that of the natural disease (CDC, 2007a).

Vaccines are classified as *live attenuated* and *inactivated*. Live attenuated vaccines are produced by modifying a disease-producing virus or bacterium in the laboratory. The altered vaccines allow production of an immune response as the organism replicates in the vaccinated person. Although the organisms in live attenuated vaccines replicate, they usually do not cause the disease, or if they do, the case is usually much milder than the natural disease (CDC, 2007a). Live attenuated vaccines must be handled and stored carefully because they may be destroyed by heat and light.

Examples of live attenuated vaccines include MMR, oral polio, varicella, and TB (*Bacille Calmette Guerin* vaccine [BCG]).

Inactivated vaccines are produced by growing the organism in a culture medium, then inactivating it with heat or chemicals. The organisms in inactivated vaccines do not replicate, and the vaccine's effectiveness depends on the body's immune system to develop protection following a second or third dose. Influenza, pertussis, HBV, tetanus, and HIB are examples of diseases that a person can be inoculated against with inactivated vaccines (CDC, 2007a).

IMMUNIZATION SCHEDULE

The recommended immunization schedule for routine pediatric vaccinations has undergone multiple major changes over the last two decades. Changes include the addition of vaccination for HIB in the early 1980s, the addition of an MMR booster in 1990, the inclusion of vaccination against HBV in 1992, addition of vaccination against varicella in 1997, addition of vaccination against hepatitis A in high-risk areas, addition of a series to protect against pneumococcal disease in 2000, recommendation for yearly vaccination of young children against influenza in 2005, and addition of rotavirus vaccine in 2007. The immunization schedule may be viewed at the CDC website at http://www.cdc.gov/vaccines/recs/schedules/child-schedule.htm. This website presents the standard immunization schedules for children and adults, as well as the schedules for "catching up" children and adults who are lacking immunizations.

The Standards for Pediatric Immunization Practices, published in 1993, focused on eliminating barriers to the reception and delivery of vaccines and avoiding missed opportunities to provide immunizations. Revised in 2003, the standards have been broadened to include the effective communication of vaccination information and the development of community partnerships to reach target populations (CDC, 2003). These standards, with numerous programs at each local, state, and federal level of the public health system, have been quite successful in improving the rates of complete immunization for U.S. children. The standards are outlined in Box 19-1.

BOX **19-1** Standards for Pediatric Immunization Practices

AVAILABILITY OF VACCINES

1. Vaccination services are readily available.
2. Vaccinations are coordinated with other health care services and provided in a medical setting when possible.
3. Barriers to vaccination are identified and minimized.
4. Patient costs are minimized.

ASSESSMENT OF VACCINATION STATUS

5. Health care professionals review the vaccination and health status of patients at every encounter to determine which vaccines are indicated.
6. Health care professionals assess for and follow only medically accepted contraindications.

EFFECTIVE COMMUNICATION ABOUT VACCINE BENEFITS AND RISKS

7. Parents/guardians and patients are educated about the benefits and risks of vaccination in a culturally appropriate manner and in easy-to-understand language.

PROPER STORAGE AND ADMINISTRATION OF VACCINES AND DOCUMENTATION OF VACCINATIONS

8. Health care professionals follow appropriate procedures for vaccine storage and handling.
9. Up-to-date, written vaccination protocols are accessible at all locations where vaccines are administered.

10. People who administer vaccines and staff who manage or support vaccine administration are knowledgeable and receive ongoing education.
11. Health care professionals simultaneously administer as many indicated vaccine doses as possible.
12. Vaccination records for patients are accurate, complete, and easily accessible.
13. Health care professionals report adverse events after vaccination promptly and accurately to the Vaccine Adverse Events Reporting System (VAERS) and are aware of a separate program, the Vaccine Injury Compensation Program (VICP).
14. All personnel who have contact with patients are appropriately vaccinated.

IMPLEMENTATION OF STRATEGIES TO IMPROVE VACCINATION COVERAGE

15. Systems are used to remind parents/guardians, patients, and health care professionals when vaccinations are due and to recall those who are overdue.
16. Office- or clinic-based patient record reviews and vaccination coverage assessments are performed annually.
17. Health care professionals practice community-based approaches.

From Centers for Disease Control and Prevention: Standards for pediatric immunization practices, *Pediatrics* 112:958-963, 2003.

CONTRAINDICATIONS

Adverse reactions to vaccines is of concern to all clinicians. Although adverse reactions to vaccines are uncommon, they do occur and may be severe. Reactions can occur because of allergies to vaccine components (e.g., eggs, egg proteins, antibiotics, preservatives, and adjuvants). Therefore patient allergies should be considered before administration of specific vaccines.

Mild illness with or without low-grade fever is not a contraindication for vaccination. However, vaccination should be postponed in cases of moderate or severe febrile illness to avoid confusion between a vaccine side effect and an unknown underlying cause.

Pregnancy is not a contraindication for immunization using inactivated vaccines, antitoxins, or immune globulins. However, pregnant women should avoid live vaccines (i.e., MMR, varicella, and yellow fever) unless the risk of infection is very high. Likewise, immunocompromised patients should not receive live vaccines, although MMR

can be administered to asymptomatic HIV-infected people and varicella can be given to people with humoral immunodeficiency and some asymptomatic HIV-infected people, as determined by their physician (CDC, 2007a).

PARENTAL EDUCATION AND CONSENT

In October 1994 the CDC instituted a requirement that all health care providers administering any vaccine for DPT, MMR, or polio provide parents with Vaccine Information Statements (VIS). The VIS were written to simplify explanations about the benefits and risks associated with MMR, polio, DPT, and tetanus/diphtheria vaccines. Since that time all providers are required to provide a copy of the relevant VIS each time a patient is vaccinated (CDC, 2007a). The VIS have been translated into Chinese, French, Spanish, and Vietnamese and can be obtained from the CDC and the state health departments. Information on vaccine administration can also be found on the CDC's website.

DOCUMENTATION

Legal documentation of vaccinations is important for both the individual and the provider for future administration and follow-up of hypersensitivity reactions. Both individual and provider immunizations should be maintained. It is the responsibility of the health care provider to maintain accurate records. These records should include the patient name, dates immunized, vaccine type, vaccine manufacturer, vaccine lot number, date of the VIS, and the name, title, and address of the person administering the vaccine (Grimes, 2007).

REPORTING ADVERSE VACCINE EVENTS

The **Vaccine Adverse Event Reporting System (VAERS)** was developed to comply with the National Childhood Vaccine Injury Act of 1986 to "provide a single system for the collection and analysis of reports on all adverse events associated with the administration of any U.S. licensed vaccine in all groups" (Chen et al., 1994, p. 542). Events such as seizures following administration of the DTAP, or paralysis following the polio vaccine are reportable to the VAERS. The VAERS is operated by the CDC and Food and Drug Administration; additional information can be obtained by calling a 24-hour toll-free telephone number (1-800-822-7967) or visiting the VAERS website at http://www.cdc.gov/od/science/iso/research_activties/vaers.htm.

ADULT IMMUNIZATION

In general, people are aware of pediatric immunizations, but most adults and many health care providers are unaware of recommended immunizations for adults. For example, the CDC reports that a median of only 70% of persons 65 years or older have received the influenza vaccine (CDC, 2007a). Appropriately vaccinating adults should be a priority for all health care providers.

Many adolescents and young adults suffer needlessly from vaccine-preventable diseases such as HBV, varicella, influenza, and meningitis. To address this problem, in 1996 a routine health care visit was recommended for adolescents 11 to 12 years of age to ensure that this group would receive HBV, varicella vaccine (if no history of the disease), a second dose of MMR vaccine, and a booster dose of tetanus and diphtheria vaccine if it had been more than 5 years since their last booster. Also, many colleges and universities are now requiring new students to provide some minimal level of proof of immunization before enrollment. In 1999 the CDC recommended that vaccination against meningococcal disease be provided to freshmen and other undergraduate students who request the vaccine, although routine vaccination is not recommended (CDC, 2000). More recently, vaccination against human papilloma virus (HPV) was recommended for all girls, starting around age 11 or 12. "Catch-up" vaccination may also be encouraged for older girls and young women (CDC, 2007a).

The recognized source for information on vaccines and management of vaccination programs is *Epidemiology and Prevention of Vaccine-Preventable Diseases*. This book, commonly known as "The Pink Book," is published by the CDC and available in its entirety at http://www.cdc.gov/vaccines/pubs/pinkbook/default.htm.

SEXUALLY TRANSMITTED DISEASES

The number and type of different sexually transmitted diseases (STDs) has increased dramatically over the last several decades. Because of this, STDs have been termed a "hidden epidemic of tremendous health and economic consequence in the United States" (USDHHS, 2000, p. 253 Indeed, it is estimated that more than 19 million cases of STDs occur each year in the United States, with almost half of them in people aged 15 to 24 years (USDHHS, CDC, 2005). Direct medical costs related to STDs in the United States are estimated to be up to $14.1 billion annually. People considered at risk for STDs and HIV infection include the following:

- Those who are contacts of, or have a previous history of, documented STD and HIV infection
- Pregnant women
- Individuals who are or were recently sexually active (especially those with multiple sexual partners)
- Individuals living in areas with high prevalence of HIV and STDs
- Homosexual and bisexual men
- Drug and alcohol abusers
- Those involved in the exchange of sex for drugs or money (USDHHS/ODPHP, 1998)

Until as recently as the early 1980s, the only STDs (also called *sexually transmitted infections [STIs]*) commonly recognized by the public were syphilis and gonorrhea. By the beginning of the century, more than a dozen STDs were recognized. In addition to syphilis and gonorrhea, the most commonly occurring include: HIV, hepatitis B and C, chlamydia, genital herpes, HPV, trichomoniasis, and bacterial vaginosis. The symptoms of STDs vary with gender, the infection present, and the severity of the infection. Nurses who work in public health, school health, and in family practice areas must be familiar with the signs, symptoms, and treatment of STDs. Visit the CDC website or refer to *The Red Book* for this information.

PRIMARY PREVENTION OF SEXUALLY TRANSMITTED DISEASES

Primary prevention of STDs is based on changing the sexual behaviors that place individuals at risk. Education and counseling on abstinence, high-risk behaviors, and safer sex strategies (e.g., the use of condoms and other barriers and spermicides) is essential in primary prevention of STDs. It is the responsibility of the health care provider to counsel and educate those at risk to change their behaviors. When counseling clients at risk for STDs, it is also important to use language and terminology that the client understands and to reassure them that treatment will be provided regardless of ability to pay, citizenship or immigration status, language spoken, or lifestyle.

Sexual intimacy in a mutually monogamous relationship between partners known to be disease-free and sexual abstinence are the only certain ways to prevent infection. To reduce the possibility of exposure, safer sex counseling should include correct use of latex condoms for each sexual encounter, avoidance of sex with high-risk partners, avoiding anal intercourse, and avoiding the use of substances that impair judgment (e.g., alcohol, cocaine, marijuana).

SECONDARY PREVENTION OF SEXUALLY TRANSMITTED DISEASES

Early diagnosis and prompt, appropriate treatment are essential in stopping the spread of STDs. Treatment must include instruction on medication compliance and referral for treatment of all sex partners. In most cases, partners of clients with STDs should be examined. Resources for referral should be identified

in advance, and information should be made available where STDs are most likely to be detected (e.g., drug treatment and HIV treatment centers).

TRENDS IN INCIDENCE AND PREVALENCE OF SELECTED COMMUNICABLE DISEASES

Nurses who work in community-based settings should continually watch for changes in rates of communicable diseases. It is particularly important to monitor trends in area populations and communities. Several diseases are discussed here because of their importance to nurses in community-based practice.

ACQUIRED IMMUNODEFICIENCY SYNDROME AND HUMAN IMMUNODEFICIENCY VIRUS

It is well known that HIV is transmitted primarily by sexual contact involving the exchange of body fluids (e.g., vaginal secretions and semen) with an infected individual. It is also transmitted by the following means: blood transfusion or exposure to blood, blood products, or tissues of an infected person; by perinatal transmission from an infected mother to the child during pregnancy, delivery, or when breastfeeding; and by sharing needles or syringes with an infected person. The infection of HIV is widespread; an estimated 47 million adults and children have AIDS worldwide. In the United States an estimated 1.2 million people are HIV positive, with 24% to 27% being unaware of their diagnosis (CDC , 2006). In recent years incidence rates have stabilized at about 40,000 cases per year (United Nations/World Health Organization [UN/WHO], 2006) The UN/WHO report on HIV/AIDS for 2006 states "The future course of the world's HIV epidemics hinges in many respects on the behaviours [*sic*] young people adopt or maintain, and the contextual factors that affect those choices" (Joint United Nations Programme on HIV/AIDS, pg. 8). This statement emphasizes the need for prevention and education among teenagers and young adults.

At the inception of the epidemic, HIV/AIDS was largely found in white men who had sex with men; however, this trend has changed over the last decade. Indeed, the proportion of cases among whites has decreased from 60% to less than half of all cases. Minorities now bear the heaviest HIV burden in the

United States, with 50% of new AIDS cases occurring among African Americans and 20% among Hispanics. Men still account for the most new diagnoses (73%), with two-thirds of those attributable to homosexual sex (UN/WHO, 2006). The prevalence of AIDS among women has also risen, and women now account for 27% of all cases (UN/WHO, 2006). Fortunately, however, because of widespread testing of pregnant women and treatment with zidovudine (formerly called *azidothymidine [AZT]*), perinatal transmission rates have declined substantially.

Treatment for HIV and AIDS has become relatively effective over the last decade, changing AIDS from a death sentence to a chronic disease for those who have access to care. Management of HIV and AIDS, however, is highly complex, very expensive, and changes frequently. In addition, side effects can be significant and debilitating. Drugs used to treat HIV infection include antiemetics, antimicrobials, antifungals, antivirals, protease inhibitors, antimycobacterials, and antiretrovirals, among others.

Prevention efforts should be targeted at creating awareness and reduction of risk behaviors in high-risk populations and preventing transmission of HIV infection by people who are infected. Periodic testing of those in high-risk groups (e.g., those practicing unprotected sex, IV drug users) should be encouraged, and referrals for treatment should be planned in advance.

TUBERCULOSIS

Although the incidence of TB in the United States has been stable for the last decade, ranging from around 18,000 cases in 1998 to less than 14,000 in 2005, the potential for outbreaks exists. In addition, many new cases are identified in immigrants and those in other high-risk groups. This trend is cause for concern, in particular because of the emergence of multiple drug-resistant strains.

Persons at risk for TB include the medically underserved (particularly those of Black, Hispanic, Asian, Native American, and Alaskan Native heritage); foreign-born individuals from high-prevalence areas (Asia, Africa, and Latin America); those in close contact with infectious TB cases; individuals with medical conditions known to increase the risk of TB (e.g., HIV, diabetes, chronic renal failure, conditions requiring prolonged corticosteroid therapy); alcoholics and IV drug users; residents of high-risk

environments (long-term care facilities, correctional institutions, and mental institutions), and health care workers who serve high-risk clients (USDHHS/ODPHP, 1998). Guidelines for TB screening are as follows:

- Screening for TB should be performed on children and adults from high-risk groups.
- The Mantoux test (intradermal injection of 0.1 ml of purified protein derivative in the long axis of the forearm) should be performed whenever possible.
- The Mantoux test should be read 48 to 72 hours after placement by palpating the margin of induration and measuring and recording the diameter. Treatment is indicated if induration is greater than 5 mm to greater than 15 mm, depending on exposure, age, risk factors, and presence of symptoms.
- It should be recognized that absence of a reaction does not exclude a diagnosis of TB infection, particularly when the individual has symptoms of active disease. Induration of less than 5 mm may occur early in the course of TB infection or in individuals with altered immune function (e.g., clients with AIDS).
- Vaccination with BCG may cause false-positive Mantoux reactions, but this decreases with time and rarely causes an induration of 15 mm or greater.
- Live vaccines such as MMR and oral polio vaccine may interfere with response to the Mantoux test. Tuberculosis testing may be administered either concurrently with these vaccines or 4 to 6 weeks afterward.

Additional testing after positive Mantoux results consists of chest radiograph and sputum smear and culture to determine if there is active disease. If the results of these tests are negative, the client is usually placed on a preventive medication regimen, typically oral isoniazid (INH) 300 mg daily for 6 to 12 months (CDC, 1994c). For clients with active TB as evidenced by radiographs and sputum cultures, therapy consists of administration of multiple drugs over a period of several months, depending on symptoms, exposure, preexisting conditions, and sputum cultures.

EMERGING INFECTIONS

Emerging infectious diseases are those diseases whose incidence in humans has increased within the past two decades or threatens to increase in the near future. They can be new or previously unrecognized infectious diseases, reemerging diseases, or infectious diseases that have developed resistance to previously effective antimicrobial drugs. Factors identified as contributing to concern over emerging infectious diseases include social and environmental changes, explosive population growth, expanding poverty, urban migration, international travel, changes in the way food is processed and distributed, and technology (CDC, 1998).

Box 19-2 lists some emerging infections of which nurses who work in community-based settings should be aware. Other potentially important emerging infections that have been the subject of concern are *Escherichia coli* 0157:H7, group A streptococcal

disease, Hantavirus pulmonary syndrome, and drug-resistant pneumococcus and avian flu. All health care providers should monitor current concerns or trends in communicable diseases in their community to assist in identification of suspect cases and provide education, prevention, and early treatment where indicated.

To address concerns about emerging infections, the CDC has developed a set of goals and objectives (CDC, 1998). These include objectives to strengthen infectious disease surveillance and response, improve methods for gathering and evaluating surveillance data, ensure the use of surveillance data to improve public health practice and medical treatment, and strengthen global capacity to monitor and

---

BOX **19-2** Emerging Infections

VARIANT CREUTZFELDT-JAKOB DISEASE

Variant Creutzfeldt-Jakob disease (vCJD) first appeared in the United Kingdom in the mid-1990s, and cases have been identified in a number of countries in northern Europe and elsewhere around the world. It is thought that vCJD is caused by a newly recognized type of transmissible agent called a *prion*. New vCJD is possibly transmitted by ingestion of beef from animals afflicted with bovine spongiform encephalopathy (mad cow disease). At least three infected cattle have been identified in the United States (one each in 2003, 2004, and 2006).

WEST NILE VIRUS

West Nile virus is a potentially serious mosquito-borne disease. The majority of people (about 80%) who are infected do not develop symptoms; some people (about 20%) experience flu-like symptoms that range in severity from mild to incapacitating and deadly. In some people, often elders, the virus can cause severe inflammation of the central nervous system leading to encephalitis or meningitis. Infections with the West Nile virus have increased dramatically in the United States since 2000: in 2002, 4156 cases; 2003, 9862 cases; 2004, 2539 cases; and 2005, 3000 cases. In these 4 years, 767 people have died from West Nile virus (CDC, 2005a; 2007c).

FOODBORNE OUTBREAKS

The United States has had several multistate foodborne outbreaks, including outbreaks caused by *Cyclospora* parasites on fresh raspberries, hepatitis A on frozen strawberries, and *Escherichia coli* 0157:H7 bacteria in apple cider, lettuce, alfalfa sprouts, tomatoes, and ground beef.

COMMUNITY-ASSOCIATED METHICILLIN-RESISTANT *S. AUREUS* (CA-MRSA)

MRSA has historically occurred almost exclusively among persons in hospitals and healthcare facilities. Recently there have been a troubling number of cases of MRSA diagnosed

in people who have not been hospitalized (CA-MRSA). The CDC has investigated clusters of CA-MRSA among athletes, military recruits, children, prisoners, and others. Factors associated with the spread of CA-MRSA include close contact, presence of cuts or abrasions, crowded living conditions, poor hygiene, and contaminated items and surfaces (CDC, 2005b).

NOROVIRUS

Noroviruses, also described as *Norwalk-like viruses* (NLV), are a leading cause of gastroenteritis in humans. NLV are highly contagious, and transmission is primarily the fecal-oral route, either by consumption of contaminated food or water or by direct person-to-person spread. The CDC estimates that 23 million cases of acute gastroenteritis each year are due to norovirus infection (at least 50% of all foodborne outbreaks of gastroenteritis). Common settings for outbreaks include restaurants (36%), nursing homes (23%), schools (13%), and cruise ships (10%) (CDC, 2006).

PERTUSSIS

U.S. incidence of pertussis has been climbing significantly in recent years. Consequently it could be considered a reemerging infection. Because vaccination to prevent pertussis has been routine since the 1950s, the number of reported cases remained around 5000 to 7000 through 2001, with periodic outbreaks. In 2002 the number of cases rose to 9770; there were 11,647 cases in 2003 and more than 25,000 cases in 2004 and 2005. The CDC reports that since 1990, there has been a disproportionate increase in the numbers of adolescents and adults affected during outbreaks (CDC, 2007d).

respond to emerging infectious diseases. The areas targeted for preventing emerging infectious diseases are the following:

- *Antimicrobial resistance:* The emergence of drug resistance in bacteria, parasites, viruses, and fungi is concerning, and many drug choices for treatment of common infections are becoming increasingly limited.
- *Foodborne and waterborne diseases:* Changes in the ways food is processed and distributed are causing more multistate outbreaks of foodborne infections; a new group of waterborne pathogens has emerged that is unaffected by routine disinfection methods.
- *Vectorborne and zoonotic diseases:* Many emerging or reemerging diseases are acquired from animals or transmitted by arthropods; environmental changes can affect the incidence of these diseases by altering the habitats of disease vectors.
- *Disease transmitted through blood transfusions or blood products:* Improvements in blood donor screening, serologic testing, and transfusion practice have helped make the U.S. blood supply relatively safe, but continued vigilance is needed.
- *Chronic diseases caused by infectious agents:* Several chronic diseases and some forms of cancer, heart disease, and ulcers might be caused or intensified by infectious agents.
- *Vaccine development and use:* Although many childhood diseases have been virtually eliminated, additional vaccines are needed to prevent diseases that are a burden in the United States or internationally (e.g., HIV, hepatitis C, malaria).
- *Diseases of persons with impaired host defenses:* Opportunistic infections are rising because of the number of persons whose defenses are impaired by illness, medical treatment, or as a result of age.
- *Diseases of pregnant women and newborns:* Some asymptomatic infections in pregnant women can increase the infant's risk of prematurity, low birth weight, long-term disability, or death; effective and accessible prenatal care is essential to preventing infection in pregnant women and babies.
- *Diseases of travelers, immigrants, and refugees:* Persons who cross international boundaries are at increased risk for contracting infectious diseases and can also disseminate diseases to new places (CDC, 2007a).

INTERNATIONAL TRAVEL

International travel may greatly increase exposure to a number of communicable diseases. Jong and McMullen (1995) state that international travelers should seek medical advice 4 to 6 weeks in advance of departure to allow "adequate time for immunizations to be scheduled, for advice and prescriptions to be given, and for specific information to be obtained when needed" (p. 3). Destinations obviously dictate travel precautions with regard to health. Of particular concern are enteric diseases, malaria, rabies and other vectorborne diseases, STDs and HIV, and other illnesses. Individual research into specific risks and careful planning of primary and secondary prevention is vitally important.

Before leaving the United States, the traveler should complete a traveler's health history, which should be carried in a safe place throughout the trip. This document should contain immunization records, a list of current medications, a list of medical problems, known drug allergies, blood type, name and telephone number of the regular doctor, and name and telephone number of the closest relative or friend in the United States.

The traveler should also prepare a medical kit to take along that includes anticipated necessary supplies and medications. To be included are any prescription and nonprescription medications (e.g., aspirin, acetaminophen or ibuprofen, antibiotic ointment, antifungal powder or cream, decongestant tablets, diarrhea prevention medications, and hydrocortisone cream). General health and first aid supplies should include antiseptic solution, Band-Aids, extra eyeglasses, insect repellent (if applicable), sunscreen, and premoistened towelettes. Women may want to take sanitary supplies and antifungal vaginal cream or suppositories.

Immunizations and prophylactic pharmacologic treatment recommendations are based on location of travel. Vaccines are available to protect against cholera, hepatitis A, HBV, Japanese encephalitis, typhoid, meningococcal disease, and yellow fever. In addition, recommendations for taking prophylactic medication for malaria should be followed. Specific information can be obtained from the local health department and from the CDC's website.

USE OF COMMUNICABLE DISEASES AS WEAPONS

The attacks of September 11, 2001, awakened Americans to their vulnerability to terrorism. The anthrax attacks that followed the World Trade Center collapse brought the specter of biologic weapons to the forefront of public attention. The CDC has placed possible agents of **bioterrorism** into three categories: Category A Agents, Category B Agents, and Category C Agents. Characteristics of each are presented in Table 19-4.

Of particular concern to health care providers are the **Category A Agents** (anthrax, botulism, plague, smallpox, tularemia, viral hemorrhagic fevers). These will be discussed briefly.

Anthrax is a spore-forming bacterium capable of producing three types of illnesses, with the type of infection depending on the mode of transmission. Skin or cutaneous anthrax is the least dangerous form of the disease, with a 1% to 20% mortality rate. Skin anthrax usually occurs as a result of contact with hides, wool, or leather from an infected animal. Cutaneous anthrax is marked by the appearance of a black, painless sore that may heal slowly without treatment. Inhalation anthrax occurs when the anthrax spores are inhaled, and is the most lethal form of the disease, with a mortality rate of 80%. Due to its high mortality rate, inhalation is the mode of transmission used in bioterrorism. Gastrointestinal anthrax is also deadly and carries a mortality rate of 25% to 60%. Severe vomiting and diarrhea follow the ingestion of contaminated meat. Anthrax is not transmissible from person to person and responds well to several antibiotics such as penicillin, doxycycline, and fluoroquinolones. Though the disease is not communicable, the lethality of inhalation anthrax, as well as the relative ease by which the spores may be delivered, makes anthrax a formidable agent of bioterrorism (CDC, 2007b).

Botulism is a paralytic disease caused by the toxin produced by *Clostridium botulinum*. Foodborne botulism results from the ingestion of the toxin from a food source, often home-canned goods. Foodborne botulism is a public health emergency due to the possibility of many exposures to the toxin through food products. Wound botulism occurs when wounds are infected with the botulism toxin. The third type, infant botulism, occurs when an infant ingests *C. botulinum*, and the toxin is released in the GI tract. Inhalation botulism occurs when the toxin is inhaled and is a result of a planned release. Inhalation botulism does not occur naturally. Botulism is not transmissible from person to person and is treated with the botulism antitoxin, which is effective in reducing the severity of the symptoms but must be administered early after exposure to the toxin to be effective. The paralysis of botulism begins with the eyelids, producing droopy eyes, and moves down the body. When the paralysis reaches the level of

TABLE **19-4** Characteristics of Bioterrorism Agents

CATEGORY OF AGENTS	CHARACTERISTICS
CATEGORY A AGENTS	Can be easily disseminated or transmitted from person to person
	Result in high mortality rates and have the potential for major public health impact
	Might cause public panic and social disruption
	Require special action for public health preparedness
CATEGORY B AGENTS	Are moderately easy to disseminate
	Result in moderate morbidity rates and low mortality rates
	Require specific enhancements of CDC's diagnostic capacity and enhanced disease surveillance
CATEGORY C AGENTS	Include emerging pathogens that could be engineered for mass dissemination in the future because of availability, ease of production and dissemination, and that have potential for high morbidity and mortality rates and major health impact

the diaphragm, death results unless the victim receives mechanical ventilation. The severity of botulism and the possibility of infecting thousands with an aerosol release makes botulism attractive as a weapon (CDC, 2007b).

Plague is caused by the *Yersinia pestis* bacteria, which exists in nature. About 5 to 15 cases of plague occur annually in the United States. The cases are rare and typically scattered among rural western regions. If used by terrorists, aerosolized *Y. pestis* could be sprayed over a city, causing plague. The two types of plague, pneumonic and bubonic, differ in communicability and symptoms. Pneumonic plague is contracted through breathing the *Y. pestis* particles from the air. The victim develops fever, weakness, and pneumonia, which can rapidly progress to shock and death. Pneumonic plague is transmissible from person to person. Bubonic plague is contracted through the bites of fleas infected with *Y. pestis*. Large swollen lymph nodes called *buboes* develop as a result of exposure to the bacteria. If untreated, bubonic plague can progress to pneumonic plague, becoming communicable from person to person. Plague is readily treated by antibiotics such as doxycycline and fluoroquinolone (CDC, 2007b).

Smallpox is caused by the variola virus and is a contagious disease that is often fatal. Smallpox has been eliminated, except for laboratory stockpiles; mass vaccination with the smallpox vaccine has ended. The smallpox vaccine is highly effective in preventing the disease and is also effective if given postexposure. After a person has become ill with smallpox, there is no known treatment. Smallpox is communicable from person to person, but prolonged face-to-face contact is necessary before the disease is contracted. In most cases the disease was transmitted to household caregivers of the victim. Smallpox is rarely transmitted by fomites such as bedding and equipment. Following an incubation period of up to 17 days, the victim becomes very ill and bedridden with high fever and malaise. After 2 days, the victim develops small red spots in the mouth and on the tongue. At this time the victim is infectious and remains so until all of the lesions have healed. The typical smallpox rash begins on the face and spreads to the arms and legs, then to the hands and feet. The lesions are painful, full-thickness lesions that are marked by an umbilication. The rash of smallpox develops slowly, making all lesions at the same stage of development. The rash may take from 3 to 4 weeks to completely resolve, leaving the person badly scarred. Due to the lack of immunity against this disease, mass exposure to smallpox could result in many deaths (CDC, 2007b).

Tularemia is a potentially deadly illness that is caused by the *Francisella tularensis* bacteria. Tularemia occurs naturally in rabbits and rodents. Tularemia disease in humans results from the bite of infected ticks or insects, handling infected animal carcasses, ingesting contaminated food or water, or by breathing in the *F. tularensis* bacteria. Tularemia is not communicable from person to person. It manifests with sudden fever, chills, diarrhea, muscle pain, dry cough, and progressive weakness. Tularemia can be fatal if not quickly treated with antibiotics. Aerosolized *F. tularensis* sprayed over a city could cause severe respiratory infection in many people. A small amount of the bacteria is capable of causing disease, making *F. tularensis* attractive as a weapon (CDC, 2007b).

Viral hemorrhagic fevers (VHFs) are a group of illnesses caused by a distinct family of viruses. Infection may lead to multisystem failure and hemorrhage, but hemorrhage is rarely the cause of death in victims of VHFs. Rather, the failure of multiple body systems results in death. The viruses that cause VHFs include four families: arenaviruses, filoviruses, bunyaviruses, and flaviviruses. VHFs are found all over the globe but are restricted to regions where the host lives. All VHFs are thought to be zoonotic, and humans are infected when they come into contact with infected animals. Some of the VHFs such as Ebola, Marburg, Lassa, and Crimean-Congo, are transmissible from person to person and are spread through contact with contaminated body fluids. VHFs vary in the signs and symptoms displayed, but generally the victim will have malaise, dizziness, and subdural bleeding. Internal bleeding and bleeding from body orifices may develop. In these cases the victim will quickly progress to shock, coma, and seizures. There is no treatment for the VHFs, only supportive care (CDC, 2007b).

The list of all the known agents of bioterrorism, fact sheets detailing each of these agents, and an image library can be found on the CDC website. As technology advances and the physiology of diseases changes, the lists of diseases and agents useful for bioterrorism will grow. It is important that all nurses have some knowledge of these agents. Nurses who work in emergency departments and public health departments will be on the front lines of a bioterror event and must remain current in their knowledge of these agents (CDC, 2007b).

SUMMARY

Prevention of communicable disease, whether primary or secondary, is one of the most important functions of nurses who work in community-based settings. This chapter has discussed several aspects of communicable disease control, including identification and reporting of suspected cases, prevention through immunization, and education and counseling efforts to reduce transmission of STDs. Encouraging monitoring of selected diseases and emerging infections and disease prevention during international travel concludes the discussion.

In the opening case study, Mark was a public health nurse responsible for investigating cases of reportable communicable diseases, and because of this he had a direct, defined role in communicable disease control. However, it is important to remember that all nurses need to be aware of communicable diseases in their area of practice and know how and when to report them.

As mentioned throughout the chapter, considerable information is available online for those wishing to learn more about any of the communicable diseases discussed here. Of primary importance is the information provided by the CDC (www.cdc.gov), particularly for information relevant to the United States. State health departments also maintain websites for more specific, regionally related information.

KEY POINTS

- Although improvement in morbidity and mortality from communicable diseases has been dramatic, particularly for vaccine-preventable diseases (measles, diphtheria, polio), a number of threats and risks still exist (HIV, TB, influenza).
- Communicable diseases may be transmitted directly (kissing, touching, sexual contact) or indirectly (through fomites, substances, or vec-

tors). Airborne transmission may be either direct or indirect.
- The CDC and the individual state legislatures have identified Reportable Communicable Diseases. Guidelines for reporting include who is responsible for reporting; what information is required; how, when, and to whom to report; and steps taken to control spread.
- Many communicable diseases are preventable through immunization. The recommended immunization schedule for infants and children is complex and has changed several times in recent years. Providers should be aware of contraindications and precautions for vaccines, parent education materials, consent requirements, and reporting of adverse vaccine events.
- The number and incidence of STDs have increased dramatically over the last several decades. The most common STDs include chlamydia, gonorrhea, herpes, HIV, human papillomavirus, and syphilis.
- Nurses working in community-based settings should watch for changes in rates of communicable diseases. Diseases that should be closely monitored include TB, HIV and AIDS, and emerging infections.
- Often, nurses in community settings are asked to advise clients on issues related to international travel. Information that might be needed includes pretravel recommendations and immunization requirements and recommendations.
- Nurses in community settings should be aware of the agents that might potentially be used in bioterrorism attacks. The ability to recognize the diseases caused by Category A Agents (e.g. anthrax, smallpox) is vital.

Learning Activities & Application to Practice
In Class

1. Discuss modes of communicable disease transmission. Identify and outline primary prevention strategies to reduce or eliminate each type of transmission.
2. Visit the local public health department to discuss surveillance and control of communicable diseases. Find out about local and regional trends in communicable diseases. Learn about the process of reporting.

3. Discuss the current pediatric immunization schedule and the Standards for Pediatric Immunization Practices with classmates. Become aware of recent changes and contraindications and precautions.

In Clinical

4. In a log or diary, compile a list of communicable illnesses encountered in the clinical setting. When possible, participate in the process of reporting of communicable diseases.
5. Participate in a pediatric immunization clinic or work with nurses who routinely immunize children. If possible, help screen children for possible contraindications. Also provide the required parent education.

REFERENCES

American Academy of Pediatrics (2006): *The red book* (website): http://aapredbook.aappublications.org/current.shtml. Accessed September 29, 2007.

Centers for Disease Control and Prevention (2007a): *Epidemiology and prevention of vaccine-preventable diseases* (pink book), ed 10, Atlanta, 2007, Public Health Foundation.

Centers for Disease Control and Prevention (2007b): *Bioterrorism agents and diseases* (website): http://www.bt.cdc.gov/agent/agentlist-category.asp. Accessed September 30, 2007.

Centers for Disease Control and Prevention (2006): *HIV and AIDS in the Unites States: A picture of today's epidemic* (website): http://www.cdc.gov/hiv/topics/surveillance/united_states.htm. Accessed April 14, 2008.

Centers for Disease Control and Prevention (2007c): *West Nile virus activity in the U.S.* (website): http://www.cdc.gov/ncidod/dvbid/westnile/surv&controlCaseCount05_detailed.htm. Accessed October 6, 2007.

Centers for Disease Control and Prevention (2007d): *Norovirus: technical fact sheet* (website): http://www.cdc.gov/ncidod/dvrd/revb/gastro/norovirus-factsheet.htm. Accessed October 6, 2007.

Centers for Disease Control and Prevention (2007e): Summary of notifiable diseases–United States, 2005, *MMWR Morb Mortal Wkly Rep* 54(53):1, 2007.

Centers for Disease Control and Prevention (2006): Surveillance for acute viral hepatitis, *MMWR Morb Mortal Wkly Rep* 56:SS-3, 2006.

Centers for Disease Control and Prevention (2005a): *West Nile virus (WNV) fact sheet* (website): http://www.cdc.gov/ncidod/dvbid/westnile/wnv_factSheet.htm. Accessed October 6, 2007.

Centers for Disease Control and Prevention (2005b): *Community-associated MRSA information for clinicians* (website): http://www.cdc.gov/ncidod/dhqp/ar_mrsa_ca_clinicians.html. Accessed October 5, 2007.

Centers for Disease Control and Prevention (2003): Standards for pediatric immunization practices, *Pediatrics* 112:958, 2003.

Centers for Disease Control and Prevention (2000): Meningococcal disease and college students, recommendations of the Advisory Committee on Immunization Practices (ACIP), *MMWR Morb Mortal Wkly Rep* 49(RR-07):11, 2000.

Centers for Disease Control and Prevention (1998): Preventing emerging infectious disease: a strategy for the 21st century, overview of the updated CDC plan, *MMWR Morb Mortal Wkly Rep* 47(RR15):1, 1998.

Centers for Disease Control and Prevention (1992): *Principles of epidemiology*, ed 2, Atlanta, 1992, Centers for Disease Control and Prevention.

Chen RT, Rastogi SC, Mullen JR et al: The vaccine adverse event reporting system (VAERS), *Vaccine* 12(6):542, 1994.

Grimes DE: Communicable disease and public health. In Nies M, McEwen M, editors: *Community/public health nursing: promoting the health of populations*, ed 4, Philadelphia, 2007, Saunders.

Jong EC, McMullen R: Sexually transmitted disease and foreign travel. In Jong EC, McMullen R, editors: *The travel and tropical medicine manual*, ed 2, Philadelphia, 1995, Saunders.

Merrill RD, Timmreck TC: *Introduction to epidemiology*, ed 4, Sudbury, 2006, Jones and Bartlett.

National Center for Health Statistics: Deaths: leading causes for 2004, *Natl Vital Stat Rep* 55(10):1, 2007, National Center for Health Statistics.

United Nations/World Health Organization (2006): *The joint United Nations programme on HIV/AIDS* (website): http://www.who.int/globalatlas/default.asp. Accessed September 10, 2007.

U.S. Department of Health and Human Services: *Healthy people 2010*: conference ed, Washington, DC, 2000, Government Printing Office.

U.S. Department of Health and Human Services (2005): *Trends in sexually transmitted diseases in the United States, 2005* (website): http://www.cdc.gov/std/stats/toc2005.htm. Accessed September 10, 2007.

U.S. Department of Health and Human Services/Office of Disease Prevention, Health Promotion (USDHHS/ODPHP): *Clinician's handbook of preventive services*, ed 2, Washington, DC, 1998, Government Printing Office.

Appendix A

Giger and Davidhizar's Transcultural Assessment Model

CULTURALLY UNIQUE INDIVIDUAL

1. Place of birth
2. Cultural definition
   What is . . .
3. Race
   What is . . .
4. Length of time in country (if appropriate)

COMMUNICATION

1. Voice quality
   A. Strong, resonant
   B. Soft
   C. Average
   D. Shrill
2. Pronunciation and enunciation
   A. Clear
   B. Slurred
   C. Dialect (geographical)
3. Use of silence
   A. Infrequent
   B. Often
   C. Length
      (1) Brief
      (2) Moderate
      (3) Long
      (4) Not observed
4. Use of nonverbal
   A. Hand movement
   B. Eye movement
   C. Entire body movement
   D. Kinesics (gestures, expression, or stances)
5. Touch
   A. Startles or withdraws when touched
   B. Accepts touch without difficulty
   C. Touches others without difficulty
6. Ask these and similar questions:
   A. How do you get your point across to others?
   B. Do you like communicating with friends, family, and acquaintances?
   C. When asked a question, do you usually respond (in words or body movement, or both)?

D. If you have something important to discuss with your family, how would you approach them?

SPACE

1. Degree of comfort
   A. Moves when space invaded
   B. Does not move when space invaded
2. Distance in conversations
   A. 0 to 18 inches
   B. 18 inches to 3 feet
   C. 3 feet or more
3. Definition of space
   A. Describe degree of comfort with closeness when talking with or standing near others
   B. How do objects (e.g., furniture) in the environment affect your sense of space?
4. Ask these and similar questions:
   A. When you talk with family members, how close do you stand?
   B. When you communicate with coworkers and other acquaintances, how close do you stand?
   C. If a stranger touches you, how do you react or feel?
   D. If a loved one touches you, how do you react or feel?
   E. Are you comfortable with the distance between us now?

SOCIAL ORGANIZATION

1. Normal state of health
   A. Poor
   B. Fair
   C. Good
   D. Excellent
2. Marital status
3. Number of children
4. Parents living or deceased?
5. Ask these and similar questions:
   A. How do you define social activities?
   B. What are some activities that you enjoy?
   C. What are your hobbies, or what do you do when you have free time?

D. Do you believe in a Supreme Being?

E. How do you worship that Supreme Being?

F. What is your function (what do you do) in your family unit/system?

G. What is your role in your family unit/system (father, mother, child, advisor)?

H. When you were a child, what or who influenced you most?

I. What is/was your relationship with your siblings and parents?

J. What does work mean to you?

K. Describe your past, present, and future jobs.

L. What are your political views?

M. How have your political views influenced your attitude toward health and illness?

TIME

1. Orientation to time
   A. Past-oriented
   B. Present-oriented
   C. Future-oriented
2. View of time
   A. Social time
   B. Clock-oriented
3. Physiochemical reaction to time
   A. Sleeps at least 8 hours a night
   B. Goes to sleep and wakes on a consistent schedule
   C. Understands the importance of taking medication and other treatments on schedule
4. Ask these and similar questions:
   A. What kind of timepiece do you wear daily?
   B. If you have an appointment at 2 PM, what time is acceptable to arrive?
   C. If a nurse tells you that you will receive a medication in "about a half hour," realistically, how much time will you allow before calling the nurses' station?

ENVIRONMENTAL CONTROL

1. Locus-of-control
   A. Internal locus-of-control (believes that the power to affect change lies within)
   B. External locus-of-control (believes that fate, luck, and chance have a great deal to do with how things turn out)
2. Value orientation
   A. Believes in supernatural forces
   B. Relies on magic, witchcraft, and prayer to affect change
   C. Does not believe in supernatural forces
   D. Does not rely on magic, witchcraft, or prayer to affect change
3. Ask these and similar questions:
   A. How often do you have visitors at your home?
   B. Is it acceptable to you for visitors to drop in unexpectedly?
   C. Name some ways your parents or other persons treated your illnesses when you were a child.
   D. Have you or someone else in your immediate surroundings ever used a home remedy that made you sick?
   E. What home remedies have you used that worked? Will you use them in the future?
   F. What is your definition of "good health"?
   G. What is your definition of illness or "poor health"?

BIOLOGICAL VARIATIONS

1. Conduct a complete physical assessment noting:
   A. Body structure (small, medium, or large frame)
   B. Skin color
   C. Unusual skin discolorations
   D. Hair color and distribution
   E. Other visible physical characteristics (e.g., keloids, chloasma)
   F. Weight
   G. Height
   H. Check lab work for variances in hemoglobin, hematocrit, and sickle cell phenomena if Black or Mediterranean
2. Ask these and similar questions:
   A. What diseases or illnesses are common in your family?

B. Has anyone in your family been told that there is a possible genetic susceptibility for a particular disease?

C. Describe your family's typical behavior when a family member is ill.

D. How do you respond when you are angry?

E. Who (or what) usually helps you to cope during a difficult time?

F. What foods do you and your family like to eat?

G. Have you ever had any unusual cravings for:
   (1) White or red clay dirt?
   (2) Laundry starch?

H. When you were a child what types of foods did you eat?

I. What foods are family favorites or are considered traditional?

NURSING ASSESSMENT

1. Note whether the client has become culturally assimilated or observes own cultural practices.

2. Incorporate data into plan of nursing care:
   A. Encourage the client to discuss cultural differences; people from diverse cultures who hold different world views can enlighten nurses.
   B. Make efforts to accept and understand methods of communication.
   C. Respect the individual's personal need for space.
   D. Respect the rights of clients to honor and worship the Supreme Being of their choice.

E. Identify a clerical or spiritual person to contact.

F. Determine whether spiritual practices have implications for health, life, and well-being (e.g., Jehovah's Witnesses may refuse blood and blood derivatives; an Orthodox Jew may eat only kosher food high in sodium and may not drink milk when meat is served).

G. Identify hobbies, especially when devising interventions for a short or extended convalescence or for rehabilitation.

H. Honor time and value orientations and differences in these areas. Allay anxiety and apprehension if adherence to time is necessary.

I. Provide privacy according to personal need and health status of the client (NOTE: the perception of and reaction to pain may be culturally related).

J. Note cultural health practices.
   (1) Identify and encourage efficacious practices.
   (2) Identify and discourage dysfunctional practices.
   (3) Identify and determine whether neutral practices will have a long-term ill effect.

K. Note food preferences.
   (1) Make as many adjustments in diet as health status and long-term benefits will allow and that dietary department can provide.
   (2) Note dietary practices that may have serious implications for the client.

From Giger J, Davidhizar R: *Transcultural nursing: assessment and intervention*, St. Louis, 2007, Mosby.

This and all other appendixes can be found on the book's Evolve website in the Assessment Tools section.

Appendix B

Healthstyle: A Self-Test

All of us want good health. But many of us do not know how to be as healthy as possible. Health experts now describe *lifestyle* as one of the most important factors affecting health. In fact, it is estimated that as many as seven of the ten leading causes of death could be reduced through common-sense changes in lifestyle. That's what this brief test, developed by the Public Health Service, is all about. Its purpose is simply to tell you how well you are doing when it comes to staying healthy. The behaviors covered in the test are recommended for most Americans. Some of them may not apply to persons with certain chronic diseases or handicaps or to pregnant women. Such individuals may require special instructions from their physicians.

	Almost Always	Sometimes	Almost Never
Cigarette Smoking			
If you *never smoke*, enter a score of 10 for this section and go to the next section on *Alcohol and Drugs*.			
1. I avoid smoking cigarettes.	2	1	0
2. I smoke only low-tar and low-nicotine cigarettes *or* I smoke a pipe or cigars.	2	1	0

Smoking Score:_____

	Almost Always	Sometimes	Almost Never
Alcohol and Drugs			
1. I avoid drinking alcoholic beverages *or* I drink no more than one or two drinks a day.	4	1	0
2. I avoid using alcohol or other drugs (especially illegal drugs) as a way of handling stressful situations or the problems in my life.	2	1	0
3. I am careful not to drink alcohol when taking certain medicines (for example, medicine for sleeping, pain, colds, and allergies), or when pregnant.	2	1	0
4. I read and follow the label directions when using prescribed and over-the-counter drugs.	2	1	0

Alcohol and Drugs Score:_____

	Almost Always	Sometimes	Almost Never
Eating Habits			
1. I eat a variety of foods each day, including fruits and vegetables, whole grain breads and cereals, lean meats, dairy products, dry peas and beans, and nuts and seeds.	4	1	0
2. I limit the amount of fat, saturated fat, and cholesterol I eat (including fat on meats, eggs, butter, cream, shortenings, and organ meats such as liver).	2	1	0
3. I limit the amount of salt I eat by cooking with only small amounts, not adding salt at the table, and avoiding salty snacks.	2	1	0

4. I avoid eating too much sugar
   (especially frequent snacks of
   candy or soft drinks).   2   1   0

Eating Habits Score:_____

Exercise/Fitness

1. I maintain a desired weight,
   avoiding overweight and
   underweight.   3   1   0
2. I do vigorous exercise for
   15 to 30 minutes at least
   three times a week
   (examples: running, swimming,
   brisk walking).   3   1   0
3. At least three times a week, I do
   15 to 30 minutes of exercise that
   enhances my muscle tone
   (examples: yoga, calisthenics).   2   1   0
4. I spend part of my leisure
   time participating in individual,
   family, or team activities that
   increase my level of fitness
   (examples: gardening, bowling,
   golf, baseball).   2   1   0

Exercise/Fitness Score:_____

Stress Control

1. I have a job or do other work
   that I enjoy.   2   1   0
2. I find it easy to relax and express
   my feelings freely.   2   1   0
3. I recognize and prepare in advance
   for events or situations likely to be
   stressful for me.   2   1   0
4. I have close friends, relatives,
   or others I can talk to about
   personal matters and call
   on for help when
   I need them.   2   1   0

5. I participate in group
   activities (examples: church
   and community organizations)
   or hobbies I enjoy.   2   1   0

Stress Control Score:_____

Safety

1. I wear a seat belt while riding in
   a car.   2   1   0
2. I avoid driving while under the
   influence of alcohol and other drugs.   2   1   0
3. I obey traffic rules and the speed
   limit when driving.   2   1   0
4. I am careful when using
   potentially harmful products
   or substances (such as household
   cleaners, poisons, and
   electrical devices).   2   1   0
5. I avoid smoking in bed.   2   1   0

Safety Score:_____

WHAT YOUR SCORES MEAN TO YOU

Scores of 9 and 10

Excellent! Your answers show that you are aware of the importance of this area to your health. Even better, you are putting your knowledge to work for you by practicing good health habits. As long as you continue to do so, this area should not pose a serious health risk. It's likely you are setting an example for your family and friends to follow. Since you got a very high test score on this part of the test, you may want to consider other areas where your scores may suggest room for improvement.

Scores of 6 to 8

Your health practices in this area are good, but there is room for improvement. Look again at the items you answered with a "Sometimes" or "Almost

Never." What changes can you make to improve your score? Even a small change can often help you achieve better health.

Scores of 3 to 5

Your health risks are showing. Would you like more information about the risks you are facing and why it is important for you to change these behaviors? Perhaps you need help in deciding how to successfully make the changes you desire. In either case, help is available.

Scores of 0 to 2

Obviously, you were concerned enough about your health to take the test, but your answers show that you may be taking serious and unnecessary risks with your health. Perhaps you are not aware of the risks and what to do about them. The information and help you need are available, if you wish. The next step toward good health habits is up to you.

YOU CAN START RIGHT NOW!

The test you just completed offered numerous suggestions to help you reduce your risk of disease and premature death. Here are some of the most significant:

AVOID CIGARETTES. Cigarette smoking is the single most important preventable cause of illness and early death. It is especially risky for pregnant women and their unborn babies. Persons who stop smoking reduce their risk of getting heart disease and cancer. So if you're a cigarette smoker, think twice about lighting up that next cigarette. If you choose to continue smoking, try decreasing the number of cigarettes you smoke and switch to a low tar and nicotine brand.

FOLLOW SENSIBLE DRINKING HABITS. Alcohol produces changes in mood and behavior. Most people who drink are able to control their intake of alcohol and avoid undesired—and often harmful—effects. Heavy, regular use of alcohol can lead to cirrhosis of the liver, a leading cause of death. Also, statistics clearly show that mixing drinking and driving is often the cause of fatal or crippling accidents. So if you drink, do it wisely and in moderation. Use care in taking drugs. Today's greater use of drugs—both prescribed and illegal—is one of our most serious health risks. Some prescription drugs can be dangerous if taken with alcohol or before driving. Excessive or continued use of tranquilizers (or "pep pills") can cause physical and mental problems. Using or experimenting with illicit drugs such as marijuana, heroin, cocaine, and PCP may lead to a number of damaging effects or even death.

EAT SENSIBLY. Overweight individuals are at greater risk for diabetes, gall bladder disease, and high blood pressure. So it makes good sense to maintain proper weight. But good eating habits also mean minimizing the amount of fat (especially saturated fat), cholesterol, sugar, and salt in your diet. If you must snack, try nibbling on fresh fruits and vegetables. You'll feel better—and look better too.

EXERCISE REGULARLY. Almost everyone can benefit from exercise—and there's some form of exercise almost everyone can do. (If you have any doubt, check first with your doctor.) Usually as little as 15 to 30 minutes of vigorous exercise three times a week will help you have a healthier heart, eliminate excess weight, tone up sagging muscles, and help you sleep better. Think how much difference all these improvements could make in the way you feel!

LEARN TO HANDLE STRESS. Stress is a normal part of living; everyone faces it to some degree. The causes of stress can be good or bad, desirable or undesirable (a promotion on the job or the loss of a spouse). Properly handled, stress need not be a permanent problem. But unhealthy responses to stress—such as driving too fast or erratically, drinking too much, or accepting prolonged anger or grief—can cause a variety of physical and mental problems. Even on a very busy day, find a few minutes to slow down and relax. Talk over a problem with someone you trust; it can often help you find a satisfactory solution. Pick your battles, and learn to distinguish between things that are "worth fighting about" and things that are less important.

BE SAFETY CONSCIOUS. Think "safety first" at home, at work, at school, at play, and on the highway. Buckle seat belts and obey traffic rules. Keep poisons and weapons out of the reach of children, and keep emergency numbers by your telephone. When the unexpected happens, you'll be prepared.

Where Do You Go From Here?

Start by asking yourself a few frank questions: "Am I really doing all I can to be as healthy as possible?" "What steps can I take to feel better?" "Am I willing to begin now?" If you scored low in one or more sections of the test, decide what changes you want to make for improvement. You might pick the aspect of your lifestyle where you feel you have the best chance for success, and tackle that one first. Once you have improved your score there, go on to other areas.

If you've already tried to change your health habits (to stop smoking or exercise regularly, for example), don't be discouraged if you haven't yet succeeded. The difficulty you're encountering may be due to influences you've never really thought about—like advertising—or to a lack of support and encouragement. Understanding these influences is an important step toward changing the way they affect you.

THERE'S HELP AVAILABLE. In addition to personal actions you can take on your own, there are community programs and groups (such as the YMCA or the local chapter of the American Heart Association) that can assist you and your family to make the changes you want to make. If you'd like to know more about these groups or about health risks, contact your local health department or the National Health Information Clearinghouse. There's a lot you can do to stay healthy or to improve your health—and there are organizations that can help you. Start a new HEALTHSTYLE today!

For assistance in locating specific information on these and other health topics, write to: National Health Information Clearinghouse, P.O. Box 1133, Washington, DC 20013. Or visit the National Health Information Center website at www.health.gov/nhic/.

From Office of Disease Prevention and Health Promotion: *Healthstyle: A self-test* (Publication No. H0012, Washington, DC, 1981, National Health Information Clearinghouse.

This and all other appendixes can be found on the book's Evolve website in the Assessment Tools section.

Appendix C

Healthy Heart I.Q.

Please answer "true" or "false" to the following questions to test your knowledge of heart disease and its risk factors. Then check the answers and explanations that follow to see how well you did.

1. The risk factors for heart disease that you *can do something about* are high blood pressure, high blood cholesterol, smoking, obesity, and physical inactivity.   T   F
2. A stroke is often the first symptom of high blood pressure, and a heart attack is often the first symptom of high blood cholesterol.   T   F
3. A blood pressure greater than or equal to 140/90 mm Hg is generally considered to be high.   T   F
4. High blood pressure affects the same number of Blacks as it does whites.   T   F
5. The best ways to treat and control high blood pressure are to control your weight, exercise, eat less salt (sodium), restrict your intake of alcohol, and take your high blood pressure medicine, if prescribed by your doctor.   T   F
6. A blood cholesterol level of 240 mg/dL is desirable for adults.   T   F
7. The most effective dietary way to lower the level of your blood cholesterol is to eat foods low in cholesterol.   T   F
8. Lowering blood cholesterol levels can help people who have already had a heart attack.   T   F
9. Only children from families at high risk of heart disease need to have their blood cholesterol levels checked.   T   F
10. Smoking is a major risk factor for four of the five leading causes of death, including heart attack, stroke, cancer, and lung diseases such as emphysema and bronchitis.   T   F
11. If you have had a heart attack, quitting smoking can help reduce your chances of having a second attack.   T   F
12. Someone who has smoked for 30 to 40 years probably will not be able to quit smoking.   T   F
13. The best way to lose weight is to increase physical activity and eat fewer calories.   T   F
14. Heart disease is the leading killer of men **and** women in the United States.   T   F

1.   TRUE   High blood pressure, smoking, and high blood cholesterol are the three most important risk factors for heart disease. On the average, each one doubles your chance of developing heart disease, so a person who has all three of these risk factors is eight times more likely to develop heart disease than someone who has none. Obesity increases the likelihood of developing high blood cholesterol and high blood pressure, both of which increase your risk for heart disease. Physical inactivity increases your risk of heart attack. Regular exercise and good nutrition are essential to reducing high blood pressure, high blood cholesterol,

and overweight. People who exercise are also more likely to cut down or stop smoking.

2. TRUE   A person with high blood pressure or high blood cholesterol may feel fine and look great; there are often no signs that anything is wrong until a stroke or heart attack occurs. To find out if you have high blood pressure or high blood cholesterol, you should be tested by a doctor, nurse, or other health professional.

3. TRUE   A blood pressure of 140/90 mm Hg or greater is generally classified as *high blood pressure*. However, blood pressures that fall below 140/90 mm Hg can sometimes be a problem. If the diastolic pressure (the second or lower number) is between 85 and 89, a person is at increased risk for heart disease or stroke and should have his/her blood pressure checked at least once a year by a health professional. The higher your blood pressure, the greater your risk of developing heart disease or stroke. Controlling high blood pressure reduces your risk.

4. FALSE   High blood pressure is more common in Blacks than in whites. It affects 29 of every 100 black adults, compared to 26 of every 100 white adults. Also, with aging, high blood pressure is generally more severe among Blacks than among whites and therefore causes more strokes, heart disease, and kidney failure.

5. TRUE   Recent studies show that lifestyle changes can help keep blood pressure levels normal, even into advanced age, and are important in treating and preventing high blood pressure. Limit high-salt foods, which include many snack foods like potato chips, salted pretzels, and salted crackers; processed foods, such as canned soups; and condiments, such as ketchup and soy sauce. Also, it is **extremely**

important to take blood pressure medication, if prescribed by your doctor, to make sure your blood pressure stays under control.

6. FALSE   A total blood cholesterol level of under 200 mg/dL is **desirable** and usually puts you at a lower risk for heart disease. A blood cholesterol level of 240 mg/dL or above is **high** and increases your risk of heart disease. If your cholesterol level is high, your doctor will want to check your levels of LDL cholesterol ("bad" cholesterol) and HDL cholesterol ("good" cholesterol). A HIGH level of LDL cholesterol increases your risk of heart disease, as does a LOW level of HDL cholesterol. A cholesterol level of 200 to 239 mg/dL is considered **borderline-high** and usually increases your risk for heart disease. If your cholesterol is borderline-high, you should speak to your doctor to see if additional cholesterol tests are needed. All adults 20 years of age or older should have their blood cholesterol level checked at least once every 5 years.

7. FALSE   Reducing the amount of cholesterol in your diet is important; however, eating foods **low in saturated fat** is the most effective dietary way to lower blood cholesterol levels, along with eating less total fat and cholesterol. Choose low-saturated-fat foods, such as grains, fruits, and vegetables; low-fat or skim milk and milk products; lean cuts of meat; fish; and chicken. Trim fat from meat before cooking; bake or broil meat rather than fry; use less fat and oil; and take the skin off chicken and turkey. Reducing overweight will also help lower your level of LDL cholesterol, as well as increase your level of HDL cholesterol.

8. TRUE   People who have had one heart attack are at much higher risk for a second attack. Reducing blood cholesterol levels can greatly slow

down (and in some people, even reverse) the buildup of cholesterol and fat in the walls of the coronary arteries and significantly reduce the chances of a second heart attack.

9. TRUE Children from "high risk" families, in which a parent has high blood cholesterol (240 mg/dL or above) or in which a parent or grandparent has had heart disease at an early age (at 55 years of age or younger), should have their cholesterol levels tested. If a child from such a family has a cholesterol level that is high, it should be lowered under medical supervision, primarily with diet, to reduce the risk of developing heart disease as an adult. For most children who are not from high-risk families, the best way to reduce the risk of adult heart disease is to follow a low-saturated-fat, low-cholesterol eating pattern. All children over the age of 2 years and all adults should adopt heart-healthy eating patterns as a principal way of reducing coronary heart disease.

10. TRUE Heavy smokers are two to four times more likely to have a heart attack than nonsmokers, and the heart attack death rate among all smokers is 70% greater than that of nonsmokers. Older male smokers are also nearly twice as likely to die from stroke than older men who do not smoke, and these odds are nearly as high for older female smokers. Further, the risk of dying of lung cancer is 22 times higher for male smokers than male nonsmokers and 12 times higher for female smokers than female non-smokers. Finally, 80% of all deaths from emphysema and bronchitis are directly related to smoking.

11. TRUE One year after quitting, ex-smokers cut their extra risk for heart attack by about half or more, and eventually the risk will return to normal in healthy ex-smokers. Even if you have already had a heart attack, you can reduce your chances of having a second attack if you quit smoking. Ex-smokers can also reduce their risk of stroke and cancer, improve blood flow and lung function, and help stop diseases like emphysema and bronchitis from getting worse.

12. FALSE Older smokers are more likely to succeed at quitting smoking than younger smokers. Quitting helps relieve smoking-related symptoms like shortness of breath, coughing, and chest pain. Many quit to avoid further health problems and to take control of their lives.

13. TRUE Weight control is a question of balance. You get calories from the food you eat. You burn off calories by exercising. Cutting down on calories, especially calories from fat, is key to losing weight. Combining this with regular physical activity, like walking, cycling, jogging, or swimming, not only can help in losing weight, but also in maintaining weight loss. A steady weight loss of 0.5 to 1 pound a week is safe for most adults, and the weight is more likely to stay off over the long run. Losing weight, if you are overweight, may also help reduce your blood pressure, lower your LDL cholesterol, and raise your HDL cholesterol. Being physically active and eating fewer calories will also help you control your weight if you quit smoking.

14. TRUE Coronary heart disease is the number one killer in the United States. Approximately 700,000 Americans died of coronary heart disease in 2002, and over half these deaths were women.

From National Heart, Lung, and Blood Institute: *Healthy heart I. Q* (NIH Publication No. 92-2724), Washington, DC, 1992, National Heart, Lung, and Blood Institute.

This and all other appendixes can be found on the book's Evolve website in the Assessment Tools section.

Appendix D

Comprehensive Older Person's Evaluation (COPE)

PROVIDER NAME (PRINT): _____ DATE OF VISIT: _____

CHIEF COMPLAINT: _____

Today I will ask you about your overall health and function and will be using a questionnaire to help me obtain this information. The first few questions are to check your memory.

PRELIMINARY COGNITION QUESTIONNAIRE: RECORD IF ANSWER IS CORRECT WITH (+). IF ANSWER IS INCORRECT WITH (−). RECORD TOTAL NUMBER OF ERRORS.

(+, −)

A. What is the date today? _____

B. What day of the week is it? _____

C. What is the name of this place? _____

D. What is your telephone number? (RECORD ANSWER) _____ _____
   IF SUBJECT DOES NOT HAVE PHONE, ASK: What is your street
   address? _____ _____

E. How old are you? (RECORD ANSWER) _____ _____

F. When were you born? (RECORD ANSWER FROM RECORDS IF PATIENT CANNOT _____
   ANSWER) _____

G. Who is the President of the United States now? _____

H. Who was the President just before him? _____

I. What was your mother's maiden name? _____

J. Subtract 3 from 20 and keep subtracting from each new number you get, all the way down _____

(CORRECT: 17, 14, 11, 8, 5, 2)
TOTAL ERRORS_____

IF MORE THAN 4 ERRORS, ASK K. IF MORE THAN 6 ERRORS, COMPLETE QUESTIONNAIRE FROM INFORMANT.

K. Do you think you would benefit from a legal guardian, someone who would be responsible for your legal and financial matters?
   4. Yes   2. Have functioning legal guardian (DESCRIBE: _____)
   3. Have legal guardian   1. No

DEMOGRAPHIC SECTION

1. PATIENT'S RACE OR ETHNIC BACKGROUND (RECORD) _____

2. PATIENT'S GENDER (CIRCLE)   Male   Female

3. How far did you go in school?
   6. 0–8 years   4. High school complete   2. Four year degree
   5. High school incomplete   3. College or technical school 1. Post-graduate education

SOCIAL SUPPORT SECTION: Now there are a few questions about your family and friends.

4. Are you now married, widowed, separated, or divorced, or have you never been married?
   1. Now Married   2. Widowed   3. Separated   4. Divorced   5. Never Married

5. Who lives with you? (CIRCLE ALL RESPONSES)
   1. Spouse   4. Live alone
   2. Other relative or friend (SPECIFY: _____)   5. Nursing home
   3. Group living situation (non-health)

6. Have you talked to any friends or relatives by phone during the last week?   1. Yes   2. No

7. Are you satisfied by seeing your relatives and friends as often as you want to, or are you somewhat dissatisfied about how little you see them?   1. Satisfied (SKIP TO #8)   2. Dissatisfied (ASK A)
   A. Do you feel you would like to be involved in a Senior Citizens Center for social events, or perhaps meals?   3. Yes   2. Am Involved (DESCRIBE: _____)   1. No

8. Is there someone who would take care of you for as long as you needed if you were sick or disabled?
    1. Yes   (SKIP TO C)   2. No   (ASK A)
    A. Is there someone who would take care of you for a short time?   1. Yes (SKIP TO C)   2. No (ASK B)
    B. Is there someone who could help you now and then?   1. Yes (ASK C)   2. No (ASK C)
    C. Whom would we call in case of an emergency? (RECORD NAME AND TELEPHONE) _____

FINANCIAL SECTION: The next few questions are about your finances and any problems you might have.
9. Do you own, or are you buying, your own home?   1. Yes (SKIP TO #10)   2. No (ASK A)
    A. Do you feel you need assistance with housing?
        3. Yes (DESCRIBE: _____)
        2. Have subsidized or other housing assistance
        1. No
10. Are you covered by private medical insurance, Medicare, Medicaid, or some disability plan? (CIRCLE ALL THAT APPLY)
        1. Private insurance (SPECIFY BELOW AND SKIP TO #11) _____
        2. Medicare   3. Medicaid
        4. Disability (SPECIFY: _____) (ASK A)
        5. None   6. Other (SPECIFY: _____)
    A. Do you feel you need additional assistance with your medical bills?   2. Yes   1. No
11. Which of these statements best describes your financial situation?
        3. My expenses are so heavy that I cannot meet my bills   (ASK A)
        2. My expenses make it difficult to meet my bills   (ASK A)
        1. My bills are no problem to me (SKIP TO #12)
    A. Do you feel you need financial assistance such as (CIRCLE ALL THAT APPLY)
        1. Food stamps   3. Assistance in paying your heating or electrical bills
        2. Social Security or disability payments   4. Other financial assistance? (DESCRIBE: _____)
PSYCHOLOGICAL HEALTH SECTION: The next few questions are about how you feel about your life in general. There are no right or wrong answers, only what best applies to you. *Please answer yes or no to each question.*
12. Is your daily life full of things that keep you interested?   1. Yes   2. No
13. Have you, at times, very much wanted to leave home?   2. Yes   1. No
14. Does it seem that no one understands you?   2. Yes   1. No
15. Are you happy most of the time?   1. Yes   2. No
16. Do you feel weak all over much of the time?   2. Yes   1. No
17. Is your sleep fitful and disturbed?   2. Yes   1. No
18. Taking everything into consideration, how would you describe your satisfaction with your life in general at the present time—good, fair, or poor?   1. Good   2. Fair   3. Poor
19. Do you feel you now need help with your mental health; for example, a counselor or psychiatrist?
        3. Yes   2. Have (SPECIFY: _____)   1. No
PHYSICAL HEALTH SECTION: The next questions are about your health.
20. During the past month (30 days), how many days were you so sick that you couldn't do your usual activities, such as working around the house or visiting with friends?   TOTAL NUMBER OF DAYS: _____
21. Relative to other people your age, how would you rate your overall health at the present time; excellent, good, fair, poor, or very poor?
        1. Excellent   (SKIP to #22)   3. Good (ASK A)   5. Poor (ASK A)
        2. Very Good   (SKIP TO #22)   4. Fair (ASK A)
    A. Do you feel you need additional medical services such as a doctor, nurse, visiting nurse, or physical therapy?   (CIRCLE ALL THAT APPLY)
        1. Doctor   2. Nurse   3. Visiting nurse   4. Physical therapy   5. None
22. Do you use an aid for walking, such as a wheelchair, walker, cane, or anything else? (CIRCLE AID USUALLY USED)   5. Wheelchair 4. Walker 3. Cane 2. Other (SPECIFY): _____ 5. None
23. How much do your health troubles stand in the way of your doing things you want to do; not at all, a little, or a great deal?
        1. Not at all (SKIP TO #24)   2. A little (ASK A)   3. A great deal (ASK A)
    A. Do you think you need assistance to do your daily activities; for example, do you need a live-in aide or choreworker?
        1. Live-in aide   3. Have aide, choreworker or other assistance (DESCRIBE: _____)
        2. Choreworker   4. None needed

24. Have you had, or do you currently have, any of the following health problems? (IF YES, PLACE AN "X" IN APPROPRIATE BOX AND DESCRIBE [MEDICAL RECORD INFORMATION MAY BE USED TO HELP COMPLETE THIS SECTION.])

	HX	CURRENT	DESCRIBE
a. Arthritis or rheumatism?			
b. Lung or breathing problem?			
c. Hypertension?			
d. Heart trouble?			
e. Phlebitis or poor circulation problems in arms or legs?			
f. Diabetes or low blood sugar?			
g. Digestive ulcers?			
h. Other digestive problem?			
i. Cancer?			
j. Anemia?			
k. Effects of stroke?			
l. Other neurological problem? (SPECIFY): _____			
m. Thyroid or other glandular problem? (SPECIFY): _____			
n. Skin disorders such as pressure sores, leg ulcers, burns?			
o. Speech problem?			
p. Hearing problem?			
q. Vision or eye problem?			
r. Kidney or bladder problems, or incontinence?			
s. A problem of falls?			
t. Problem with eating or your weight? (SPECIFY): _____			
u. Problem with depression or your nerves? (SPECIFY): _____			
v. Problem with your behavior? (SPECIFY): _____			
w. Problem with your sexual activity?			
x. Problem with alcohol?			
y. Problem with pain?			
z. Other health problems? (SPECIFY): _____			

25. What medications are you currently taking, or have been taking, in the last month? (May I see your medication bottles?) (IF PATIENT CANNOT LIST, ASK CATEGORIES A–R AND NOTE DOSAGE AND SCHEDULE, OR OBTAIN INFORMATION FROM MEDICAL OR PHARMACY RECORDS AND VERIFY ACCURACY WITH THE PATIENT.)

	Rx (DOSAGE AND SCHEDULE)
a. Arthritis medication	
b. Pain medication	
c. Blood pressure medication	
d. Water pills or pills for fluid	
e. Medication for your heart	
f. Medication for your lungs	
g. Blood thinners	
h. Medication for your circulation	
i. Insulin or diabetes medication	
j. Seizure medication	
k. Thyroid pills	
l. Steroids	
m. Hormones	
n. Antibiotics	
o. Medicine for nerves or depression	
p. Prescription sleeping pills	
q. Other prescription drugs	
r. Other non-prescription drugs	

26. Many people have problems remembering to take their medications, especially ones they need to take on a regular basis. How often do you forget to take your medications? Would you say you forget often, sometimes, rarely, or never?   4. Often   3. Sometimes   2. Rarely   1. Never

ACTIVITIES OF DAILY LIVING: The next set of questions ask whether you would need help with any of the following activities of daily living.

27. I would like to know whether you can do these activities without any help at all, or if you need assistance to do them. Do you need help to: (IF YES, DESCRIBE, INCLUDING PATIENT NEEDS)

	Yes	No	DESCRIBE (INCLUDE NEEDS)
a. Use the telephone?			
b. Get to places out of walking distance? (Use transportation?)			
c. Shop for clothes and food?			
d. Do your housework?			
e. Handle your money?			
f. Feed yourself?			
g. Dress and undress yourself?			
h. Take care of your appearance?			
i. Get in and out of bed?			
j. Take a bath or shower?			
k. Prepare your meals?			
l. Have any problem getting to the bathroom on time?			

28. During the past six months, have you had any help with such things as shopping, housework, bathing, dressing, and getting around?
    2. Yes (SPECIFY: _____)
    1. No

Pearlman RA: Development of a functional assessment questionnaire for geriatric patients: The Comprehensive Older Person's Evaluation (COPE), *Journal of Chronic Diseases* 40(suppl)1: 85S-98S, 1987.

This and all other appendixes can be found on the book's Evolve website in the Assessment Tools section.

Appendix E

Family Health Assessment

Family surname: _____
Household members (name, age, and relationship to head of household): _____
_____
_____
_____

Family composition: _____
_____

Genogram:

Family health tree (include health problems of individual members):

Ecomap (for social and health agencies include hours of service, distance and transportation, availability of interpreters, and criteria for receiving services such as age, sex, and income barriers):

Family characteristics	Source(s) of information	Date
Extended family		
Relatives living outside household		
Location of relatives		
Frequency and duration of contact		
Means of communication		
Family mobility		
Length of time living in residence		
Location of previous residence		
Frequency of geographic moves		
Country/area of origin		
Family structure		
Educational experiences		
Employment history		
Financial resources		
Leisure time interests		
Division of labor		
Allocation of roles		
Distribution of authority and power		

Family characteristics	Source(s) of information	Date
Family cohesion		
Emotional bonding of family members		
Degree of individual autonomy		
Family adaptation		
Flexibility in role change		
Flexibility in power structures		
Family processes		
How members communicate		
How decisions are made		
How problems are solved		
How conflict is handled		
Family social integration		
Language(s) and/or dialect(s) spoken; where		
Literacy; ability to read or write in language(s)		
Degree of racial or cultural identity		
Degree of social network with neighbors, friends, and other family members		
Network with religious organizations		
Network with social organizations		
Degrees of stress experienced by the family		
Combinations of stressors:		
1.		
2.		
3.		
Family health behavior		
Activities of daily living (how family spends typical day)		
Health history		
Health status (i.e., problems and priorities)		
Risk behaviors		
Self-care (health promotion and prevention)		
Health care resources		
Professionals and lay healers		
Working with family and agencies		
Family strengths		
Family priorities		

Family characteristics	**Source(s) of information**	**Date**
Family–nurse contract(s)		

Family cultural influences
Values, attitudes, and beliefs about

   Spirituality

   Rituals (holidays and celebrations)

   Customs

   Dietary habits

   Child-rearing practices

   Health

   Folk diseases and folk medicine

   Cultural healers

   Care of ill family member

   Role of spiritual leader in care of ill family member

Family environment	**Source(s) of information**	**Date**
Family residence Adequacy of size		
Structurally safe		
Sanitation: water, sewage, and garbage		
Adequacy of sleeping arrangement		
Cooking and refrigeration		
Storage of medicines and cleaning agents		
Loose rugs		
Smoke alarm		
Emergency numbers		
Family neighborhood Location (e.g., urban or rural)		
Type (e.g., semicommercial)		
Age composition		
Safety Traffic patterns		
Lighting		
Security (i.e., police)		
Density (i.e., noise, crowding, poverty, and crime)		

Family environment	Source(s) of information	Date
Modes of transportation		
Resources Grocery shopping		
Pharmacy		
Recreational (e.g., parks)		
Educational		
Religious		
Emergency (i.e., fire and hospital)		
Neighborhood interaction		
Family community Industry and business		
Leadership		
Government		
Migration (i.e., in and out of community)		
Community memberships/interaction		
Social services		
Health services Primary care		
Institutions (e.g., hospital or nursing home)		

Siegrist BC: Family health. In Nies MA, McEwen M, editors: *Community/public health nursing: Promoting the health of populations*, ed 4, St. Louis, 2007, Saunders.

This and all other appendixes can be found on the book's Evolve website in the Assessment Tools section.

Glossary

The number in parentheses after each term represents the chapter in which that term is found.

12-step programs (18): mutual help groups that provide supportive interaction to help individuals meet a goal of recovery from use and abuse of drugs, alcohol, or compulsive behavior patterns. Participation in 12-step groups (e.g., Narcotics Anonymous and Alcoholics Anonymous) gives social support and structure that assists in the recovery process.

A

Active immunity (19): protection against a communicable disease that is produced by the person's own immune system. Active immunity occurs following the stimulation of the body's immune system to produce antibodies and cellular immunity, often after a person has had a disease. Active immunity can also be achieved through administration of a vaccine that produces an immunological memory similar to that of the natural disease.

Activities of daily living (15): normal activities of living that generally include bathing, dressing, eating, getting in and out of bed and chairs, walking, going outside, and toileting.

Adult immunization (15): recommendations of the Immunization Practices Advisory Committee that all older adults should have completed a primary series of diphtheria and tetanus toxoids, a single dose of pneumococcal polysaccharide vaccine, and annual vaccination against influenza.

Advocate (2): someone who acts on behalf of, or intercedes for, the client. Advocates ensure that clients receive necessary care and services.

Agent (6): a factor, such as a microorganism, chemical substance, or form of radiation, whose presence, excessive presence, or (in deficiency diseases) relative absence is essential for the occurrence of a disease.

Agoraphobia (18): literally, fear of the marketplace or open places. About one third of all people who experience panic attacks eventually develop agoraphobia. Persons with agoraphobia frequently progress to the point where they cannot leave their homes without experiencing anxiety.

Alzheimer's disease (15): a degenerative mental disorder characterized by progressive brain deterioration, resulting in impaired memory and changes in thought patterns and behaviors. Approximately 4 million Americans have Alzheimer's disease, and it is a leading cause of death among adults.

Ambulatory care (10): personal health care or health services (e.g., outpatient surgery and chemotherapy, diagnostic tests, and procedures) provided to noninstitutionalized patients. Ambulatory care includes care, procedures, and services provided in settings such as home, work, church, and school.

American Red Cross (ARC) (9, 14): a voluntary support agency founded in 1881 by Clara Barton. The ARC has more than 1300 local chapters throughout the United States and provides disaster relief services to people around the clock.

Ambulatory nursing practice (10): the provision of comprehensive nursing care for individuals or families in community-based settings. Ambulatory nursing care is largely focused on health promotion, primary prevention, screening for early identification of disease, and assisting in treatment regimens for both acute and chronic illnesses (e.g., colds, influenza, ear infection, hypertension, diabetes).

Ambulatory oncology nursing practice (10): nursing care provided in oncology clinics, physician's offices, and 23-hour and 24-hour clinics and day hospitals. Ambulatory oncology nursing practice includes patient counseling, health care maintenance, primary care, patient education, therapeutic care, normative care, nonclient-centered care, and telephone triage.

Ambulatory surgery (10): the process in which patients have surgery, recover, and are discharged home the same day. Nurses who work in outpatient surgical centers may provide preoperative care, intraoperative care, or postanesthesia care.

Analytical epidemiology (6): investigation of the etiology of disease.

Anemia screening (12): recommended routine screening of hemoglobin or hematocrit levels during infancy (6 to 9 months) and early childhood to detect iron deficiency anemia. Screening for adolescent females is also recommended.

Anorexia nervosa (18): an eating disorder that occurs when a person becomes obsessed with a fear of fat and with losing weight. Anorexia nervosa usually begins in early adolescence and often develops with a fairly gradual decrease in caloric intake. However, the decrease in caloric intake continues until the anorexic is consuming almost nothing.

Anxiety disorders (18): a group of mental disorders characterized by feelings of severe anxiety, resulting symptoms, and efforts to avoid those symptoms. Anxiety disorders are the most common of all of the mental disorders, affecting as many as 13% of the general population at any time. Some of the more commonly encountered anxiety disorders are generalized anxiety disorder (GAD), panic disorder, phobias, obsessive-compulsive disorder, and posttraumatic stress disorder (PTSD).

Assisted reproductive technology (14): therapies that have been developed to treat infertility. Some of the available options include in vitro fertilization, gamete intrafallopian transfer (GIFT), zygote intrafallopian transfer, donor ovum transfer, donor embryo, and therapeutic donor insemination.

Atmospheric quality (7): the purity of the air available for breathing purposes. Atmospheric quality is threatened by air pollutants such as ozone, carbon monoxide, nitrogen dioxide, particulates, sulfur dioxide, and lead, which can cause lung damage, inflammatory responses, and respiratory symptoms.

Attention deficit hyperactivity disorder (ADHD) (18): a disorder that affects 3% to 5% of all children and is characterized by inattention, hyperactivity, and impulsivity.

B

Behavioral therapy (18): the use of learning principles to change thought patterns and behaviors systematically. Behavior therapy is used to encourage the individual to learn specific skills to obtain rewards and satisfaction.

Stress management, biofeedback, and relaxation training are examples of behavior therapy.

Bioterrorism (19): the use of communicable diseases as weapons.

Blended family (16): a family made up of one divorced or widowed adult with all or some of his or her children and a new spouse with all or some of his or her children; may include the children born to this union so that parents, stepparents, children, and stepchildren or stepsiblings live together.

Body Mass Index (BMI) (12): a reliable indicator of body fatness; correlates well with direct measures of body fatness such as underwater weighing.

Bottle mouth syndrome (12): the destruction of teeth in older infants and toddlers who are allowed to fall asleep with a bottle of formula, milk, or another sweetened fluid in their mouths.

Breast cancer (14): the most common cancer among women in the United States (excluding skin cancer) and the second leading cause of cancer deaths in women. In the United States a woman's average lifetime risk for developing breast cancer is approximately one in eight.

Bulimia nervosa (18): an eating disorder characterized by binge eating and "purging" (self-induced vomiting, use of laxatives, diuretics, fasting, and excessive exercise) to prevent weight gain.

C

Capitation (5): in managed care, a negotiated, prepaid fixed fee for each covered individual or family. For the capitation fee, the managed care organization agrees to provide the services stipulated in the contract for a specified time period.

Carbon monoxide (CO) (7): a colorless, odorless gas that results from burning of fossil fuels. More than 200 deaths each year are caused by accidental carbon monoxide poisoning.

Case management (4, 11): the process of identifying needs for and arranging, coordinating, monitoring, and evaluating prevention services (primary, secondary, and tertiary) to achieve designated health outcomes and ensure quality and cost-effectiveness. In case management, one professional is responsible for assessing needs, targeting services to meet the needs, and monitoring and evaluating client status to ensure that needs are met adequately.

Category A Agents (19): anthrax, botulism, plague, smallpox, tularemia, and viral hemorrhagic fevers. They can be easily disseminated or transmitted from person to person, result in high mortality rates, and have the potential for major public health impact.

Child abuse (12): any physical or mental injury, sexual abuse or exploitation, negligent treatment or maltreatment of a child by a person who is responsible for the child's welfare.

Child safety (12): efforts to protect children from injury. Potential threats targeted by childhood safety measures include motor vehicle accidents, bicycle accidents, violence, poisoning, drowning, burns, sports-related accidents, asphyxiation, and falls.

Chlorofluorocarbons (CFCs) (7): gases found in refrigerants, aerosols, and some solvent cleaning agents; theorized to contribute to stratospheric ozone depletion.

Chunking (3): the ability to read and understand an entire sentence or idea at one time.

Clinical pathway (4): specific goals and expected outcomes, which are measured on an ongoing basis, and a method to record care given.

Cognitive impairment (15): mental impairment that is common among older individuals and often increases with age. An estimated 5% to 10% of individuals older than 65 years of age and almost 50% of those over 85 years of age experience some degree of cognitive impairment. Alzheimer's disease, vascular infarctions, and pharmaceuticals are frequently implicated as inducing cognitive changes.

Coinsurance (5): a predetermined amount or percentage of the cost of covered services that the beneficiary will pay. The coinsurance may be an agreed-upon percentage of the fee or the balance of the total for fixed-price services.

Collaborator (2): someone who participates in the process of making health care management decisions with individuals from various professions. Collaborators work with the client and the family or caregivers to jointly determine the course of care.

Community-based nursing (1): the application of the nursing process in caring for individuals and families in community settings. Community-based nursing emphasizes all levels of prevention (i.e., primary, secondary, and tertiary), but focuses more on secondary and tertiary levels. Home health nursing and nursing in outpatient or ambulatory settings are examples of community-based nursing.

Community health nursing (1): a synthesis of nursing practice and public health practice applied to promoting and preserving the health of populations. Community health nursing practice is continuous and comprehensive and considers the impact of the environment on health. Public health nursing, school nursing, and occupational health nursing are examples of community health nursing.

Conditions of participation (11): regulations that must be met by home health care agencies to be eligible for Medicare reimbursement. Conditions of participation consist of explicit rules and standards that outline requirements for virtually all aspects of home health care and detail such areas as personnel qualifications, notifying patients of their rights, acceptance of patients, plan of care, medical supervision, types of services offered by the agency, and the duties of each service provider.

Contraception (14): actions or interventions to prevent pregnancy. Several methods of contraception are available, including abstinence, barriers (e.g., condoms, diaphragm), hormonal methods (e.g., oral contraceptives, Depo-Provera, Norplant), intrauterine devices (IUDs), sterilization, and natural family planning.

Coordination of community resources (11): referral by a nurse to other services; requires the nurse to be knowledgeable about services offered by his or her own agency and any resources available in the community that would benefit clients. To coordinate care the nurse must understand the referral process, determine if the client is eligible for the services offered by the agency or organization, have an understanding of how to refer a client for a particular service, know the costs of services and payment mechanism, and be aware of the location, telephone number, hours of operation, and contact person.

Copayments (5): specified flat fees per units of service or time that the individual pays; the insurer pays the remaining costs.

Correctional nursing (10): provision of primary care and emergency services for inmates in correctional facilities. Correctional nursing typically includes screening activities, direct health care services, analysis of individual health behaviors, and teaching, counseling, and assisting individuals in assuming responsibility for their own health.

Counselor (2): a professional who listens to clients and their families and encourages them to explore issues and options. Counselors assist with identification of problems and possible solutions and provide guidance through the problem-solving process.

Crisis (9): a turning point for the worse, when the incident has gotten out of control, leading to multiple casualties, severe destruction, or both.

Culture (8): the knowledge, beliefs, art, morals, laws, and other capabilities and habits acquired by man as a member of society. Culture includes nonphysical traits, such as values, attitudes, and customs that are shared by a group of people and passed from one generation to the next. Culture provides the organizational structure or basis for behavior within the group.

D

Deductibles (5): sums that must be paid each calendar year before the insurance policy becomes active. Deductible amounts vary greatly, from almost nothing to several thousand dollars.

Depression (18): mental illness that affects almost 19 million people in the United States each year. The most prevalent types of depression are major depression, dysthymia, and bipolar disorder.

Descriptive epidemiology (6): examination of the amount and distribution of a disease interms of person, place, and time to distinguish characteristics of individuals who have a specic disease from those who do not.

Developmental screening (12): monitoring of the progression of infants, children, and adolescents through developmental tasks. Assessment of developmental level can be accomplished by using screening tools, a thorough history, physical assessment, and/or direct observation.

Diagnosis-related groups (DRGs) (5): classification system that groups patients into categories, based on the coding system of the International Classification of Disease, Ninth Revision-Clinical Modification (ICD-9-CM). DRGs are used to establish health care payments under Medicare.

Direct care provider (2): a professional who is involved in the direct delivery of care. This role includes performing tasks or skills for which the nurse has been trained and that are typically associated with nursing practice (e.g., client assessment, taking vital signs, medication administration, changing dressings, and inserting catheters).

Direct transmission (19): transmission of a disease-causing organism through physical contact, including biting, kissing, and touching or sexual contact. Airborne transmission through dust and droplet and droplet nuclei may also be direct.

Direct victims (9): those who suffer the immediate effects of a disaster; they may be injured, dead, an evacuee, or refugee.

Disability (17): any restriction on or lack of ability resulting from a physical or psychological limitation that disrupts the performance of an activity in a normal manner or within the normal range. Limitations in functional activities, activities of daily living (ADL), and instrumental activities of daily living (IADL) determine disability.

Disaster (9, 17): any event that causes destruction and devastation that cannot be alleviated without assistance. Disasters may be the result of "natural" occurrences (e.g., hurricanes, tornadoes, floods, droughts) or they may be "manmade" (e.g., war, terrorism, civil disasters, accidents).

Disaster triage (9): triage allows health care personnel to identify the most salvageable clients so that treatment can be initiated immediately. The focus of disaster triage is to do as little as possible for the greatest number in the shortest period of time.

Discharge planning (11): the process of determining and planning to meet client needs following release from a health care facility. Discharge planning ensures that the client and family needs are identified and evaluated, with responsibility for meeting those needs being transferred to the client, the client's caregiver or significant others, or other health care providers.

Disease management (4): the provision of care necessary to minimize health care expenditures through integrating activities that target chronic and costly disease conditions (e.g., AIDS, diabetes) by coordinating care across the continuum of care settings or delivery systems. Disease management addresses the entire cycle of a disease process, incorporating primary, secondary, and tertiary care interventions and promoting self-care management. It is usually population based and requires active involvement by the client as well as various health care providers.

Disempowerment (17): the loss of power or control over one's circumstances.

Disenfranchisement (17): a feeling of separation from mainstream society in which the individual does not have an emotional connection with any group in particular or the larger social fabric in general.

Domestic violence (14): pattern of abusive behavior perpetrated by someone who is or was in an intimate relationship with the victim. Domestic violence is the major cause of injury to women.

E

Early and Periodic Screening, Diagnosis and Treatment (EPSDT) Program (12): a comprehensive and preventive health care program for Medicaid-eligible individuals up to age 21. Services provided by EPSDT include a comprehensive health and developmental history; a comprehensive unclothed physical examination; designated laboratory tests; appropriate immunizations; health education; dental, hearing, and vision services; and any other necessary health care to correct or ameliorate illnesses and conditions found during screenings.

Ecomap (16): a tool that can be used to explain a family's linkages to their suprasystems or the larger environment. The ecomap visually illustrates the dynamic family-environment interactions and shows the connections between the family and the world.

Education for All Handicapped Children Act (PL 94-142) (10): law enacted by Congress in 1975 that gives all students between the ages of 3 and 18 years the right to a free and appropriate public education in the least restrictive environment possible, regardless of physical or mental disabilities. Handicapping conditions covered by this Act include auditory impairment, visual imparment, mental retardation, orthopedic impairment, serious emotional disturbance (e.g., inability to build interpersonal relationships, inappropriate behavior or feelings, depression), and specific learning disability (e.g., dyslexia).

Educator (2): a nurse who teaches individuals, families, and groups about maintenance of health, threats to health, and relevant lifestyle choices that affect health. The information presented should allow clients to make informed decisions on health matters and to direct self-care to follow treatment regimens.

Elder abuse (15): neglect, physical injury, or exploitation that results in harm to an older adult. Elder abuse can take one of several forms, including physical abuse, confinement, psychological or emotional abuse, financial or material abuse, neglect, or abandonment.

Emergency (9): an unforeseen event or condition requiring immediate action. Emergencies can occur internally or externally.

Emergency contraception (14): use of high doses of standard birth control pills as postcoital contraception or "morning after pills." Emergency contraception averts pregnancy by preventing ovulation or preventing fertilization of the egg or transportation of the egg to the uterus.

Emerging infectious diseases (19): those diseases whose incidence in humans has increased within the past two decades or threatens to increase in the near future. Emerging infections can be new or previously unrecognized infectious diseases, reemerging diseases, or infectious diseases that have developed resistance to previously effective antimicrobial drugs. Examples of emerging infections include new Variant Creutzfeldt-Jakob Disease (vCJD); a virulent strain of influenza; foodborne outbreaks, including outbreaks caused by *Cyclospora* parasites, hepatitis A virus, and *Escherichia coli* 0157:H7 bacteria; and multidrug-resistant tuberculosis–strain W.

Enterostomal care (11): nursing interventions specifically related to wound care and specialized care for clients with a colostomy, an ileostomy, or a urostomy. Enterostomal care involves assessment of the wound and evaluation of the efficacy of treatment, cleaning, and debridement and includes obtaining cultures and teaching the patient and/or caregiver how to change the dressing using sterile technique.

Epidemiology (6): the study of the distribution and determinants of health-related states or events in a specified population, and the application of this study to the control of health problems.

Ethnic group (8): designated or basic division of groups of individuals distinguished by customs, characteristics, or language; group of persons who possess common physical and mental traits as a result of heredity, cultural traditions, language, customs, and common history.

Extended family (16): a family comprising the nuclear family plus other relatives of one or both spouses; relatives may or may not live with the nuclear family and may include great-grandparents and great-great-grandparents.

External emergencies (9): hazardous or harmful events that occur somewhere in the community outside of a defined business, industrial complex, residence, or other facility.

F

Family (16): social units or systems composed of two or more persons in a committed relationship. The family provides protection, nourishment, and socialization for family members.

Family assessment (16): the basic step for promoting the health of a family. A family health assessment may help the nurse identify the health status of individual members of the family and aspects of family composition, function, and process.

Family crises (16): serious problems experienced in all families. There are two basic types of family crises, the maturational crisis and the situational crisis. A maturational crisis is a normal transition point (e.g., adolescence, marriage, parenthood) when old patterns of communication and old roles must be exchanged for new patterns and roles. A situational crisis can occur when the family experiences an event that is sudden, unexpected, and unpredictable and may lead to disorganization, tension, and severe anxiety. Examples of situational crises include illness, accidents, death, and natural disasters.

Family health tree (16): a method to record pertinent data about a family's medical and health histories. The family health tree typically includes causes of death of deceased family members, genetically linked diseases (i.e., heart disease, cancer, diabetes, hypertension, sickle cell anemia, allergies, asthma), environmental and occupational diseases, psychosocial problems (i.e., mental illness), obesity, and infectious disease.

Family planning services (14): health care and counseling that provides women and men information and care they need to make informed choices about whether and when to become parents. Comprehensive family planning includes consideration of a number of factors regarding childbearing, adoption, use of contraceptives, natural family planning, treatment of infertility, and preconception counseling.

Family roles (16): socially expected behavior patterns that are determined by a person's position or status. In families, roles are the assigned or assumed parts that members play during day-to-day living; they are bestowed and defined by the family.

Federal Emergency Management Agency (FEMA) (9, 14): the federal agency that assesses and responds to disaster events in the United States; responsibilities include emergency planning, preparedness, mitigation, response, and recovery.

First responders (9): fire, police, and ambulance services.

Foodborne pathogens (7): microbiological contamination of food that is usually caused by improper storage, handling, and/or preparation of food. Several foodborne pathogens have been cited as being of primary concern with regard to foodborne illnesses. These include *Salmonella*, *Campylobacter*, *Escherichia coli* 0157:H7, and *Listeria monocytogenes*.

Functional independence (15): the extent to which the individual is able to complete "normal" and "instrumental" activities of daily living without assistance from others.

G

Gatekeeper (5): The primary care physician within managed care plans is frequently referred to as the "gatekeeper." Usually the gatekeeper is a family practitioner, internist, pediatrician, or gynecologist who is responsible for all primary care for the enrolled patient. To avoid duplication of services and overuse of specialists, the gatekeeper coordinates all care and determines when to refer the client to a specialist.

Genogram (16): a tool that helps the nurse outline or diagram the family's structure to view family patterns. The genogram details births, deaths, divorces, and remarriages and may also identify other characteristics (race, social class), occupations, and places of family residence.

H

Handicap (17): a disadvantage resulting from an impairment or disability.

Hazardous waste (7): approximately 10% of industrial wastes, which include poisons, inflammable materials, infectious contaminants, explosives, and radionuclides. Some of the most common hazardous wastes include lead, mercury, polychlorinated biphenyls [PCBs], chromium, trichloroethane or trichloroethylene, and benzene. Medical waste, including cultures, items contaminated with human blood and blood products, contaminated animal carcasses, wastes from patients isolated with highly communicable diseases, and all used sharps are also hazardous wastes.

Hazards (9): sources of danger that need to be identified both within and outside the facility.

Head Start (12): a federally funded, comprehensive preschool program for children who are at risk for academic problems associated with poverty and lack of sufficient social stimulation. Low-income children 3 to 5 years of age are eligible for Head Start programs.

Health education (3): any planned combination of learning experiences designed to predispose, enable, and reinforce voluntary behavior conducive to health in individuals, groups, or communities.

Health maintenance organization (HMO) (5): a managed care organization that contracts with an individual, group, or organization to provide health care for enrollees. The HMO agrees to provide a set of services for a set fee (typically a capitated fee). HMOs attempt to provide services to clients at a cost lower than the fee paid and thereby profit by (1) delivering less costly care and less total services and (2) minimizing referrals to other providers. HMOs provide care to clients with no or minimal deductibles and copayments.

Health promotion (13): activities or actions related to encouraging individual lifestyles or personal choices that positively influence health (e.g., encouraging physical activity and fitness, good nutrition, substance abuse prevention).

Healthy People 2010 (1): the national prevention initiative of the U.S. Department of Health and Human Services (USDHHS). *Healthy People 2010* has two goals: (1) to increase quality and years of healthy life for U.S. residents and (2) to eliminate health disparities. There are 467 objectives divided among 28 focus areas, and the objectives may be used as framework to guide health-promotion activities in schools, clinics, worksites, and for community-wide initiatives.

Hearing deficit (15): some degree of hearing impairment that may affect up to 33% of individuals aged 65 years and over. The most common types of hearing loss and associated factors are presbycusis (slow decline in hearing ability), tinnitus, conductive hearing loss, and sensorineural hearing loss.

Hearing screening (12): early detection of hearing disorders. Hearing screening includes questioning to determine auditory responsiveness and speech and language development, physical examination to detect abnormalities of the ear canal and tympanic membrane, and pure-tone audiometry testing. Individuals with abnormal results should be referred to a specialist for further testing and treatment.

Homeless (17): a person who regularly sleeps in a supervised shelter, an institution that provides a temporary residence, or in a public or private place not designated for sleeping.

Home health care (11): that component of health care in which services are provided to individuals and families in their places of residence for the purpose of promoting, maintaining, or restoring health, or maximizing the level of independence, while minimizing the effects of disability and illness.

Home health nursing (11): integrates medical/surgical, community health, parent-child, gerontological, and psychiatric-mental health nursing into home health care practice. It refers to comprehensive nursing care provided to individuals and families in their place of residence, focusing on the environmental, psychosocial, economic, cultural, and personal health factors affecting health status.

Hospice care (11): palliative care provided to the terminally ill; it is frequently provided in the home. Hospice care focuses on the family and the patient and provides assistance in dealing with emotional, spiritual, and medical problems; coordinating professional and volunteer services; and making the patient as comfortable as possible through pain and symptom management.

Host (6): a person or other living organism that can be infected by an infectious agent under natural conditions.

I

Illness prevention (13): lessening or removal of risk factors for specific diseases and early identification of diseases through screening and prompt remediation.

Immunity (19): protection from infectious disease. There are two basic mechanisms for acquiring immunity: active and passive.

Immunization schedule (19): recommended immunizations for infants and children. Includes a schedule of 11 childhood vaccines by age 18 months, including four doses of DTP, three doses of polio vaccine, one dose of MMR, three or four doses of HIB conjugate vaccine, three doses of hepatitis B vaccine, one dose of varicella vaccine, and four doses of pneumococcal vaccine. Booster immunizations of DTP, polio, and MMR are given to older children.

Impairment (17): an anatomical, mental, or psychological loss or another abnormality that results in an individual experiencing deviation from normal structure, function, or development.

Incidence rate (6): a measure of the frequency with which an event, such as a new case of illness, occurs in a population over a period. The denominator is the population at risk; the numerator is the number of new cases occurring during a given time.

Incontinence (15): the involuntary loss of urine. Incontinence is a significant cause of disability and dependency in older adults and contributes to social isolation, embarrassment, feelings of loss of control, and low self-esteem.

Independent practice association (IPA) (5): a managed care model in which the fiscal agent contracts with a range of physicians who are not associated with each other and work in independent practices to provide services on a capitated basis.

Indirect transmission (16): the transmission of an agent carried from a reservoir to a susceptible host by suspended air particles or by animate (vector) or inanimate (vehicle) intermediaries.

Indirect victims (9): the family and friends of the direct victim or first responders.

Indoor biological contaminants (7): mold, mildew, bacteria, viruses, dust mites, and other potential health threats that may result from contaminated central air and heating units that become breeding grounds. Biological contaminates can trigger allergic reactions, including asthma, and spread infectious illnesses (i.e., colds, influenza, and chicken pox).

Infertility (14): the inability to conceive after 1 year of regular sexual intercourse without contraception. In women the most common causes of infertility are problems in ovulation, blocked or scarred fallopian tubes, and endometriosis. In men, abnormal or too few sperm is the most frequent cause of infertility.

Infusion therapy (11): the delivery of antibiotics, pain medication, total parenteral nutrition, hydration, and chemotherapy in the home.

Instrumental activities of daily living (IADL) (15): the ability to perform necessary functions of life, such as taking transportation, preparing meals, shopping, managing money, routine housework, and using the telephone.

Intentional food additives (7): those substances added to food during processing to enhance the nutritional content, improve flavor, enhance color, improve consistency, or increase the shelf life.

Interdisciplinary collaboration (11): initiation and maintenance of a collegial and collaborative relationship with all health care providers working with the client. Professionals involved in interdisciplinary collaboration for health care planning and delivery include nurses, physicians, physical therapists, occupational therapists, speech therapists/speech pathologists, social workers, registered dietitians/nutritionists, home health aides, pharmacists, phlebotomists, laboratory technicians, respiratory therapists, enterostomal therapists, chaplains, and massage therapists.

Internal emergencies (9): events that initiate within a facility.

L

Leader (2): an individual with the ability to influence the behavior of others. Nurse leaders work with others to identify and assess threats to health and intervene to remove or lessen these threats.

Lead poisoning (7): excessive levels of lead in the blood. Lead poisoning in children can adversely affect intelligence, behavior, and development. Lead-based paint in homes and buildings built before 1960 has been identified as the major source of lead poisoning. Anemia, central nervous system disorders, and renal involvement may result from lead exposure.

Literacy (3): "using printed and written information and material to function in society, to achieve one's goals, and to develop one's knowledge and potential" (Kutner et al, 2007, p. 2; complete reference information available in Chapter 3).

M

Managed care (4, 5): the "umbrella," or generic, term that describes a variety of prepaid and managed fee-for-service health care plans. Managed care plans are designed to encourage greater control over the use and cost of health care services through (1) providing incentives to contain costs, (2) providing barriers to inappropriate use of specialists, (3) administrative management of the use of services, and (4) facilitating the paperwork required on the part of consumers.

Manager (2): role that includes planning, organizing, coordinating, marketing, controlling, and evaluating care and care delivery. The role includes management of time, available resources, other personnel, and program organization and coordination, in addition to management of the client's care.

Marginalization (17): persons who are marginalized live on the "margins" or edges of society rather than in the mainstream; marginalization limits control and power.

Mass casualty incident (9): a situation with a large number of casualties (100 or greater) that significantly overwhelms available emergency services.

Medicaid (5): a national and state-sponsored public assistance (welfare) health program. Enacted by Title XIX of the Social Security Act of 1965, Medicaid is financed jointly by the states and federal government, with the federal contributions matching 50% to 77% of state contributions.

Medicare (5): a national health insurance plan begun in 1965 under Title XVIII of the Social Security Act. Those eligible for Medicare are (1) persons 65 years of age and older, (2) disabled individuals who are entitled to Social Security benefits, and (3) end-stage renal disease patients. Medicare uses indirect financing and service delivery administered by the Centers for Medicare and Medicaid Services (CMS) (formerly known as the HCFA) branch of the U.S. Department of Health and Human Services (USDHHS), which contracts with independent providers.

Mental health (18): a state of successful performance of mental function, resulting in productive activities, fulfilling relationships with other people, and the ability to adapt to change and to cope with adversity. Mental health refers not only to the absence of mental disorders but also to the ability of an individual to negotiate daily challenges and social interactions of life without experiencing cognitive, emotional, or behavioral dysfunction.

Mental illness (18): maladaptive responses to distress and an inability to mobilize resources. The mentally ill person is often dependent, has low self-esteem, and has difficulty forming interpersonal relationships.

Migrant health centers (MHCs) (17): health clinics funded by the Migrant Health Act (1962) that serve migrant and agricultural workers and families. MHCs typically offer environmental health services (e.g., rodent control, field sanitation, sewage treatment), infectious and parasitic disease screening and control, and accident prevention programs.

Migrant workers (17): individuals whose principal employment is in agriculture on a seasonal basis and who establish a temporary residence for such employment while traveling from location to location.

Minority group (8): a segment of the population that differs from the majority, based on physical or cultural characteristics.

Mitigation (9): measures taken before an emergency or disaster event.

Morbidity rates (6): measure of the frequency of occurrence of disease in a defined population during a specified time interval.

Mortality rates (6): measure of the frequency of occurrence of death in a defined population during a specified time interval.

Multiple casualty incident (9): an incident in which between 2 and 100 persons are injured.

N

NA-TECH disasters (9): natural disaster incidents that cause a technological problem.

Natural history of disease (6): the temporal course of disease from onset (inception) to resolution.

Newborn screenings (12): state-mandated requirement that all newborns be tested for congenital diseases. Tests are conducted for hypothyroidism, phenylketonuria, galactosemia, hemoglobinopathies (e.g., sickle cell disease, thalassemia), maple syrup urine disease, congenital adrenal hyperplasia, cystic fibrosis, and other conditions.

Norms (8): the rules by which human behavior is governed that are the result of the cultural values held by the group.

Nuclear dyad (16): husband and wife or other couple living alone without children.

Nuclear family (16): mother, father, and child(ren) living together but apart from both sets of the father's and mother's parents; the nuclear family is composed of a married husband and wife and children. The children may be either biological offspring or adopted.

Nursing case management (4): redefinition and restructuring of an already existing practice strategy in which nurses assume overall responsibility for client care management, oversee coordination of care, and serve as client advocates.

Nursing Interventions Classification (NIC) system (2): a taxonomy of more than 540 nursing interventions that have been defined and developed to include examples of appropriate nursing activities (behaviors or actions that implement the intervention). The identified nursing interventions are divided into seven "domains": (1) physiological: basic (care that supports physical functioning), (2) physiological: complex (care that supports homeostatic regulation), (3) behavioral (care that supports psychosocial functioning and facilitates lifestyle changes), (4) safety (care that supports protection against harm), (5) family (care that supports the family unit), (6) health system (care that supports effective use of the health care delivery system), and (7) community (care that supports the health of the community).

O

Obesity (13): weight 20% or more above desirable weight. Obesity is associated with hypertension, type 2 diabetes, hypercholesterolemia, coronary artery disease, some types of cancer, gallbladder disease, arthritis, sleep apnea, and stroke.

Objectives (3): specific steps that one takes to arrive at the destination.

Obsessive-compulsive disorder (OCD) (18): mental disorder in which an individual is overcome with the urge to engage in some ritual to avoid a persistent frightening thought, idea, image, or event—the obsession. Compulsions are the rituals or behaviors repeatedly performed to prevent, neutralize, or dispel the dreaded obsession. When the individual tries to resist the compulsion, anxiety increases. Common compulsions include handwashing, counting, checking, or touching.

Occupational health nursing (10): the specialty nursing practice that focuses on promotion, prevention, and restoration of health within the context of a safe and healthy work environment. It includes the prevention of adverse health effects from occupational and environmental hazards and provides for and delivers occupational and environmental health and safety services to workers and worker populations.

Occupational health risk (7): workplace risks and hazards related to use of heavy equipment, exposure to chemicals and biohazards, sunlight, cold, and noise, and potential for assault or violence. Occupations with relatively higher rates of occupational risk include mining, logging, agriculture, construction, manufacturing, trucking, and warehousing.

Occupational Safety and Health Act (PL 91-596) (10): federal legalization passed in 1970 to promote safe and healthful working conditions and to preserve human resources. Among other things, the Occupational Safety and Health Act formed the Occupational Safety and Health Administration (OSHA), which sets and enforces standards of occupational safety and health and the National Institute for Occupational Safety and Health (NIOSH), which researches and recommends occupational safety and health standards to OSHA and funds educational centers for the training of occupational health professionals; established federal occupational safety and health standards; and created a mechanism for imposition of fines and other punitive measures for violation of federal occupational safety and health regulations.

Osteoporosis (14): skeletal disease characterized by decreased bone mass, which leads to increased skeletal fragility and subsequent tendency to fracture. Osteoporosis affects about 8 million U.S. residents, including an estimated 18% of women older than 50 years and 90% of women older than 75.

Ozone (7): gas that occurs in two layers in the atmosphere. In the stratosphere, ozone acts to shield the earth from harmful effects of ultraviolet radiation given off by the sun. But at ground level, high concentrations of ozone are a major health concern because ozone is one of the primary problem gases in air pollution.

Ozone depletion (7): refers to evidence that the Earth's stratospheric ozone layer is being destroyed by chlorofluorocarbons (CFCs). Theoretically, radiation from the sun elicits a chemical reaction between the CFCs and ozone, resulting in thinning of the ozone layer.

P

Panic disorder (18): mental disorder in which individuals progressively experience anxiety attacks. Often the first attack or cluster of attacks follows a variety of life stresses. The initial attack may occur suddenly and unexpectedly while the patient is performing everyday tasks. During an anxiety attack the individual experiences tachycardia, dyspnea, dizziness, chest pain, nausea, numbness or tingling of the hands and feet, trembling or shaking, sweating, choking, or a feeling that he or she is going to die, go crazy, or do something uncontrolled. A diagnosis of panic disorder is made when attacks occur with some degree of frequency or regularity.

Parish nursing (10): nursing care that serves to promote the health of a faith community (churches or synagogues) through working with the pastor and staff to integrate the theological, psychological, sociological, and physiological perspectives of health and healing into the work, sacrament, and services of the congregation. Parish nursing interventions include organization of support groups, provision of referrals to community resources, health education, counseling, and acting as a liaison within the larger health care system.

Passive immunity (19): protection against a communicable disease produced by an animal or human and transferred to another human. Passive immunity often provides effective protection, but this protection wanes over time—usually a few weeks or months. Examples of passive immunity include transplacental transfer of immunity from a mother to her infant and injection of constituents of blood products from human donors (e.g., homologous pooled human antibody, immune globulin).

Perceived seriousness (3): One's belief regarding the seriousness of a given condition.

Perceived susceptibility (3): One's belief regarding the chance of getting a given condition.

Perinatal home care (11): care for pregnant and postpartum clients in the home. Perinatal home care includes technologically advanced care for high-risk pregnancies (e.g., uterine monitoring, fetal monitoring, ultrasound, infusion therapy, and hypertension monitoring) and care for neonates with complications (e.g., apnea monitoring). Postpartum care for uncomplicated clients following shortened hospital stays is also a component.

Phobia (18): an irrational fear of something (an object or situation). As many as 8% of Americans are affected by phobias at any given time. Adults with phobias realize their fears are irrational, but facing the feared object or situation might bring on severe anxiety or a panic attack.

Physical activity and fitness (13): regular exercise to promote health. Physical activity helps control blood lipid abnormalities, diabetes, and obesity and can help lower blood pressure. In addition, regular activity helps control weight, increases lean body mass, decreases body fat percentage, produces relief from some symptoms of depression, improves flexibility, increases muscle strength and endurance, and increases bone density.

Polypharmacy (15): the prescribing of multiple drugs for a patient; commonly occurs among older people. Both prescription and nonprescription medications contribute to problems encountered in polypharmacy.

Posttraumatic stress disorder (PTSD) (18): a debilitating condition that follows a terrifying event. Individuals with PTSD have recurring, persistent, frightening thoughts and memories of their ordeal. Traumatic incidents that trigger PTSD may have threatened that individual's life or the life of someone else. Incidents include "shell shock" or "battle fatigue" common to war veterans, violent attack (e.g., kidnapping, rape, mugging), serious accidents, or natural disasters (e.g., earthquake, tornado) or witnessing mass destruction or injury, such as after an airplane crash.

Poverty (17): to have few or no material possessions and to have inadequate access to family and community resources.

Poverty threshold (17): a predetermined index established yearly by the Census Bureau; provides a set of income thresholds that vary by family size and composition to determine who is poor. If a family's total income is less than the federally defined poverty threshold, then that family is considered poor. In 2006 the poverty threshold for a family of four with two children was $20,614.

Preferred provider organizations (PPOs) (5): business arrangements or contracts between a panel of health care providers, usually hospitals and physicians, and purchasers of health care services (e.g., self-insured employers or health insurance companies). The providers agree to supply services to a defined group of patients on a discounted fee-for-service basis. In PPOs the organization, usually a health insurer, contracts to provide health services for a set fee using selected physicians. The physician agrees to the fee structure of the PPO in return for the PPO providing patients.

Prenatal care (14): health care for pregnant women, which reduces complications of pregnancy and promotes a healthy delivery and infant. Prenatal care should include initial and ongoing risk assessment, individualized care based on case management principles, nutritional counseling, education to reduce or eliminate unhealthy habits, stress reduction, social support services, and health education.

Prevalence rate (6): The proportion of persons in a population who have a particular disease or attribute at a specified point in time or over a specified period of time.

Primary health care (1): health promotion and illness prevention activities, such as well child checkups, routine physical examinations, prenatal care, and diagnosis and treatment of common acute or episodic illnesses. Primary health care is traditionally conducted in convenient, community-based settings.

Psychiatric home health care (11): home care provided for individuals with diagnoses of suspected mental illnesses; these individuals need psychiatric services but cannot use traditional outpatient mental health services. Psychiatric home care can prevent hospitalization for clients with diagnoses such as severe depression, schizophrenia, and Alzheimer's disease.

Psychotherapeutic medications (18): are used to treat mental illnesses by controlling symptoms. As with medications for physical health problems, the appropriateness of psychotherapeutic medications and their prescribed regimen depends on the diagnosis, side effects, and patient response. Psychotherapeutic medications include antipsychotics, antimanic medications, anticonvulsants, antidepressants, antianxiety agents, and stimulants.

Psychotherapy (18): treatment for mental disorders that relies primarily on structured conversation aimed at changing a patient's attitudes, feelings, beliefs, defenses, personality, and behavior. In psychotherapy the therapist's procedures vary across schools of psychotherapy and with the nature of the patient's problem. Various types of psychotherapy include individual or interpersonal therapy, family therapy, couples therapy, group therapy, play therapy, and cognitive therapy.

Public health nursing (10): nursing practice in public health departments. The focus of public health nursing often includes prevention and control of communicable diseases through provision of immunizations, provision of easily accessible (affordable) treatment for sexually transmitted diseases (STDs), and screening, diagnosis, and treatment of certain communicable diseases (e.g., tuberculosis, AIDS, and Hansen disease). In addition, many public health departments provide prenatal and family planning services, well-baby care, community mental health services, and home health care.

Q

Qualifications for home care (11): Medicare requirements for coverage of home health care services. To qualify for Medicare reimbursement (1) the person to whom the services are provided must be eligible for Medicare; (2) services must be "reasonable and necessary" in relation to the patient's health status and medical needs; (3) the client's care must require intermittent skilled nursing care, physical therapy, or speech therapy; (4) the client must be homebound; (5) the client must be under the care of a physician who develops and monitors a home health plan; and (6) the home health agency must be certified to participate in Medicare.

R

Race (8): classification or grouping of humans primarily based on physical characteristics (e.g., skin color, hair color and texture, eye shape and color, height). Anthropologically, individuals from a given race have a common geographic origin of their ancestors.

Racism (8): excessive belief in the superiority of one's own racial group.

Radon (7): a colorless, odorless, radioactive gas resulting from the natural breakdown (radioactive decay) of uranium. Radon enters buildings through cracks in solid floors, through construction joints, and in other ways, and dangerously high levels can be found in many homes.

Reportable diseases (19): those communicable diseases that require notification of authorities whenever encountered by a health care professional. There are a large number of reportable diseases, and they include AIDS, anthrax, hepatitis A, hepatitis B, most vaccine-preventable diseases, STDs, malaria, and Lyme disease.

Researcher (2): a professional who identifies problems or questions for investigation,

participates in approved research studies, and disseminates research findings to clients and other professionals. As researchers, nurses should remain informed of developments relative to their individual practice.

Role model (2): a person who demonstrates an action or behavior that is learned by others. Role modeling is both conscious and unconscious, and nurses in all settings demonstrate to others both positive and negative actions and attitudes related to health and health care.

Rural nursing (10): nursing care provided to residents in nonurban settings. Rural nursing practice must consider issues and barriers such as distance, isolation, and sparse resources. Rural nurses most often practice in clinic settings, home health, or a combination. Rural nurses must be clinically competent in a very broad number of areas and are typically cross-trained to manage client needs in areas including trauma, routine obstetrical care, care of children and elders, and care of clients with mental health needs.

S

School nursing (10): nursing care provided to students in school settings. Care typically focuses on prevention and control of communicable diseases, care of ill or injured students, administration or oversight of procedures for students with special health needs, administration of screening programs, provision and monitoring for a safe and healthful environment, health promotion, health counseling, and school program management.

Screening (13): interventions to assess the presence of signs of disease in the period of early pathogenesis before symptoms occur. Health screenings should be based on age and risk factors.

Secondary health care (1): relatively serious or complicated care that has historically been provided to patients in hospitals. Recent changes in techniques, procedures, and medical practice have moved much of secondary health care into community settings. Examples of community-based secondary health care include outpatient surgery for complex procedures that would have required hospitalization just a few years ago (e.g., cholecystectomy, hysterectomy, appendectomy, herniorrhaphy), treatment of serious illnesses (e.g., chemotherapy, radiotherapy), and a wide variety of diagnostic testing procedures (e.g., computed tomography, magnetic resonance imaging, angiography).

Secondhand smoke (7): the combination of smoke given off by the burning of a cigarette, pipe, or cigar and the smoke exhaled from the lungs of smokers. The Environmental Protection Agency (EPA) has classified secondhand smoke as a known carcinogen. Secondhand smoke is estimated to cause approximately 3000 lung cancer deaths in nonsmokers each year.

Self-efficacy (3): one's confidence in one's ability to take action to reduce health risks.

Sexually transmitted diseases (STDs) (19): communicable diseases directly transmitted during sexual contact. The number and type of different STDs has increased dramatically over the last several decades. Of the top 10 infections reported to the CDC in 1998, 5 were STDs (chlamydia, gonorrhea, AIDS, syphilis, and hepatitis B), and it is estimated that more than 15 million cases of STDs occur each year in the United States.

Single-parent family (13): mother or father living with either biological or adopted children; they may be tied emotionally but not legally to a partner.

Skilled nursing services (11): those nursing services that are reimbursable by Medicare. Covered nursing services include observation and assessment of a patient's condition, management and evaluation of a patient care plan, teaching and training activities for the patient and the patient's family or caregivers, tube feedings, tracheotomy aspiration, wound care, ostomy care, rehabilitation care, and venipuncture.

Smoking cessation (13): programs, tools, medications, and various interventions to help tobacco users quit. Interventions include self-help groups, videos and written materials, nicotine chewing gum, nicotine patches, hypnosis, and acupuncture.

Stages of family development (16): evolution of a normal family through a series of several stages. The stages include beginning or establishment, early childbearing, families with young children, families with school-age children, families with adolescents, families as launching centers, middle-age families, and aging families.

State Children's Health Insurance Program (SCHIP) (12): program created in 1997 to provide health insurance coverage for uninsured children. Most children covered by SCHIP are from working families with incomes too high to qualify for Medicaid but too low to afford private health insurance. Covered services include inpatient and outpatient hospital care, physician's surgical and medical care, laboratory and x-ray services, and well-baby/well-child care, including immunizations. Prescription drugs, mental health services, vision care, and hearing-related care may be provided in some states.

Stereotyping (8): the belief or notion that all people from a given group are the same.

Subculture (8): a fairly large aggregate of individuals who share characteristics that are not common to all members of the culture and allow them to be considered a distinguishable subgroup; a group of persons within a culture of the same age, socioeconomic level, ethnic origin, education, or occupation who have an identity of their own but are related to the total culture.

Substance abuse (18): patterns of use of alcohol and/or other drugs that result in health consequences or impairment in social, psychological, and occupational functioning.

Suicide (18): the most serious potential outcome of mental disorders and a leading cause of death in the United States. Each year, more than 30,000 U.S. residents take their own lives. Depression, schizophrenia, panic disorder, and alcohol and other drug abuse have been implicated in both attempted and completed suicides.

T

Teenage pregnancy (14): pregnancy in young women under the age of 19 years; 95% are unintended. Each year about 10% of teenage girls become pregnant and about 500,000 give birth. Teenage pregnancy is associated with complications of pregnancy (both fetal and maternal), failure of the mother to complete high school, unemployment, poverty, and reliance on government assistance.

Terrorism (9, 14): the unlawful use of force or violence against persons or property to intimidate or coerce a government or civilian population in the furtherance of political or social objectives. In most cases, terrorists use explosives or incendiary devices against their targets, but there is growing concern over the potential for terrorists' use of biologic organisms (i.e., anthrax or smallpox) or chemical agents (i.e., sarin gas, mustard gas).

Tertiary health care (1): management of chronic, complicated, long-term health problems. Tertiary care includes home health care, hospice care, and care provided in rehabilitation centers.

Third party reimbursement (5): fiscal payment by an intermediary or "third party" such as an insurance company (e.g., Blue Cross, Aetna), Medicare, or Medicaid. This third party insures beneficiaries against health expenses. The individual pays a premium for coverage, and the insurer then pays health care bills on his or her behalf.

Transcultural nursing (8): nursing practice focused on the provision of nursing care in a manner that is sensitive to the cultural beliefs and values of individuals, families, and groups. In transcultural nursing, culturally sensitive nursing interventions show an appreciation of and respect for differences and an attempt to decrease the possibility of stress or conflict arising from cultural misunderstanding.

U

Ultraviolet radiation (7): radiation given off from the sun; contributes to skin cancer, which is the most common form of cancer in the United States. Exposure to ultraviolet radiation is believed to cause more than 90% of basal and squamous cell carcinomas.

Unintentional food additives (7): substances that enter and remain in food as a result of their use as pesticides, after being added to animal food, or from packaging.

Utilization management (4): the formal and comprehensive review of services used by a patient to ensure that they are: (1) medically necessary, (2) provided in the most appropriate care setting, and (3) at or above quality standards.

Utilization review (5): a process of monitoring and evaluating the quality of health care, including necessity, appropriateness, and efficiency. The goal of utilization review is to monitor and provide incentives to influence the use of health care services through examination of hospitalization rates, admissions, length of stay,

frequency of diagnostic and therapeutic procedures, and appropriateness and efficacy of practice patterns.

V

Vaccine Adverse Event Reporting System (VAERS) (19): system developed to provide a single system for the collection and analysis of reports on all adverse events associated with the administration of any U.S. licensed vaccine. The VAERS is operated by the CDC and Food and Drug Administration.

Vaccine-preventable disease (19): those communicable diseases for which effective vaccines are available. The incidence of vaccine-preventable diseases (e.g., measles, mumps, diphtheria, pertussis) has dropped dramatically over the last three to four decades because of active immunization.

Values (8): personal perceptions of what is good or useful; desirable beliefs and standards.

Vector (6): an animate intermediary in the indirect transmission of an agent that carries the agent from a reservoir to a susceptible host.

Vehicle (6): an inanimate intermediary in the indirect transmission of an agent that carries the agent from a reservoir to a susceptible host.

Vision deficit (15): loss of vision in adults, which increases with age. It is estimated that more than 90% of older people require the use of corrective lenses and approximately 18% of all older people have significant visual deficits. Cataracts, glaucoma, macular degeneration, and diabetic retinopathy often cause visual problems in the elderly.

Vision screening (12): early detection and referral for treatment of vision disorders. Vision screening includes a careful history, thorough examination, vision testing, and referral of abnormal or asymmetrical results for further testing and treatment.

Vulnerability (17): situation in which a person or group is more likely to develop a health-related problem or problems and to have more serious outcomes stemming from their exposure to multiple risks. Vulnerability is exacerbated by the combined effects of limited resources and contributing factors such as disempowerment, disenfranchisement, and marginalization.

Vulnerable groups (17): those people who have an increased risk or susceptibility to adverse health outcomes. Vulnerable groups include disabled persons, homeless persons, migrant workers, persons in extreme poverty, persons who are HIV positive, persons with serious health problems, pregnant adolescents, refugees and recent immigrants, severely mentally ill individuals, substance abusers, very young or very old individuals, victims of disasters, and victims of violence.

W

Women, Infants, and Children (WIC) (12): federally funded program that provides food, nutrition counseling, and access to health services for low-income women, infants, and children. Pregnant or postpartum women, infants, and children up to age 5 years who meet income guidelines and residency requirements and who are determined to be at "nutritional risk" are eligible. Most WIC programs provide vouchers that participants use at authorized stores to purchase nutritious foods.

Workers' compensation (10): a nationwide state-operated insurance system, with each state having its own law and program. Workers' compensation benefits are awarded to individuals who sustain physical or mental injuries from their employment, regardless of who or what was the cause of the injury or illness. Workers' compensation generally provides ongoing payment of wages and benefits to the injured or disabled worker or dependent survivor for wages lost, medical care and related costs, funeral and burial costs, and some rehabilitation expenses.

Workplace violence (9): "violent acts against a person at work or on duty, including physical assaults (rape and sexual assault and aggravated and simple assault) and robbery" (Warchol, 1998, p.1; for full reference information, see Chapter 9).

Index

Note: Entries followed by "b" indicate boxes; "f" figures; "t" tables.